Atlas of
HUMAN
ANATOMY

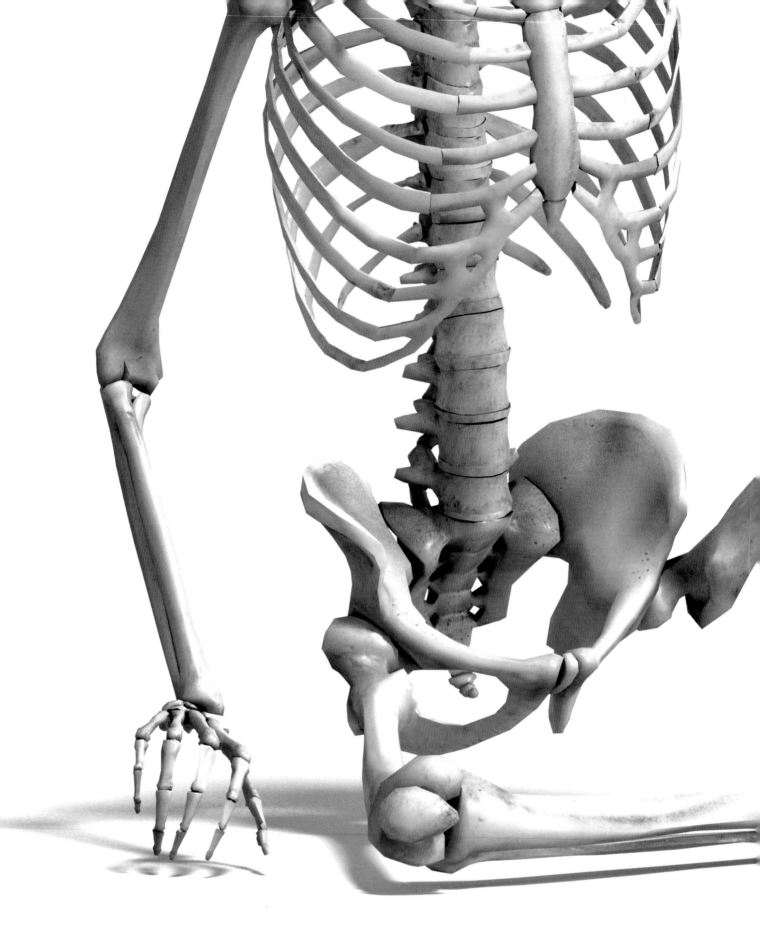

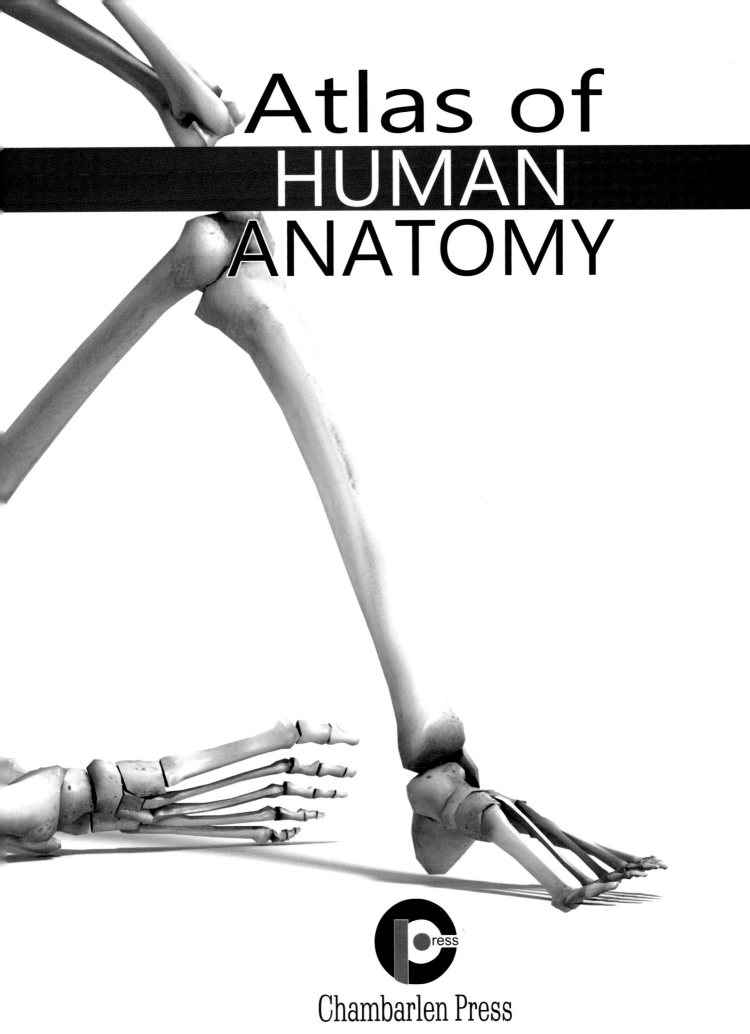

Atlas of
HUMAN
ANATOMY

Chambarlen Press

Author
Jordi Vigué
Director of Medical Scientific Team
Asklepios Medical Atlas

Redaction team
Medical Scientific Team
Asklepios Medical Atlas

Collaborators
Dr. Joaquim Claret
Dra. Rosa Gratacòs
Dra. Teresa Oriol
Dr. Jordi Aymerich
Dra. Joaquima d'Abadal i Puig-rafagut
Dr. Màrius Puigserinanell
Dra. Lluïsa Terricabras

Scientific advisors
An overview of the human body
Ricard Ramos Izquierdo
Specialist in Thoracic Surgery, Associate
Professor ofHuman Anatomy and
Embryology. Universitat deBarcelona

Skin
Rosa María Penín Mosquera
Specialist in Pathological Anatomy
Pathological Anatomy Service, H.U.B
l'Hospitalet de Llobregat, Barcelona

Muscular system
Xavier Rius i Moreno
Specialist in Orthopedic Surgery and
Traumatology, H.U.B. IHospitalet de
Llobregat, Barcelona

ISBN: 978-19107-0300-7

First published : 2015

Copyright © 2015, Chambarlen International

Published by:
Chambarlen International
Third Floor, 207 Regent Street, W1B3HH

Skeletal system
Marc Blasi i Brugué
Associate Professor of Human Anatomy
Infirmary Grade, Universitat de Barcelona
Echographic Anatomy Laboratoire,
Medical Department. Universitat
de Barcelona

Joints
Xavier Rius i Moreno
Specialist in Orthopedic Surgery
and Traumatology, H.U.B. IHospitalet
de Llobregat, Barcelona

Cardiovascular system
Mònica Buxeda Rodríguez
Licenciate in Medicine, Universitat de
Barcelona, Docent Collaborator and
Research Worker by Human Anatomy
Medical Department, H.U.B. l'Hospitalet
deLlobregat, Barcelona

Digestive system
Ivan Macía Vidueira
Specialist in Thoracic Surgery, Hospital
Universitari deBellvitge. Associate
Professor, Nursery School, Universitat
de Barcelona

Respiratory system
Anna Ureña i Lluveras
Specialist in Thoracic Surgery, H.U.B
L'Hospitalet deLlobregat,
Barcelona.

Nephro-urinary system
Albert Francès i Comalat
Specialist in Urology, Hospital del Mar
Barcelona. Associate Professor of Urology
Universitat Autònoma de Barcelona,
Universitat Pompeu Fabra

Genital system
Carla Rojas Bautista
Specialist in Obstetrics and Gynecology,
Zita West Assisted Fertility, Londres

Immune system
Montserrat Arnán Sangermán
Specialist in Hematology, Clinical
Hematology
Service, Hospital Duran i Reynals, Institut
Català d'Oncologia. L'Hospitalet
de Llobregat, Barcelona

Endocrine system
Núria Vilarrasa i Garcia
Specialist in Endocrinology and Nutrition
Hospital Universitari de Bellvitge
l'Hospitalet
de Llobregat, Barcelona

Nervous system
Mònica Buxeda Rodríguez
Licenciate in Medicine, Universitat de
Barcelona, Docent Collaborator and
Research Worker by Human Anatomy
Medical Department, H.U.B. l'Hospitalet
deLlobregat,
Barcelona

Organs of the senses
Ignacio Viza i Puiggròs
Departament of Otorinolaryngology.
Hospital Universitari Dexeus, Barcelona

Documentation
Archivo Asklepios Medical Atlas
Narcisa Mallol
Ramon Ciutadella
Josep Coromina
Concepció Santmartí
Victôria Santmarc
Montse Segueró

Terminology and index
Dr. Jordi Balandrau
Dra. M. Dolors Caldera

Correction
Dra. Carolina Dalmau
Dra. Alexandra Deulofeu
Dr. Guillem Adrall

Illustration team
Chief
Myriam Ferrón i Viñas
Illustrators
Marina Bona
Eugeni Fernández
Miquel Ferrón i Geis
Ali Garousi
Jordi Giménez
Alex Luengo
Pedro Moreno Gil
Pere Ruiz Grima
Jorge Rodrigo
Francisco Sánchez
Jordi Segú
Pablo Villafrade Blanco

Editorial team
Chief
Miquel Ridola

General coordination
Josep Graell Malars

Informatic treatment of images
Llorenç Torrent
Joaquim Serna
Raquel Compayó
Dolors Martínez
Olga Zgustovà

General documentation
Asklepios Medical Atlas

Graphic design and diagramation
Estudi gràfic APEX
Chief
Alba Lucía Suárez Cristancho
Graphic designers
Libia Yolanda Bernal Parada
Gloria Ximena Rodríguez López
Iohann Vargas Sotomayor

SCIENTIFIC ADVISORS OF ATLAS of HUMAN ANATOMY

GENERAL COORDINATOR
Dr. Ricard Ramos Izquierdo
Specialist in Thoracic Surgery, Associate
Professor ofHuman Anatomy and
Embryology. Universitat deBarcelona

**SCIENTIFIC ADVISORS AND
COLLABORATORS**

Andrés Alvarado Segovia
Sports Medicine Specialist. Bodytech, Bogotá

Josep Maria de Anta Vinyals
Associate Profesor of Anatomy and Human
Embryology, Campus de Ciències de la Salut
de Bellvitge. Universidad de Barcelona

Montse Arnán Sangermán
Specialist in Hematology, Clinical Hematology
Service, Hospital Duran i Reynals, Institut
Català d'Oncologia. L'Hospitalet de
Llobregat, Barcelona

Lorenzo Balagueró Lladó
Former Chief of the Gynecology Unit
Hospital Universitari de Bellvitge, lHospitalet
de Llobregat, Barcelona. Tenured Professor of
Obstetrics and Gynecology. Faculty of
Medicine, Universitat de Barcelona

Carme Baliellas i Comellas
Specialist of the Digestive Unit. Hospital
Universitari de Bellvitge. Barcelona

Cristina Berdié i Rabanaque
Specialist in Obstetrics and Gynecology
Hospital General de l'Hospitalet de Llobregat
Barcelona

Jordi Bermúdez Mas
Professor of Biophysics, Department of
Physiological Sciences II. Universitat de
Barcelona

Marc Blasi i Brugué
Associate Professor of Human Anatomy
Infirmary Grade, Universitat de Barcelona
Echographic Anatomy Laboratoire, Medical
Department. Universitat de Barcelona

Enric Buendía i Gràcia
Former Chief of the Immunology Unit
Hospital Universitari de Bellvitge. lHospitalet
de Llobregat, Barcelona

Mònica Buxeda Rodríguez
Licenciate in Medicine, Universitat de
Barcelona, Docent Collaborator and Research
Worker by Human Anatomy, Medical
Department, H.U.B. l'Hospitalet deLlobregat
Barcelona

Xavier Cabo Cabo
Specialist in Orthopedic Surgery and
Traumatology, Head of the Septics Functional
Unit, H.U.B. lHospitalet de Llobregat
Barcelona. Associate Professor of Orthopedic
Surgery and Traumatology. Universitat de
Barcelona

Josep M. Caminal i Mitjana
Specialist in Ophthalmology, H.U.B
lHospitalet deLlobregat, Barcelona
Associate Professor of Ophthalmology
Universitat de Barcelona

Anna Carrera Burgaya
Tenured Professor of Human Anatomy and
Embryology, Medical Sciences Department
Universitat de Girona

María Lluïsa Catasús i Clavé
Specialist in Rehabilitation, H.U.B. lHospitalet
de Llobregat, Barcelona

Manuel Chiva Royo*
Tenured Professor of the Department of
Physiology, Universidad de Barcelona

Josep Ramon Ferreres i Riera
Specialist in Dermatology, H.U.B. lHospitalet
de Llobregat, Barcelona

Albert Francès i Comalat
Specialist in Urology, Hospital del Mar
Barcelona. Associate Professor of Urology
Universitat Autònoma de Barcelona
Universitat Pompeu Fabra. Barcelona

Eladio Franco Miranda
Specialist in Urology.H.U.B. lHospitalet de
Llobregat, Barcelona. Associate Professor of
Urology, Universitat de Barcelona

Xavier Fulladosa Oliveras
Specialist in Nephrology. H.U.B. lHospitalet
de Llobregat, Barcelona.

José Manuel Gómez Sáez
Chief of the Endocrinology and Nutrition
Section, H.U.B. lHospitalet de Llobregat
Barcelona.
Associate Professor of Endocrinology
Universitat
de Barcelona

Jordi Guardiola Capó
Chief of the Gastro-intestinal Section,H.U.B
l'Hospitalet de Llobregat, Barcelona.

José Antonio Hernández Hermoso
Chief of the Service de Orthopaedic Surgery
and Traumatology. Hospital Germans Trias i
Pujol. Badalona, Barcelona

Francisco Jara Sureda
Specialist in Cardiology. H.U.B. lHospitalet de
Llobregat, Barcelona

Casimiro Fco. Javierre Garcés
Specialist in Medicine of Sport. Aggregate
Professor, Unitat de Fisiologia Departament
de Ciències Fisiològiques II, Universitat de
Barcelona

Xavier Juanola i Roura
Chief of the Rheumatology Section. H.U.B
lHospitalet de Llobregat, Barcelona.
Professor ofRheumatology, Universitat
de Barcelona.

Jerky Krupinski
Specialist in Neurology, Hospital Mútua de
Terrassa. Terrassa, Barcelona

Iván Macía Vidueira
Specialist in Thoracic Surgery, Hospital
Universitari deBellvitge. Associate Professor
Nursery School, Universitat de Barcelona

Frederic Manresa i Presas
Chief of the Pneumology Service. H.U.B
lHospitalet de Llobregat, Barcelona. Tenured
Professor ofPneumology. Universitat de
Barcelona

Mª Cristina Manzanares Céspedes
Tenured Professor of Human Anatomy and
Embryology, Campus de Ciències de la Salut
deBellvitge. Universitat de Barcelona

Mª Isabel Miguel Pérez
Tenured Professor of Human Anatomy and
Embryology, Campus de Ciències de la Salut
deBellvitge. Universitat de Barcelona

Júlia Miró i Lladó
Specialist in Neurology, Unidad de Epilepsias
H.U.B. lHospitalet de Llobregat, Barcelona

Juan Moya Amorós
Chief of the Thoracic Surgery Service, H.U.B
LHospitalet de Llobregat, Barcelona. Tenured
Professor of Surgery. Universitat de
Barcelona

Rosa María Penín Mosquera
Specialist in Pathological Anatomy
Pathological Anatomy Service, H.U.B
l'Hospitalet de Llobregat, Barcelona

Joan Pericas Bosch
Specialist in Pediatrics

Elena Pina Pascual
Specialist in Hematology, Haemostasis and
Thrombosis Area, H.U.B. lHospitalet de
Llobregat. Barcelona

Albert Prats Galino
Professor of Human Anatomy and
Embryology. Universitat de Barcelona

Manuel Ramos Izquierdo
DO Osteopathic. Physiotherapy of Sport
Grade Physiotherapy Professor, Universitat
Ramon Llull. Institut Ramos Izquierdo
Barcelona

Emilio Ramos Rubio
Chief of the General and Gastro-intestinal
Surgery Section, Hepatic Transplant Unit
H.U.B. lHospitalet de Llobregat, Barcelona
Tenured Professor of Surgery. Universitat de
Barcelona

Jordi Rancaño Ferreiro
Former Chief of the Angiology and Vascular
Surgery Section, H.U.B. lHospitalet de
Llobregat, Barcelona. Associate Professor of
Vascular Surgery. Universitat deBarcelona.

Purificación Regueiro Espín
Specialist in Obstetrics and Gynecology.
Hospital General de l'Hospitalet de Llobregat,
Barcelona.

Xavier Rius i Moreno
Specialist in Orthopaedic Surgery and
Traumatology, H.U.B. l Hospitalet de
Llobregat, Barcelona.

Francesc Rivas Doyague
Specialist in Thoracic Surgery, H.U.B.
l'Hospitalet de Llobregat, Barcelona.

Josep Rodríguez Tolrá
Specialist in Urology, Head of the
Andrology, Erectile Dysfunction
and Urethral Pathology Unit, H.U.B.
l Hospitalet de Llobregat,
Barcelona.

Carla Rojas Bautista
Specialist in Obstetrics and Gynecology,
Zita West Assisted Fertility,
Londres.

Antonio Romera Villegas
Specialist in Angiology and Vascular
Surgery, H.U.B. l Hospitalet de Llobregat,
Barcelona.

Francisco Rubio Borrego
Chief of the Neurology Service, H.U.B.
l Hospitalet de Llobregat, Barcelona. Tenured
Professor of Neurology, Universitat de
Barcelona.

Xavier Sabaté de la Cruz
Chief of the Cardiology Section, Arrhythmia
Unit, H.U.B. l Hospitalet de Llobregat,
Barcelona. Associate Professor of Cardiology.
Universitat de Barcelona.

Ramon Segura Cardona
Professor Emeritus of Physiology. Universitat
de Barcelona.

Octavi Servitje Bedate
Specialist in Dermatology, H.U.B. l Hospitalet
de Llobregat, Barcelona. Associate Professor
of Dermatology. Universitat de Barcelona.

Antoni Surós i Batlló
Former Chief of the Digestive Unit, Hospital
Universitari de Bellvitge. l Hospitalet de
Llobregat, Barcelona.

Sandra Torra Alsina
Specialist in Digestive System, Digestive Unit,
Hospital Parc Sanitari Sant Joan de Déu,
Universitat de Barcelona.

Anna Ureña Lluveras
Specialist in Thoracic Surgery, Hospital
Universitari de Bellvitge.
L'Hospitalet de Llobregat,
Barcelona.

Magín Valls Porcel
Former Chief of the Gynecology Section,
Hospital Universitari de Bellvitge l Hospitalet
de Llobregat. Barcelona.

Antonio Vidaller Palacín
Former Chief of the Internal Medicine
Section. H.U.B. l Hospitalet de Llobregat.
Barcelona. Associate Professor of Medicine.
Universitat de Barcelona.

Núria Vilarrasa i Garcia
Specialist in Endocrinology and Nutrition,
Hospital Universitari de Bellvitge l'Hospitalet
de Llobregat, Barcelona.

Ignacio Viza i Puiggròs
Department of Otorinolaryngology. Hospital
Universitari Dexeus, Barcelona.

 * Deceased
** H. U. B. Hospital Universitari de Bellvitge
(Barcelona)

Anatomy is the science that deals in a comprehensive way and completes the study of macroscopic structures of the human body. In this aspect it differs from the Cytology; that is dedicated to cell study, or the histology that studies the tissues.

By its absolute obviousness, it is considered slightly less that is useless to insist in the need of knowing our own body, because it is the most next and constitutional that has to deal with the human being. Neither we think that it is necessary to insist in the interest that, since the most remote epochs of human beings, man has shown that he obtains to save his body, the struggle for survival, the belief in extraterrestrial forces, in divinity, witchcraft, at the bottom it wasn't another thing that a manifestation of the absolute interest in which our ancestors use to take everything that had as final object to save our own body.

Surely was the fear, reverential fear, a certain mystery to universal reality and solemn to death, in which repeatedly impinged without exception the ancient popular beliefs and traditions that considerate one unforgivable desecration the dissection of corpses for study, which explains the experimental ignorance of human body and a lot of aspects of its anatomy, as internal organs, blood circulation, the nervous system, etc.

In west culture, the practice of embalming of corpses let to ancient Egyptians the acquisition of some knowledge about human anatomy, so the Ebers papyrus (which has been dated from the year 1500 bC and that constitutes one of the most ancient medical texts and that was found between the rests of a mummy in the tomb of Assassif in the year 1862 by Edwin Smith and that was acquired after by the German Egyptologist Georg Ebers, from which comes the name) it contents some anatomical descriptions, specially the chapter C, where the hearth is studied and blood vessels.

The properly scientists origins of anatomy go back to the ancient classic Greece. So both the anatomy and physiology were addressed by Alcmeon of Crotona (500 years bC) that use to dissect animals, who described the optic nerve and differentiated the veins from arteries. Democritus of Abdera (470 to 370 bC), disciple of Socrates and Anaxagoras and contemporary friend of Hippocrates, and Diogenes of Apolonia (V century bC), disciple of Anaxagoras and as Aristotle's, author of a veins description, performed important contributions to the study of human anatomy.

It was the Greek philosopher and scientist Aristotle's (384 bC-322 bC) who used for the first time the word anatomy, that means to cut from the bottom to the top, to refer to dissection.

The colonization of Egypt by means of Greek culture and the prestigious School of Alexandria behaved the increase of the anatomy study. In that epoch appeared very important names as Herofilus (IV century bC) and Erasistratus (304-240 bC). As said by Celsus and Tertullian, Herofilus had practiced the vivisection in more than 600 corpses of criminals that Ptolomeus Lagos had sent to him for "greater glorious of science", this period was closed with Galenus (129-199), one of the most important Greek physicians of classic ancient Greece besides Hippocrates, that spent most of his life in Rome. Although they are riddled with errors, his 9 books of anatomy were used as base of knowledge and learning of anatomy during many centuries. Its treaty of anatomical administration probably constitutes the first text of dissection. Their mistakes were unavoidable, because they came in a great measure in fact that for studies for human anatomy, they used animals as apes and pigs, which anatomy is in many cases substantially different from that of the human being.

After a middle Age characterized by obscurantism, the prohibitions and all kinds of threats and punishments to whom dissected corpses, the renaissance supposed a substantial change toward another things order in many senses. It should be stated that it was in that epoch when it were established the bases of what it would be the modern studies of anatomy, it should be noted in this sense of humanistic labor, the many-sided Italian anatomist Leonardo da Vinci (1452-1519) who performed more than one thousand artistic sheets with drawings and sketches in which it was amplified the named man of Vitruvius, famous drawing accompanied of various anatomic annotations that Leonardo made in 1490, in which are studied the proportions of human body, beginning of texts of roman architect Marcus Vitruvius Pollion (I century bC) who took his name. But the great renaissance figure of anatomy was the physician Andries van Wezel (lat. Andreas Vesalius) (1514-1564), whose work De humani corporis fabrica *(1453), in which it is included a meritory collection of illustrations of Italian painter Johan Stefan Van Kalkar (~1499-1546), disciple of Tizianus, who marked an inflection point that broke with the past, based in the direct study of human body, which let in evidence the mistakes of Galenus.*

The tradition of Wezel was continued by the Italian physician and surgeon Gabrielle Fallopio (1523-1562) whom was dedicated at most to the study of head anatomy and contributed greatly to the knowledge of inner ear and eardrum and also studied the genital organs of both sex and described the uterine tubes, known as Fallopian tubes *in his honor) and the Italian physician Bartolomeo Eustachio (1520-1574), author of different studies of bones anatomy, muscles, veins, middle ear and the rear of the buccal cavity. His work* Romanae Archetypae Tabulae Anatomicae, *published in 1783, many years after his dead by Giovanni Maria Lancisi, is an excellent text and specially interesting by its precision.*

In the XVII century the invention of microscopy opened a new path to the study of anatomic science, which provided the appearance of figures as the Italian physician Marcelo Malpighi (1628-1694), who discovered the blood capillaries, the alveolar structure of lungs, different morphological details of spleen, kidney and liver and with whom there were established the bases of microscopic anatomy.

Since then, the studies about anatomy performed by means of rigorous scientifical methods hasn't been ceased. Science and research advance without stopping and technology provides day by day sophisticated means thanks to them nowadays it can be achieved knowledge that only a few years ago were unimaginable.

After this brief tour through the anatomy history, to continue with the conductive thread of this discourse and get in another facet essential and determinant for the physician professional, I would like to contribute with a phrase of the Catalan catedratic Josep de Letamendi (1828-1897) which I have always considered convincing and true: "The physician that only knows medicine, only knows a poor medicine". *His intentionality is clear and what he wants to say this illustrious master doesn't need any comment.* Intelligenti pauca. *In medicine, as in other sciences, the professional knowledge always has to be conjugated armonically with psychology and human sensibility for the patient that goes to him.*

In the context of all what it has been said formerly, it has been prepared this Atlas of General Anatomy. *Anatomy is an special science, because it constitutes at the same time the foundation and an necessary and irreplaceable vehicle, through which the physician, who could be a researcher or a practitioner whom attends patients in consultation or at the operating room, he will have the path more accessible and easy to his special branch. The same could be said for the student, and for the overall health and any person that works professionally in the human body care, his health, his maintenance and everything that goes toward a better quality of life.*

Fortunately in one important part of nowadays young generations it is advised a great sensibility for human body care, doing physical exercise, worrying about the body mass index (BMI), practicing sports, going regularly to the gym, taking care of the diet, etc.

There is no doubt that, by one side, the own body constitutes the partner, the travel companion, the most faithful friend that every human being has, because he/she is going to live with this body all days of his life and by other hand, by the fact that it is an unitary whole, the human being functions in such a way that body and mind go always at unison. Thus, when some part of the body has a problem, it damages or suffers, is all the human being that finds himself bad, sad, pessimistic. The same as, when the individual has a good or bas new or passes through a good or bad moment, is all the body that for good or bad resents. From here comes the interest when not the obligation to take care of this body and as first step, to know it piece by piece to guarantee its maintenance and welfare.

Any professional of medicine knows that the patient that attends to consulting room, as least has not one but two problems: One healthy problem (the phatology or affection that suffers) and a physicological problem (fear, sadness, depression), according to each patient situation, to these problems there are added others: familiar, economic, social problems, etc. Knowing how to attend cordially the patient, try to put in his own situation, gain the trust, equals to hit in more than the 50% in the problem solving.

While it has been prepared with modern criteria and using the most advanced technologies for the built of sheets that are provided in this Atlas of General Anatomy, *the presentation of each organ or any of its parts has been done, as it not could be done in another way, at classic way, although it has been privileged all of these that could contribute to a better comprehension of what is given. The sketches, the diagrams and some brief explanations precisely have been given attending to this interest.*

Also it has been used anytime the international consensual anatomical terminology. From all of this comes our trust to get this work to offer to the reader a modern work, useful and with a sense eminently didactic and functional.

It is obvious that any work, and also this Atlas of General Anatomy, *as very complete that could be, never will exhaust the subject. Being conscious of that, we let the door opened to other works that achieve going farther and farther. In any person dedicated to his job, the study, the anxiety and the effort joined to the permanent eagerness of getting the achievements never stop. In any case the goal of this* Atlas of General Anatomy *is to offer to the reader a compendium about human body. In this sense we expect that this Atlas be useful to everybody that uses it and to constitute a good foundation for the professional practice, to strength the knowledge and to complete the answer to many questions and concerns.*

Jordi Vigué
General Anatomy Atlas *Author*
Director of Medical Scientific Team
Asklepios Medical Atlas

SUMMARY

SKELETAL SYSTEM 157

XIV

XX

ORGANS OF THE SENSES **655**

BIBLIOGRAPHY **679**

XXI

Atlas of
HUMAN
ANATOMY

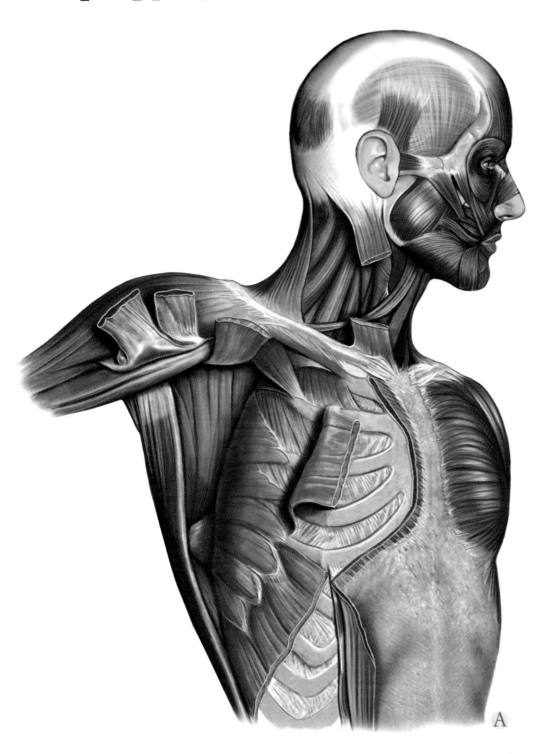

AN OVERVIEW
of the HUMAN BODY

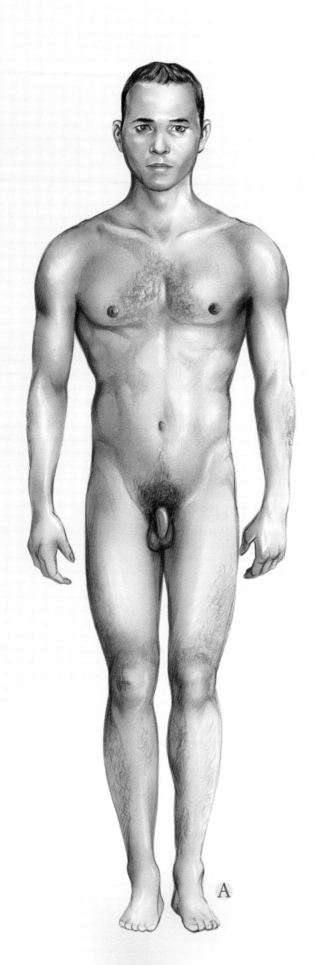

A

As for the other living beings, the human body is the result of an evolutionary process that began millions of years ago when life started on the Earth and that is still taking place. The group of organs forming the human body, the constitution, morphology and physiology of each one of them, the structures and functional units that participate in the assembling of the body and the interconnection among all these units and the other elements in order to form a multi-functional organism, a unit, make its study a hard work entailing some difficulties. This investigation gets even harder because, despite all that we already know about the organism, there are still many secrets to be unveiled. For that reason is a must to have a working methodology characterized by a logical order and a meticulous systematization of each one of the discrete elements and also of the system it belongs to, all the time having in mind the existence of a homeostasis among all the organs and systems.

There are some aspects to take into account when trying to understand the human body and, far from being neglected, they must be considered as essential. The above mentioned aspects referred to the knowledge of the anatomic external elements, the different regions they are divided into, the cavities they present, the basic vocabulary normally used when describing and defining the organs, positions or movements, etc. This chapter is exactly devoted to offer this information.

It is essential to have available this knowledge, even more in nowadays society where there is a constant updating in topics like sports, new findings in medicine, diseases, accidents, beauty, and in general, everything pertaining to the human body; this explains the reason why day by day life is being progressively altered in each one of its different aspects; whether it be the medical science, health and fitness, or the cosmetic treatments and the care of the body appearance. Having available this knowledge about the human body becomes a solid foundation upon which a complete understanding about Anatomy and Physiology can be consolidated, and this is also valid for Cytology, and for the Medical Science in general and all its specialties.

It is crucial not to forget that although when considering the human body as a unit, each of its external elements is devoted to accomplish a specific function and has a particular name.

EXTERNAL ANATOMICAL ELEMENTS (I)

FEMALE SEX. ANTERIOR GENERAL VIEW

4

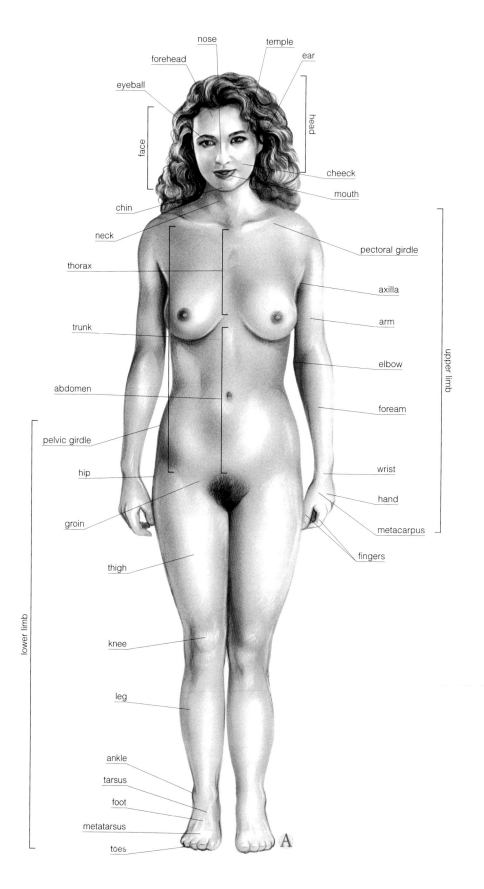

nose

temple

ear

forehead

eyeball

head

face

cheeck

mouth

chin

neck

pectoral girdle

thorax

axilla

arm

trunk

elbow

abdomen

foream

pelvic girdle

upper limb

hip

wrist

hand

groin

metacarpus

fingers

thigh

lower limb

knee

leg

ankle

tarsus

foot

metatarsus

toes

A

EXTERNAL ANATOMICAL ELEMENTS (II)
MALE SEX. POSTERIOR GENERAL VIEW

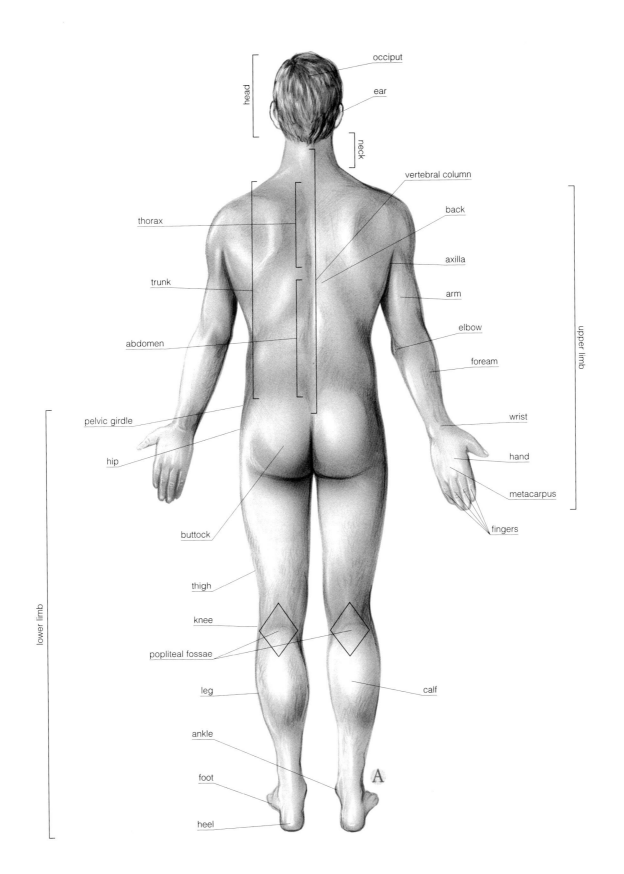

head

occiput

ear

neck

vertebral column

thorax

back

axilla

trunk

arm

elbow

abdomen

foream

upper limb

pelvic girdle

wrist

hip

hand

metacarpus

fingers

buttock

thigh

knee

popliteal fossae

leg

calf

lower limb

ankle

foot

heel

A

5

SUPERFICIAL ANATOMY (I)

MALE SEX. ANTERIOR VIEW

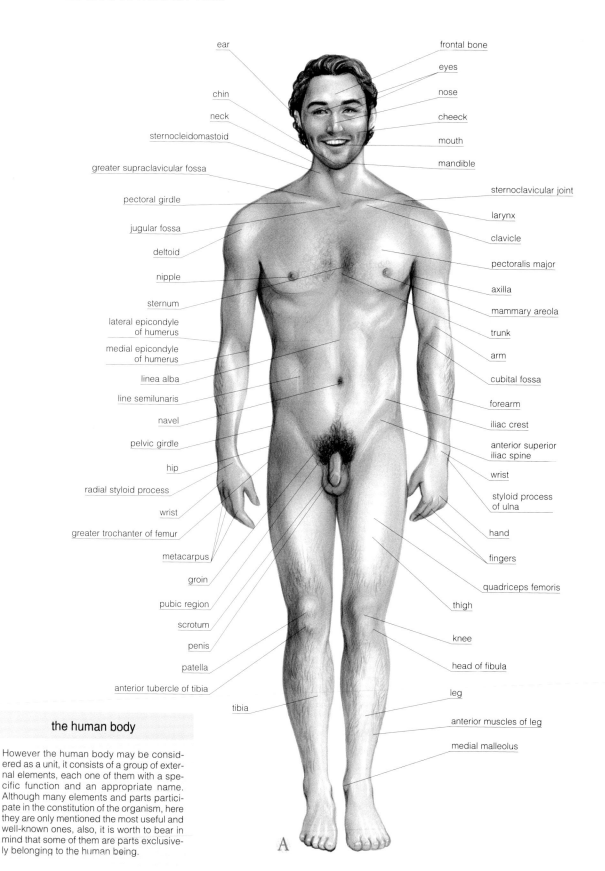

ear — frontal bone
eyes
chin — nose
neck — cheeck
sternocleidomastoid — mouth
greater supraclavicular fossa — mandible
pectoral girdle — sternoclavicular joint
jugular fossa — larynx
deltoid — clavicle
nipple — pectoralis major
sternum — axilla
lateral epicondyle of humerus — mammary areola
medial epicondyle of humerus — trunk
linea alba — arm
line semilunaris — cubital fossa
navel — forearm
pelvic girdle — iliac crest
hip — anterior superior iliac spine
radial styloid process — wrist
wrist — styloid process of ulna
greater trochanter of femur — hand
metacarpus — fingers
groin — quadriceps femoris
pubic region — thigh
scrotum — knee
penis — head of fibula
patella — leg
anterior tubercle of tibia — anterior muscles of leg
tibia — medial malleolus

A

the human body

However the human body may be considered as a unit, it consists of a group of external elements, each one of them with a specific function and an appropriate name. Although many elements and parts participate in the constitution of the organism, here they are only mentioned the most useful and well-known ones, also, it is worth to bear in mind that some of them are parts exclusively belonging to the human being.

6

SUPERFICIAL ANATOMY (II)

MALE SEX. POSTERIOR VIEW

the shapes of the human body

The shapes that appear along the different parts of the human body are not of a capricious type, but they basically obey three separate principles: the hormone action, specific for male and for female individuals; the fact that they are conditioned by various structures (bones, muscles, intestines, etc.) they contain; and finally, the shapes are also conditioned by the function these structures are intended to accomplish (movement, locomotion, prehensility, etc.). When the human body is attentively examined it appears that all its shapes can be logically explained.

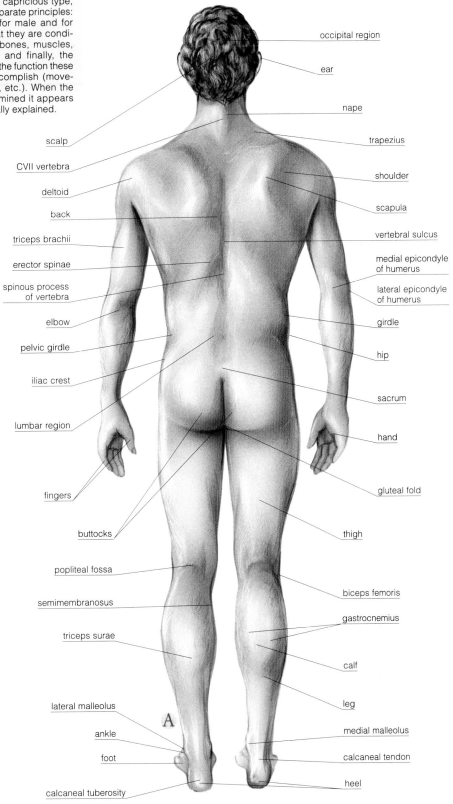

occipital region

ear

nape

trapezius

shoulder

scapula

vertebral sulcus

medial epicondyle of humerus

lateral epicondyle of humerus

girdle

hip

sacrum

hand

gluteal fold

thigh

biceps femoris

gastrocnemius

calf

leg

medial malleolus

calcaneal tendon

heel

scalp

CVII vertebra

deltoid

back

triceps brachii

erector spinae

spinous process of vertebra

elbow

pelvic girdle

iliac crest

lumbar region

fingers

buttocks

popliteal fossa

semimembranosus

triceps surae

lateral malleolus

ankle

foot

calcaneal tuberosity

A

7

REGIONS of the HUMAN BODY (I)

FEMALE SEX. ANTERIOR GENERAL VIEW

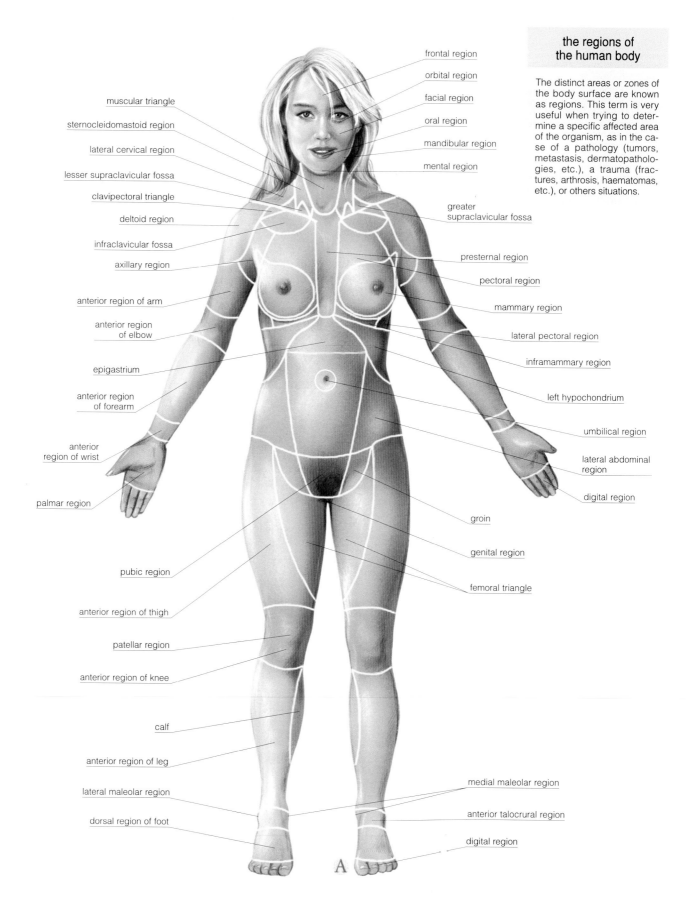

muscular triangle

sternocleidomastoid region

lateral cervical region

lesser supraclavicular fossa

clavipectoral triangle

deltoid region

infraclavicular fossa

axillary region

anterior region of arm

anterior region of elbow

epigastrium

anterior region of forearm

anterior region of wrist

palmar region

pubic region

anterior region of thigh

patellar region

anterior region of knee

calf

anterior region of leg

lateral maleolar region

dorsal region of foot

frontal region

orbital region

facial region

oral region

mandibular region

mental region

greater supraclavicular fossa

presternal region

pectoral region

mammary region

lateral pectoral region

inframammary region

left hypochondrium

umbilical region

lateral abdominal region

digital region

groin

genital region

femoral triangle

medial maleolar region

anterior talocrural region

digital region

A

the regions of the human body

The distinct areas or zones of the body surface are known as regions. This term is very useful when trying to determine a specific affected area of the organism, as in the case of a pathology (tumors, metastasis, dermatopathologies, etc.), a trauma (fractures, arthrosis, haematomas, etc.), or others situations.

8

REGIONS of the HUMAN BODY (II)
FEMALE SEX. POSTERIOR GENERAL VIEW

the regions of the human body

Assigning a region to each one of the areas of the body surface is a precision gaining strategy, however is not easy to exactly determine the different regions because sometimes the limits are not very clear. Also, it is worth to bear in mind the fact that a region can be divided into various sub-regions; or the same zone may present various names according to the criteria of different anatomists.

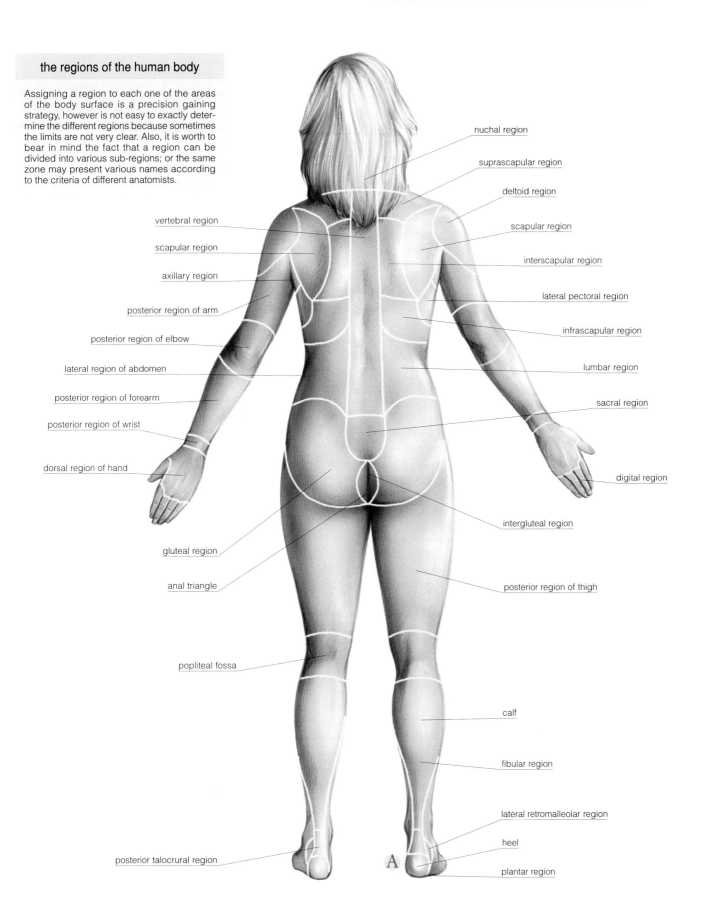

nuchal region

suprascapular region

deltoid region

scapular region

interscapular region

lateral pectoral region

infrascapular region

lumbar region

sacral region

digital region

intergluteal region

posterior region of thigh

calf

fibular region

lateral retromalleolar region

heel

plantar region

vertebral region

scapular region

axillary region

posterior region of arm

posterior region of elbow

lateral region of abdomen

posterior region of forearm

posterior region of wrist

dorsal region of hand

gluteal region

anal triangle

popliteal fossa

posterior talocrural region

A

9

REGIONS of the HUMAN BODY (III). HEAD (I)

MALE SEX. ANTERIOR VIEW

the head

Besides being an anatomic area of the human body used to identify individuals, and of containing a group of organs corresponding to various apparatuses that accomplish different functions (digestive, respiratory, visual, olfactory, phonatory, etc.), the head is also the receptacle of one of the most vital elements of the human being, the brain. The brain and all its appendages have an important role in the utter control of the whole organism.

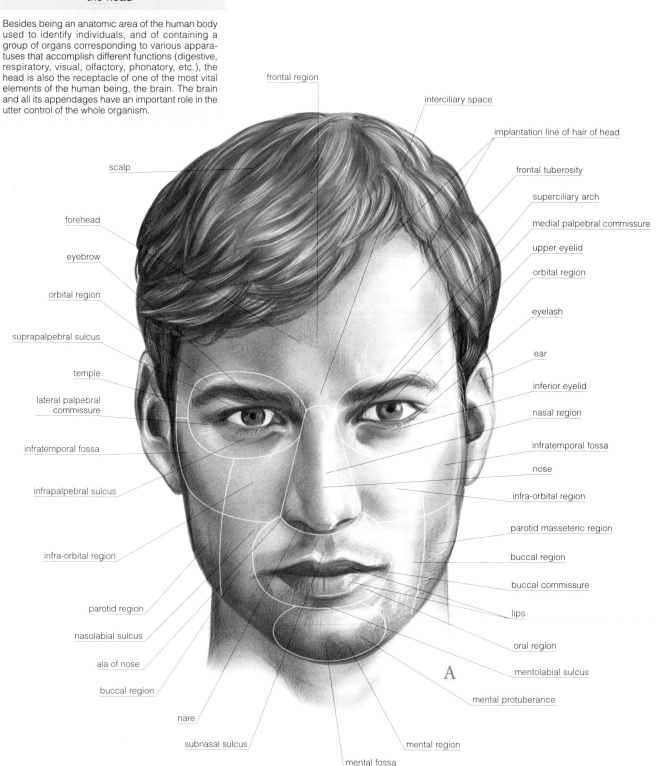

frontal region

interciliary space

implantation line of hair of head

frontal tuberosity

superciliary arch

medial palpebral commissure

upper eyelid

orbital region

eyelash

ear

inferior eyelid

nasal region

infratemporal fossa

nose

infra-orbital region

parotid masseteric region

buccal region

buccal commissure

lips

oral region

mentolabial sulcus

mental protuberance

mental region

mental fossa

scalp

forehead

eyebrow

orbital region

suprapalpebral sulcus

temple

lateral palpebral commissure

infratemporal fossa

infrapalpebral sulcus

infra-orbital region

parotid region

nasolabial sulcus

ala of nose

buccal region

nare

subnasal sulcus

A

10

REGIONS of the HUMAN BODY (IV). HEAD (II)

MALE SEX. LATERAL VIEW

the head

The head is normally defined as the upper portion of the human body. It is made up for two basic components: the skull, located at the superior-posterior section, and the face, located at the inferior- anterior section. It contains many elements and it presents specific characteristics; sometimes just slight alterations in them can make the difference between one individual from another, in terms of appearance, health conditions, state of mind or personal identity. It also contains a group of muscular and nervous structures which movement participates in the definition of the facial expression in every moment.

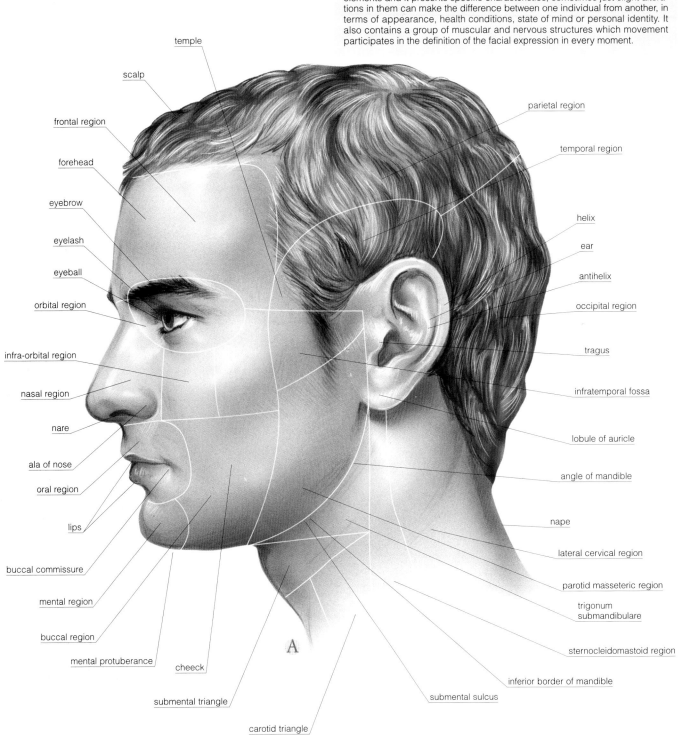

temple
scalp
frontal region
forehead
eyebrow
eyelash
eyeball
orbital region
infra-orbital region
nasal region
nare
ala of nose
oral region
lips
buccal commissure
mental region
buccal region
mental protuberance
cheeck
submental triangle
carotid triangle

parietal region
temporal region
helix
ear
antihelix
occipital region
tragus
infratemporal fossa
lobule of auricle
angle of mandible
nape
lateral cervical region
parotid masseteric region
trigonum submandibulare
sternocleidomastoid region
inferior border of mandible
submental sulcus

A

11

REGIONS of the HUMAN BODY (V). HAND

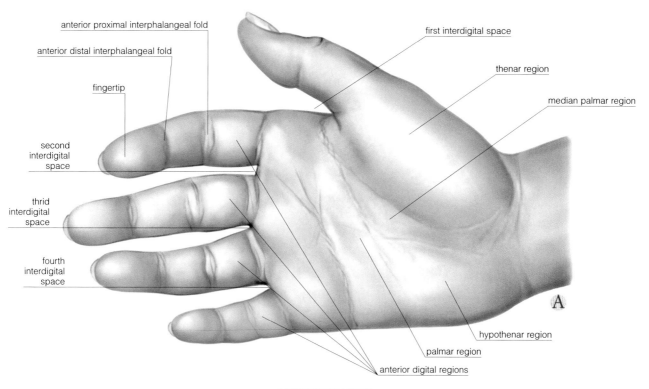

anterior proximal interphalangeal fold

anterior distal interphalangeal fold

fingertip

second interdigital space

thrid interdigital space

fourth interdigital space

first interdigital space

thenar region

median palmar region

hypothenar region

palmar region

anterior digital regions

ANTERIOR VIEW

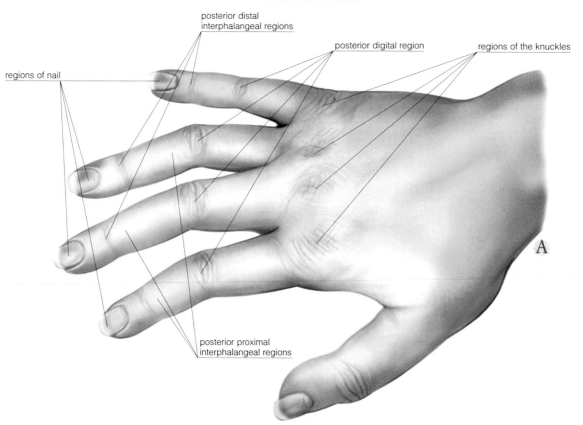

posterior distal interphalangeal regions

posterior digital region

regions of the knuckles

regions of nail

posterior proximal interphalangeal regions

DORSAL VIEW

12

REGIONS of the HUMAN BODY (VI). FOOT

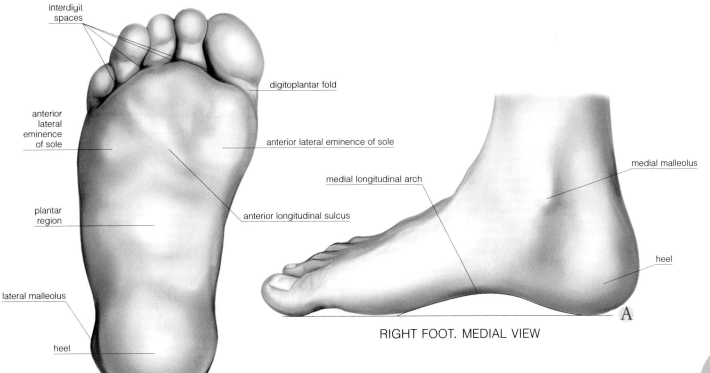

interdigit spaces

digitoplantar fold

anterior lateral eminence of sole

anterior lateral eminence of sole

medial longitudinal arch

medial malleolus

plantar region

anterior longitudinal sulcus

lateral malleolus

heel

heel

RIGHT FOOT. MEDIAL VIEW

RIGHT FOOT. PLANTAR VIEW

13

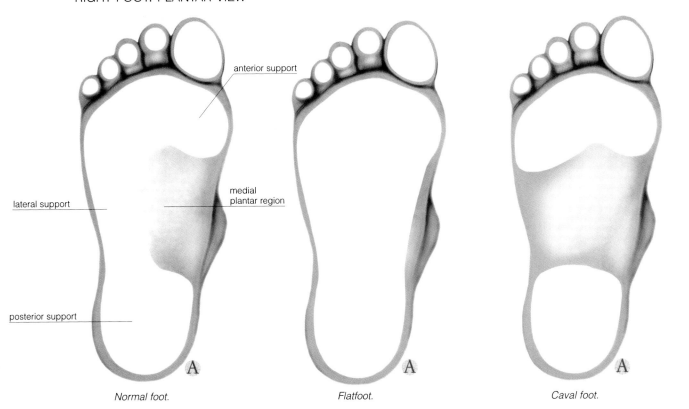

anterior support

lateral support

medial plantar region

posterior support

Normal foot.

Flatfoot.

Caval foot.

FOOTPRINTS. REGIONS OF SUPPORT

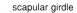

EXTERNAL ANATOMICAL ELEMENTS (I)
MAIN DIFFERENCES BETWEEN SEXES

FEMALE SEX. ANTERIOR VIEW

scapular girdle
Due to the important muscular development in this region, men's scapular girdle is wider than women's.

breasts
As a result of the mammary gland the development during puberty, female breasts are more voluminous than male. After giving birth, the mammary gland secretes milk in order to feed the newborn. During pregnancy the breast increase in size and may become more sensitive. The areola and the nipple turns darker. These changes could also happen during a woman's menstrual cycle.

mammary areoles
This area is more prominent in women than men in order to facilitate breastfeeding.

pubic hair
In women, the distribution of the hair takes the shape of an inverted triangle, while in men a rhomboidal shape.

thighs
Women's thighs and buttocks are more voluminous than men's because of the deposit of fatty tissue in these sites.

height
An average of height, a woman's stature is 5-7% smaller than men's.

facial hair
The woman's face barely has hair, while men's is covered by abundant hair, especially in the area of the chin and upper lip.

pectoral hair
The women's chest does not have hair while the man's chest usually does.

nipple
Women's nipples are more prominent than men's because the canals that originate in the mammary gland at the end in the nipple, to facilitate the suction of the milk, while breastfeeding.

pelvic girdle
It's adapted for the reproductive functions (pregnancy and birth); the group of bones that form it (ileum, isqueon and pubis) are wider in women than in men.

external genitalia
These are very different in men and women. The woman has vulva, barely prominent and hidden between the thighs. Man has penis and scrotum (containing the testicles), perfectly visible and exposed.

hair
In general, women's legs and arms are covered by a small amount of thin hair.

14

the body according to gender

The human body, either female or male, has many elements identical in shape and function (mouth, eyes, hands, feet, etc.) However, some elements are specific for each gender, mainly due to the changes in hormonal concentrations, and more important to the reproductive functions that each one must play. Primary; sexual characteristics (testicles in men, ovaries in women), secondary (penis, prostate in men, and vagina, uterus and uterine tubes in women) and also certain morphologic characteristics (height, figure and proportions), hormonal (estrogens, progesterone, etc.) and psychological (character, emotions, etc.)

A

EXTERNAL ANATOMICAL ELEMENTS (II)
MAIN PARTS of the HUMAN BODY

FEMALE SEX. POSTERIOR VIEW

head

Upper section of the body, which contains two basic elements: the cranium, which occupies the upper posterior section and is a bone cavity where the brain-the central section of the nervous system- and its annexes is located, and the face, located in the lower anterior section, which is the place where the digestive and respiratory system tracts section off from. The lower anterior section also includes the external components of most of the main sense organs: eyes, ears, nose, mouth, all of which play important roles.

neck

Section of the body, of a cylindrical shape, located between the head (hyoid bone) and the thorax (collarbone), which joins them. Its inner section contains many tracts: respiratory, digestive, circulatory, lymphatic, nervous, etc., in addition to the spinal cord.

thorax

Upper section of the trunk, between the neck and the abdomen. With it, it constitutes the trunk, which is the central section of the body. It contains an osteocartilaginous structure (thoracic cavity), where the lungs, heart and other structures are located. It is separated from the lower section of the trunk (abdomen) by the diaphragm muscle.

trunk

It is the central section of the body where the upper central area of the head, the superior lateral sections of the upper limbs, and the inferior lateral sections of the lower limbs join together. It contains two parts: thorax and abdomen; the abdomen also includes the pelvis.

upper limbs

Refers to two appendixes which section, one on each side, from the upper section of the trunk. They contain a group of bones, muscles and joints which can make gestures, lift weights, etc. They have four basic parts (arm; its skeleton is made up of the humerus-,elbow-where joint with the same name is located-, forearm-which bone structure is made up of the radius and the ulna-and the hand-where the carpal and metacarpal bones and the phalanges of the fingers- are located), which have a bone structure and a muscle coverage. Its respective joints possess great mobility, especially the hands.

abdomen

Constitutes the trunk, along with the thorax. The inside of the abdomen contains most of the organs of the digestive system (stomach, intestines, liver and pancreas), as well as the spleen and the urinary organs. Its lower region (or pelvis) contains the urogenital organs and the final section of the digestive system.

15

lower limbs

Refers to two appendixes which section from the lower and lateral sections of the abdomen, one from each side. They are made up of four basic parts (thigh; its skeleton is made up of the femur-, knee-where the joints structures with the same name are gathered-, leg; its bone structure is made up of the tibia, the fibula, and the patella-, and the foot-where the tarsus and metatarsus bones, as well as the phalanges of the fingers are located-); its bone structure and muscle coverage develop great mobility through its limbs. These limbs enable to sustain the entire body structure (maintain a biped posture). It also enables walking.

general distribution of the human body

Despite of having various apparatuses, systems and other functional structures that in its turn contain specific organs and elements, the human body presents a general and basic structure, with specific functions assigned to each one of its parts. Thus, while some are responsible of bipedal posture, making possible all movements and locomotion, others act as receptacles and house organs and structures with vital functions.

EXTERNAL PROJECTION of INTERNAL ORGANS (I)

MALE SEX. ANTERIOR VIEW

internal organs

The internal organs are sited inside the cavities of the human body, so all of them are housed and fill up the organism. The human body contains a large amount of organs and each one of them plays a specific role. Moreover, their shapes adapt and therefore one organ perfectly fits another one to take advantage of the available space without interfering in the normal functioning of the adjoining organ.

larynx

The larynx, specifically the thyroid cartilage, is projected on the anterior and central regions of the neck, where it forms a shape called the laryngeal prominence.

thyroid gland

Located in the anterior section of the neck. It is not prominent. It is adherent to anterior tracheal surface.

heart

Its external projection corresponds to the anterior side of the thorax, called region n precordial, even though the vertex of the heart is projected on the left side of the anterior thoracic wall.

liver

The largest section of the liver corresponds to an area called right hypochondrium, in the right superior angle of the abdominal cavity, below the diaphragm.

gallbladder

Refers to a pear shaped bag which is located in the inferior section of the right lobule of the liver. In it, the bile which has been poured by the hepatic biliary tracts is stored. This bile ends up in the duodenum in order to help to emulsify the fats and to stimulate the movements of the digestive tube (peristalsis).

ascending colon

First section of the large intestine. It occupies the right lateral region of the abdominal cavity. It is projected on the right anterior side and in the right iliac fossa.

caecum

Initial section of the large intestine. It is projected on the lower right part of the abdominal wall, below the ileum opening, in the region which corresponds to the left iliac fossa.

vermiform appendix

Elongated diverticulum, narrow and in the shape of a worm (which is where the name comes from), which hangs from the cecum. This appendix communicates with the cecum.

urinary bladder

Organ in the shape of a bag, located in the lower central section of the abdomen. It is projected in this region, above and behind the symphysis of the pubis.

trachea

Refers to the lower extension of the larynx. It is a cylindrical and cartilaginous tube which is projected on the central section of the neck, through its anterior side, immediately below the laryngeal prominence.

lungs

The lungs are two organs, right and left, with a spongy consistency. Their external projection corresponds to the anterior, lateral and posterior walls of the thorax.

spleen

Lymph organ with an oval shape which projects on the upper left section of the abdomen, known as left hypochodrium.

stomach

Wide bag which is a section of the digestive tube. It is projected on the central, left, and upper regions of the abdomen, in the epigastrium.

transverse colon

Section of the large intestine, located between the ascending colon (where it starts), and the descending colon (where it continues). It is projected from right to left, like a band below the stomach, dividing the abdomen in two.

descending colon

Last section of the large intestine. In its inception, it is projected on the left lateral region of the abdominal cavity, in the anterior side. It subsequently occupies the retroperitoneal compartment.

small intestine

Long tube which sections from the stomach and curls inside the anterior central area of the abdominal cavity.

A

16

EXTERNAL PROJECTION of INTERNAL ORGANS (II)

MALE SEX. POSTERIOR VIEW

external projection of the internal organs

Knowing the location of the different organs within the great cavities of the human body (cranial, thoracic, abdominal, and pelvic) is important. In case of an accident or a surgical intervention, the doctor needs to know exactly where to find each organ in order to access to these organs by a track.

vertebral column
The vertebrae that form it project along the middle region of the back. The spinous process may be palpated through the skin covering this region.

scapula
Flat bone, shaped as a triangle that may be palpated through the skin on the back on both sides of the dorsum. Its superior external border may be palpated through the shoulders musculature.

ribs
These are flat, curved bones, which are palpable through the thoracic wall. They form a cage that protects the thoracic cavity.

heart
its external projection corresponds to the anterior surface of the thorax, known as the precordial region. The vertex of the heart projects onto the anterior thoracic wall.

lungs
There are two lungs, a right lung and a left lung. Both have a spongy consistence. Their external projections correspond to the anterior, lateral and posterior regions of the thorax.

liver
It occupies most of the right hipochodrium. It is located at the right superior angle of the abdominal cavity underneath of the diaphragm.

spleen
Lymphoid organ located on the superior left side of the abdominal cavity, also known as left hypochondrium.

kidneys
Two organs shaped as a half moon that are projected onto the middle posterior region of the trunk on both sides of the back bone in the retroperineal region.

stomach
Wide muscular bag located in the central superior region of the abdomen in the epigastric region.

ascending colon
It is the first portion of the large intestine and occupies the right lateral area of the abdominal cavity.

descending colon
Last part of the large intestine. Its first portion projects into the left lateral region of the abdominal cavity, and latter occupies the retroperitonem.

iliac crests
Forms the superior edge of the hipbone. They may be palpated through the skin of the lateral region of the abdominal cavity.

sigmoid colon
Part of the descending colon, its inferior prolongation is located inside the peritoneum, and inside the pelvic cavity where it continues as the rectum.

rectum
Last portion of the large intestine, it connects the final portion of the sigmoid colon with the anus. Its projection is located in the perineal region.

sacrum and coccyx
Bones located at the end of the backbone. They may are palpated on the superior region of the intergluteal region, known as sacral region.

A

17

EXTERNAL PROJECTION of INTERNAL ORGANS (III)

MALE SEX

18

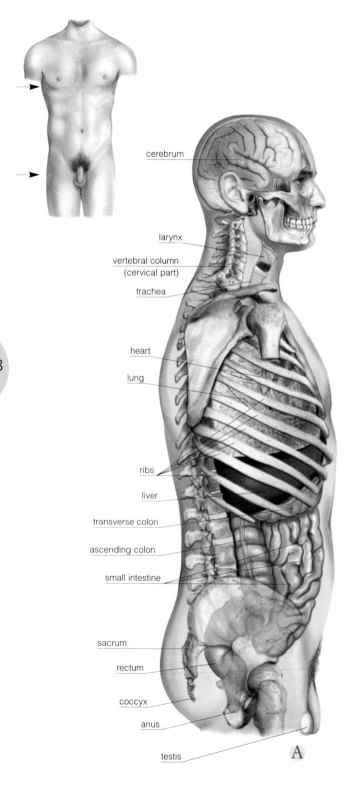

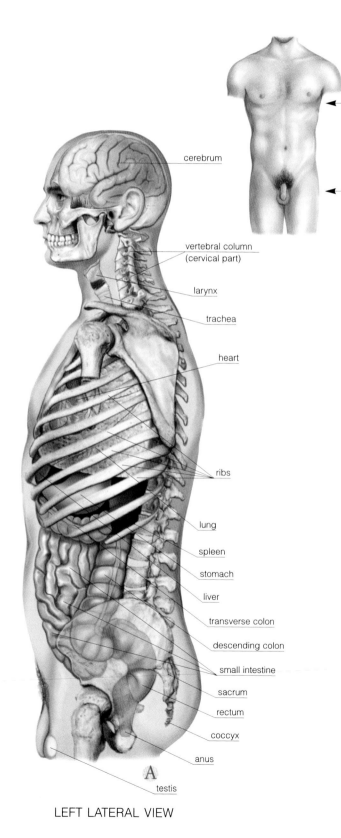

cerebrum

larynx

vertebral column
(cervical part)

trachea

heart

lung

ribs

liver

transverse colon

ascending colon

small intestine

sacrum

rectum

coccyx

anus

testis

A

RIGHT LATERAL VIEW

cerebrum

vertebral column
(cervical part)

larynx

trachea

heart

ribs

lung

spleen

stomach

liver

transverse colon

descending colon

small intestine

sacrum

rectum

coccyx

anus

testis

A

LEFT LATERAL VIEW

EXTERNAL PROJECTION of INTERNAL ORGANS (IV)

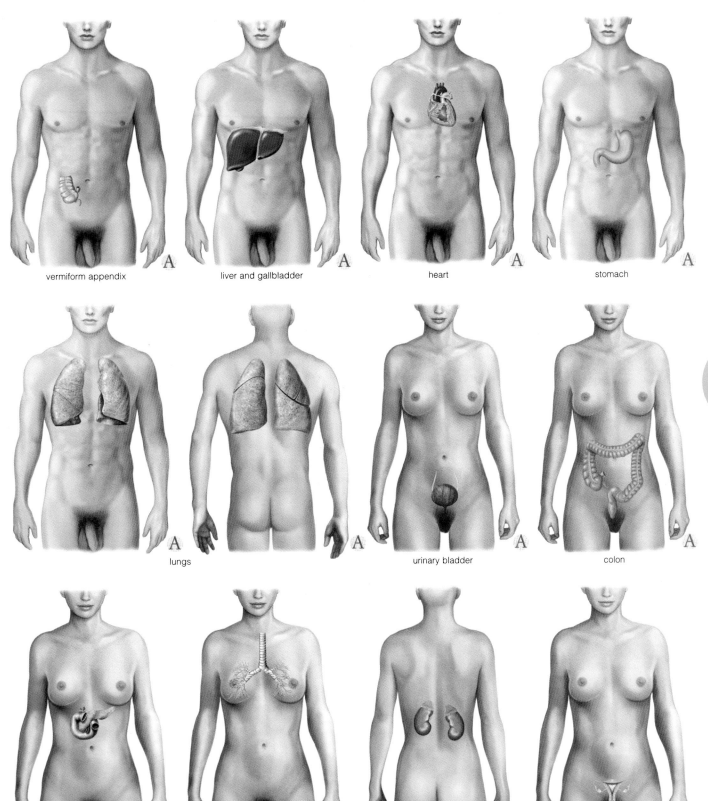

19

vermiform appendix

liver and gallbladder

heart

stomach

lungs

urinary bladder

colon

pancreas

trachea and bronchi

kidneys

uterus and ovaries

TRANSVERSE SECTIONS (I)

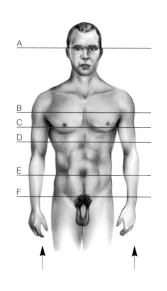

A
B
C
D
E
F

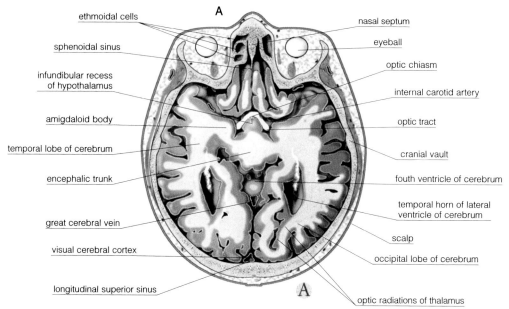

A

ethmoidal cells

nasal septum

sphenoidal sinus

eyeball

infundibular recess
of hypothalamus

optic chiasm

internal carotid artery

amigdaloid body

optic tract

temporal lobe of cerebrum

cranial vault

encephalic trunk

fouth ventricle of cerebrum

temporal horn of lateral
ventricle of cerebrum

great cerebral vein

scalp

visual cerebral cortex

occipital lobe of cerebrum

longitudinal superior sinus

optic radiations of thalamus

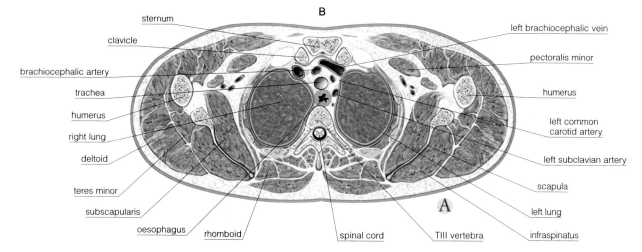

B

sternum

left brachiocephalic vein

clavicle

pectoralis minor

brachiocephalic artery

humerus

trachea

left common
carotid artery

humerus

right lung

left subclavian artery

deltoid

scapula

teres minor

left lung

subscapularis

infraspinatus

oesophagus   rhomboid   spinal cord   TIII vertebra

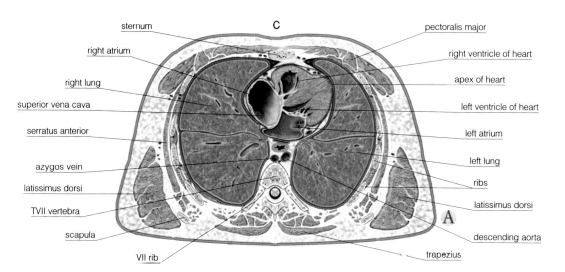

C

sternum

pectoralis major

right atrium

right ventricle of heart

right lung

apex of heart

superior vena cava

left ventricle of heart

serratus anterior

left atrium

azygos vein

left lung

latissimus dorsi

ribs

TVII vertebra

latissimus dorsi

scapula

descending aorta

VII rib

trapezius

TRANSVERSE SECTIONS (II)

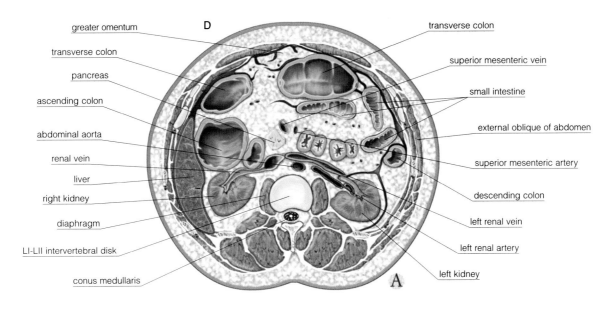

greater omentum — D — transverse colon
transverse colon — superior mesenteric vein
pancreas — small intestine
ascending colon — external oblique of abdomen
abdominal aorta — superior mesenteric artery
renal vein — descending colon
liver — left renal vein
right kidney — left renal artery
diaphragm — left kidney
LI-LII intervertebral disk
conus medullaris

A

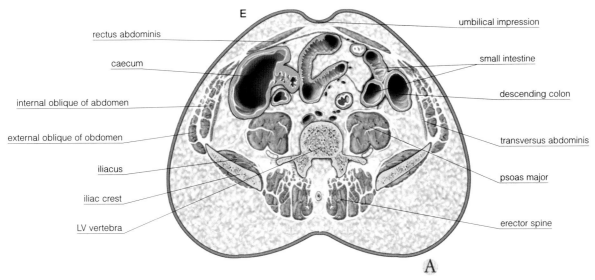

— E —
rectus abdominis — umbilical impression
caecum — small intestine
internal oblique of abdomen — descending colon
external oblique of obdomen — transversus abdominis
iliacus — psoas major
iliac crest
LV vertebra — erector spine

A

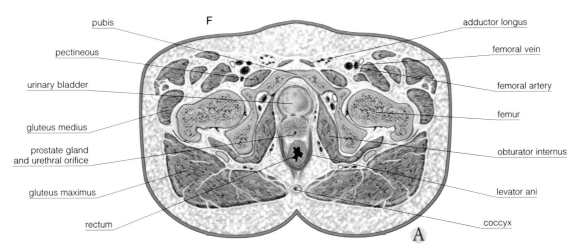

pubis — F — adductor longus
pectineous — femoral vein
urinary bladder — femoral artery
gluteus medius — femur
prostate gland and urethral orifice — obturator internus
gluteus maximus — levator ani
rectum — coccyx

A

DESCRIPTIVE TERMINOLOGY. ORIENTATION. PLANES

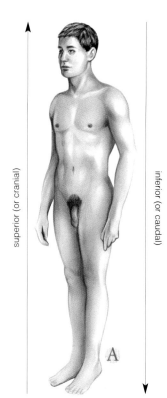

superior (or cranial)

inferior (or caudal)

A

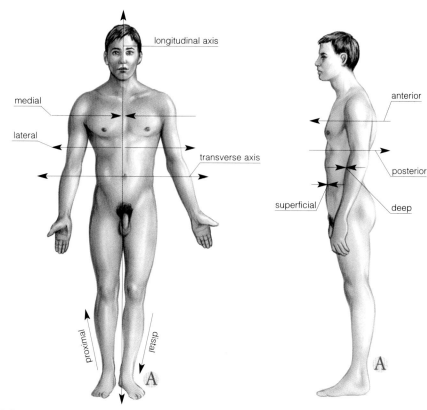

longitudinal axis

medial

lateral

transverse axis

proximal

distal

A

anterior

posterior

superficial

deep

A

ORIENTATION, RELATION and COMPARISON TERMINOLOGY

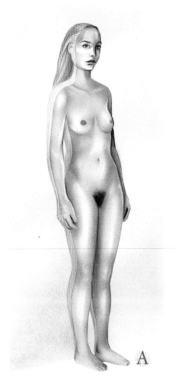

frontal plane (or coronal plane)

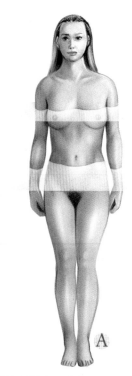

horizontal planes (o transverse planes)

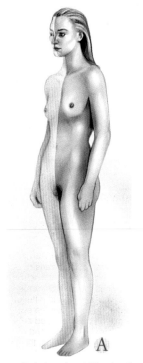

sagittal plane (or middle plane)

BODY PLANES

GLANDS. FUNCTIONAL CLASSIFICATION

merocrine glands

Refers to cells which pour their secretions to the corresponding tubule or alveolus through exocytosis (the substance to be secreted passes through the cell membrane of the apical pole, immediately after it has been synthesized). Salivary and sweat glands belong to this group. Unlike holocrine glands, this does not lead to the destruction or a loss of integrity for these cells.

holocrine glands

Refers to cells that need to break down in order to pour their secretion substances to the corresponding tubule or alveolus. Cell debris or even whole cells may be part of these secretions. These glands need to constantly renew themselves. Sebaceous cells are included in these glands.

apocrine glands

Refers to secretion products that are stored in the inner part of the cells, close to the apical pole, up to the moment when the cell membrane opens and frees up the secretion, after which the cell membrane closes up again. Mammary glands belong to this group, as well as some sweat glands, which activity starts up during puberty and secrete a very dense sweat, mainly located in the armpit, anus, perineum, groin, etc.

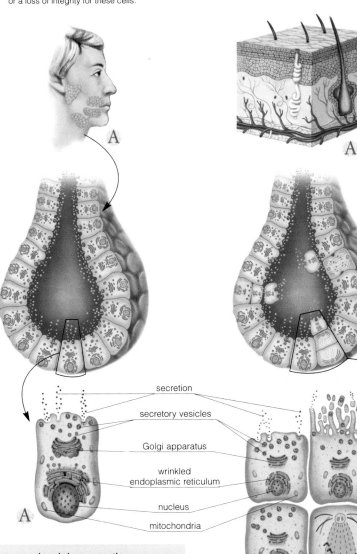

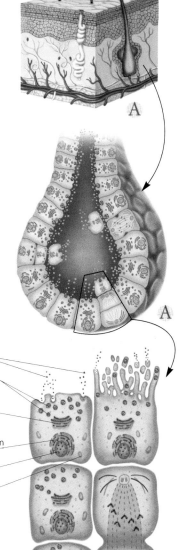

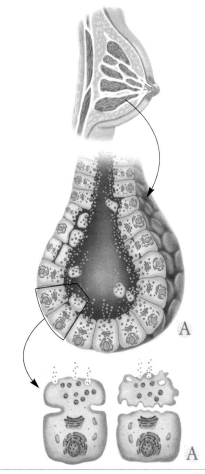

secretion

secretory vesicles

Golgi apparatus

wrinkled endoplasmic reticulum

nucleus

mitochondria

23

glandular secretion

It is the process of elaboration of a specific product or substance as a result of the activity of a gland. This activity goes from the separation of a specific substance coming from the bloodstream, by means of chemical selection, to the obtainment of a new substance after a previous process of transformation. This process may be done in different ways. Thus, according to the place the secretion is poured the glands are classified as endocrines, or with internal secretion, and exocrines, or with external secretion. Also, the exocrine glands, coming from epithelial tissue and according to the mechanism of secretion, may be classified as merocrines, holocrine, and apocrine glands.

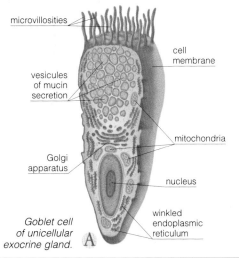

microvillosities

cell membrane

vesicles of mucin secretion

mitochondria

Golgi apparatus

nucleus

winkled endoplasmic reticulum

Goblet cell of unicellular exocrine gland.

THE BODY SYSTEMS (I)

organization of the human body

The human body has a structure that includes apparatuses and systems accomplishing specific functions each one of them. These functions can be classified according to different tasks: supporting and movement (skeleton, muscles and joints), maintenance and nutrition (cardiovascular, respiratory and digestive), cleansing and defense (skin, urinary system, blood and immunologic system), general control (nervous system and endocrine secretion), relation with the outer of the body (senses) and the perpetuation of the human species (genital). All the above mentioned functions allow all the normal activities and they also work in obtaining all that the body needs, and also participate in avoiding and/or defending the organism from any possible harmful agent.

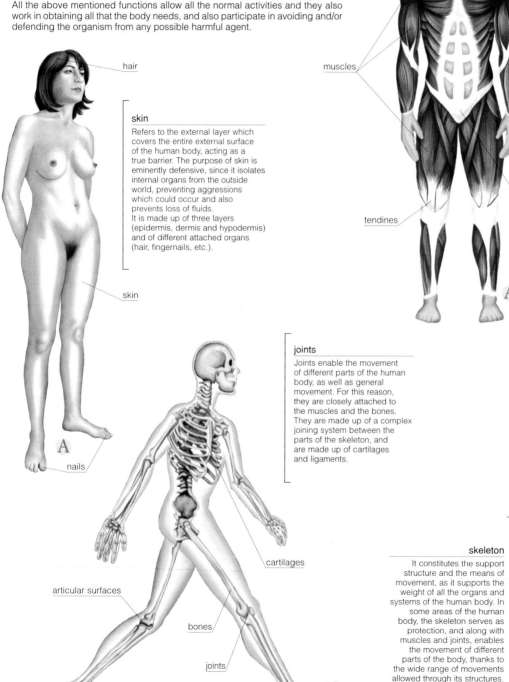

hair

skin

Refers to the external layer which covers the entire external surface of the human body, acting as a true barrier. The purpose of skin is eminently defensive, since it isolates internal organs from the outside world, preventing aggressions which could occur and also prevents loss of fluids.
It is made up of three layers (epidermis, dermis and hypodermis) and of different attached organs (hair, fingernails, etc.).

skin

nails

muscles

muscles

Refers to the complex muscular set which supports the human body and joins many of its elements. Muscles also allow the movement of different joints. It provides the necessary motor force to enable the movement of bones and joints. Muscles are organized in different layers around the skeleton.

tendines

fasciae

joints

Joints enable the movement of different parts of the human body, as well as general movement. For this reason, they are closely attached to the muscles and the bones. They are made up of a complex joining system between the parts of the skeleton, and are made up of cartilages and ligaments.

cartilages

articular surfaces

bones

joints

skeleton

It constitutes the support structure and the means of movement, as it supports the weight of all the organs and systems of the human body. In some areas of the human body, the skeleton serves as protection, and along with muscles and joints, enables the movement of different parts of the body, thanks to the wide range of movements allowed through its structures.

bones

THE BODY SYSTEMS (II)

systems

The apparatuses and systems of the organism are in charge of supplying it, in every moment, with the necessary conditions to survive but also to enjoy and appropriate quality of life. The basic functions each apparatus or system accomplishes are intended to satisfy all the needs within an apparatus or system when it is required that satisfactorily fulfills a specific function of the organism. On the other hand, each apparatus or system consist of a group of organs and elements that are very well synchronized one to the other and to the appropriate function they are appointed to. All this assembly of parts is also an interdependent unit.

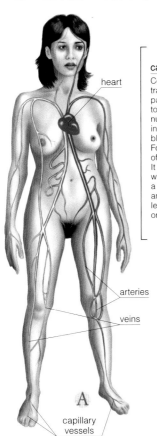

heart

arteries

veins

capillary
vessels

cardiovascular system

Conduction method which transports blood to any part of the body, in order to provide the necessary nutritional elements contained in blood. In the return trip, blood carries waste products. For these reasons, the role of blood is primarily nutritious. It is made up of the heart, which acts as a center and a motor for the entire system, and blood vessels which leave the heart (arteries) or enter the heart (veins).

mouth

oesophagus

stomach

liver

small
intestine

large
intestine

rectum

anus

digestive system

Its role is eminently digestive, since it is in charge of ingesting food, running it through the digestive process, facilitating its absorption to the blood, and eliminating waste substances which result from the entire process. In order to carry out this role, the digestive system has different organs and two very important complementary elements: the liver and the pancreas.

25

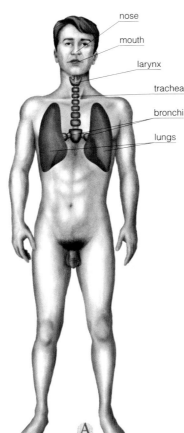

nose

mouth

larynx

trachea

bronchi

lungs

kidney

ureters

urinary
bladder

urethra

respiratory system

Its role is both nutritional and purifying, since it has two purposes: make sure the blood receives oxygen, which is fundamental for human cell metabolism, and ease the expulsion of carbon dioxide, which is a residual product of said metabolism. It includes airways and two terminal structures, which are the lungs. Its functioning is closely related to the heart.

nephro-urinary system

This system is in charge of filtering blood and extracting damaging products or products which cannot be used, exiting them through urine. Therefore, it is the natural purifying method of the human body. It is made up of two organs, the kidneys, which play a strictly purifying role, and other structures, which function is to transport urine to the outside through the urethra.

THE BODY SYSTEMS (III)

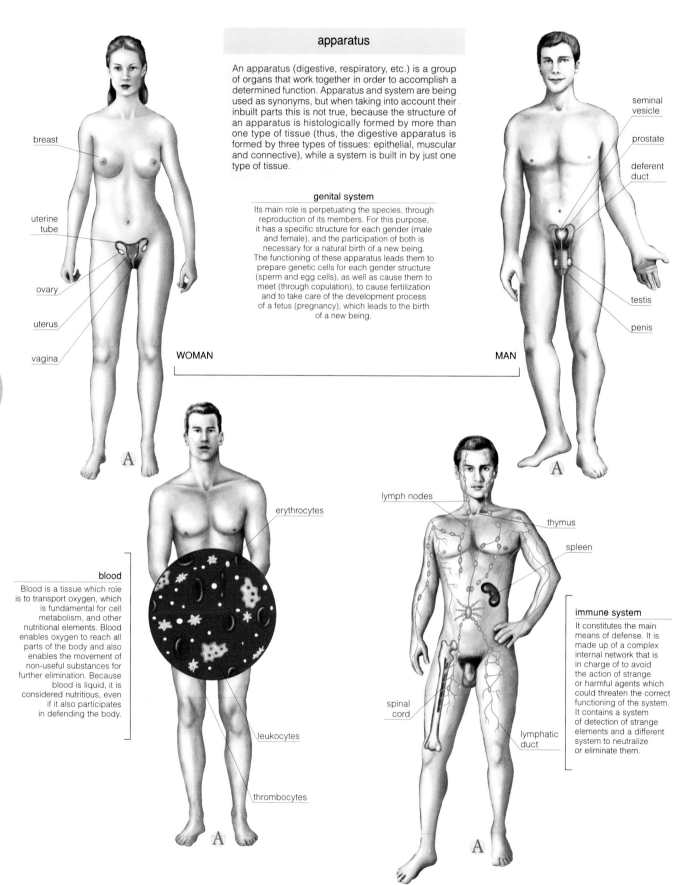

apparatus

An apparatus (digestive, respiratory, etc.) is a group of organs that work together in order to accomplish a determined function. Apparatus and system are being used as synonyms, but when taking into account their inbuilt parts this is not true, because the structure of an apparatus is histologically formed by more than one type of tissue (thus, the digestive apparatus is formed by three types of tissues: epithelial, muscular and connective), while a system is built in by just one type of tissue.

genital system

Its main role is perpetuating the species, through reproduction of its members. For this purpose, it has a specific structure for each gender (male and female), and the participation of both is necessary for a natural birth of a new being. The functioning of these apparatus leads them to prepare genetic cells for each gender structure (sperm and egg cells), as well as cause them to meet (through copulation), to cause fertilization and to take care of the development process of a fetus (pregnancy), which leads to the birth of a new being.

breast

uterine tube

ovary

uterus

vagina

WOMAN

seminal vesicle

prostate

deferent duct

testis

penis

MAN

26

blood

Blood is a tissue which role is to transport oxygen, which is fundamental for cell metabolism, and other nutritional elements. Blood enables oxygen to reach all parts of the body and also enables the movement of non-useful substances for further elimination. Because blood is liquid, it is considered nutritious, even if it also participates in defending the body.

erythrocytes

leukocytes

thrombocytes

lymph nodes

thymus

spleen

spinal cord

lymphatic duct

immune system

It constitutes the main means of defense. It is made up of a complex internal network that is in charge of to avoid the action of strange or harmful agents which could threaten the correct functioning of the system. It contains a system of detection of strange elements and a different system to neutralize or eliminate them.

THE BODY SYSTEMS (IV)

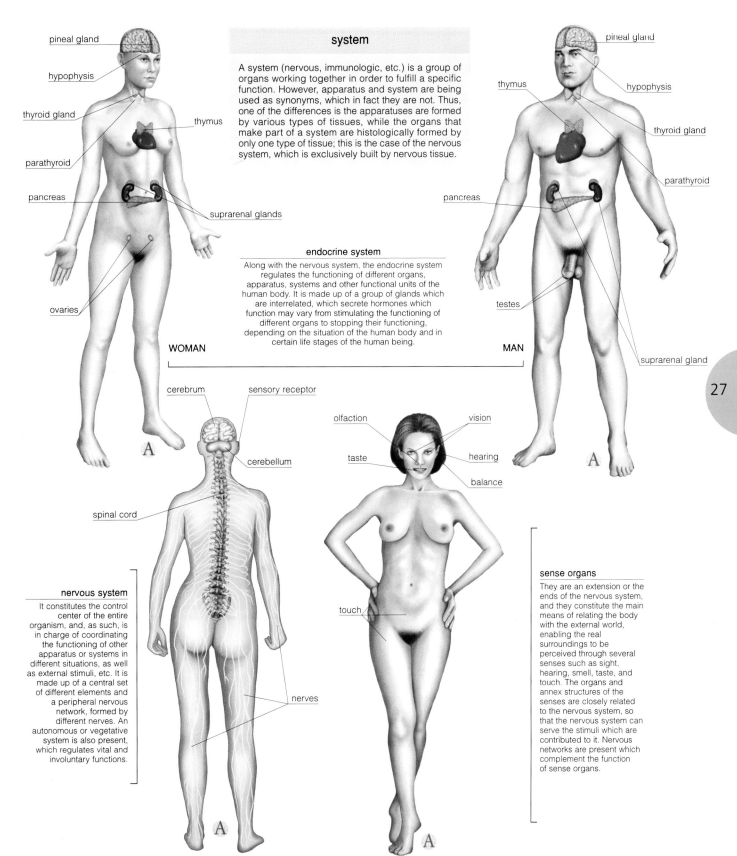

pineal gland

hypophysis

thyroid gland

thymus

parathyroid

pancreas

suprarenal glands

ovaries

WOMAN

system

A system (nervous, immunologic, etc.) is a group of organs working together in order to fulfill a specific function. However, apparatus and system are being used as synonyms, which in fact they are not. Thus, one of the differences is the apparatuses are formed by various types of tissues, while the organs that make part of a system are histologically formed by only one type of tissue; this is the case of the nervous system, which is exclusively built by nervous tissue.

pineal gland

thymus

hypophysis

thyroid gland

parathyroid

pancreas

testes

suprarenal gland

MAN

endocrine system

Along with the nervous system, the endocrine system regulates the functioning of different organs, apparatus, systems and other functional units of the human body. It is made up of a group of glands which are interrelated, which secrete hormones which function may vary from stimulating the functioning of different organs to stopping their functioning, depending on the situation of the human body and in certain life stages of the human being.

27

cerebrum

sensory receptor

cerebellum

spinal cord

nerves

olfaction

vision

taste

hearing

balance

touch

nervous system

It constitutes the control center of the entire organism, and, as such, is in charge of coordinating the functioning of other apparatus or systems in different situations, as well as external stimuli, etc. It is made up of a central set of different elements and a peripheral nervous network, formed by different nerves. An autonomous or vegetative system is also present, which regulates vital and involuntary functions.

sense organs

They are an extension or the ends of the nervous system, and they constitute the main means of relating the body with the external world, enabling the real surroundings to be perceived through several senses such as sight, hearing, smell, taste, and touch. The organs and annex structures of the senses are closely related to the nervous system, so that the nervous system can serve the stimuli which are contributed to it. Nervous networks are present which complement the function of sense organs.

MUCOUS and SEROUS MEMBRANES

mucous
membrane of nose

mucous
membrane of mouth

mucous membrane
of oesophagus

mucous membrane of bronchus

A

mucous membrane

It is a membranous coating of the cavities and ducts of the body which are communicated with the exterior and segregate mucus. It consists of a superficial layer, epithelium, and a deep one, dermis, which is separated from the epithelial one by a basement membrane and from the submucous tunic by a layer of smooth muscular fibers, the muscular layer of the mucous membrane. This is the case of the hollow cavities of the digestive tract and also of the respiratory, urinary and genital ducts. In any case, they are always membranes which have been dampen by some type of secretion, for example, in the case of the urinary ducts, by the urine. The mucosas normally accomplish two functions, absorption and secretion. Most of the mucosas (like the ones in the digestive tract or the respiratory ducts) contain goblet cells which secrete lubricant and protector mucus, but some (like the ones on the urinary ducts) lack this type of cells.

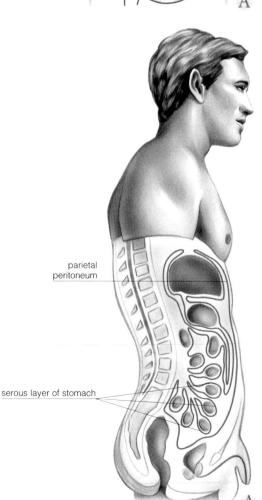

parietal pleura

visceral pleura

visceral layer
of serous pericardium

parietal layer
of serous
pericardium

A

parietal
peritoneum

serous layer of stomach

A

serous membrane

It is a membrane lining the exterior part of the closed cavities of the body (perineum, pleura and pericardium) and it also appears on the surface of some organs or viscus. It corresponds to the wet membrane of the closed anterior cavity of the body. It consists of various thin layers of loose connective tissue that are covered by the mesothelium at the free surfaces. The serosas contain a parietal layer lining the wall of a cavity that folds and becomes the visceral layer, which is the one coating the external surface of the organs or entrails contained in a cavity. The serous cavities always contain an amount of white and translucent liquid, a serous exudate, which is secreted by the mesothelium cells and it contains macrophages, mesothelium cells and small size lymphocytes. This liquid lubricates parietal and visceral layers, facilitating the slipping of one layer over the other and reducing friction, thus avoiding organs and entrails get stuck one to the other or to the wall of the cavity.

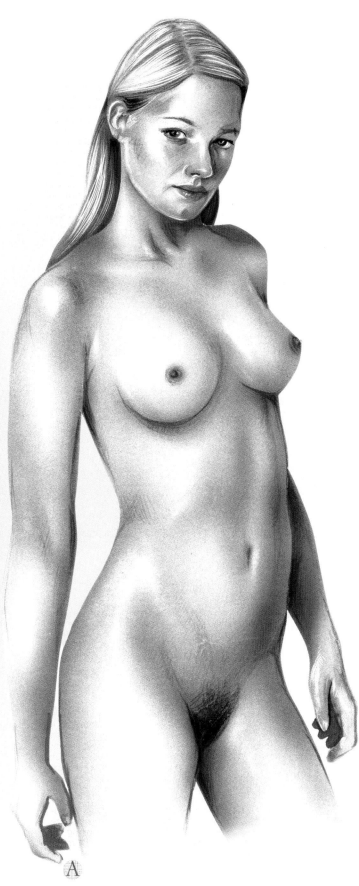

SKIN

The skin is the integumentary tissue resistant and flexible which covers the entire body surface and in natural orifices, continues with mucous membranes. It is basically made up of the epidermis, which is an epithelial ectodermal layer, and by the dermis or layer of mesodermal origin. The skin surface of an adult individual measures about 2m^2 and corresponds approximately to 5% of the total weight.

Skin is the largest organ of the body and also is the one that more functions performs, to the point of be essential for the subsistence of human beings:

- It acts as a defense barrier against external aggressions of different types: microorganisms, several chemical attacks, accidents, fire, sun ultraviolet rays, weather, etc.
- It constantly keeps an own polyvalent activate immune system.
- It retains substances into the organism which are essential,
  as blood, lymph, spinal fluid, hormones, etc.
- It is provided with a thermoregulation system, based on secretion and evaporation water, to maintain a proper body heat.
- It exchanges solar energy into vitamin D, essential in absorption of calcium and phosphorus.
- It maintains a narrow homeostasis with inner corporal organs, which makes that its aspect, color, texture, etc. help to define the state of the individual health.
- It is the main organ of sense of touch. Not even miniscule, any of its parts contain nervous ends and sensitive receptors related to temperature, pain, pressure, friction, etc.
- It represents an excellent way to know of human being and about particular situations and how the person feels both mood or emotionally (flushed face when feeling shame, goose bumps with the fear, radiant about happiness, etc.).
- It shows in each individual forms and specific characteristics that becomes skin the main sign of physical identity.

In spite of appearing at first sight as a simple organ, is enough what it has been stated to certify the importance of this functional unit for human being's life.

SKIN STRUCTURE

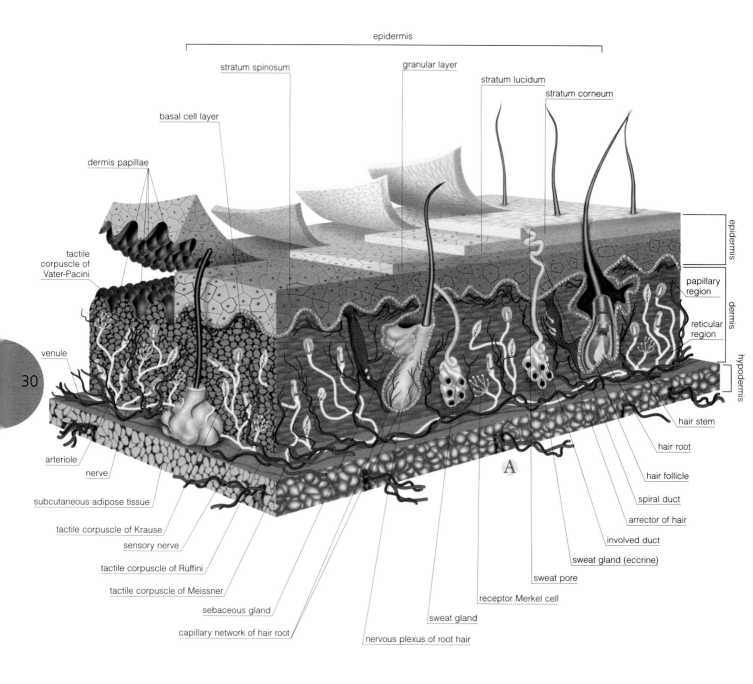

epidermis

stratum spinosum

granular layer

stratum lucidum

stratum corneum

basal cell layer

dermis papillae

tactile corpuscle of Vater-Pacini

venule

30

arteriole

nerve

subcutaneous adipose tissue

tactile corpuscle of Krause

sensory nerve

tactile corpuscle of Ruffini

tactile corpuscle of Meissner

sebaceous gland

capillary network of hair root

nervous plexus of root hair

sweat gland

receptor Merkel cell

sweat pore

sweat gland (eccrine)

involved duct

arrector of hair

spiral duct

hair follicle

hair root

hair stem

epidermis

papillary region

dermis

reticular region

hypodermis

A

skin

The skin is the external layer that covers the whole surface of the human body. A few elements from the body fulfill as many functions as the skin does. Many of these functions are so important that became the skin an essential organ. It acts as a protective barrier with an eminent defensive function against the external elements and aggressions; through the skin it is manifested the general state of the individual, both the health and mood; it is the primary tactile organ, it is the characteristic and identity organ of each individual. The skin gives much information about the external environment: cold, heat, humidity, stimulus, and a long etcetera. It has three layers and has different annex organs.

HAND. FOLDS and FINGERPRINTS

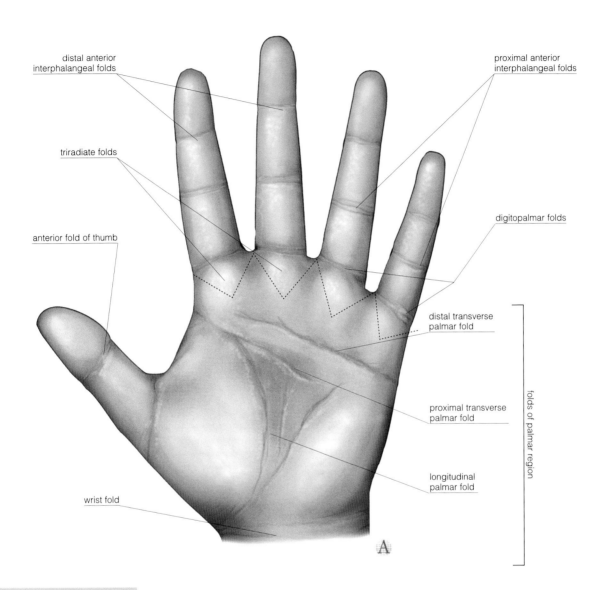

distal anterior interphalangeal folds

proximal anterior interphalangeal folds

triradiate folds

anterior fold of thumb

digitopalmar folds

distal transverse palmar fold

proximal transverse palmar fold

folds of palmar region

longitudinal palmar fold

wrist fold

Ⓐ

31

fingerprints

These are a set of ridges and crests that are disposed in a singular and particular way for each individual. They are observed in the skin of the anterior surface of the hand and foot. When ink is used on these surfaces and then put on paper, are printed on it a set of characteristic drawings that are known as palm prints (if they are from the whole hand), plantar prints (if they are from the foot) or fingerprints (if they are from the fingers). Taking these prints is very common in medicine, especially to identify the newborn (pediatric medicine) or deceased individuals in special circumstances (forensic and judicial medicine).

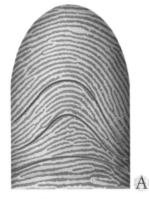

Simple arch.

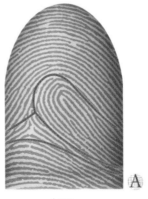

Loop.

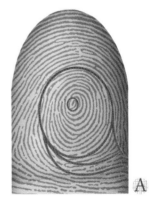

Simple spiral.

FINGERPRINT TYPES

CUTANEOUS FOLDS

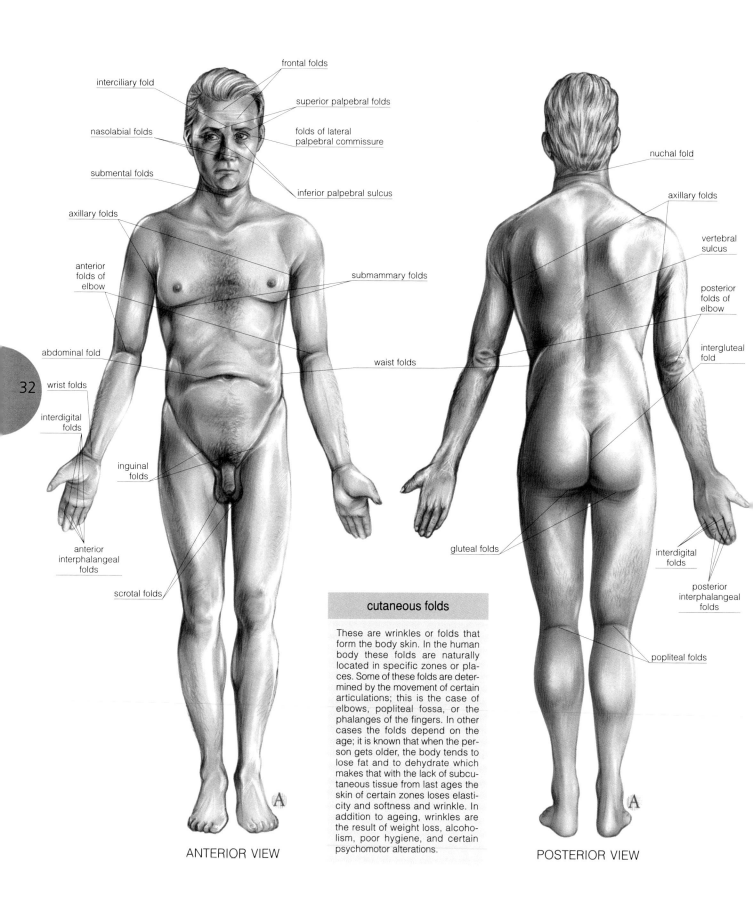

frontal folds

interciliary fold

superior palpebral folds

nasolabial folds

folds of lateral palpebral commissure

submental folds

inferior palpebral sulcus

axillary folds

anterior folds of elbow

submammary folds

abdominal fold

waist folds

wrist folds

interdigital folds

inguinal folds

anterior interphalangeal folds

scrotal folds

nuchal fold

axillary folds

vertebral sulcus

posterior folds of elbow

intergluteal fold

gluteal folds

interdigital folds

posterior interphalangeal folds

popliteal folds

32

ANTERIOR VIEW

POSTERIOR VIEW

cutaneous folds

These are wrinkles or folds that form the body skin. In the human body these folds are naturally located in specific zones or places. Some of these folds are determined by the movement of certain articulations; this is the case of elbows, popliteal fossa, or the phalanges of the fingers. In other cases the folds depend on the age; it is known that when the person gets older, the body tends to lose fat and to dehydrate which makes that with the lack of subcutaneous tissue from last ages the skin of certain zones loses elasticity and softness and wrinkle. In addition to ageing, wrinkles are the result of weight loss, alcoholism, poor hygiene, and certain psychomotor alterations.

TENSION LINES of SKIN

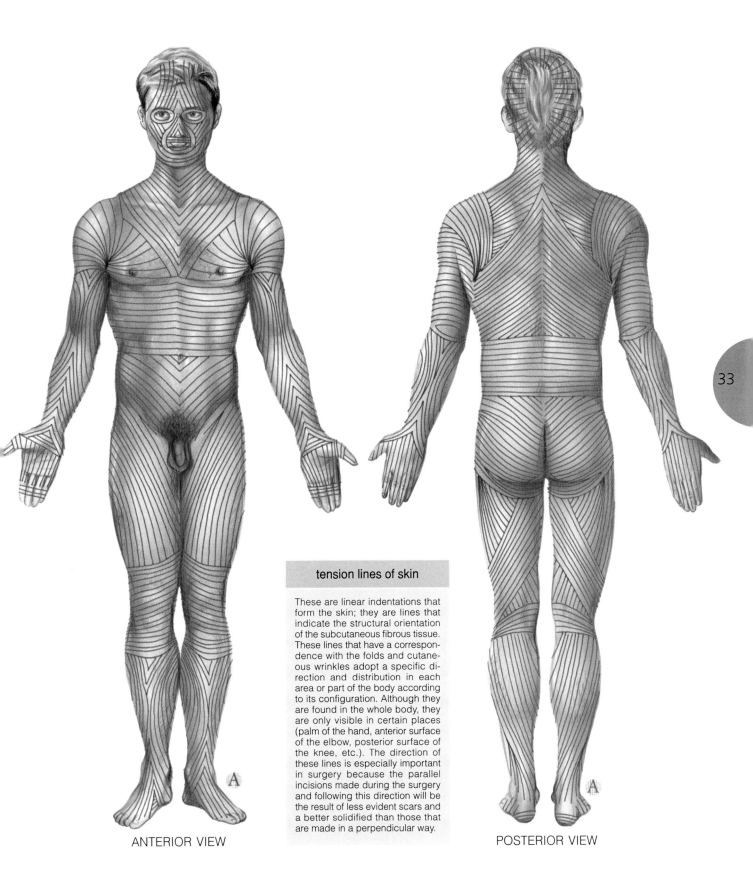

tension lines of skin

These are linear indentations that form the skin; they are lines that indicate the structural orientation of the subcutaneous fibrous tissue. These lines that have a correspondence with the folds and cutaneous wrinkles adopt a specific direction and distribution in each area or part of the body according to its configuration. Although they are found in the whole body, they are only visible in certain places (palm of the hand, anterior surface of the elbow, posterior surface of the knee, etc.). The direction of these lines is especially important in surgery because the parallel incisions made during the surgery and following this direction will be the result of less evident scars and a better solidified than those that are made in a perpendicular way.

ANTERIOR VIEW

POSTERIOR VIEW

33

CALCULATION of BODILY SURFACE

calculation of bodily surface

The calculation of bodily surface is complex because the human body has many prominences, concavities, crannies and several shapes. In certain occasions, especially when burns are produced, it is said about the percentage of the affected area. In order to establish this calculation, it is often used as a method the so called nine formula, slang that has been applied because adopts the number 9 as the base. Thus in adults, the head represents 4.5%, each upper limb is the equivalent of 4.5%, the anterior and posterior parts of the trunk are calculated each one as 18 percent, and it is also calculated in 9% each lower limp, and the remaining 1% for the genitalia.

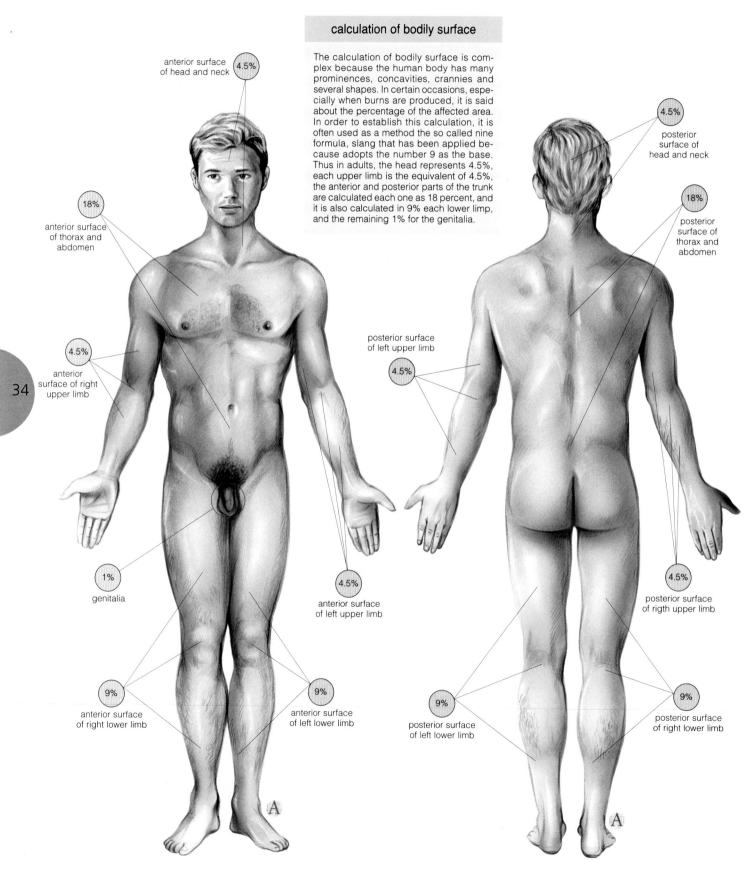

anterior surface of head and neck — 4.5%

posterior surface of head and neck — 4.5%

anterior surface of thorax and abdomen — 18%

posterior surface of thorax and abdomen — 18%

posterior surface of left upper limb — 4.5%

anterior surface of right upper limb — 4.5%

genitalia — 1%

anterior surface of left upper limb — 4.5%

posterior surface of rigth upper limb — 4.5%

anterior surface of right lower limb — 9%

anterior surface of left lower limb — 9%

posterior surface of left lower limb — 9%

posterior surface of right lower limb — 9%

34

ACCESSORY ORGANS of the SKIN (I). FINGERNAIL

fingers

The fingers of the hand are each one of the extensions where end the most distal extreme of the upper limb. Each finger has three bones called phalanges (the distal, middle, and proximal), except the thumb which only has two (proximal and distal). Therefore, the fingers of each hand form a set of fourteen bones. Each finger of the hand is singular and all of them are much more developed than toes and they are primarily uset to allow the individual to do many movements; some of these are exclusive of the human being.

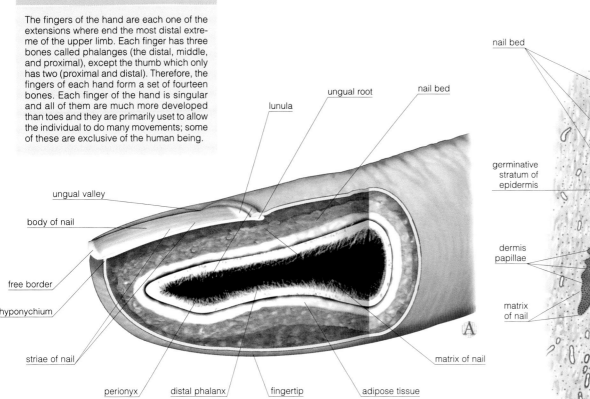

DISTAL EXTREMITY of FINGER. SECTION

Labels: lunula, ungual root, nail bed, ungual valley, body of nail, free border, hyponychium, striae of nail, perionyx, distal phalanx, fingertip, adipose tissue, matrix of nail

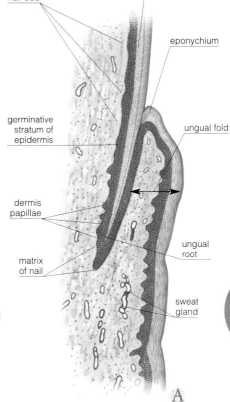

NAIL
LONGITUDINAL SECTION

Labels: nail bed, body of nail, eponychium, germinative stratum of epidermis, ungual fold, dermis papillae, ungual root, matrix of nail, sweat gland, dermis

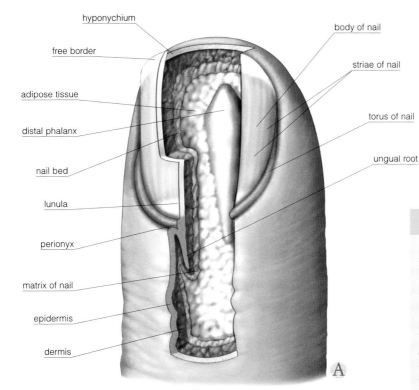

NAIL. SECTIONS at VARIOUS LEVELS

Labels: hyponychium, free border, adipose tissue, distal phalanx, nail bed, lunula, perionyx, matrix of nail, epidermis, dermis, body of nail, striae of nail, torus of nail, ungual root

nails

Nails are epidermis formations that are constituted by keretanized cells of hard consistency and corneum nature that cover and protect the dorsal surface of the fingers free extreme, both the nails of the hands and feet. Nails consist of three main strata: ungual matrix (it is inserted into a proximal ungual and it is coated by the proximal ungual fold), the ungual lamina and the ungual body. The nail is flanked by two ungual lateral furrows. The free border of the nail is separated from the skin of the finger through the hyponychium which is a narrow band with a half moon shape.

ACCESSORY ORGANS of the SKIN (II). HAIR FOLLICLE

hair follicle

The hair follicle is a tube like structure that ends in a sack shape, inside this are found the hair and the sebaceous glands. These glands pour their secretion, the sebum, within the interior canal of the hair follicle. The hair is an epidermis filamentous formation that commonly covers the skin of mammals in order to protect it. The hair caves into the skin and vertically moves across the epidermis and dermis and then the base widens; into this base takes place the formation process.

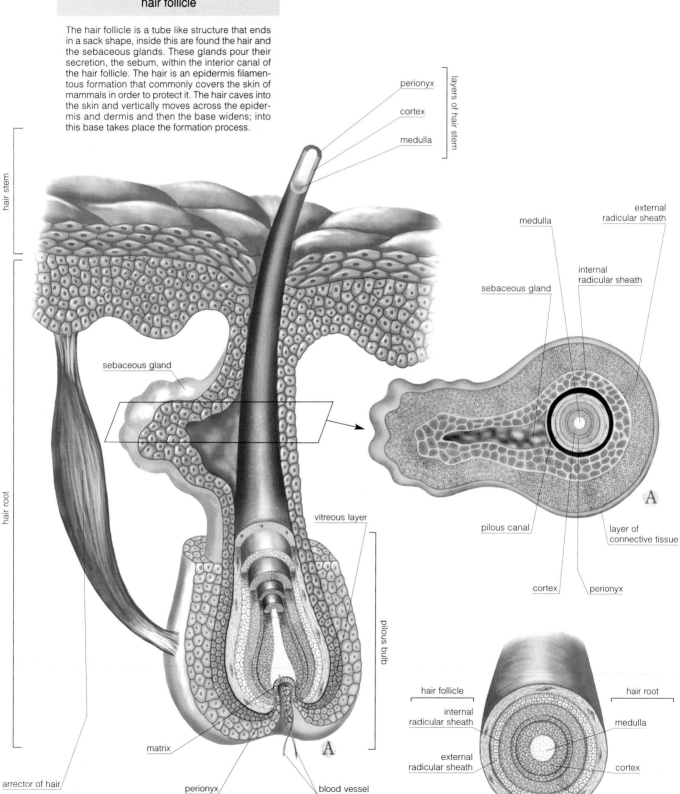

36

hair stem

hair root

layers of hair stem
- perionyx
- cortex
- medulla

sebaceous gland

vitreous layer

pilous bulb

matrix

arrector of hair

perionyx

blood vessel

medulla

external radicular sheath

internal radicular sheath

sebaceous gland

pilous canal

cortex

perionyx

layer of connective tissue

A

hair follicle

internal radicular sheath

external radicular sheath

dermic radicular sheath

hair root

medulla

cortex

perionyx

A

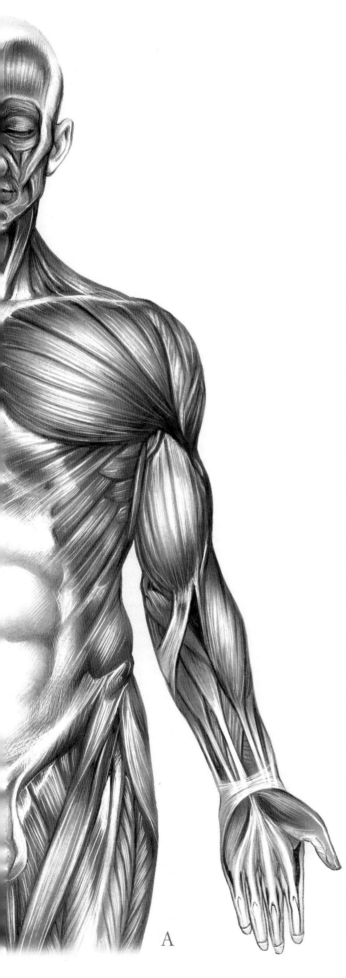

A

MUSCULAR SYSTEM

T he muscles, a specially important component of the locomotor system, are fleshy organs that thanks to their contraction ability become the immediate tool to produce or to counteract all the movements of the human body.

The organism can make many and very different movements, and all of them are vitally important: the movement of the legs when walking, the heartbeat of the cardiac muscle in order to bump blood, the movement of the eyes to see what happens in another point, the peristaltic movements of intestines which make possible that food moves forward through the digestive system, the movements of the face to express certain states of mind or any health condition, the movements of the thoracic muscles which make respiration possible, etc.

Muscles may be divided into two groups: striated muscles –or skeletal muscles, with voluntary contraction, that cover the skeleton and are responsible for the movement of this osseous structure-, and smooth muscles -or visceral muscles, which contraction is not voluntary, are responsible for the movements of the viscera, and can be found in the blood vessels, the digestive tube, the genital, urinary, and respiratory tracts, etc.

Muscles are made up of numerous muscle bundles or fascicles of tiny fibers, myofibrils, which size, shape and distribution depends on the specific muscles they belong to.

Muscles are arranged in various layers around the skeleton and they are the responsible for all the movements to that extend that in their absence is impossible to walk, heart would not be able to beat, it would not be possible for the eyes to turn, neither be the peristaltic movements, or the movements of the face, not respiration, etc. All of this turn them into absolutely indispensable.

Contraction or relaxation of skeletal muscles and of some smooth muscles, that are responsible for most of the different types of movements, is the consequence of nervous impulses ordered by the brain. In the case of skeletal muscles, it is the individual volition that arouses an order from the central nervous system, through the somatic nerves, which are then sent to the muscles that this individual wants to move. In the case of the smooth muscles, it is the nervous system itself, through the vegetative nerves, the one that automatically sends the order to produce the movement of certain muscular structures.

The whole group of muscles of the body, that besides being a support to the organism, are also responsible for getting together many of its elements, and moreover, it provides the motor power needed to let the bones and joints to move.

The interrelation between nerves and muscles, between the nerve pulses that are transmitted from the nerves and the movements of the muscles, have their common ground in the motor plate. It is the system that puts together the nerve endings and the muscle fibers. By means of a very complex process, the electrical nerve impulses coming from the nervous central system get the muscle and cause the muscle to contract or relax, this way producing functional muscular movements. Physiologically speaking, there is an absolute collaboration between muscles and nerves in order to produce any movement.

MUSCULAR TISSUE

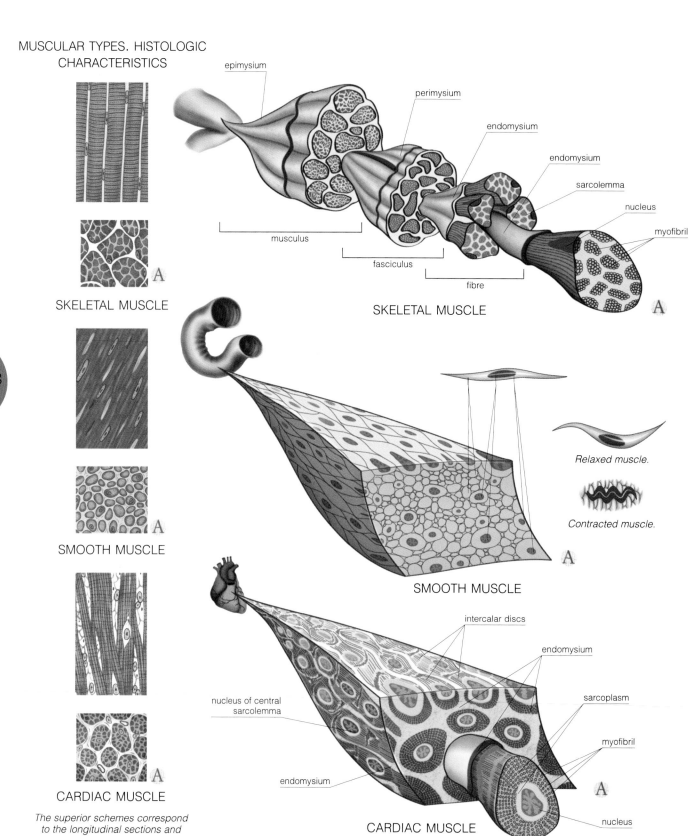

MUSCULAR TYPES. HISTOLOGIC CHARACTERISTICS

SKELETAL MUSCLE

SMOOTH MUSCLE

CARDIAC MUSCLE

The superior schemes correspond to the longitudinal sections and the inferior schemes correspond to the transversal sections.

epimysium

perimysium

endomysium

endomysium

sarcolemma

nucleus

myofibril

musculus

fasciculus

fibre

SKELETAL MUSCLE

Relaxed muscle.

Contracted muscle.

SMOOTH MUSCLE

intercalar discs

endomysium

nucleus of central sarcolemma

sarcoplasm

myofibril

endomysium

nucleus

CARDIAC MUSCLE

Source: Gartner, Hiatt, Colour Atlas of Histology, 4th ed, 2006.

38

SKELETAL MUSCLE. STRUCTURE and ORGANIZATION (I)

the structure of skeletal muscle

The structure of the skeletal muscle has a repetitive pattern as we go deeper into the smaller components. Thus, the muscle is formed by a bundle of fascicles that are wrapped up in a layer of connective tissue (epimisyum). Each one of the fascicles is formed by a bundle of muscle fibers, and for their part, they are wrapped up in a layer of connective tissue (perimysium). The muscle fibers that formed the fascicle, for their part, are formed by bundles of myofibrils, and they are wrapped up in a thin layer of connective tissue (endomysium). Each one of the myofibrils, for its part, is formed by a bundle of threads that are wrapped up in a thin layer. That is, it is the same structure all the time, even though with smaller dimensions as we go gradually deeper (muscle, fascicle, myofibril, etc.).

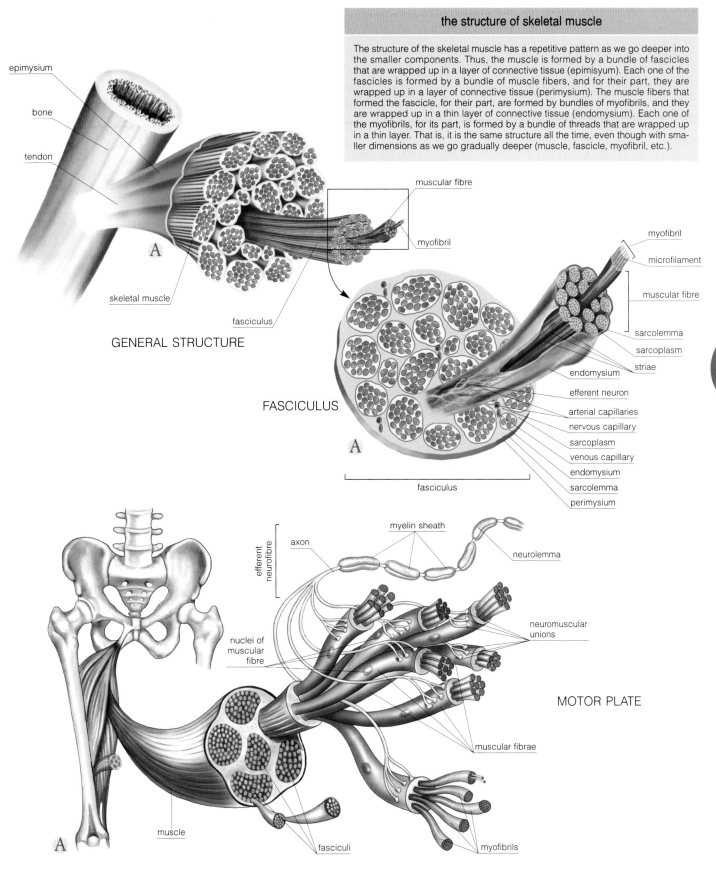

GENERAL STRUCTURE

FASCICULUS

MOTOR PLATE

SKELETAL MUSCLE. STRUCTURE and ORGANIZATION (II)

muscular contraction

Structure of skeletal muscles make possible contraction when stimuli are received from the nervous pulses. They are placed one opposite to the other and for that reason they can just pull but not push. When a muscle is relaxed, a thick or thin thread places slightly on top of another thick or thin thread. When a muscle is contracted, thick threads slide a little bit more in the middle of the thin threads and get nearer the Z-bands, the same way the fingers of one hand interweave with the fingers of the other hand.

STRUCTURE and ORGANIZATION

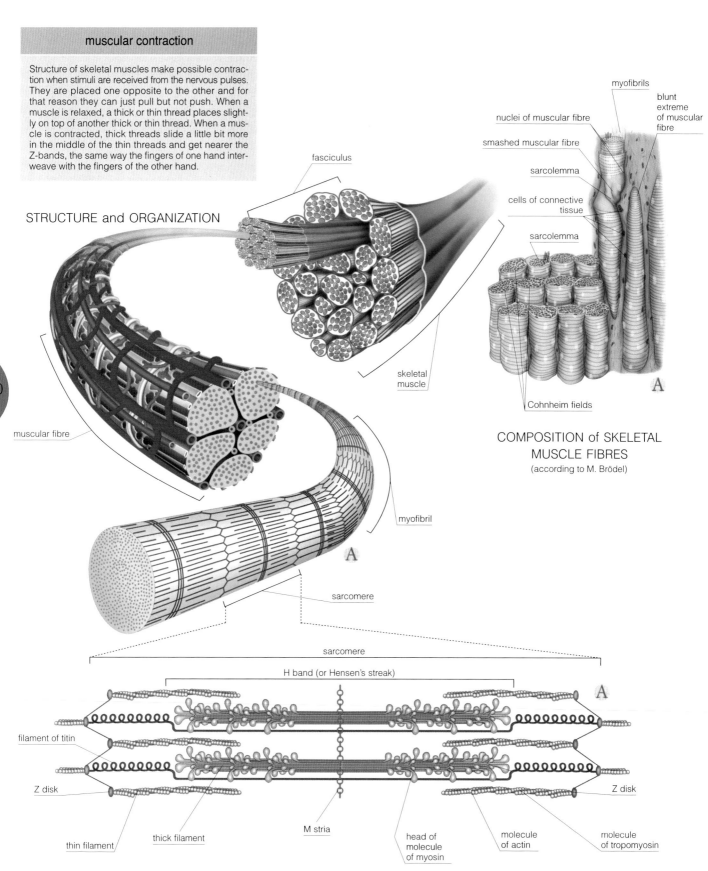

fasciculus

myofibrils

blunt extreme of muscular fibre

nuclei of muscular fibre

smashed muscular fibre

sarcolemma

cells of connective tissue

sarcolemma

skeletal muscle

Cohnheim fields

muscular fibre

COMPOSITION of SKELETAL MUSCLE FIBRES
(according to M. Brödel)

myofibril

sarcomere

sarcomere

H band (or Hensen's streak)

filament of titin

Z disk

Z disk

thin filament

thick filament

M stria

head of molecule of myosin

molecule of actin

molecule of tropomyosin

40

SKELETAL MUSCLE. STRUCTURE and ORGANIZATION (III)

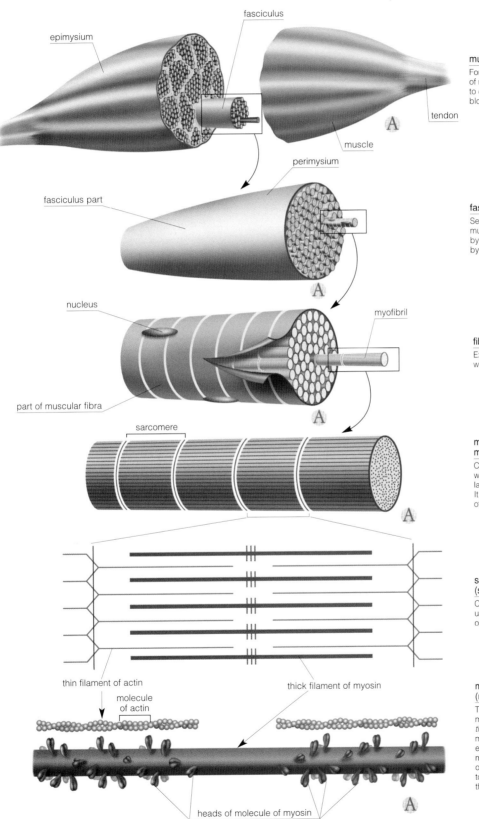

muscle (organ)

Formed by thousands
of muscle cells, in addition
to connective tissue sheaths,
blood vessels and neurofibers.

fasciculus (part of a muscle)

Set of perfectly assembled
muscle cells, separated
by the rest of the muscle
by a connective tissue sheath.

fibre (muscle cell)

Extended multi-nuclear cell
with a grooved appearance.

**myofibrils (complex organelle
made up of sets of filaments)**

Cylindrical contractile element
which, as a group, occupies the
largest area of the muscle cell.
It contains a large amount
of aligned stretch marks.

**sarcomere
(segment of a myofibrils)**

Contractile unit made
up of microfilaments
of contractile proteins.

**myofilament or filament
(macromolecular structure)**

There are two types of myofilaments,
made up of contractile proteins:
thin, which encompass actin
molecules, and *thick*, which
encompass a parallel set of
myosin molecules. The shrinkage
of muscles is achieved thanks
to the slippage of thin filaments
through the length of thick filaments.

Labels in figure: fasciculus, epimysium, tendon, muscle, perimysium, fasciculus part, nucleus, myofibril, part of muscular fibra, sarcomere, thin filament of actin, molecule of actin, thick filament of myosin, heads of molecule of myosin

41

MUSCULAR STRUCTURE

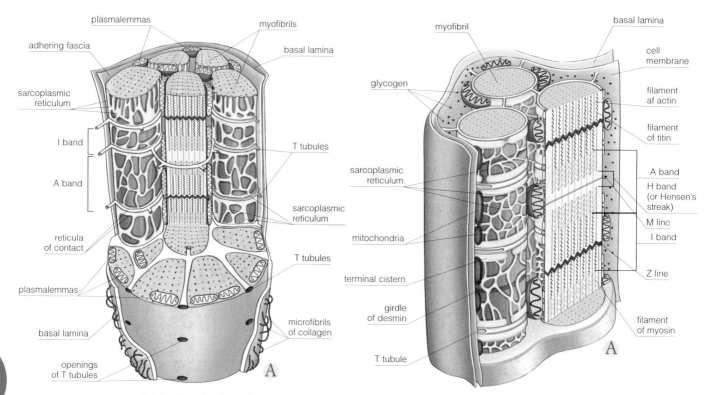

plasmalemmas

myofibrils

adhering fascia

basal lamina

sarcoplasmic reticulum

I band

A band

T tubules

sarcoplasmic reticulum

reticula of contact

T tubules

plasmalemmas

basal lamina

microfibrils of collagen

openings of T tubules

SKELETAL MUSCLE
STRUCTURE of the FIBRE

myofibril

basal lamina

glycogen

cell membrane

filament af actin

filament of titin

sarcoplasmic reticulum

A band

H band (or Hensen's streak)

M linc

I band

mitochondria

terminal cistern

girdle of desmin

Z line

T tubule

filament of myosin

SKELETAL MUSCLE
CONTRACTILE APPEARANCE
and STRUCTURE of CELL MEMBRANE

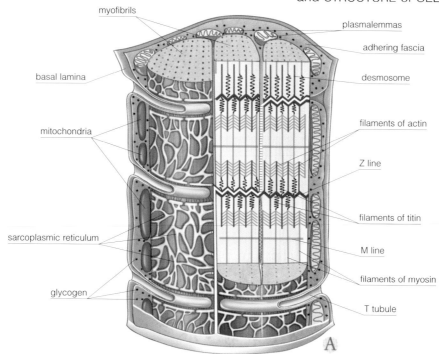

myofibrils

plasmalemmas

adhering fascia

basal lamina

desmosome

mitochondria

filaments of actin

Z line

filaments of titin

sarcoplasmic reticulum

M line

filaments of myosin

glycogen

T tubule

CARDIAC MUSCLE
CONTRACTILE APPEARANCE
and STRUCTURES of CELL MEMBRANE

SMOOTH MUSCLE. STRUCTURE

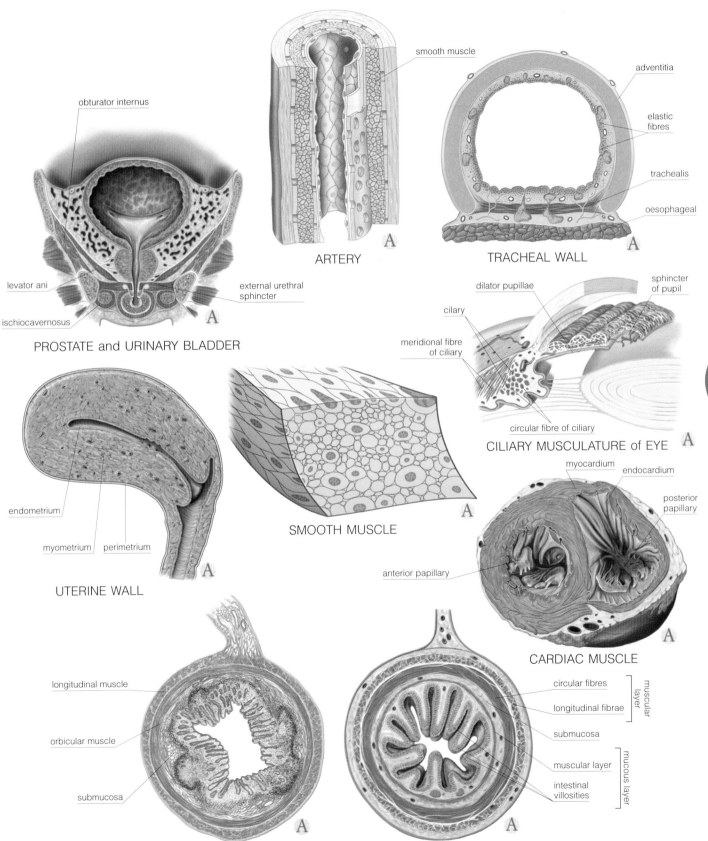

obturator internus

smooth muscle

adventitia

elastic fibres

trachealis

oesophageal

ARTERY

TRACHEAL WALL

levator ani

external urethral sphincter

ischiocavernosus

PROSTATE and URINARY BLADDER

dilator pupillae

sphincter of pupil

cilary

meridional fibre of ciliary

circular fibre of ciliary

CILIARY MUSCULATURE of EYE

endometrium

myometrium perimetrium

UTERINE WALL

SMOOTH MUSCLE

myocardium endocardium

posterior papillary

anterior papillary

CARDIAC MUSCLE

longitudinal muscle

orbicular muscle

submucosa

circular fibres

longitudinal fibrae

muscular layer

submucosa

muscular layer

intestinal villosities

mucous layer

SMALL INTESTINE WALL

MUSCULAR SYSTEM (I)

GENERAL ANTERIOR SUPERFICIAL VIEW

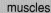

muscles

Muscles are responsible for all the movements to that extend that in their absence is impossible to walk, heart would not be able to beat, it would not be possible for the eyes to turn, neither be the peristaltic movements, or the movements of the face, not respiration, etc. All of this turn them into absolutely indispensable.

epicranial aponeurosis

occipitofrontalis

orbicularis oculi

nasalis

zygomaticus minor

levator labii superioris alaeque nasi

levator labii superioris

depresor anguli oris and depresor labii inferioris

mentalis

sternocleidomastoid

pectoralis major

serratus anterior

external oblique of abdomen

rectus abdominis

tensor fasciae latae

sartorius

pectineous

quadriceps femoris (rectus femoris)

quadriceps femoris (vastus lateralis)

adductor longus

gracilis

quadriceps femoris (vastus medialis)

tendon of quadriceps femoris

gastrocnemius (lateral head)

fibularis tertius

zygomaticus major

masseter

orbicularis oris

risorius

deltoid

trapezius

sternohyoid

biceps brachii

linea alba

brachialis

brachioradialis

pronator teres

flexor carpi radialis

palmaris longus

thenar eminence muscles

flexor carpi ulnaris

hypothenar eminence muscles

iliopsoas

tibialis anterior

fibularis longus

fibularis brevis

extensor hallucis longus

extensor digitorum longus of foot

44

A

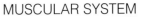

MUSCULAR SYSTEM (II)
GENERAL POSTERIOR SUPERFICIAL VIEW

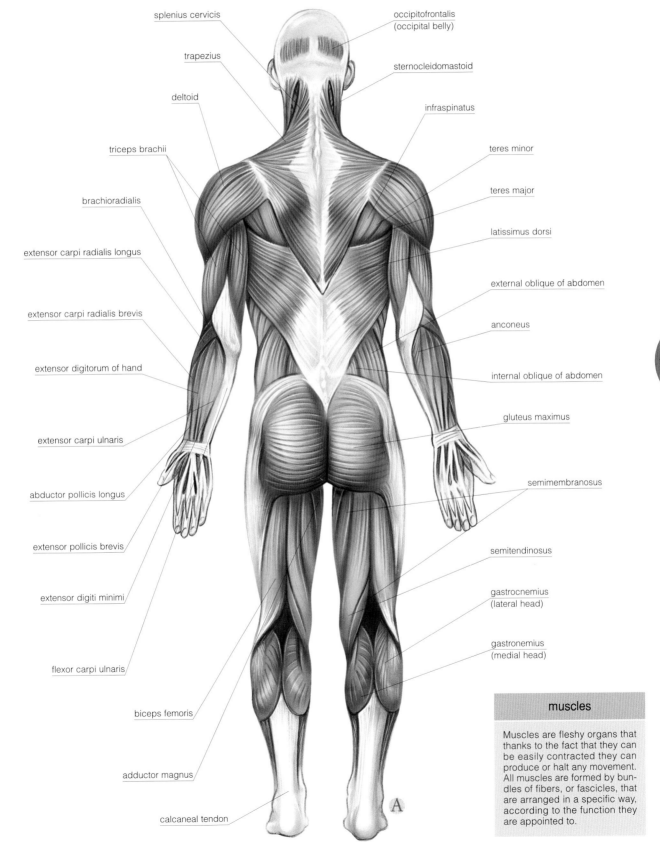

splenius cervicis

trapezius

deltoid

triceps brachii

brachioradialis

extensor carpi radialis longus

extensor carpi radialis brevis

extensor digitorum of hand

extensor carpi ulnaris

abductor pollicis longus

extensor pollicis brevis

extensor digiti minimi

flexor carpi ulnaris

biceps femoris

adductor magnus

calcaneal tendon

occipitofrontalis
(occipital belly)

sternocleidomastoid

infraspinatus

teres minor

teres major

latissimus dorsi

external oblique of abdomen

anconeus

internal oblique of abdomen

gluteus maximus

semimembranosus

semitendinosus

gastrocnemius
(lateral head)

gastronemius
(medial head)

A

45

muscles

Muscles are fleshy organs that thanks to the fact that they can be easily contracted they can produce or halt any movement. All muscles are formed by bundles of fibers, or fascicles, that are arranged in a specific way, according to the function they are appointed to.

MUSCULAR SYSTEM (III)

GENERAL LATERAL SUPERFICIAL VIEW

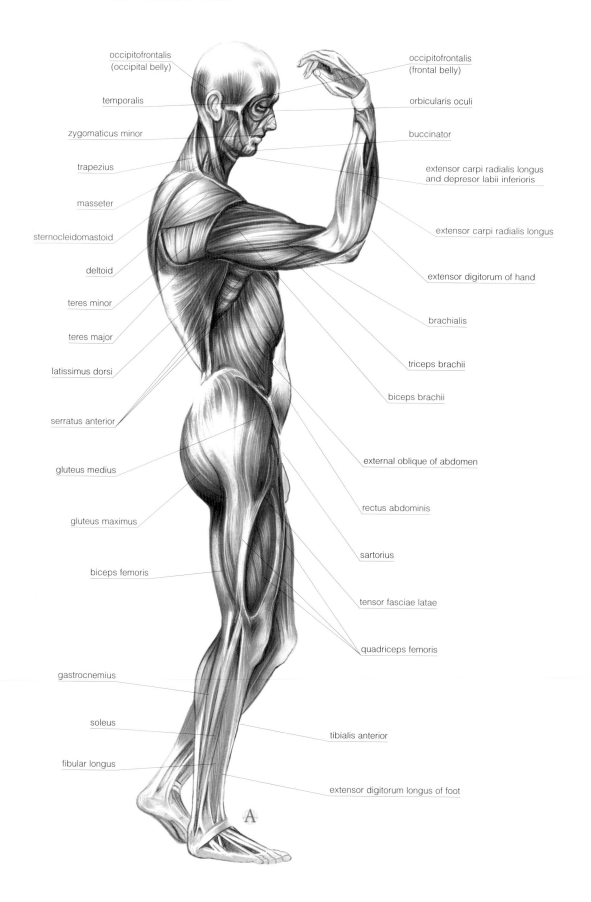

occipitofrontalis
(occipital belly)

temporalis

zygomaticus minor

trapezius

masseter

sternocleidomastoid

deltoid

teres minor

teres major

latissimus dorsi

serratus anterior

gluteus medius

gluteus maximus

biceps femoris

gastrocnemius

soleus

fibular longus

occipitofrontalis
(frontal belly)

orbicularis oculi

buccinator

extensor carpi radialis longus
and depresor labii inferioris

extensor carpi radialis longus

extensor digitorum of hand

brachialis

triceps brachii

biceps brachii

external oblique of abdomen

rectus abdominis

sartorius

tensor fasciae latae

quadriceps femoris

tibialis anterior

extensor digitorum longus of foot

A

MUSCULAR TYPES

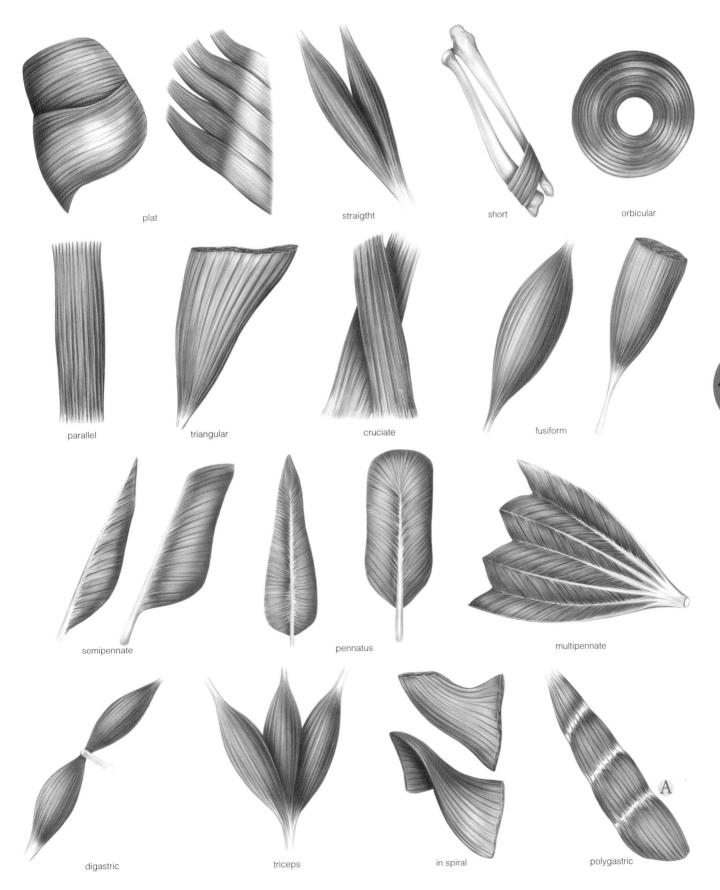

plat

straigtht

short

orbicular

parallel

triangular

cruciate

fusiform

47

semipennate

pennatus

multipennate

digastric

triceps

in spiral

polygastric

A

MUSCULAR GROUPS (I). HEAD and TRUNK (I)

ANTERIOR VIEW

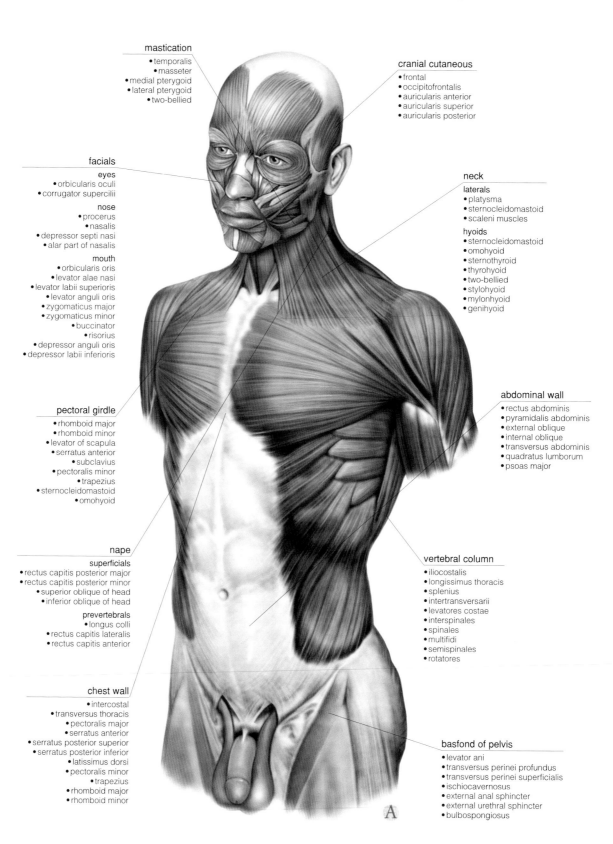

mastication
- temporalis
- masseter
- medial pterygoid
- lateral pterygoid
- two-bellied

cranial cutaneous
- frontal
- occipitofrontalis
- auricularis anterior
- auricularis superior
- auricularis posterior

facials

eyes
- orbicularis oculi
- corrugator supercilii

nose
- procerus
- nasalis
- depressor septi nasi
- alar part of nasalis

mouth
- orbicularis oris
- levator alae nasi
- levator labii superioris
- levator anguli oris
- zygomaticus major
- zygomaticus minor
- buccinator
- risorius
- depressor anguli oris
- depressor labii inferioris

neck

laterals
- platysma
- sternocleidomastoid
- scaleni muscles

hyoids
- sternocleidomastoid
- omohyoid
- sternothyroid
- thyrohyoid
- two-bellied
- stylohyoid
- mylonhyoid
- genihyoid

pectoral girdle
- rhomboid major
- rhomboid minor
- levator of scapula
- serratus anterior
- subclavius
- pectoralis minor
- trapezius
- sternocleidomastoid
- omohyoid

abdominal wall
- rectus abdominis
- pyramidalis abdominis
- external oblique
- internal oblique
- transversus abdominis
- quadratus lumborum
- psoas major

nape

superficials
- rectus capitis posterior major
- rectus capitis posterior minor
- superior oblique of head
- inferior oblique of head

prevertebrals
- longus colli
- rectus capitis lateralis
- rectus capitis anterior

vertebral column
- iliocostalis
- longissimus thoracis
- splenius
- intertransversarii
- levatores costae
- interspinales
- spinales
- multifidi
- semispinales
- rotatores

chest wall
- intercostal
- transversus thoracis
- pectoralis major
- serratus anterior
- serratus posterior superior
- serratus posterior inferior
- latissimus dorsi
- pectoralis minor
- trapezius
- rhomboid major
- rhomboid minor

basfond of pelvis
- levator ani
- transversus perinei profundus
- transversus perinei superficialis
- ischiocavernosus
- external anal sphincter
- external urethral sphincter
- bulbospongiosus

A

48

MUSCULAR GROUPS (II). HEAD and TRUNK (II)

POSTERIOR LATERAL VIEW

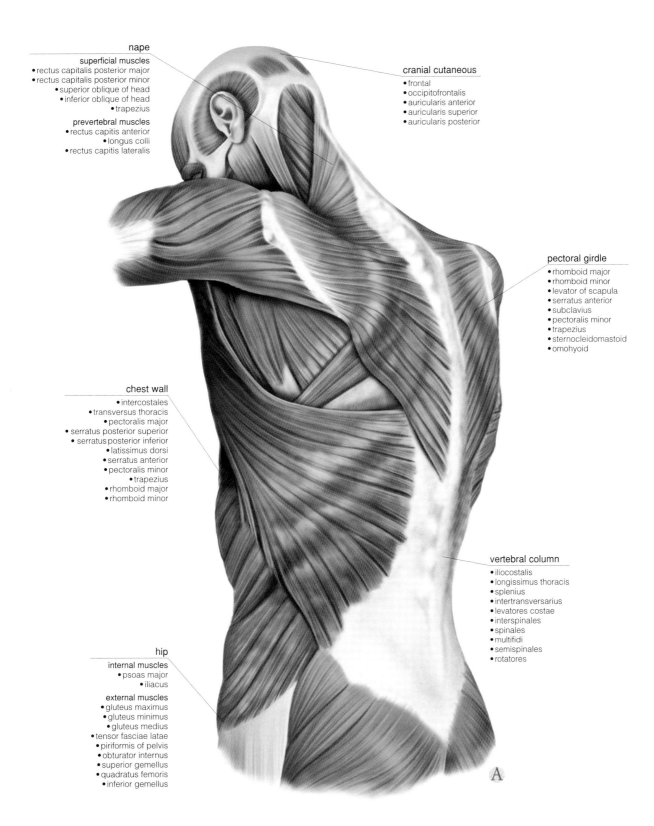

nape

superficial muscles
- rectus capitalis posterior major
- rectus capitalis posterior minor
- superior oblique of head
- inferior oblique of head
- trapezius

prevertebral muscles
- rectus capitis anterior
- longus colli
- rectus capitis lateralis

cranial cutaneous
- frontal
- occipitofrontalis
- auricularis anterior
- auricularis superior
- auricularis posterior

pectoral girdle
- rhomboid major
- rhomboid minor
- levator of scapula
- serratus anterior
- subclavius
- pectoralis minor
- trapezius
- sternocleidomastoid
- omohyoid

chest wall
- intercostales
- transversus thoracis
- pectoralis major
- serratus posterior superior
- serratus posterior inferior
- latissimus dorsi
- serratus anterior
- pectoralis minor
- trapezius
- rhomboid major
- rhomboid minor

vertebral column
- iliocostalis
- longissimus thoracis
- splenius
- intertransversarius
- levatores costae
- interspinales
- spinales
- multifidi
- semispinales
- rotatores

hip

internal muscles
- psoas major
- iliacus

external muscles
- gluteus maximus
- gluteus minimus
- gluteus medius
- tensor fasciae latae
- piriformis of pelvis
- obturator internus
- superior gemellus
- quadratus femoris
- inferior gemellus

A

49

MUSCULAR GROUPS (III). LIMBS
POSTERIOR LATERAL VIEW

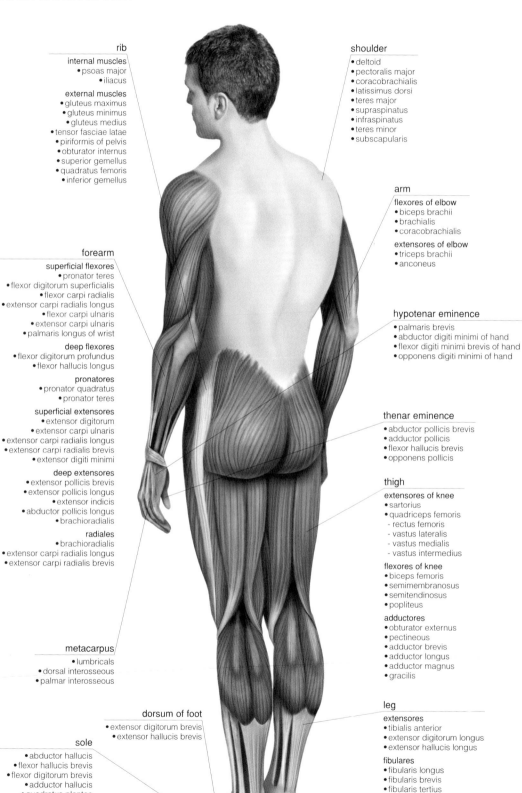

rib

internal muscles
- psoas major
  - iliacus

external muscles
- gluteus maximus
  - gluteus minimus
  - gluteus medius
- tensor fasciae latae
- piriformis of pelvis
- obturator internus
- superior gemellus
- quadratus femoris
- inferior gemellus

forearm

superficial flexores
- pronator teres
- flexor digitorum superficialis
- flexor carpi radialis
- extensor carpi radialis longus
- flexor carpi ulnaris
- extensor carpi ulnaris
- palmaris longus of wrist

deep flexores
- flexor digitorum profundus
- flexor hallucis longus

pronatores
- pronator quadratus
- pronator teres

superficial extensores
- extensor digitorum
- extensor carpi ulnaris
- extensor carpi radialis longus
- extensor carpi radialis brevis
- extensor digiti minimi

deep extensores
- extensor pollicis brevis
- extensor pollicis longus
- extensor indicis
- abductor pollicis longus
- brachioradialis

radiales
- brachioradialis
- extensor carpi radialis longus
- extensor carpi radialis brevis

metacarpus
- lumbricals
- dorsal interosseous
- palmar interosseous

dorsum of foot
- extensor digitorum brevis
- extensor hallucis brevis

sole
- abductor hallucis
- flexor hallucis brevis
- flexor digitorum brevis
- adductor hallucis
- quadratus plantae
- lumbricals
- plantar interosseous
- dorsal interosseous
- abductor digiti minimi of foot
- opponens digiti minimi of foot

shoulder
- deltoid
- pectoralis major
- coracobrachialis
- latissimus dorsi
- teres major
- supraspinatus
- infraspinatus
- teres minor
- subscapularis

arm

flexores of elbow
- biceps brachii
- brachialis
- coracobrachialis

extensores of elbow
- triceps brachii
- anconeus

hypotenar eminence
- palmaris brevis
- abductor digiti minimi of hand
- flexor digiti minimi brevis of hand
- opponens digiti minimi of hand

thenar eminence
- abductor pollicis brevis
- adductor pollicis
- flexor hallucis brevis
- opponens pollicis

thigh

extensores of knee
- sartorius
- quadriceps femoris
  - rectus femoris
  - vastus lateralis
  - vastus medialis
  - vastus intermedius

flexores of knee
- biceps femoris
- semimembranosus
- semitendinosus
- popliteus

adductores
- obturator externus
- pectineous
- adductor brevis
- adductor longus
- adductor magnus
- gracilis

leg

extensores
- tibialis anterior
- extensor digitorum longus
- extensor hallucis longus

fibulares
- fibularis longus
- fibularis brevis
- fibularis tertius

superficial flexores
- soleus
- gastrocnemius
- small plantaris

deep flexores
- tibialis posterior
- flexor digitorum longus
- flexor hallucis longus

A

50

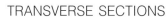

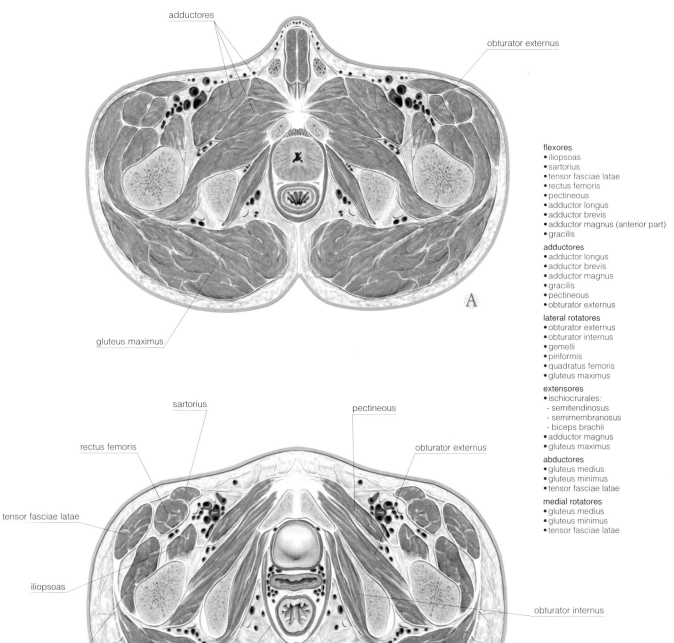

adductores

obturator externus

flexores
• iliopsoas
• sartorius
• tensor fasciae latae
• rectus femoris
• pectineous
• adductor longus
• adductor brevis
• adductor magnus (anterior part)
• gracilis

adductores
• adductor longus
• adductor brevis
• adductor magnus
• gracilis
• pectineous
• obturator externus

lateral rotatores
• obturator externus
• obturator internus
• gemelli
• piriformis
• quadratus femoris
• gluteus maximus

extensores
• ischiocrurales:
  - semitendinosus
  - semimembranosus
  - biceps brachii
• adductor magnus
• gluteus maximus

abductores
• gluteus medius
• gluteus minimus
• tensor fasciae latae

medial rotatores
• gluteus medius
• gluteus minimus
• tensor fasciae latae

gluteus maximus

51

sartorius

pectineous

rectus femoris

obturator externus

tensor fasciae latae

iliopsoas

obturator internus

vastus lateralis

gluteus maximus

levator ani

HEAD (I)
ANTERIOR SUPERFICIAL VIEW

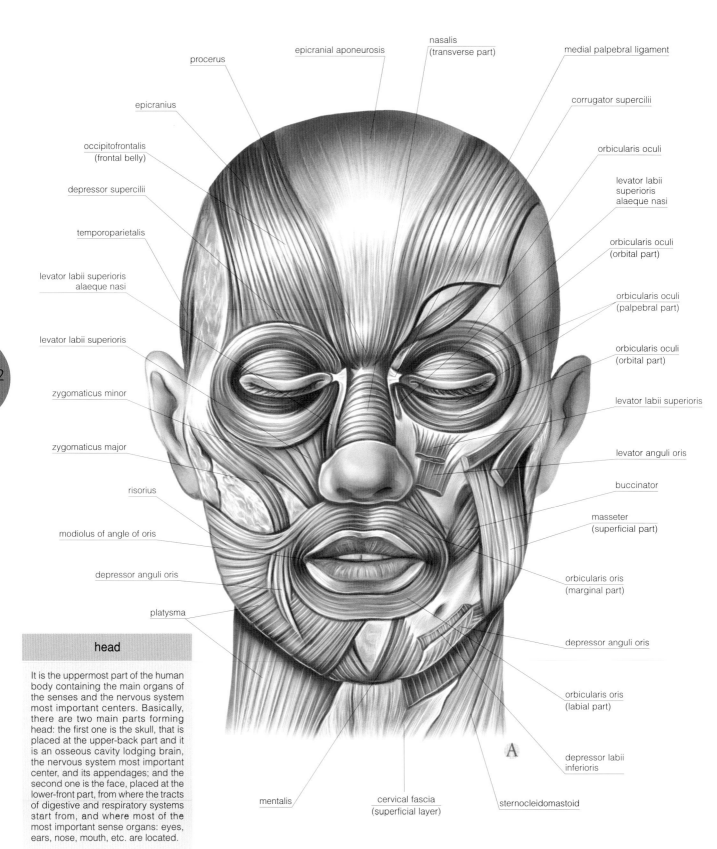

procerus

epicranial aponeurosis

nasalis
(transverse part)

medial palpebral ligament

epicranius

corrugator supercilii

occipitofrontalis
(frontal belly)

orbicularis oculi

depressor supercilii

levator labii
superioris
alaeque nasi

temporoparietalis

orbicularis oculi
(orbital part)

levator labii superioris
alaeque nasi

orbicularis oculi
(palpebral part)

levator labii superioris

orbicularis oculi
(orbital part)

zygomaticus minor

levator labii superioris

zygomaticus major

levator anguli oris

risorius

buccinator

modiolus of angle of oris

masseter
(superficial part)

depressor anguli oris

orbicularis oris
(marginal part)

platysma

depressor anguli oris

orbicularis oris
(labial part)

depressor labii
inferioris

mentalis

cervical fascia
(superficial layer)

sternocleidomastoid

A

head

It is the uppermost part of the human body containing the main organs of the senses and the nervous system most important centers. Basically, there are two main parts forming head: the first one is the skull, that is placed at the upper-back part and it is an osseous cavity lodging brain, the nervous system most important center, and its appendages; and the second one is the face, placed at the lower-front part, from where the tracts of digestive and respiratory systems start from, and where most of the most important sense organs: eyes, ears, nose, mouth, etc. are located.

52

HEAD (II)
LEFT LATERAL SUPERFICIAL VIEW

muscles of head

The head is covered by a great number of muscles, each one of them belongs to a specific group, according to the function it accomplishes. From this group of muscles we can mention the ones taking part in the expression of certain feelings (fear, unhappiness, laugh, etc.), also, the ones helping out during the masticatory process or swallowing food after it has been put into the mouth; others, they take part in the movement of the head, eyelids, or lips; that is, all of them cooperate in a wide range of different movements corresponding to thousands of different functions.

epicranius

occipitofrontalis
(frontal belly)

epicranial aponeurosis

temporalis

temporal fascia
(superficial layer)

corrugator supercilii

pericranium

orbicularis oculi
(palpebral part)

orbicularis oculi
(orbital part)

depressor supercilii

auricularis
superior

procerus

53

levator labii
superioris
alaeque nasi

nasalis
(transverse part)

occipitofrontalis
(occipital belly)

levator labii superioris

zygomaticus minor

buccinator

masseter

nasalis
(alar part)

sternocleidomastoid

orbicularis oris

trapezius

mentalis

depressor labii inferioris

risorius

A

depressor anguli oris

infrahyoid

splenius cervicis

zygomaticus major

HEAD (III). FACIAL EXPRESSION (I)

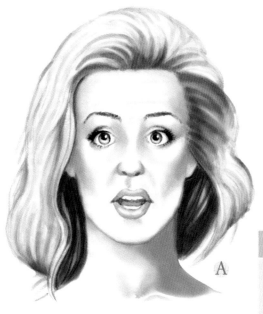

surprise

Commotion felt by the person when he/she sees or notices something completely unexpected or unpredictable. The facial gesture of surprise occurs thanks to the bilateral action of the frontal and orbicular muscles of the eyes, which raises both eyebrows until horizontal creases appear, opening the palpebral openings in an exaggerated manner.

facial expression

Facial expression is the mean an individual has to convey, using the face, the sensations he or she undergoes (happiness, horror, pleasure, bitterness, etc.). The human being is the logical conclusion of joining (mind and body) a completely inseparable unit, whose constituent elements are closely interwoven. Muscles, bones, eyes, intestines, etc. can not be easily separated from the realm of will, feelings or sensations. For that reason, a sorrow may give rise to disorders in the intestines, a depression may involve a cephalalgia, a good or bad news may sharply alter nervous tension or blood pressure. Face has been renamed as the mirror of the soul, because it reflects the mood of an individual. Here, they are displayed some basic sensations and the muscles the human body uses to reflect them by means of the facial expression.

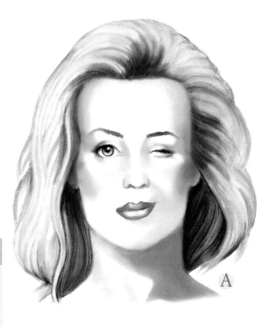

wink

Act of winking, that is to say, the temporary closing of one eye while the other one remains open. It is a voluntary action which is carried out thanks to the unilateral action of the orbicular muscle of the eye and the parotid fascia of that side of the eye.

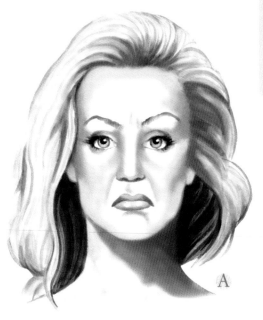

anger

Refers to the manifestation of the feeling when a person is faced with an unpleasant or troublesome situation. It is characterized by a furrowed brow and by vertical creases in the eyebrows, which is achieved thanks to the action of the corrugator muscles of the eyebrows (or supercilium corrugators) and procerus, as well as the parotid fascia.

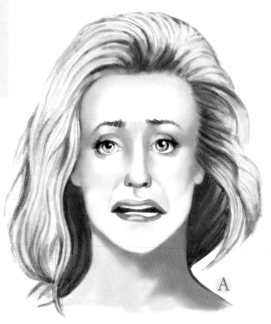

revulsion

Refers to the aversion or tedium of a person when faced with an unpleasant vision or when faced with a fact which generates complete opposition or revulsion. The facial expression shows a contraction of the depressor muscles of the edges of the mouth and the lower lip, as well as the cutaneous muscle of the neck, which move the corners of the mouth downwards.

HEAD (IV). FACIAL EXPRESSION (II)

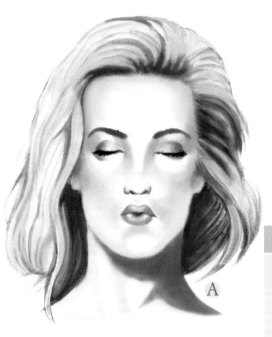

kiss

Action of kissing, that is to say, touch or press another person's lips with your own lips, in order to show love or affection. It is an intelligent expression, which is carried out thanks to the contraction of the orbicular muscle of the mouth.

facial expression muscles

Scalp
- Occipitofrontalis.
  - Frontal belly.
  - Occipital belly.

Mouth
- Orbicularis oris.
- Zygomaticus major.
- Zygomaticus minor.
- Levator labii superioris.
- Depressor labii inferioris.
- Depressor anguli oris.
- Levator anguli oris.
- Buccinator.
- Risorius.
- Mentalis.

Neck
- Platysma.

Orbit and eyebrow
- Orbicularis oculi.
- Corrugator supercilii.
- Levator palpebrae superioris.

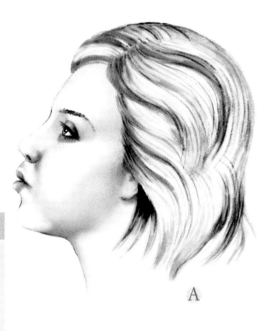

blowing

To vigorously expel air from the mouth, lengthening the lips (which are slightly opened) through the central area, and inflating the laterals in order to increase the capacity of the mouth. This action is performed thanks to the orbicular muscles of the mouth, as well as the buccinators.

55

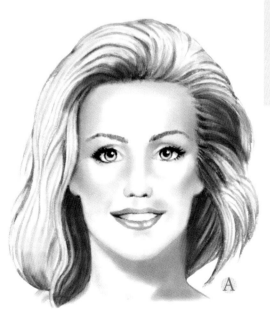

smile

Smile is to laugh slightly and without making noise. It shows a positive or pleasant sensation when faced with a certain action, person, vision, etc. This action only occurs in the human species. It is performed as a consequence of the voluntary and combined contraction of the risorius, zygomaticus and levator muscles of the mouth.

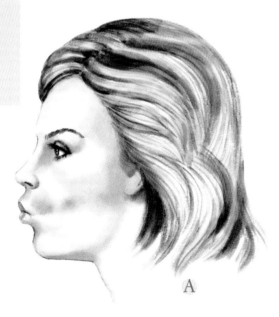

suction

To suction is to suck, extract air, juice or a similar substance with the lips. The suction of a substance from the exterior to the interior of the mouth is performed through the action of the orbicular muscle of the mouth, which frowns, as well as the buccinators, which enable the existence of a negative pressure in the inner part of the oral cavity.

HEAD (V)
LATERAL SUPERFICIAL VIEW

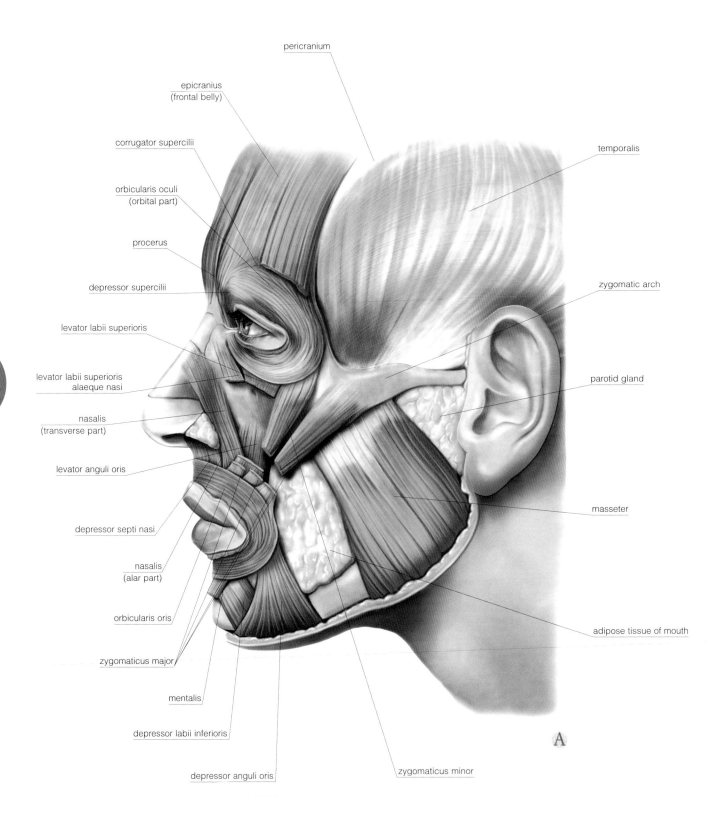

pericranium

epicranius
(frontal belly)

corrugator supercilii

orbicularis oculi
(orbital part)

procerus

depressor supercilii

levator labii superioris

levator labii superioris
alaeque nasi

nasalis
(transverse part)

levator anguli oris

depressor septi nasi

nasalis
(alar part)

orbicularis oris

zygomaticus major

mentalis

depressor labii inferioris

depressor anguli oris

temporalis

zygomatic arch

parotid gland

masseter

adipose tissue of mouth

zygomaticus minor

A

HEAD (VI). MASTICATORY MUSCLES

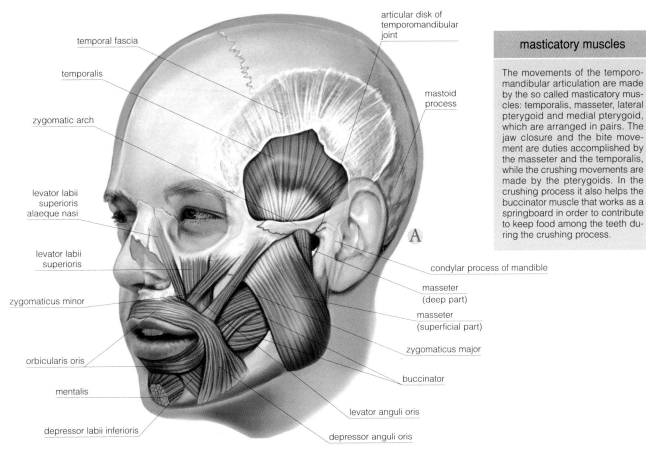

temporal fascia

temporalis

zygomatic arch

levator labii
superioris
alaeque nasi

levator labii
superioris

zygomaticus minor

orbicularis oris

mentalis

depressor labii inferioris

articular disk of
temporomandibular
joint

mastoid
process

condylar process of mandible

masseter
(deep part)

masseter
(superficial part)

zygomaticus major

buccinator

levator anguli oris

depressor anguli oris

masticatory muscles

The movements of the temporomandibular articulation are made
by the so called masticatory muscles: temporalis, masseter, lateral
pterygoid and medial pterygoid,
which are arranged in pairs. The
jaw closure and the bite movement are duties accomplished by
the masseter and the temporalis,
while the crushing movements are
made by the pterygoids. In the
crushing process it also helps the
buccinator muscle that works as a
springboard in order to contribute
to keep food among the teeth during the crushing process.

A

57

LEFT ANTERIOR LATERAL VIEWS

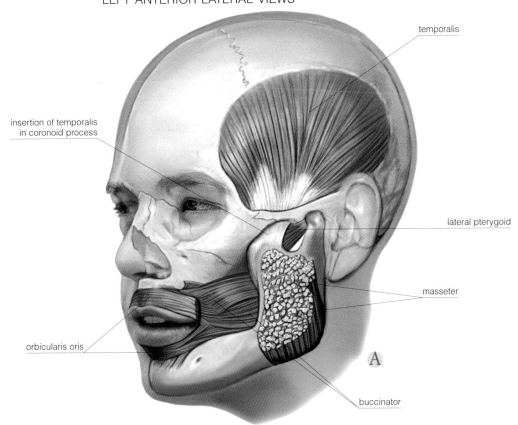

temporalis

insertion of temporalis
in coronoid process

lateral pterygoid

masseter

orbicularis oris

buccinator

A

HEAD (VII). TONGUE and FLOOR of MOUTH
LATERAL VIEW

tongue and floor of mouth

Mouth, and within the mouth, the tongue, is one of the elements of human body with a lot of functions to be accomplished: digestive, respiratory, phonatory, etc. In order to carry out these duties it needs a wide range of movements, and that is the reason there is an enormous number of muscles in the tongue to have the ability enough to fulfill all these requirements. The most important muscles belonging to this group are: the genioglossus, the styloglossus, the hyoglossus, we can also include within this group, that is in hyoid bone, the next muscles: geniohyoid, mylohyoid, digastric, thyrohyoid, stylohyoid, etc.

58

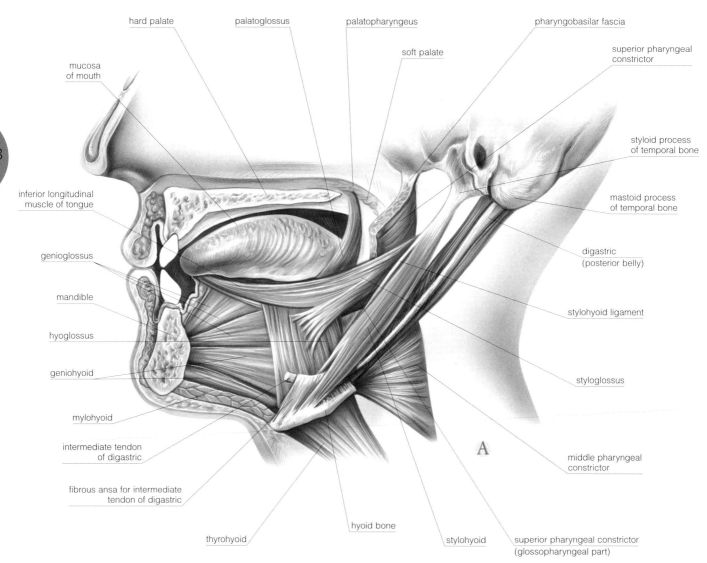

hard palate

palatoglossus

palatopharyngeus

soft palate

pharyngobasilar fascia

superior pharyngeal constrictor

mucosa of mouth

styloid process of temporal bone

mastoid process of temporal bone

inferior longitudinal muscle of tongue

digastric (posterior belly)

genioglossus

stylohyoid ligament

mandible

hyoglossus

geniohyoid

styloglossus

mylohyoid

intermediate tendon of digastric

A

fibrous ansa for intermediate tendon of digastric

middle pharyngeal constrictor

thyrohyoid

hyoid bone

stylohyoid

superior pharyngeal constrictor (glossopharyngeal part)

HEAD (VIII). FLOOR of MOUTH

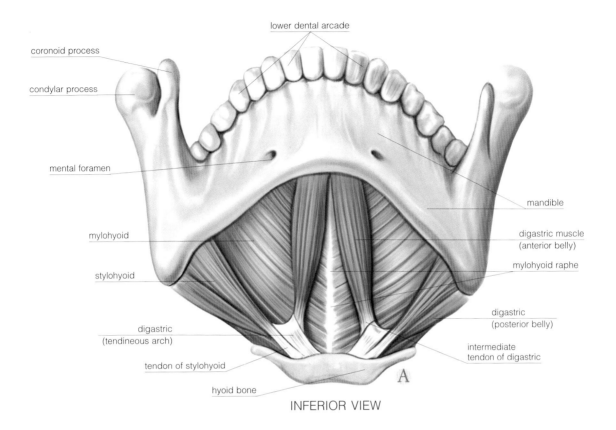

lower dental arcade

coronoid process

condylar process

mental foramen

mylohyoid

stylohyoid

digastric
(tendineous arch)

tendon of stylohyoid

hyoid bone

mandible

digastric muscle
(anterior belly)

mylohyoid raphe

digastric
(posterior belly)

intermediate
tendon of digastric

INFERIOR VIEW

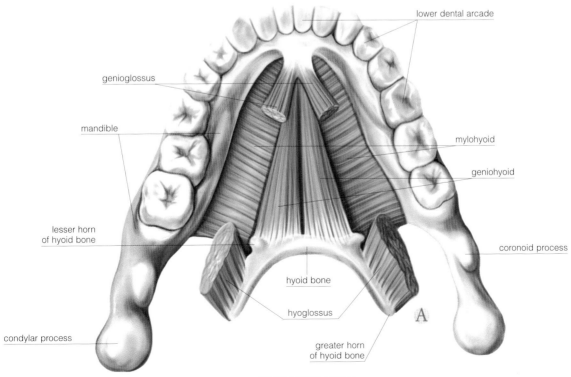

lower dental arcade

genioglossus

mandible

lesser horn
of hyoid bone

condylar process

mylohyoid

geniohyoid

coronoid process

hyoid bone

hyoglossus

greater horn
of hyoid bone

SUPERIOR VIEW

NECK (I)

POSTERIOR PREVERTEBRAL VIEW

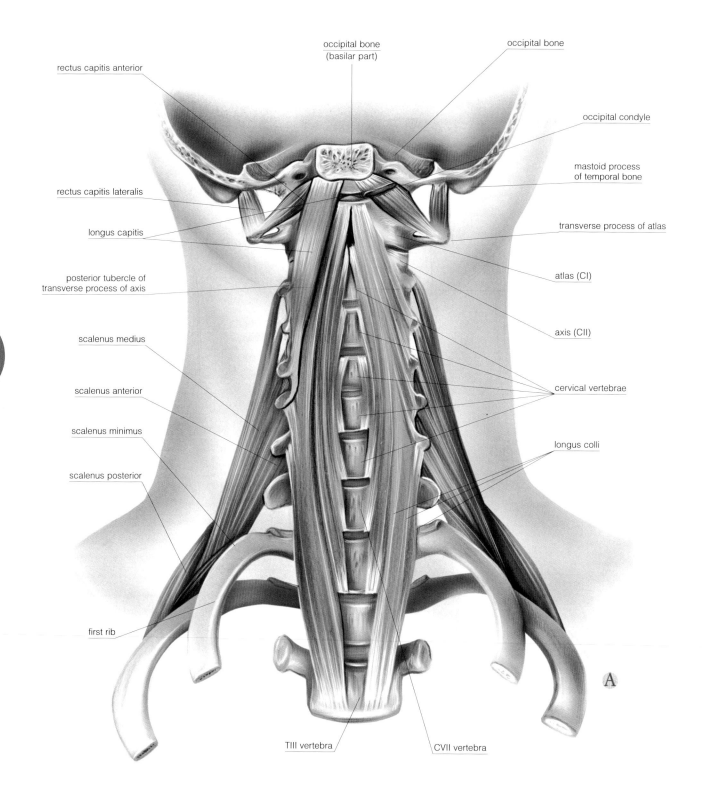

occipital bone
(basilar part)

occipital bone

rectus capitis anterior

occipital condyle

mastoid process
of temporal bone

rectus capitis lateralis

longus capitis

transverse process of atlas

posterior tubercle of
transverse process of axis

atlas (CI)

axis (CII)

scalenus medius

cervical vertebrae

scalenus anterior

scalenus minimus

longus colli

scalenus posterior

first rib

TIII vertebra

CVII vertebra

60

A

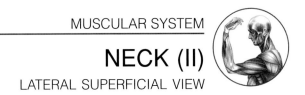

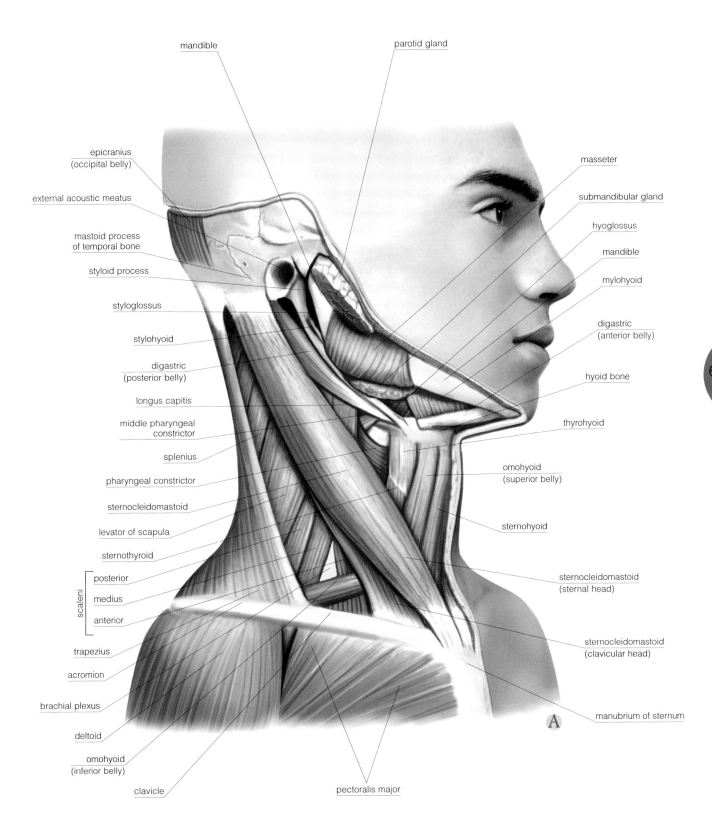

mandible

parotid gland

masseter

epicranius
(occipital belly)

submandibular gland

external acoustic meatus

hyoglossus

mastoid process
of temporal bone

mandible

styloid process

mylohyoid

styloglossus

digastric
(anterior belly)

stylohyoid

digastric
(posterior belly)

hyoid bone

longus capitis

thyrohyoid

middle pharyngeal
constrictor

splenius

omohyoid
(superior belly)

pharyngeal constrictor

sternohyoid

sternocleidomastoid

levator of scapula

sternocleidomastoid
(sternal head)

sternothyroid

scaleni
posterior

medius

anterior

sternocleidomastoid
(clavicular head)

trapezius

acromion

brachial plexus

manubrium of sternum

deltoid

omohyoid
(inferior belly)

clavicle

pectoralis major

61

A

NECK (III)

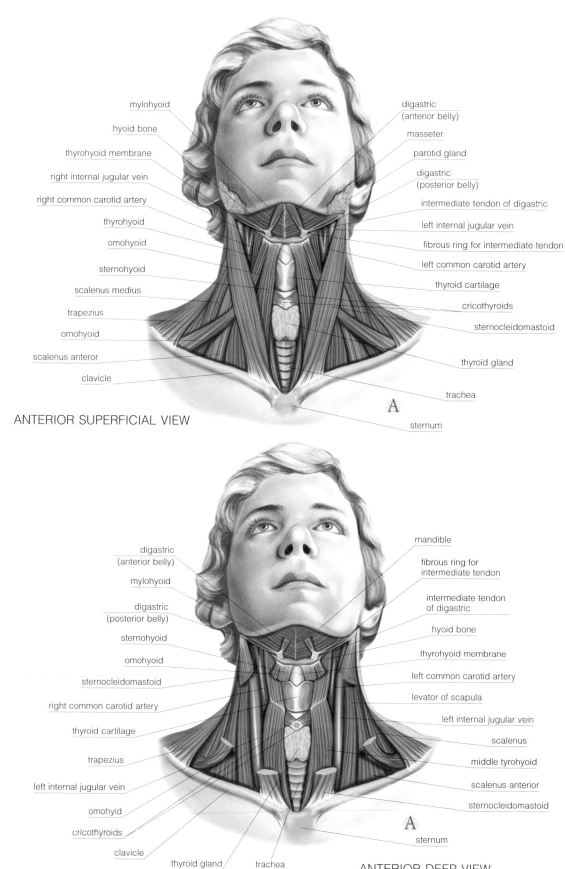

mylohyoid

hyoid bone

thyrohyoid membrane

right internal jugular vein

right common carotid artery

thyrohyoid

omohyoid

sternohyoid

scalenus medius

trapezius

omohyoid

scalenus anteror

clavicle

digastric
(anterior belly)

masseter

parotid gland

digastric
(posterior belly)

intermediate tendon of digastric

left internal jugular vein

fibrous ring for intermediate tendon

left common carotid artery

thyroid cartilage

cricothyroids

sternocleidomastoid

thyroid gland

trachea

sternum

ANTERIOR SUPERFICIAL VIEW

digastric
(anterior belly)

mylohyoid

digastric
(posterior belly)

sternohyoid

omohyoid

sternocleidomastoid

right common carotid artery

thyroid cartilage

trapezius

left internal jugular vein

omohyid

cricothyroids

clavicle

thyroid gland

trachea

mandible

fibrous ring for
intermediate tendon

intermediate tendon
of digastric

hyoid bone

thyrohyoid membrane

left common carotid artery

levator of scapula

left internal jugular vein

scalenus

middle tyrohyoid

scalenus anterior

sternocleidomastoid

sternum

ANTERIOR DEEP VIEW

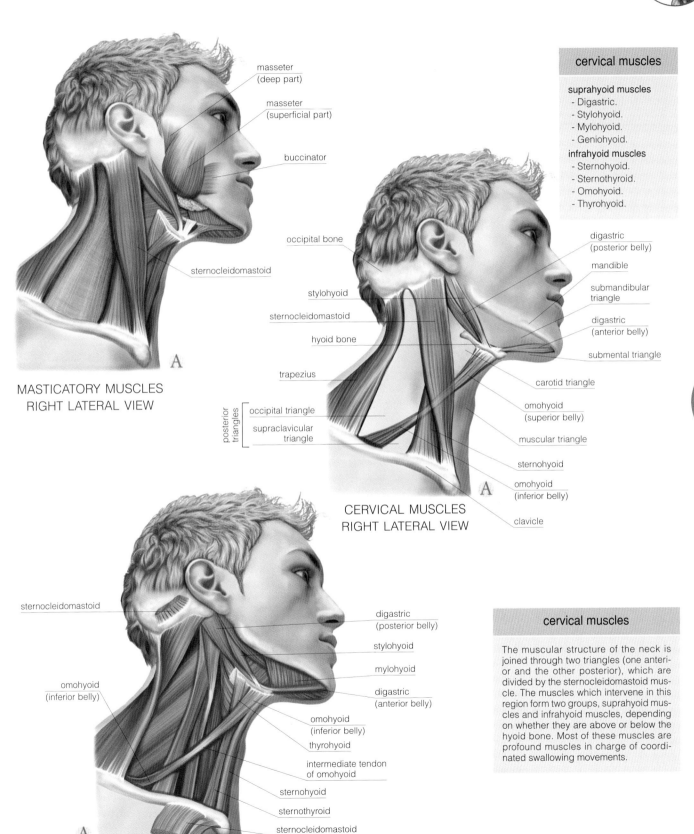

masseter
(deep part)

masseter
(superficial part)

buccinator

occipital bone

sternocleidomastoid

stylohyoid

sternocleidomastoid

hyoid bone

trapezius

posterior triangles
occipital triangle

supraclavicular
triangle

**MASTICATORY MUSCLES
RIGHT LATERAL VIEW**

A

cervical muscles

suprahyoid muscles
- Digastric.
- Stylohyoid.
- Mylohyoid.
- Geniohyoid.

infrahyoid muscles
- Sternohyoid.
- Sternothyroid.
- Omohyoid.
- Thyrohyoid.

digastric
(posterior belly)

mandible

submandibular
triangle

digastric
(anterior belly)

submental triangle

carotid triangle

omohyoid
(superior belly)

muscular triangle

sternohyoid

omohyoid
(inferior belly)

clavicle

63

**CERVICAL MUSCLES
RIGHT LATERAL VIEW**

A

sternocleidomastoid

digastric
(posterior belly)

stylohyoid

mylohyoid

omohyoid
(inferior belly)

digastric
(anterior belly)

omohyoid
(inferior belly)

thyrohyoid

intermediate tendon
of omohyoid

sternohyoid

sternothyroid

sternocleidomastoid

A

**HYOID MUSCLES
RIGHT LATERAL VIEW**

cervical muscles

The muscular structure of the neck is joined through two triangles (one anterior and the other posterior), which are divided by the sternocleidomastoid muscle. The muscles which intervene in this region form two groups, suprahyoid muscles and infrahyoid muscles, depending on whether they are above or below the hyoid bone. Most of these muscles are profound muscles in charge of coordinated swallowing movements.

NAPE (I)

POSTERIOR SUPERFICIAL and INTERMEDIATE VIEWS

muscles of nape

This group of muscles can be found under the insertion of the superficial muscles of the back, between the levator muscle of scapula and the cervical vertebrae. Their main function is to flex, to turn lateral way and to rotate neck, and therefore, all the head. The lateral movements of the head are executed by the sterno-cleidomastoid muscles and by some deeper muscles of the neck, among them the scalenus, and also by various muscles in the shape of a diamond located in the back line of the neck. On the other hand, the extension of the neck is produced by the superficial trapezius at the back, even though the splenius, located under the trapezius, are the main ones responsible for the extension of the head.

64

epicranial aponeurosis

occipitofrontalis (occipital belly)

semispinalis capitis

superior oblique of head

atlas (CI)

inferior oblique of head

splenius capitis

CIII vertebra

CIV vertebra

longissimus capitis

semispinalis capitis

splenius cervicis

splenius capitis

rectus capitis posterior minor

semispinalis capitis

rectus capitis posterior major

splenius capitis

semispinalis cervicis

sternocleidomastoid

spinous process of cervical vertebrae

trapezius

superficial layer of cervical fascia

A

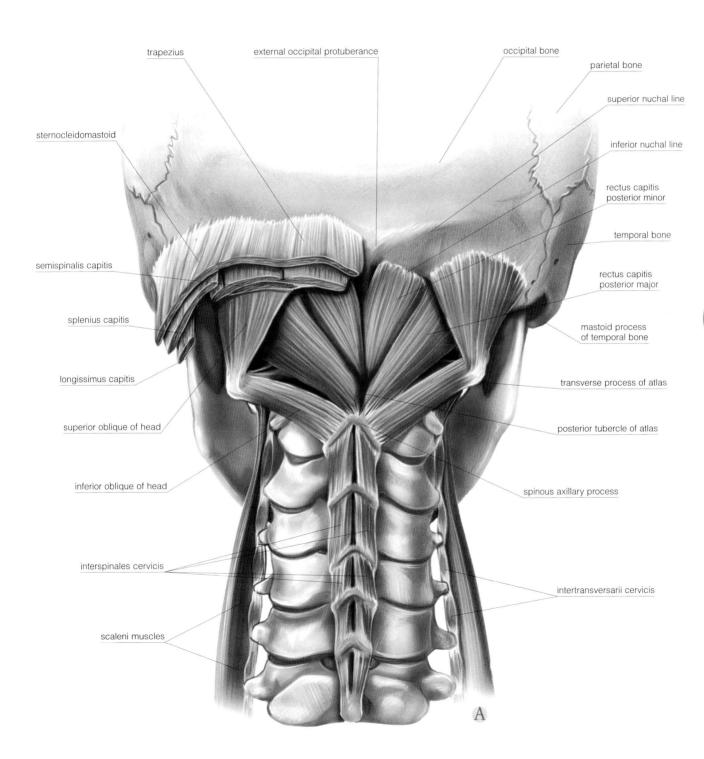

trapezius

external occipital protuberance

occipital bone

parietal bone

superior nuchal line

sternocleidomastoid

inferior nuchal line

rectus capitis posterior minor

temporal bone

semispinalis capitis

rectus capitis posterior major

splenius capitis

mastoid process of temporal bone

longissimus capitis

transverse process of atlas

superior oblique of head

posterior tubercle of atlas

inferior oblique of head

spinous axillary process

interspinales cervicis

intertransversarii cervicis

scaleni muscles

A

65

BUCCOPHARYNGEAL REGION (I)

LATERAL VIEW

66

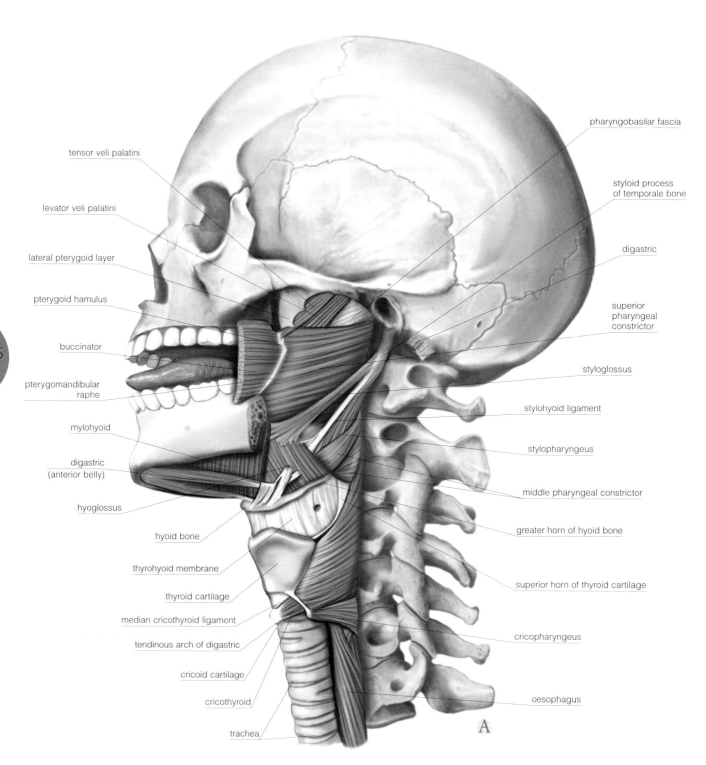

tensor veli palatini

levator veli palatini

lateral pterygoid layer

pterygoid hamulus

buccinator

pterygomandibular raphe

mylohyoid

digastric (anterior belly)

hyoglossus

hyoid bone

thyrohyoid membrane

thyroid cartilage

median cricothyroid ligament

tendinous arch of digastric

cricoid cartilage

cricothyroid

trachea

pharyngobasilar fascia

styloid process of temporale bone

digastric

superior pharyngeal constrictor

styloglossus

stylohyoid ligament

stylopharyngeus

middle pharyngeal constrictor

greater horn of hyoid bone

superior horn of thyroid cartilage

cricopharyngeus

oesophagus

A

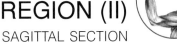
BUCCOPHARYNGEAL REGION (II)
SAGITTAL SECTION

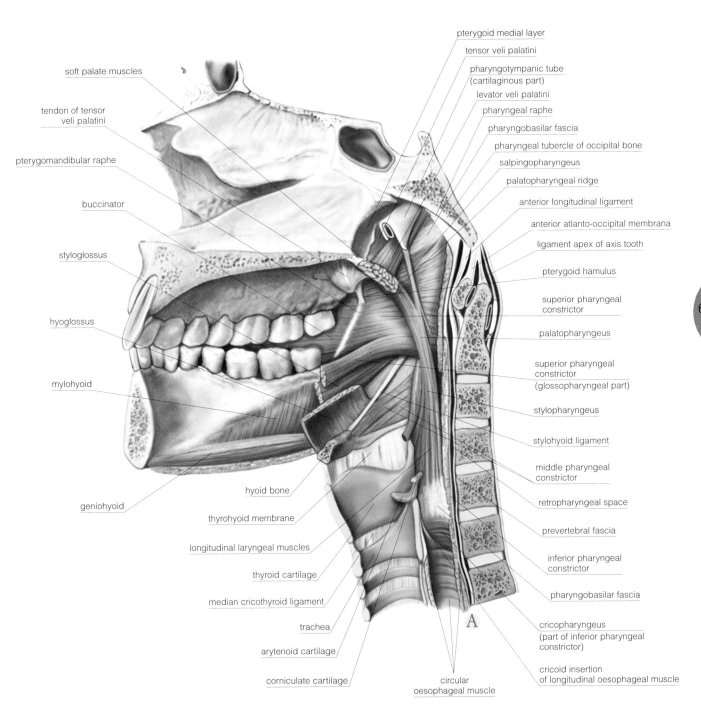

soft palate muscles

tendon of tensor
veli palatini

pterygomandibular raphe

buccinator

styloglossus

hyoglossus

mylohyoid

geniohyoid

hyoid bone

thyrohyoid membrane

longitudinal laryngeal muscles

thyroid cartilage

median cricothyroid ligament

trachea

arytenoid cartilage

corniculate cartilage

pterygoid medial layer

tensor veli palatini

pharyngotympanic tube
(cartilaginous part)

levator veli palatini

pharyngeal raphe

pharyngobasilar fascia

pharyngeal tubercle of occipital bone

salpingopharyngeus

palatopharyngeal ridge

anterior longitudinal ligament

anterior atlanto-occipital membrana

ligament apex of axis tooth

pterygoid hamulus

superior pharyngeal
constrictor

palatopharyngeus

superior pharyngeal
constrictor
(glossopharyngeal part)

stylopharyngeus

stylohyoid ligament

middle pharyngeal
constrictor

retropharyngeal space

prevertebral fascia

inferior pharyngeal
constrictor

pharyngobasilar fascia

cricopharyngeus
(part of inferior pharyngeal
constrictor)

cricoid insertion
of longitudinal oesophageal muscle

circular
oesophageal muscle

A

67

THORAX (I)
ANTERIOR SUPERFICIAL VIEW

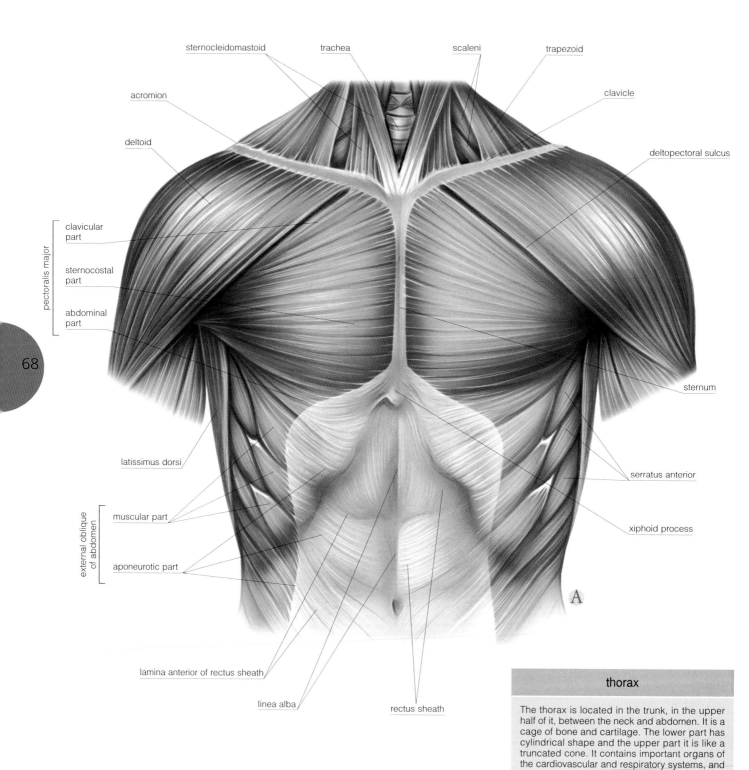

sternocleidomastoid

trachea

scaleni

trapezoid

acromion

clavicle

deltoid

deltopectoral sulcus

clavicular part

pectoralis major

sternocostal part

abdominal part

68

sternum

latissimus dorsi

serratus anterior

external oblique of abdomen

muscular part

xiphoid process

aponeurotic part

lamina anterior of rectus sheath

linea alba

rectus sheath

A

thorax

The thorax is located in the trunk, in the upper half of it, between the neck and abdomen. It is a cage of bone and cartilage. The lower part has cylindrical shape and the upper part it is like a truncated cone. It contains important organs of the cardiovascular and respiratory systems, and it is crossed by many structures of the digestive apparatus, lymphatic and nervous systems. This osseous structure is covered by a powerful group of very important muscles: deltoid, pectoralis major, latissimus dorsi, obliquus externus abdominis, rectus abdominis, etc.

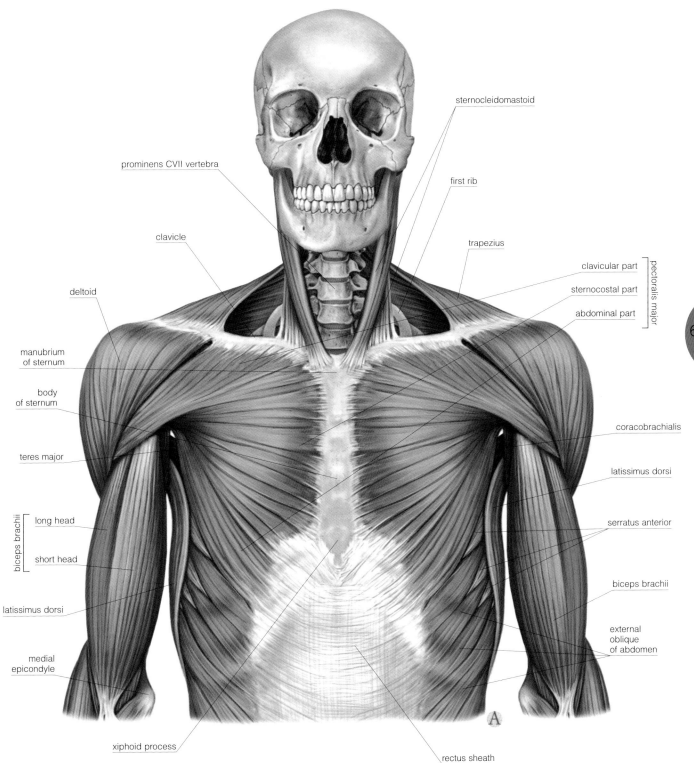

sternocleidomastoid

prominens CVII vertebra

first rib

clavicle

trapezius

clavicular part

sternocostal part

abdominal part

pectoralis major

deltoid

manubrium of sternum

body of sternum

coracobrachialis

teres major

latissimus dorsi

biceps brachii

long head

short head

serratus anterior

biceps brachii

latissimus dorsi

external oblique of abdomen

medial epicondyle

xiphoid process

rectus sheath

69

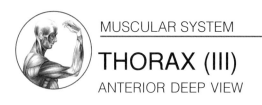

THORAX (III)
ANTERIOR DEEP VIEW

muscles of trunk

The movements of the trunk are realized by deep muscles that are joined to the vertebral column. They are responsible to keep the normal curvature of the spine (kyphosis and lordosis conditions). Muscles of the thorax embracing the adjoining sides and the diaphragm are very important to do the respiratory movements. The superficial dorsi muscles, in its turn, play a very important role in the movements of both, the shoulder girdle and the upper limbs.

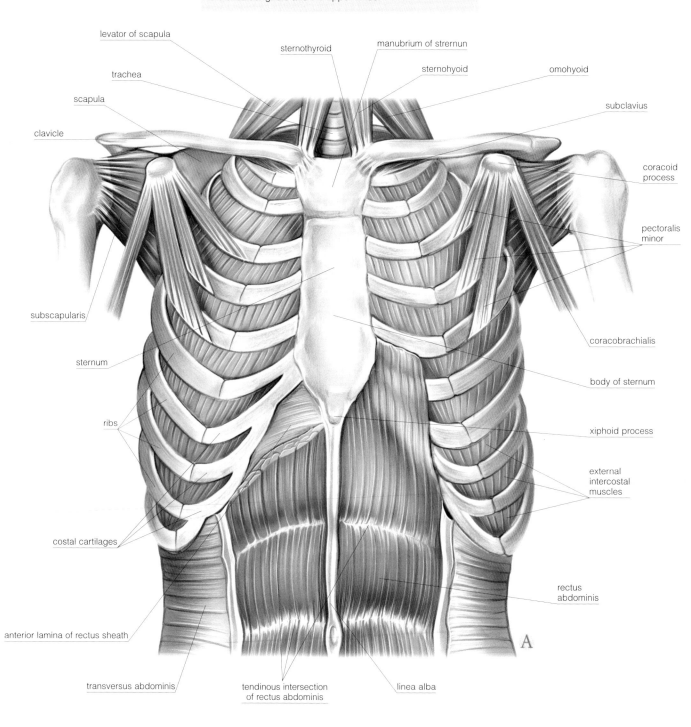

levator of scapula

sternothyroid

manubrium of strernun

trachea

sternohyoid

omohyoid

scapula

subclavius

clavicle

coracoid process

pectoralis minor

subscapularis

coracobrachialis

sternum

body of sternum

ribs

xiphoid process

external intercostal muscles

costal cartilages

rectus abdominis

anterior lamina of rectus sheath

transversus abdominis

tendinous intersection of rectus abdominis

linea alba

A

70

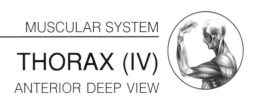

THORAX (IV)
ANTERIOR DEEP VIEW

muscles of thoracic wall

Many of the muscles of the upper limbs are linked to the thoracic cage. It is the case of the muscles perctoralis minor, subclavius, serratus anterior (front view) and latissimus dorsi (back view), and also the front and side muscles of the abdomen and some back and neck muscles. Pectoralis major and pectoralis minor muscles play an important role in the respiratory movements, insofar as they elevate the ribs to enlarge the thoracic cavity during a deep and forced inspiration.

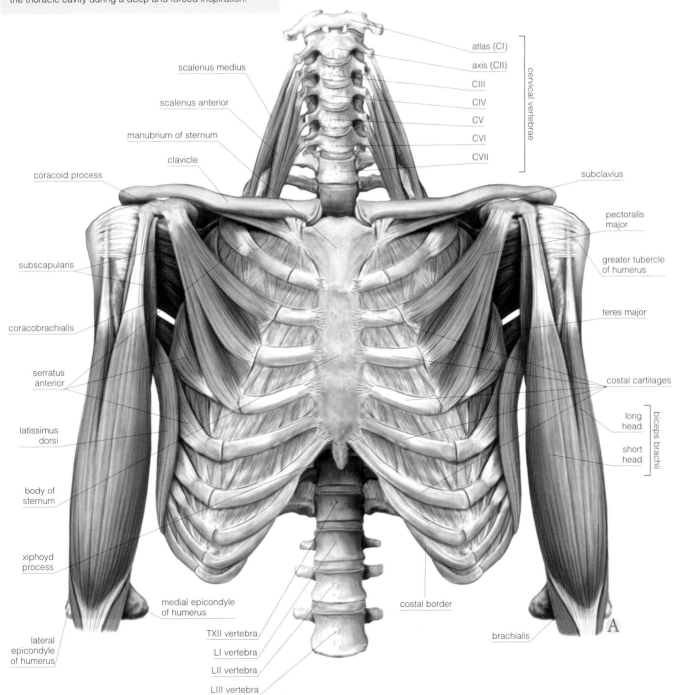

atlas (CI)
axis (CII)
CIII
CIV
CV
CVI
CVII
cervical vertebrae

scalenus medius
scalenus anterior
manubrium of sternum
clavicle
coracoid process

subclavius
pectoralis major
greater tubercle of humerus
teres major

subscapularis

coracobrachialis

serratus anterior

latissimus dorsi

body of sternum

xiphoyd process

medial epicondyle of humerus

lateral epicondyle of humerus

TXII vertebra
LI vertebra
LII vertebra
LIII vertebra

costal border

costal cartilages
long head
short head
biceps brachii

brachialis

71

A

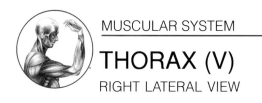

THORAX (V)
RIGHT LATERAL VIEW

muscles of thorax

The muscles of the thorax have different locations, present different shapes and make various movements that allow the human body to breath, and consequently purify blood. Among this group of muscles, it is worth mentioning the inspiratory group, which are the ones responsible for the enlargement of the volume of the thoracic cage, that way producing the expansion of the lungs and letting the outside air get into them; and also, we can mention the expiratory group, which is responsible for the shrinking in the space of the thoracic cage, causing the expulsion to the exterior of the air contained inside the lungs.

72

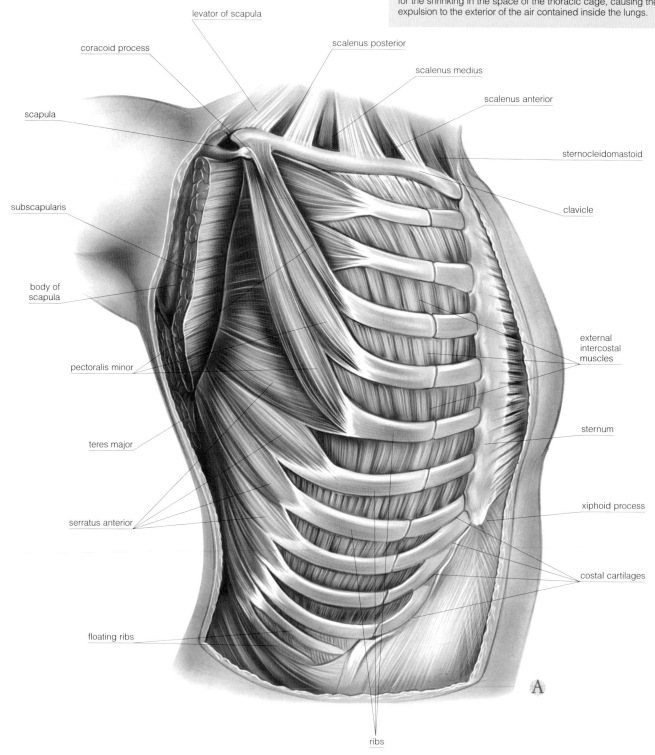

levator of scapula

coracoid process

scalenus posterior

scalenus medius

scalenus anterior

scapula

sternocleidomastoid

subscapularis

clavicle

body of scapula

external intercostal muscles

pectoralis minor

teres major

sternum

serratus anterior

xiphoid process

costal cartilages

floating ribs

ribs

A

THORAX (VI)
LEFT ANTERIOR LATERAL VIEW

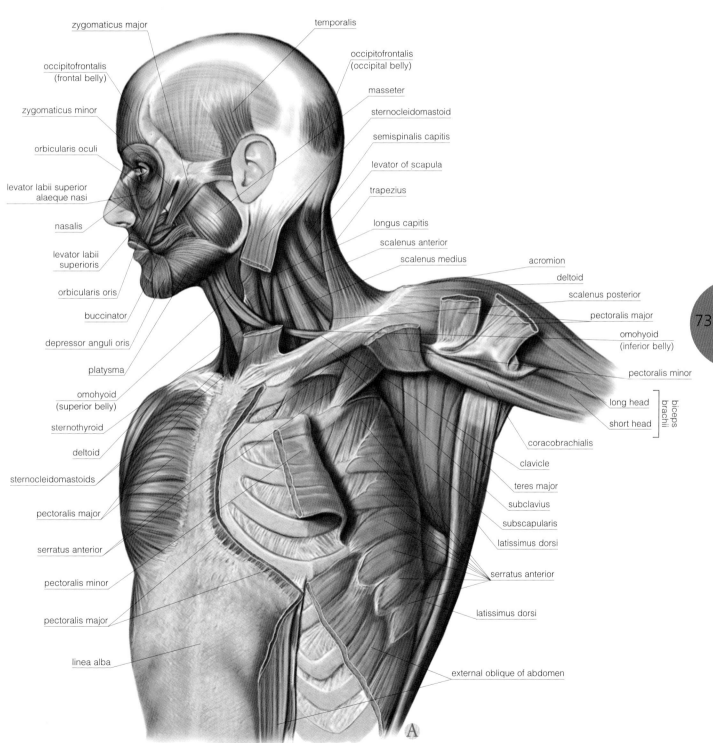

zygomaticus major

temporalis

occipitofrontalis
(occipital belly)

occipitofrontalis
(frontal belly)

masseter

zygomaticus minor

sternocleidomastoid

semispinalis capitis

orbicularis oculi

levator of scapula

levator labii superior
alaeque nasi

trapezius

longus capitis

nasalis

scalenus anterior

levator labii
superioris

scalenus medius

acromion

deltoid

orbicularis oris

scalenus posterior

pectoralis major

buccinator

omohyoid
(inferior belly)

depressor anguli oris

platysma

pectoralis minor

omohyoid
(superior belly)

long head
short head

biceps
brachii

sternothyroid

deltoid

coracobrachialis

clavicle

sternocleidomastoids

teres major

pectoralis major

subclavius

subscapularis

serratus anterior

latissimus dorsi

pectoralis minor

serratus anterior

pectoralis major

latissimus dorsi

linea alba

external oblique of abdomen

A

THORAX (VII). ANTERIOR THORACIC WALL

POSTERIOR VIEW

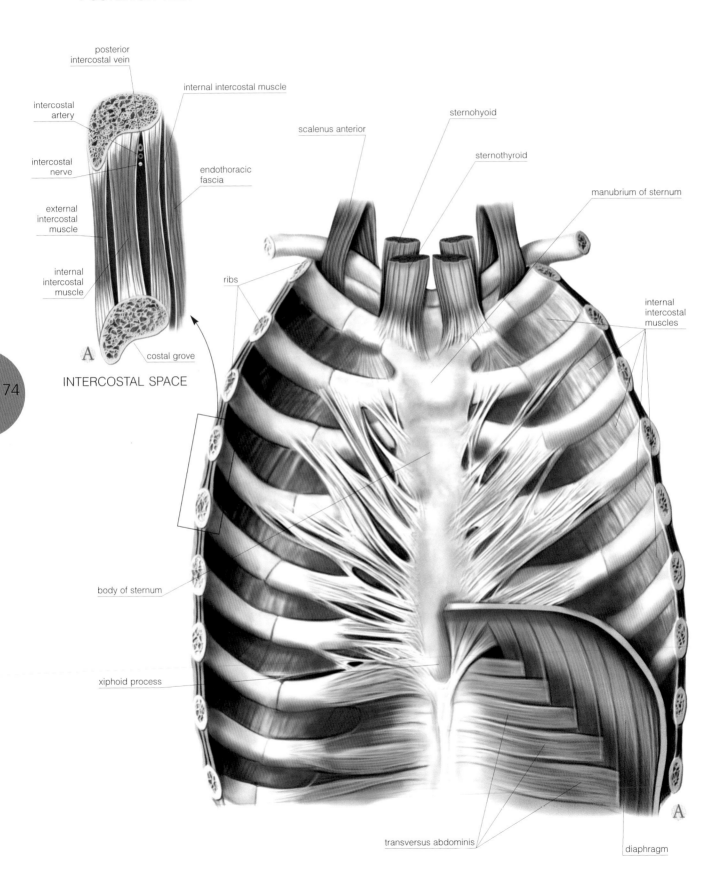

posterior
intercostal vein

internal intercostal muscle

intercostal
artery

intercostal
nerve

endothoracic
fascia

external
intercostal
muscle

internal
intercostal
muscle

A

costal grove

INTERCOSTAL SPACE

scalenus anterior

sternohyoid

sternothyroid

manubrium of sternum

ribs

internal
intercostal
muscles

body of sternum

xiphoid process

A

transversus abdominis

diaphragm

74

THORAX (VIII). POSTERIOR THORACIC WALL

ANTERIOR VIFW

intercostal muscles

The external intercostal muscles are located in the space between the ribs and they go from the back part, where the tubercules of the ribs are located, to the front part, where the chondrocostal articulations are. In the front part the muscular fibers are replaced by the external intercostal membrane. They go along from the upper rib to the next one in the lower position. The internal intercostal muscles pass in angle under the external intercostal muscles obliquely disposed. The muscular fibers go back lower sense from the inferior ridge of the rib to the border of the next rib just below. In the posterior part, between the ribs and medial to the angles, the internal intercostal muscles are replaced by the internal intercostal membrane.

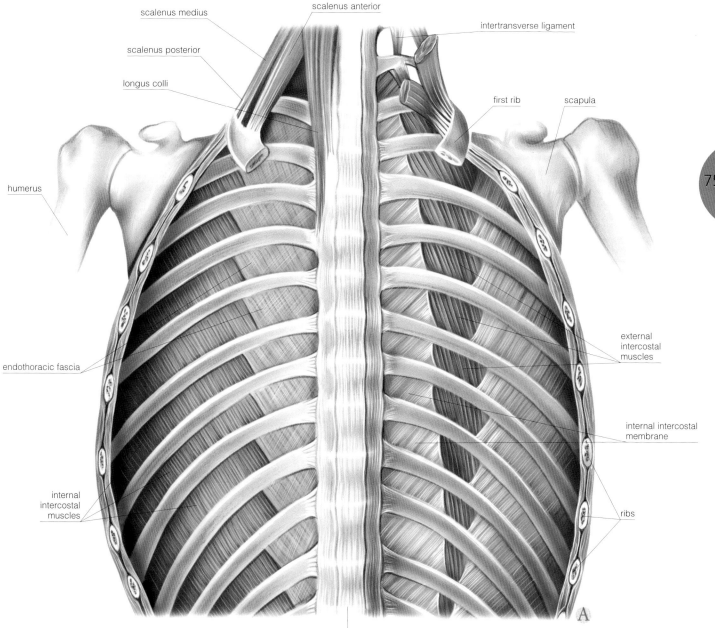

scalenus medius

scalenus anterior

intertransverse ligament

scalenus posterior

longus colli

first rib

scapula

humerus

endothoracic fascia

external intercostal muscles

internal intercostal membrane

internal intercostal muscles

ribs

75

anterior longitudinal ligament

TRUNK and ABDOMEN (I)

MALE SEX. ANTERIOR SUPERFICIAL VIEW

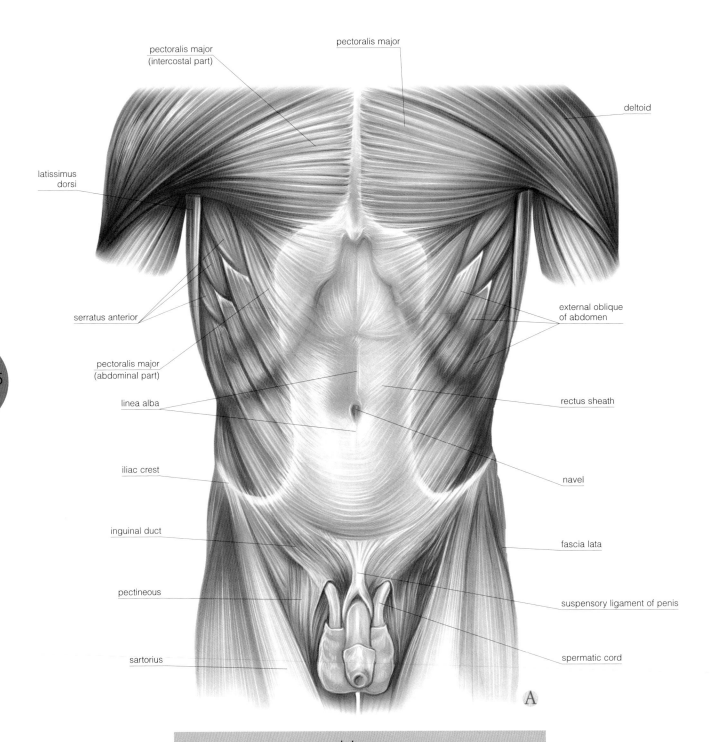

pectoralis major
(intercostal part)

pectoralis major

deltoid

latissimus
dorsi

serratus anterior

external oblique
of abdomen

pectoralis major
(abdominal part)

rectus sheath

linea alba

navel

iliac crest

inguinal duct

fascia lata

pectineous

suspensory ligament of penis

sartorius

spermatic cord

76

abdomen

Altogether with the thorax and the pelvis, located between them, the abdomen makes part of the lower part the trunk of the human body. In the front and lateral sides, abdomen wall are formed by muscles, fascias and skin. The uppermost part is limited by the diaphragm, upon which lungs and heart are resting. Inside the abdomen, there are the most part of the organs of the digestive system (stomach, intestines, liver and pancreas), spleen and urinary organs. In the lowest part of the abdomen (pelvis) the urogenital organs and the ending part of the digestive system are also contained.

TRUNK and ABDOMEN (II)
MALE SEX. ANTERIOR VIEW

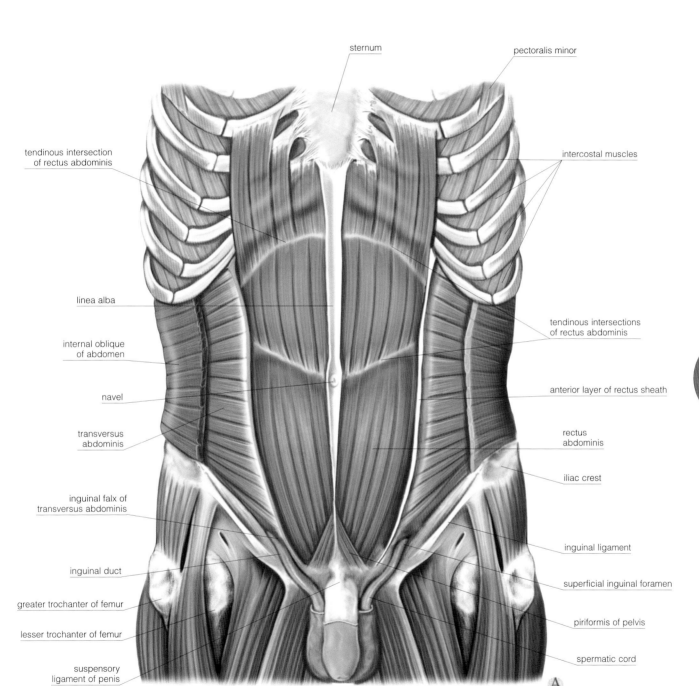

sternum

pectoralis minor

tendinous intersection of rectus abdominis

intercostal muscles

linea alba

tendinous intersections of rectus abdominis

internal oblique of abdomen

anterior layer of rectus sheath

navel

transversus abdominis

rectus abdominis

inguinal falx of transversus abdominis

iliac crest

inguinal duct

inguinal ligament

greater trochanter of femur

superficial inguinal foramen

lesser trochanter of femur

piriformis of pelvis

suspensory ligament of penis

spermatic cord

muscles of abdomen

The muscles of the abdomen are made up by four pairs of flat muscles (rectus abdominis, obliquus externus abdominis, obliquus internus abdominis and transversus abdominis), with the very decisive function of holding up and protecting the abdominal viscus and also an important role in the movement of the vertebral column (flexion and lateral bending). The holding up function is much better accomplished if the muscle tone is the appropriate; otherwise, the abdomen becomes distended. During a soft inhalation, the muscles of the abdomen become distended and the lowering of the diaphragm push the viscera down to the pelvis. When the muscles of the abdomen contract along with the diaphragm and the glottis closes, there is an increasing in the abdominal pressure which facilitates actions like defecation, urination, vomit, cough and delivery. The joint contraction of the internal muscles of the back helps in the prevention of the hyperextension of the vertebral column and also in the forming of a protective case for the whole torso.

TRUNK and ABDOMEN (III)

ANTERIOR VIEW. FRONTAL SECTION

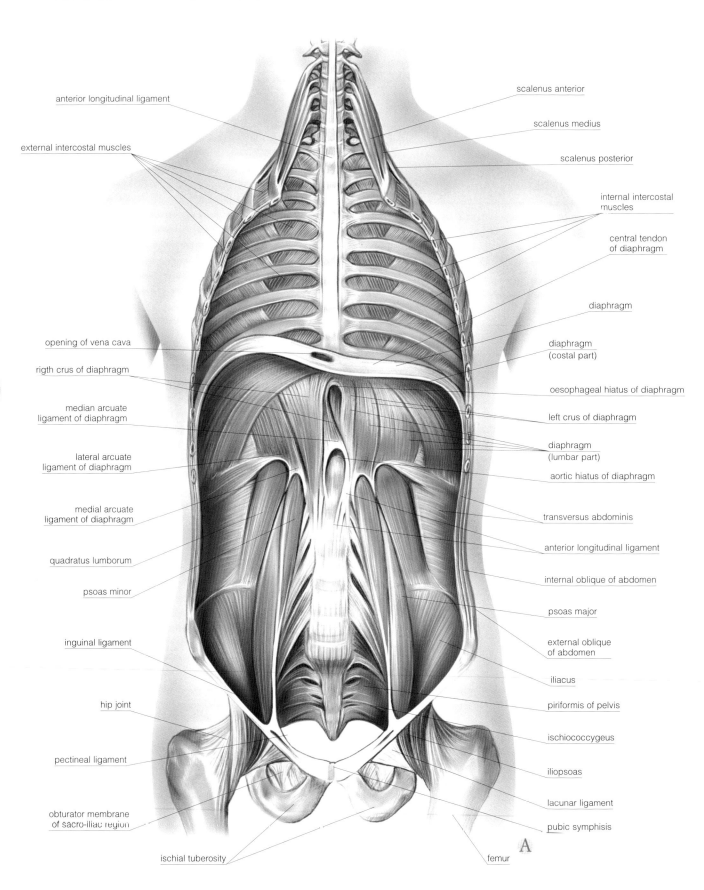

anterior longitudinal ligament

external intercostal muscles

opening of vena cava

rigth crus of diaphragm

median arcuate
ligament of diaphragm

lateral arcuate
ligament of diaphragm

medial arcuate
ligament of diaphragm

quadratus lumborum

psoas minor

inguinal ligament

hip joint

pectineal ligament

obturator membrane
of sacro-iliac region

ischial tuberosity

scalenus anterior

scalenus medius

scalenus posterior

internal intercostal
muscles

central tendon
of diaphragm

diaphragm

diaphragm
(costal part)

oesophageal hiatus of diaphragm

left crus of diaphragm

diaphragm
(lumbar part)

aortic hiatus of diaphragm

transversus abdominis

anterior longitudinal ligament

internal oblique of abdomen

psoas major

external oblique
of abdomen

iliacus

piriformis of pelvis

ischiococcygeus

iliopsoas

lacunar ligament

pubic symphisis

femur

78

A

TRUNK and ABDOMEN (IV)
ANTERIOR WALL. INTERNAL VIEW

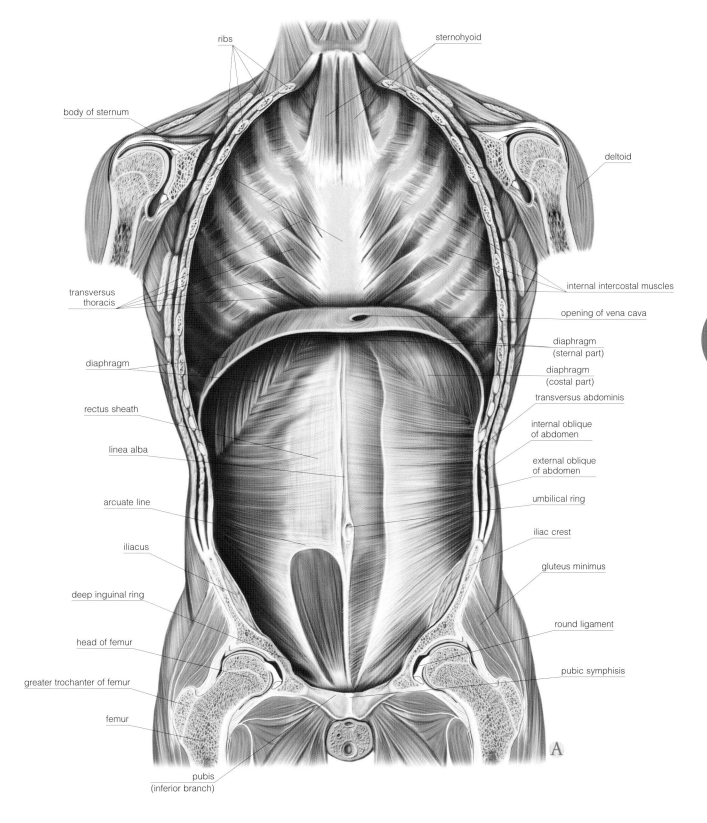

ribs

sternohyoid

body of sternum

deltoid

transversus
thoracis

internal intercostal muscles

opening of vena cava

diaphragm

diaphragm
(sternal part)

diaphragm
(costal part)

transversus abdominis

rectus sheath

internal oblique
of abdomen

linea alba

external oblique
of abdomen

arcuate line

umbilical ring

iliacus

iliac crest

gluteus minimus

deep inguinal ring

head of femur

round ligament

greater trochanter of femur

pubic symphisis

femur

pubis
(inferior branch)

A

TRUNK (I). BACK (I)
SUPERFICIAL VIEW

muscles of back

There is a double function of the muscles of the back, some of them very important: to keep upright the vertebral column and to facilitate the movements of the upper limbs (extremities) in relation to the trunk: flexion, rotation, adduction, etc.

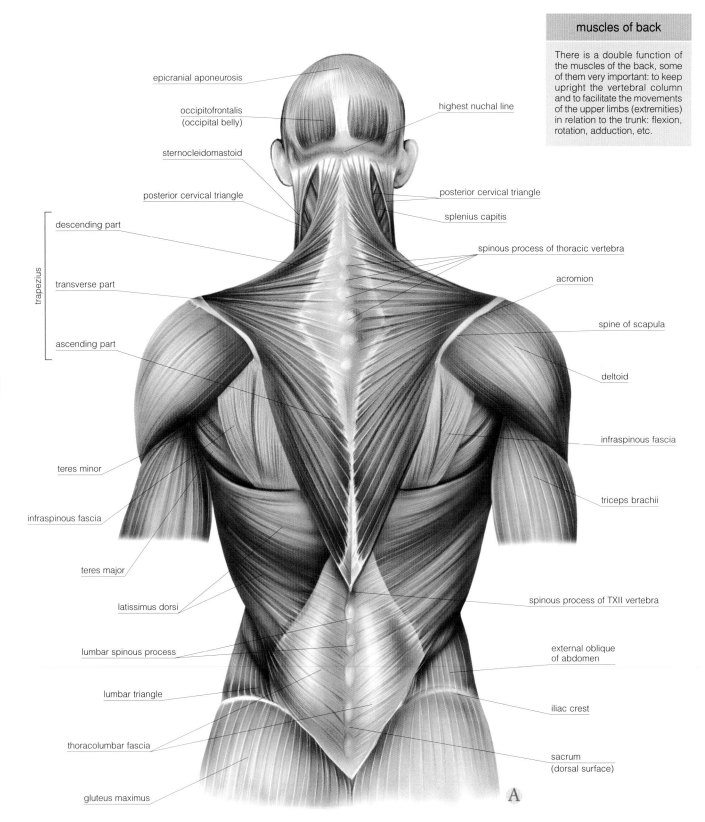

epicranial aponeurosis

occipitofrontalis (occipital belly)

sternocleidomastoid

posterior cervical triangle

trapezius
- descending part
- transverse part
- ascending part

teres minor

infraspinous fascia

teres major

latissimus dorsi

lumbar spinous process

lumbar triangle

thoracolumbar fascia

gluteus maximus

highest nuchal line

posterior cervical triangle

splenius capitis

spinous process of thoracic vertebra

acromion

spine of scapula

deltoid

infraspinous fascia

triceps brachii

spinous process of TXII vertebra

external oblique of abdomen

iliac crest

sacrum (dorsal surface)

A

TRUNK (II). BACK (II)

INTERMEDIATE VIEW

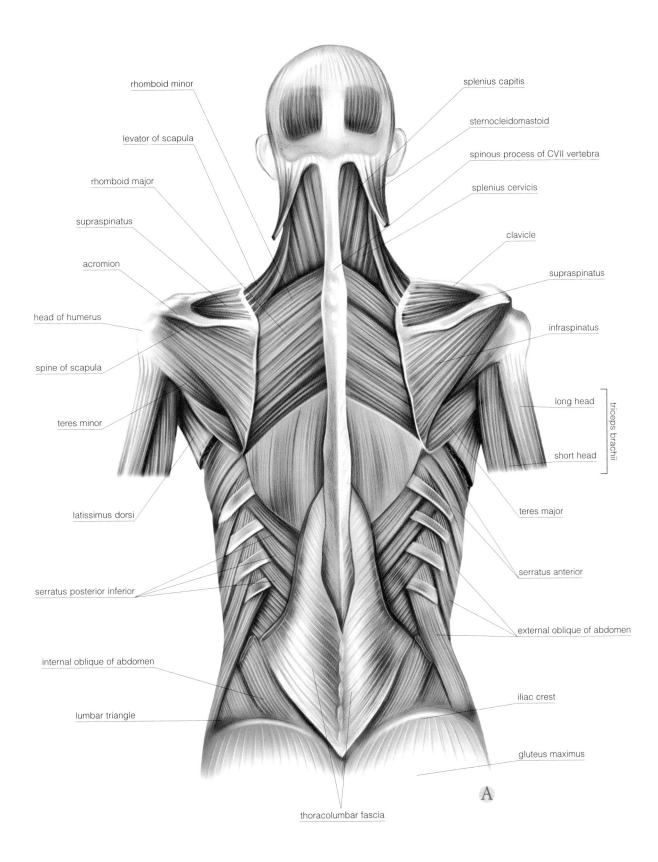

rhomboid minor

levator of scapula

rhomboid major

supraspinatus

acromion

head of humerus

spine of scapula

teres minor

latissimus dorsi

serratus posterior inferior

internal oblique of abdomen

lumbar triangle

splenius capitis

sternocleidomastoid

spinous process of CVII vertebra

splenius cervicis

clavicle

supraspinatus

infraspinatus

long head
short head
triceps brachii

teres major

serratus anterior

external oblique of abdomen

iliac crest

gluteus maximus

thoracolumbar fascia

Ⓐ

TRUNK (III)

CROSS-SECTION at the HEIGT of the TV VERTEBRA

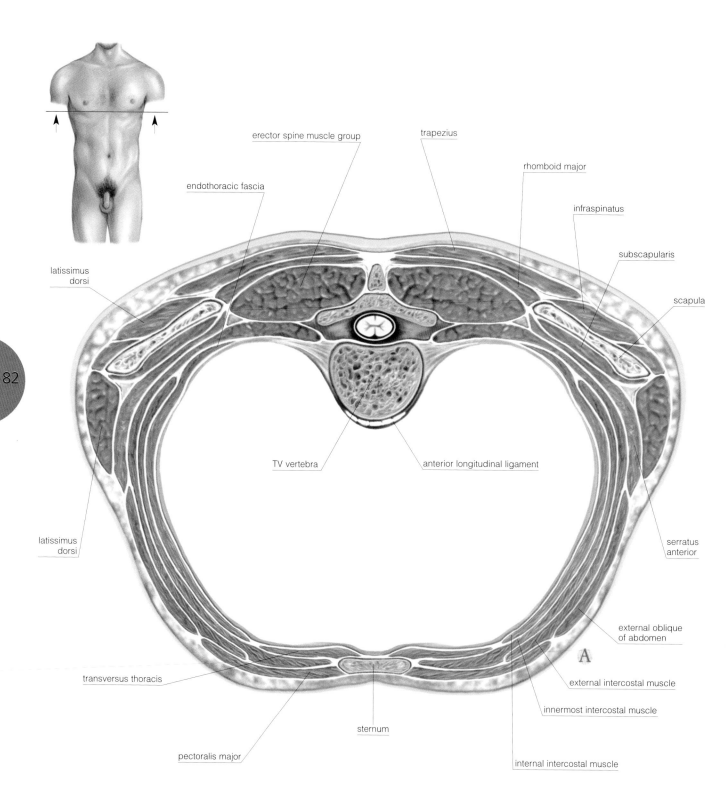

erector spine muscle group

trapezius

rhomboid major

endothoracic fascia

infraspinatus

subscapularis

scapula

latissimus dorsi

latissimus dorsi

TV vertebra

anterior longitudinal ligament

serratus anterior

external oblique of abdomen

A

transversus thoracis

external intercostal muscle

innermost intercostal muscle

sternum

internal intercostal muscle

pectoralis major

82

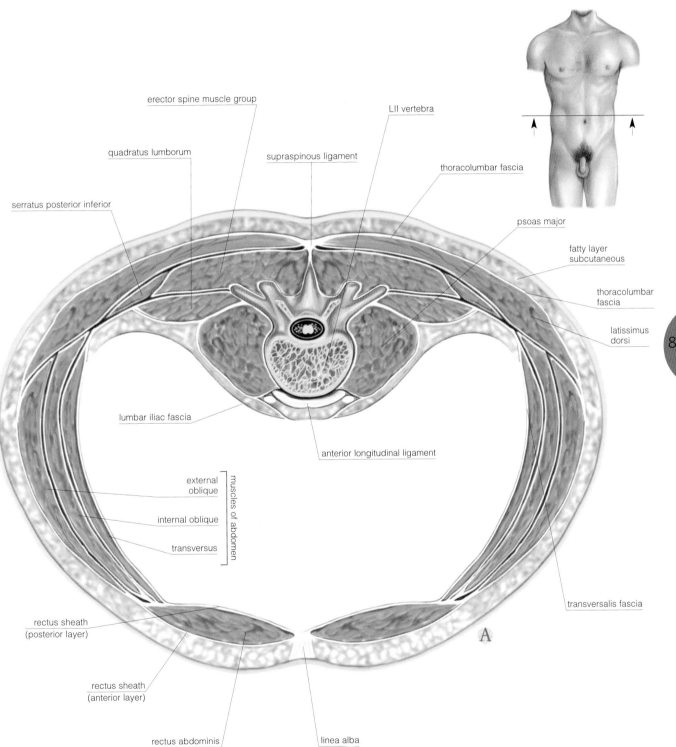

erector spine muscle group

LII vertebra

quadratus lumborum

supraspinous ligament

thoracolumbar fascia

serratus posterior inferior

psoas major

fatty layer
subcutaneous

thoracolumbar
fascia

latissimus
dorsi

83

lumbar iliac fascia

anterior longitudinal ligament

external
oblique

muscles of abdomen

internal oblique

transversus

transversalis fascia

rectus sheath
(posterior layer)

rectus sheath
(anterior layer)

rectus abdominis

linea alba

A

TRUNK (V). DIAPHRAGM (I)
SUPERIOR VIEW

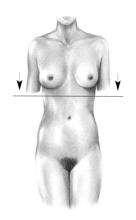

diaphragm

The diaphragm is a flat musculomebranous septum, dome-shaped and with an upper convexity, that separates the thoracic from the abdominal cavity, its concave under (abdominal) surface is covered by the parietal peritoneum. It is pierced by thee apertures: the oesophagus, the thoracic portion of the aorta artery and the inferior vena cava. It is an essential muscle during breathing, insofar as its contraction or relaxation enlarges or reduces the volume of the thoracic wall to facilitate the air inhalation and exhalation during breathing. It also has others functions, whether, involuntary actions (hiccup, vomit, etc.) or voluntary ones (laughter, expulsion of feces, etc).

During pregnancy, as the foetus grows larger, the pressure over the abdominal cavity also increases and this makes that the organs inside the abdomen have to adapt to the less available space. All this makes very difficult to the diaphragm to move, and for that reason, breathing becomes a more difficult process during pregnancy to the limit of producing the feeling of breathlessness. It is innervated by the phrenic nerve, sending a branch to the convex upper (thoracic) surface, and other one to the concave under surface. It also receives innervation from the intercostal nerves. It is irrigated by the internal thoracic arterial branches, posterior and disphagmatic arterial branches.

84

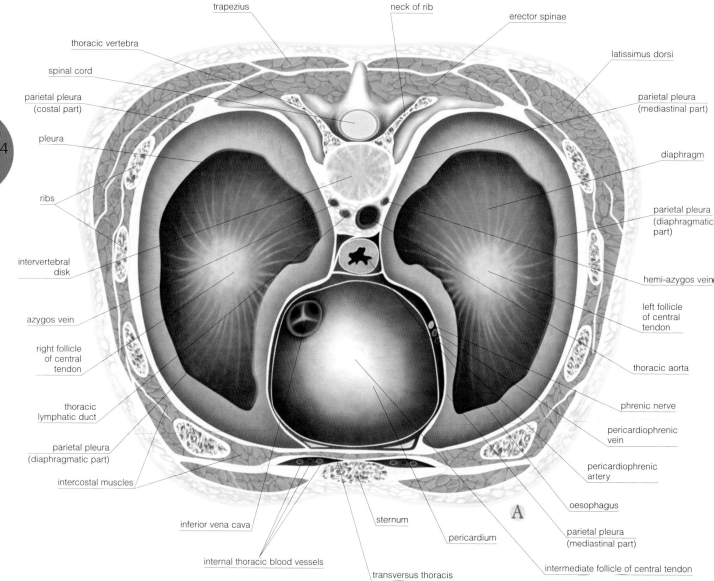

trapezius

neck of rib

erector spinae

thoracic vertebra

latissimus dorsi

spinal cord

parietal pleura (costal part)

parietal pleura (mediastinal part)

pleura

diaphragm

ribs

parietal pleura (diaphragmatic part)

intervertebral disk

hemi-azygos vein

azygos vein

left follicle of central tendon

right follicle of central tendon

thoracic aorta

thoracic lymphatic duct

phrenic nerve

parietal pleura (diaphragmatic part)

pericardiophrenic vein

intercostal muscles

pericardiophrenic artery

inferior vena cava

oesophagus

sternum

parietal pleura (mediastinal part)

pericardium

internal thoracic blood vessels

intermediate follicle of central tendon

transversus thoracis

A

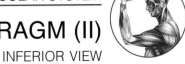

TRUNK (VI). DIAPHRAGM (II)

INFERIOR VIEW

diaphragm

In relaxation, the diaphragm is a dome-shape structure, but when it contracts it moves down to the abdomen and becomes flat-shape. Alternation between contraction and relaxation causes changes in the pressure suffered by the abdominal cavity, which facilitates the return of venous blood to the heart. On the other hand, the rhythmic contractions taken place during breathing enable the diaphragm to extremely contract in order to increase, according to volition, the intra-abdominal pressure and help in the evacuation of the contents of the organs located in the pelvis (urine, feces, or the fetus).

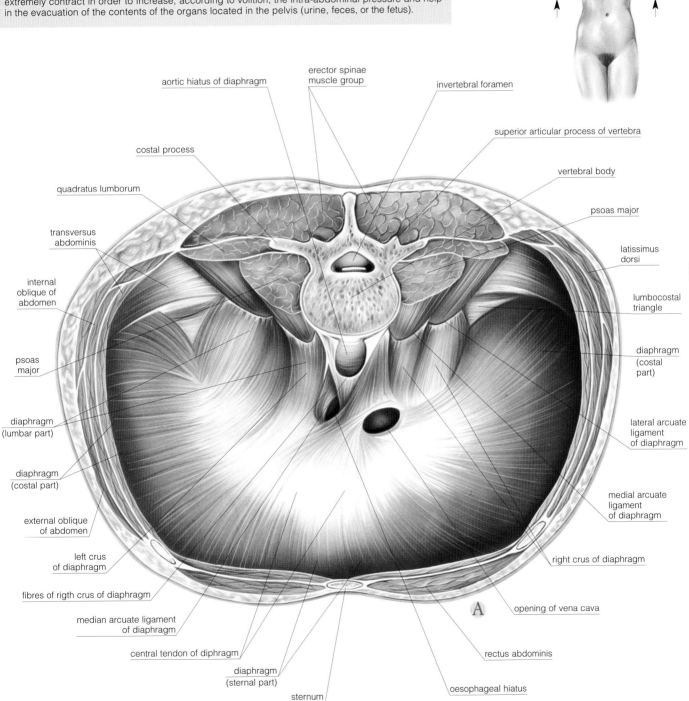

aortic hiatus of diaphragm

erector spinae muscle group

invertebral foramen

superior articular process of vertebra

costal process

vertebral body

quadratus lumborum

psoas major

transversus abdominis

latissimus dorsi

internal oblique of abdomen

lumbocostal triangle

psoas major

diaphragm (costal part)

diaphragm (lumbar part)

lateral arcuate ligament of diaphragm

diaphragm (costal part)

medial arcuate ligament of diaphragm

external oblique of abdomen

left crus of diaphragm

right crus of diaphragm

fibres of rigth crus of diaphragm

median arcuate ligament of diaphragm

opening of vena cava

central tendon of diphragm

diaphragm (sternal part)

rectus abdominis

sternum

oesophageal hiatus

PELVIS (I). MALE PELVIC FLOOR

TRANSVERSE SECTION. CRANIAL VIEW

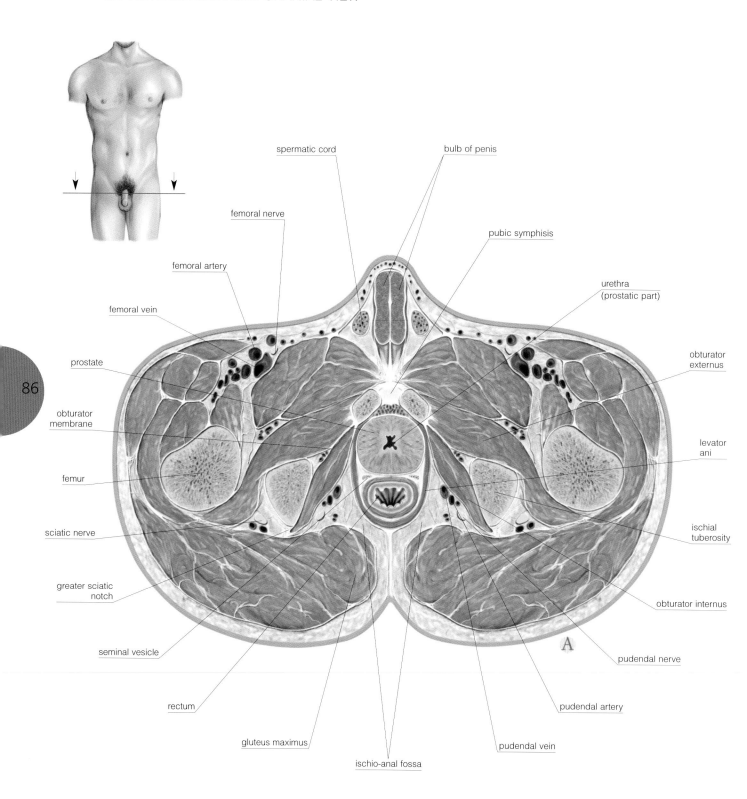

spermatic cord

bulb of penis

femoral nerve

pubic symphisis

femoral artery

urethra
(prostatic part)

femoral vein

prostate

obturator
externus

obturator
membrane

levator
ani

femur

sciatic nerve

ischial
tuberosity

greater sciatic
notch

obturator internus

seminal vesicle

pudendal nerve

rectum

pudendal artery

gluteus maximus

pudendal vein

ischio-anal fossa

86

A

PELVIS (II). FEMALE PELVIC FLOOR

TRANSVERSE SECTION. CRANIAL VIEW

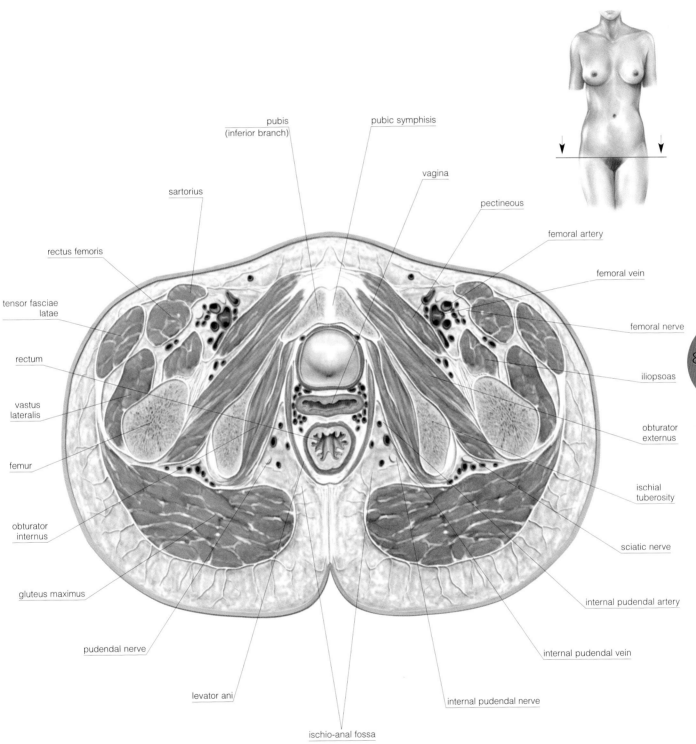

pubis
(inferior branch)

pubic symphisis

vagina

sartorius

pectineous

femoral artery

rectus femoris

femoral vein

tensor fasciae
latae

femoral nerve

87

rectum

iliopsoas

vastus
lateralis

obturator
externus

femur

ischial
tuberosity

obturator
internus

sciatic nerve

gluteus maximus

internal pudendal artery

pudendal nerve

internal pudendal vein

levator ani

internal pudendal nerve

ischio-anal fossa

PERINEUM (I). MALE SEX

perineum

Referring to perineum means two things: an external surface area and a deep compartment within the body. The perineum area is the narrowest region between the proximal thirds of the muscles. But, when the lower limbs are in abduction it is a diamond-shape area going, in the front view, from the mons pubis and the lateral medial surfaces of the thighs to the winkles of the gluteal muscles and the upper end of the gluteal fissure, in the back view. The perineum compartment is bounded by the lower strait if the pelvis and split from the pelvic cavity by the pelvic diaphragm, which is formed by the levator ani and coccygeus muscles. The osseofibrous structures bounding the perineum, or perineum compartment, are: symphysis pubis (front), pubis inferior ramus and ischial ramus (front-lateral), tuberosities of the ischium (lateral), sacro-tuberous ligaments (back-lateral) and inferior margin sacrum and coccyx (back).

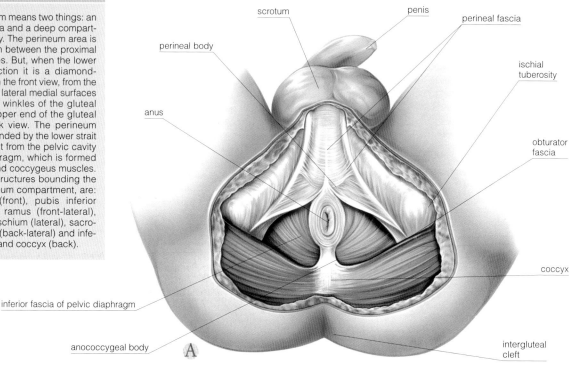

SUPERFICIAL FASCIA (UROGENITAL REGION)

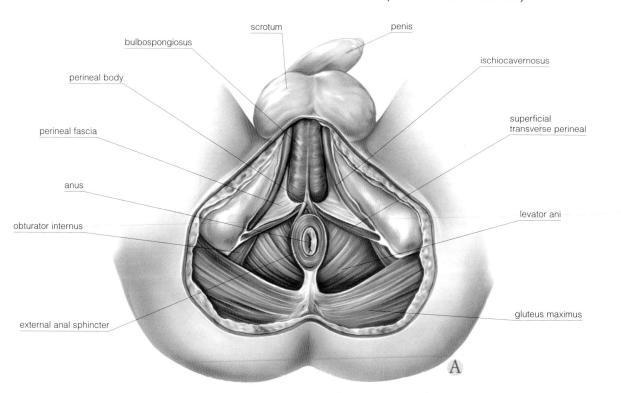

DIAPHRAGMATIC FASCIA (ANAL REGION)

PERINEUM (II). FEMALE SEX

muscles of pelvic floor

Two pairs of muscles, levator ani and ilio-coccygeus, form the floor of the pelvis, funnel-shaped, that it is also known as pelvic diaphragm. These group of muscles close the lower strait of the pelvic cavity, they hold and raise the floor of the pelvis, and support and regulate the intraabdominal pressure, by this means regulating the expulsion of the contents of the urinary bladder, the rectum and the uterus. The pelvic diaphragm contains two orifices: the anus and the urethra, and in the case of women, also the vagina. The lower part of the pelvic diaphragm is the perineum. Under the muscles of the floor of the pelvis and in the anterior half of the perineum, between both sides of the pubic arch, it is the pelvic diaphragm, made up by a small triangular bed, where it is located the external urethrae sphincter. In the posterior half of the perineum is located the external anal sphincter. In front of this sphincter muscle is located the tendinous arch of the pelvis fascia, a very strong muscle in which many perineum muscles get inserted.

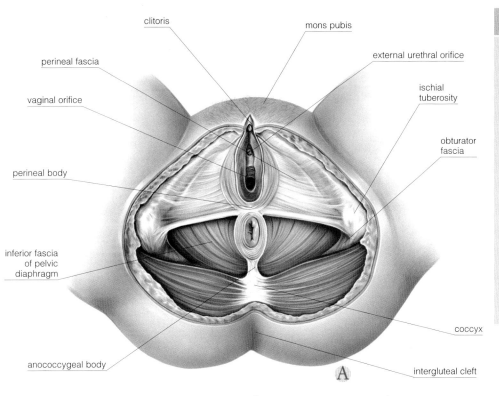

Labels: clitoris, mons pubis, external urethral orifice, perineal fascia, vaginal orifice, ischial tuberosity, obturator fascia, perineal body, inferior fascia of pelvic diaphragm, coccyx, anococcygeal body, interngluteal cleft

SUPERFICIAL FASCIA (UROGENITAL REGION)

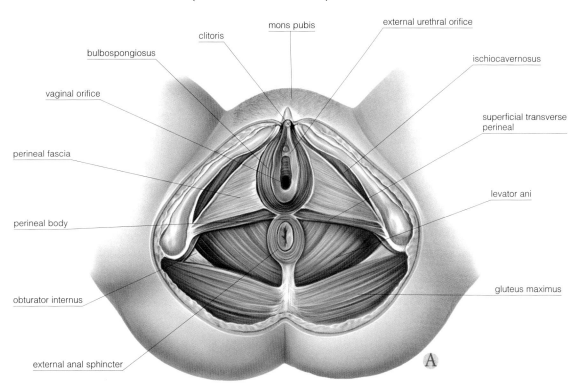

Labels: bulbospongiosus, clitoris, mons pubis, external urethral orifice, vaginal orifice, ischiocavernosus, superficial transverse perineal, perineal fascia, perineal body, levator ani, obturator internus, gluteus maximus, external anal sphincter

DIAPHRAGMATIC FASCIA (ANAL REGION)

PERINEUM (III). MALE SEX
PERINEAL VIEW

90

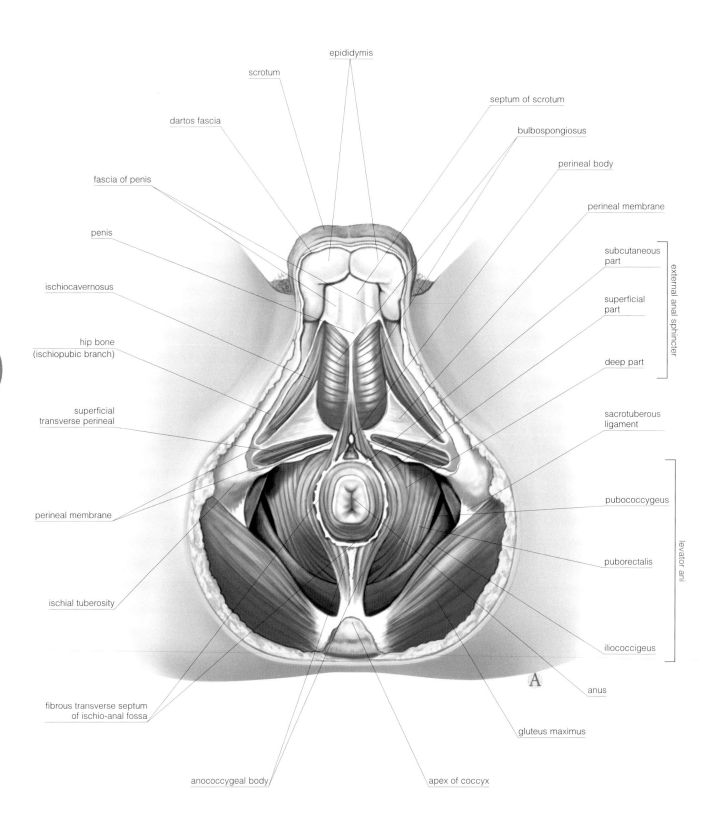

epididymis

scrotum

septum of scrotum

dartos fascia

bulbospongiosus

perineal body

fascia of penis

perineal membrane

penis

subcutaneous part

ischiocavernosus

superficial part

external anal sphincter

hip bone
(ischiopubic branch)

deep part

sacrotuberous ligament

superficial
transverse perineal

pubococcygeus

perineal membrane

levator ani

puborectalis

ischial tuberosity

iliococcigeus

A

anus

fibrous transverse septum
of ischio-anal fossa

gluteus maximus

anococcygeal body

apex of coccyx

PERINEUM (IV). FEMALE SEX

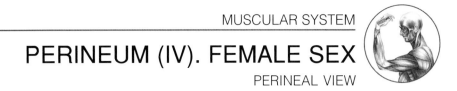

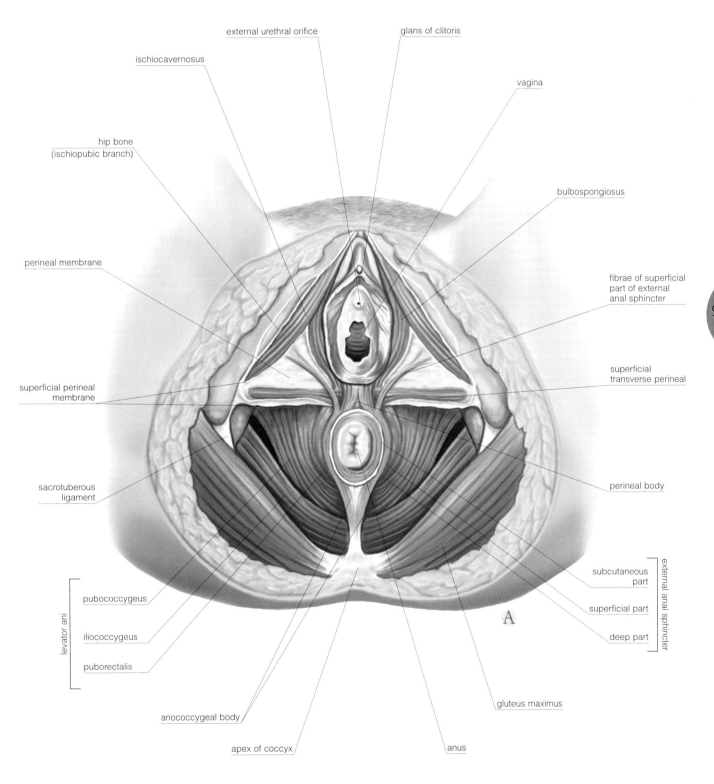

external urethral orifice

glans of clitoris

ischiocavernosus

vagina

hip bone
(ischiopubic branch)

bulbospongiosus

perineal membrane

fibrae of superficial
part of external
anal sphincter

91

superficial transverse perineal

superficial perineal
membrane

sacrotuberous
ligament

perineal body

levator ani

pubococcygeus

iliococcygeus

puborectalis

subcutaneous
part

superficial part

deep part

external anal sphincter

gluteus maximus

anococcygeal body

apex of coccyx

anus

A

UPPER LIMB (I)

RIGHT UPPER LIMB. LATERAL GENERAL SUPERFICIAL VIEW

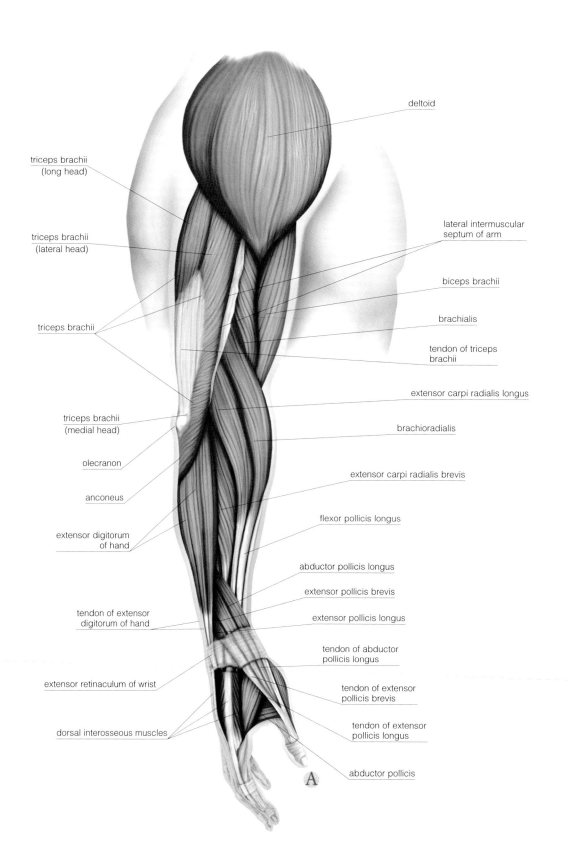

deltoid

triceps brachii
(long head)

triceps brachii
(lateral head)

triceps brachii

triceps brachii
(medial head)

olecranon

anconeus

extensor digitorum
of hand

tendon of extensor
digitorum of hand

extensor retinaculum of wrist

dorsal interosseous muscles

lateral intermuscular
septum of arm

biceps brachii

brachialis

tendon of triceps
brachii

extensor carpi radialis longus

brachioradialis

extensor carpi radialis brevis

flexor pollicis longus

abductor pollicis longus

extensor pollicis brevis

extensor pollicis longus

tendon of abductor
pollicis longus

tendon of extensor
pollicis brevis

tendon of extensor
pollicis longus

abductor pollicis

A

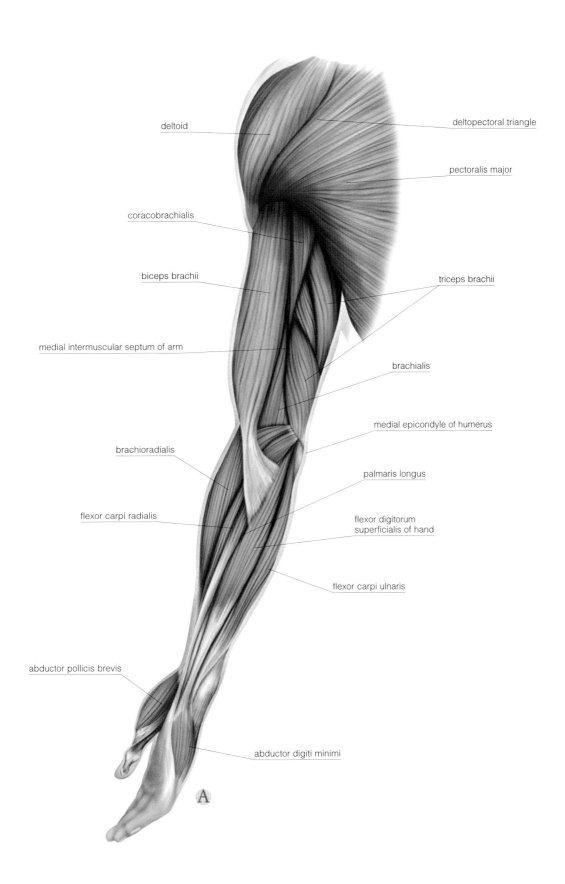

deltoid

deltopectoral triangle

pectoralis major

coracobrachialis

biceps brachii

triceps brachii

medial intermuscular septum of arm

brachialis

medial epicondyle of humerus

brachioradialis

palmaris longus

flexor carpi radialis

flexor digitorum
superficialis of hand

flexor carpi ulnaris

abductor pollicis brevis

abductor digiti minimi

A

UPPER LIMB (III)

RIGHT UPPER LIMB. LATERAL SUPERFICIAL VIEW

upper limb

The upper limbs are two appendages that start at each side of the upper part of the trunk. They contain a group of bones, muscles and joints to be used to gesticulate, lift weights, etc. Each one of them consist of four basic parts (arm -whose skeletal part is formed by the humerus-, elbow -where there are the structures of the elbow joint-, forearm -whose skeletal structure is made up by the radius and the ulna- and hand -where they come all together the carpal bones, metacarpal bones and the phalanges of the fingers-), all of them with osseous structure, muscular casing and joints (elbow joints, radioulnar articulation, radiocarpal, intercarpal, intermetacarpal, metacarpophalangeal, interphalangeal, etc.), which gives them great mobility, specially in the case of hands. One of the most characteristic functions of these muscles is allowing the performance of a wide range of movements, some of them specific of human species.

94

deltoid

deltopectoral triangle

pectoralis major

triceps brachii
(long head)

biceps brachii
(short head)

medial intermuscular septum of arm

brachialis

triceps brachii
(medial head)

tendon of biceps brachii

medial epicondyle
of humerus

pronator teres

bicipital aponeurosis

brachioradialis

antebrachial fascia

extensor carpi radialis longus

flexor carpi ulnaris

extensor carpi radialis brevis

palmaris longus

abductor pollicis longus

flexor carpi radialis

flexor pollicis longus

flexor superficialis digitorum manus

tendon of brachioradialis

tendon of flexor digitorum
superficialis of hand

pronator quadratus

flexor carpi ulnaris

tendon of abductor
pollicis longus

tendon of flexor carpi ulnaris

tendon of palmaris longus

flexor retinaculum of wrist

tendon of flexor carpi radialis

A

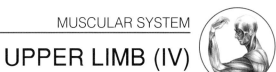

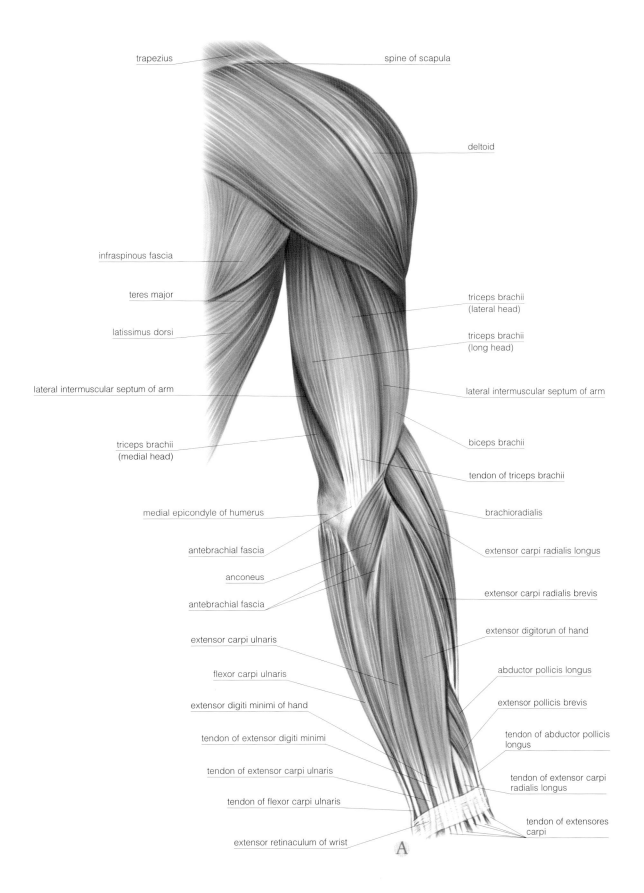

trapezius

spine of scapula

deltoid

infraspinous fascia

teres major

triceps brachii (lateral head)

latissimus dorsi

triceps brachii (long head)

lateral intermuscular septum of arm

lateral intermuscular septum of arm

triceps brachii (medial head)

biceps brachii

tendon of triceps brachii

medial epicondyle of humerus

brachioradialis

antebrachial fascia

extensor carpi radialis longus

anconeus

extensor carpi radialis brevis

antebrachial fascia

extensor digitorun of hand

extensor carpi ulnaris

abductor pollicis longus

flexor carpi ulnaris

extensor pollicis brevis

extensor digiti minimi of hand

tendon of abductor pollicis longus

tendon of extensor digiti minimi

tendon of extensor carpi ulnaris

tendon of extensor carpi radialis longus

tendon of flexor carpi ulnaris

tendon of extensores carpi

extensor retinaculum of wrist

A

UPPER LIMB (V)

RIGHT UPPER LIMB. ANTERIOR DEEP VIEW

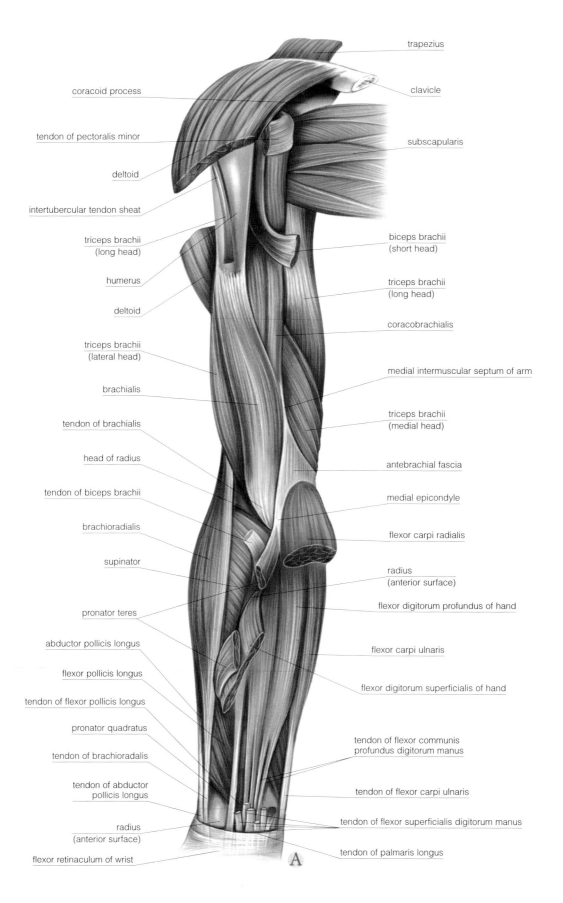

trapezius

coracoid process

clavicle

tendon of pectoralis minor

subscapularis

deltoid

intertubercular tendon sheat

triceps brachii
(long head)

biceps brachii
(short head)

humerus

triceps brachii
(long head)

deltoid

coracobrachialis

triceps brachii
(lateral head)

medial intermuscular septum of arm

brachialis

triceps brachii
(medial head)

tendon of brachialis

head of radius

antebrachial fascia

tendon of biceps brachii

medial epicondyle

brachioradialis

flexor carpi radialis

supinator

radius
(anterior surface)

pronator teres

flexor digitorum profundus of hand

abductor pollicis longus

flexor carpi ulnaris

flexor pollicis longus

tendon of flexor pollicis longus

flexor digitorum superficialis of hand

pronator quadratus

tendon of brachioradalis

tendon of flexor communis
profundus digitorum manus

tendon of abductor
pollicis longus

tendon of flexor carpi ulnaris

radius
(anterior surface)

tendon of flexor superficialis digitorum manus

flexor retinaculum of wrist

tendon of palmaris longus

A

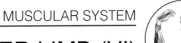

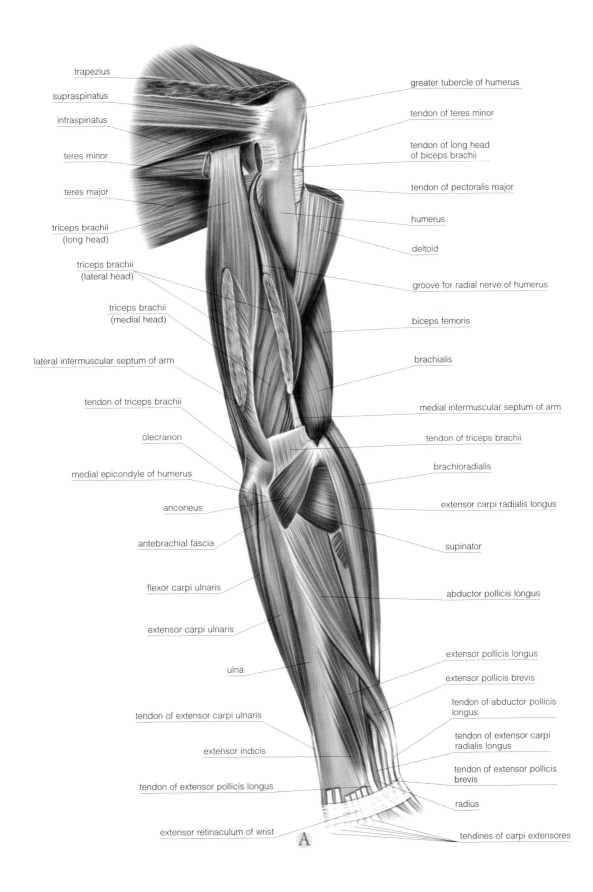

trapezius

supraspinatus

infraspinatus

teres minor

teres major

triceps brachii
(long head)

triceps brachii
(lateral head)

triceps brachii
(medial head)

lateral intermuscular septum of arm

tendon of triceps brachii

olecranon

medial epicondyle of humerus

anconeus

antebrachial fascia

flexor carpi ulnaris

extensor carpi ulnaris

ulna

tendon of extensor carpi ulnaris

extensor indicis

tendon of extensor pollicis longus

extensor retinaculum of wrist

greater tubercle of humerus

tendon of teres minor

tendon of long head
of biceps brachii

tendon of pectoralis major

humerus

deltoid

groove for radial nerve of humerus

biceps femoris

brachialis

medial intermuscular septum of arm

tendon of triceps brachii

brachioradialis

extensor carpi radialis longus

supinator

abductor pollicis longus

extensor pollicis longus

extensor pollicis brevis

tendon of abductor pollicis
longus

tendon of extensor carpi
radialis longus

tendon of extensor pollicis
brevis

radius

tendines of carpi extensores

A

97

UPPER LIMB (VII). SHOULDER (I)
RIGHT UPPER LIMB

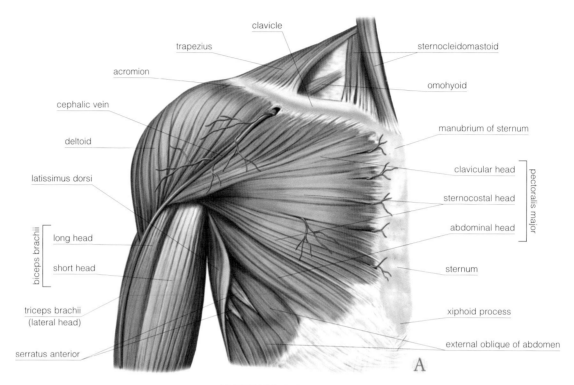

clavicle

trapezius

acromion

cephalic vein

deltoid

latissimus dorsi

biceps brachii
long head
short head

triceps brachii
(lateral head)

serratus anterior

sternocleidomastoid

omohyoid

manubrium of sternum

pectoralis major
clavicular head
sternocostal head
abdominal head

sternum

xiphoid process

external oblique of abdomen

ANTERIOR VIEW

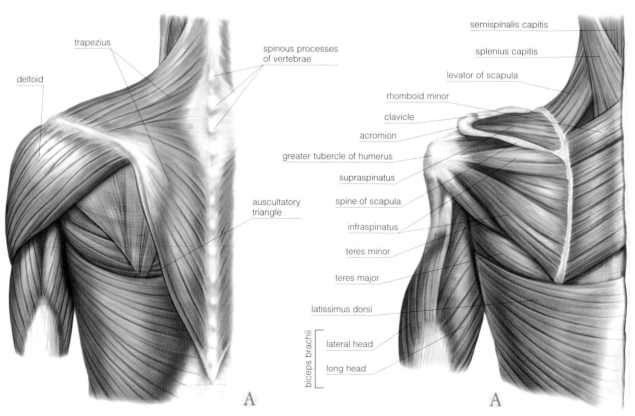

trapezius

deltoid

spinous processes
of vertebrae

auscultatory
triangle

POSTERIOR SUPERFICIAL VIEW

semispinalis capitis

splenius capitis

levator of scapula

rhomboid minor

clavicle

acromion

greater tubercle of humerus

supraspinatus

spine of scapula

infraspinatus

teres minor

teres major

latissimus dorsi

biceps brachii
lateral head
long head

SUPERIOR DEEP VIEW

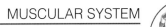

UPPER LIMB (VIII). SHOULDER (II)

RIGHT UPPER LIMB. ANTERIOR VIEW

muscles of the shoulder joint

The spheroidal articulation of the shoulder is the most flexible of the human body. There are nine muscles that cross this articulation and fall within the humerus (pectoralis major, latissimus dorsi, deltoid, subscapularis, supraspinatus, infraspinatus, teres major, teres minor, coracobrachial). All of them originated from the shoulder girdle, except the latissimus dorsi and the pectoralis major which originated from the axial skeleton.

Among all these nines muscles only the superficial ones (pectoralis major, pectoralis minor and deltoid) are agonists of the movements of the arm. A group of four of these muscles (supraspinnatus, infraspinatus, teres minor and subscapularis) is known as muscles of the rotator cuff. They are born in the scapula and its tendons go to the humerus and disappear into the fibrous capsule of the articulation of the shoulder.

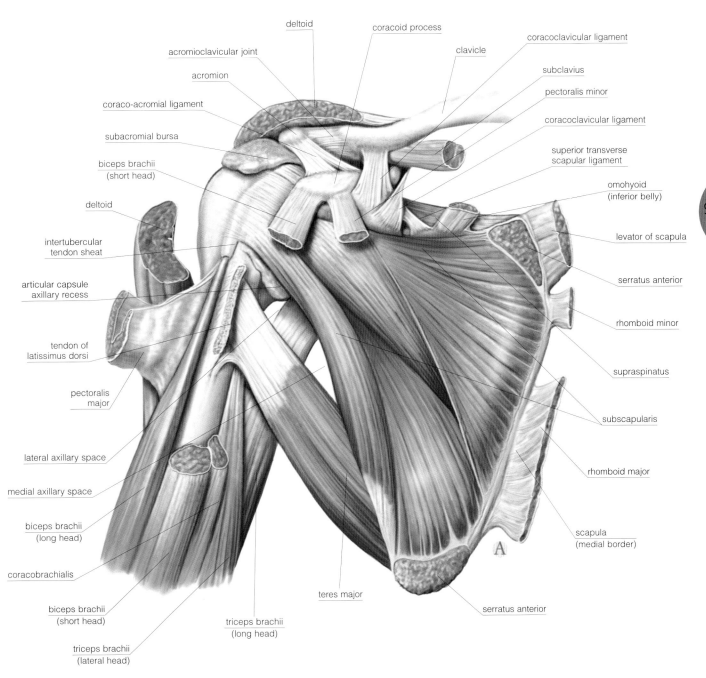

deltoid

coracoid process

clavicle

coracoclavicular ligament

acromioclavicular joint

acromion

subclavius

pectoralis minor

coraco-acromial ligament

coracoclavicular ligament

subacromial bursa

superior transverse
scapular ligament

biceps brachii
(short head)

omohyoid
(inferior belly)

deltoid

levator of scapula

intertubercular
tendon sheat

serratus anterior

articular capsule
axillary recess

rhomboid minor

tendon of
latissimus dorsi

supraspinatus

pectoralis
major

subscapularis

lateral axillary space

rhomboid major

medial axillary space

biceps brachii
(long head)

scapula
(medial border)

coracobrachialis

A

biceps brachii
(short head)

triceps brachii
(long head)

teres major

serratus anterior

triceps brachii
(lateral head)

UPPER LIMB (IX). SHOULDER (III)

RIGHT UPPER LIMB. POSTERIOR VIEW

deltoid

It is a powerful and thick muscle with a rough texture. It covers the shoulder and shapes the round form it has. As its name suggests, it is shaped like a Greek capital delta, Δ. It is divided into different parts: front and back (unipennate fibers) and middle (multipennate). When all the three portions contract at the same time it happens the abduction process of the arm. It is the agonist of the pectoralis major and latissimus dorsi muscles that participate in the abduction of the arm. If only the front fibers contract, it can work out the strong flexion and the median rotation of the humerus, becoming therefore the synergistic combination of the pectoralis major muscle. If only the back fibers contract, it extends and laterally rotates the arm. It also participates while walking in the swinging of the arms to help in this process.

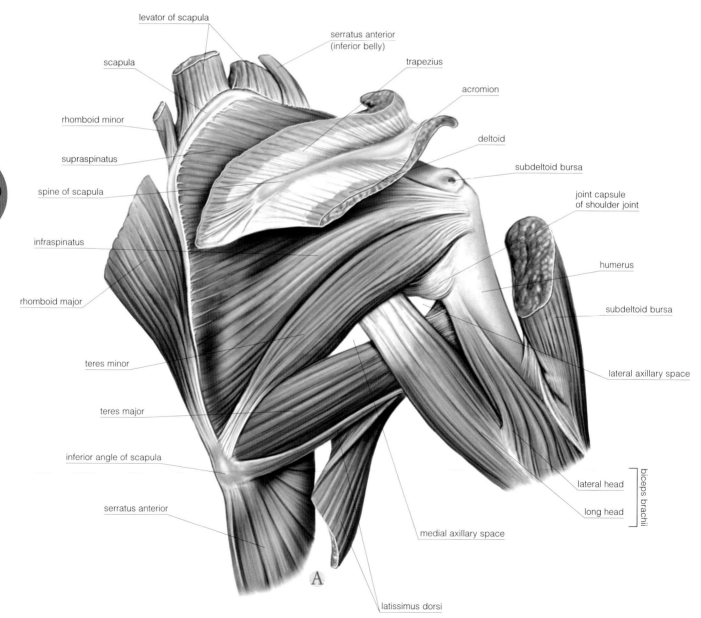

levator of scapula

serratus anterior
(inferior belly)

scapula

trapezius

acromion

rhomboid minor

deltoid

supraspinatus

subdeltoid bursa

spine of scapula

joint capsule
of shoulder joint

infraspinatus

humerus

rhomboid major

subdeltoid bursa

teres minor

lateral axillary space

teres major

inferior angle of scapula

lateral head

long head

biceps brachii

serratus anterior

medial axillary space

A

latissimus dorsi

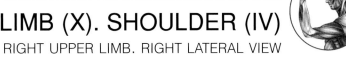

UPPER LIMB (X). SHOULDER (IV)

RIGHT UPPER LIMB. RIGHT LATERAL VIEW

muscular sheath of rotators

Although the rotator cuff works in a synergistic combination during the angular and circular movements of the arm, its main function is to keep the head of the humerus inside the glenoid socket of the scapula and to reinforce the joint capsule. Teres major and coracobrachial muscles are small and cross the shoulder joint, though they do not belong to the anatomy of the shoulder.

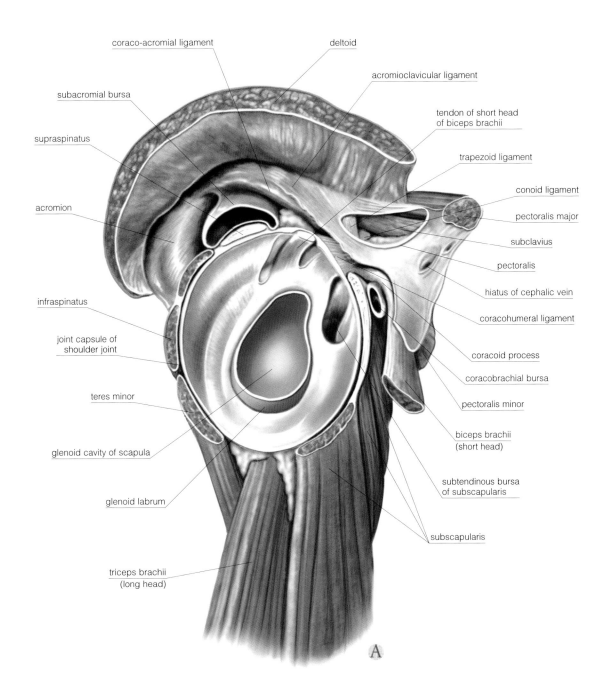

coraco-acromial ligament

deltoid

acromioclavicular ligament

subacromial bursa

tendon of short head of biceps brachii

supraspinatus

trapezoid ligament

conoid ligament

acromion

pectoralis major

subclavius

pectoralis

hiatus of cephalic vein

infraspinatus

coracohumeral ligament

joint capsule of shoulder joint

coracoid process

coracobrachial bursa

teres minor

pectoralis minor

biceps brachii (short head)

glenoid cavity of scapula

subtendinous bursa of subscapularis

glenoid labrum

subscapularis

triceps brachii (long head)

A

UPPER LIMB (XI). SHOULDER (V)

RIGHT UPPER LIMB. ANTERIOR VIEWS

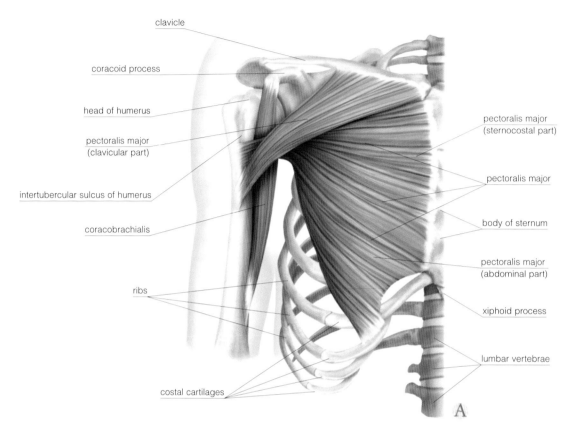

clavicle

coracoid process

head of humerus

pectoralis major
(clavicular part)

intertubercular sulcus of humerus

coracobrachialis

ribs

costal cartilages

pectoralis major
(sternocostal part)

pectoralis major

body of sternum

pectoralis major
(abdominal part)

xiphoid process

lumbar vertebrae

A

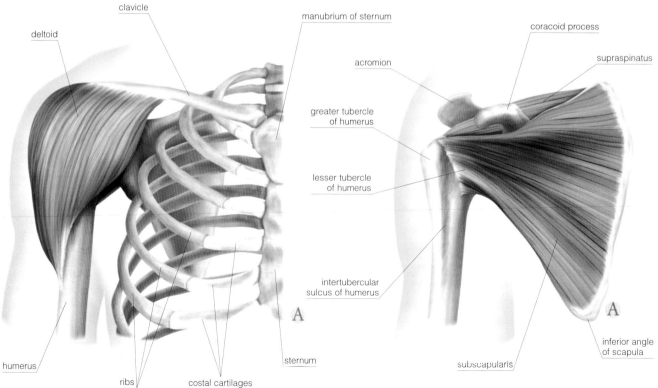

deltoid

clavicle

manubrium of sternum

coracoid process

acromion

supraspinatus

greater tubercle
of humerus

lesser tubercle
of humerus

intertubercular
sulcus of humerus

humerus

ribs

costal cartilages

sternum

subscapularis

inferior angle
of scapula

A

A

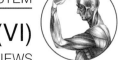

UPPER LIMB (XII). SHOULDER (VI)

RIGHT UPPER LIMB. POSTERIOR VIEWS

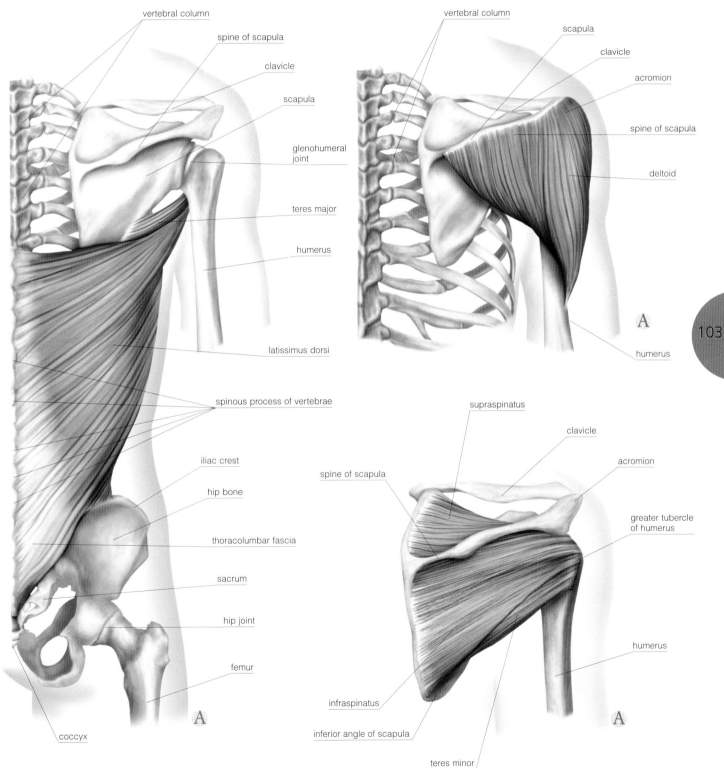

vertebral column

spine of scapula

clavicle

scapula

glenohumeral joint

teres major

humerus

latissimus dorsi

spinous process of vertebrae

iliac crest

hip bone

thoracolumbar fascia

sacrum

hip joint

femur

coccyx

A

vertebral column

scapula

clavicle

acromion

spine of scapula

deltoid

humerus

A

supraspinatus

clavicle

spine of scapula

acromion

greater tubercle of humerus

humerus

infraspinatus

inferior angle of scapula

teres minor

A

UPPER LIMB (XIII). ARM (I)

RIGHT UPPER LIMB. ANTERIOR VIEW

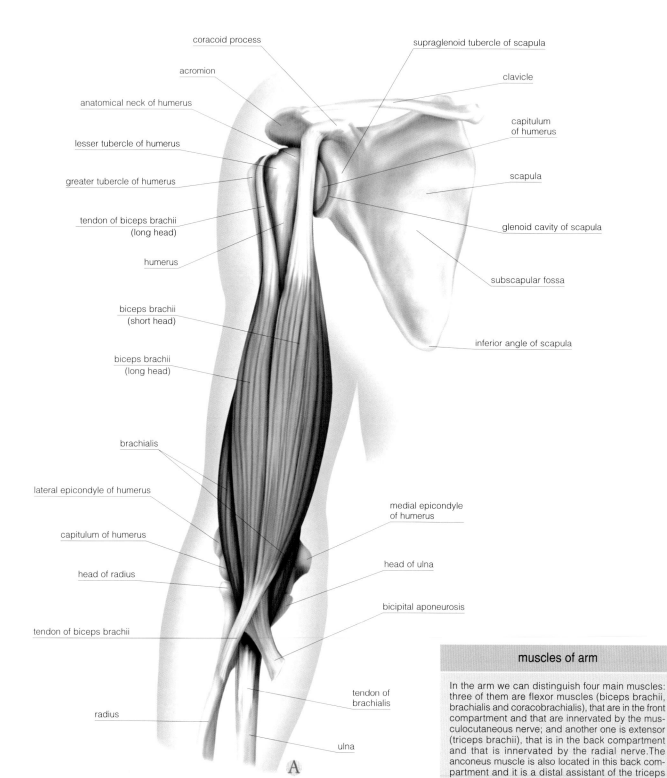

coracoid process

supraglenoid tubercle of scapula

acromion

clavicle

anatomical neck of humerus

capitulum
of humerus

lesser tubercle of humerus

greater tubercle of humerus

scapula

tendon of biceps brachii
(long head)

glenoid cavity of scapula

humerus

subscapular fossa

biceps brachii
(short head)

biceps brachii
(long head)

inferior angle of scapula

brachialis

lateral epicondyle of humerus

medial epicondyle
of humerus

capitulum of humerus

head of ulna

head of radius

bicipital aponeurosis

tendon of biceps brachii

tendon of
brachialis

radius

ulna

A

muscles of arm

In the arm we can distinguish four main muscles: three of them are flexor muscles (biceps brachii, brachialis and coracobrachialis), that are in the front compartment and that are innervated by the musculocutaneous nerve; and another one is extensor (triceps brachii), that is in the back compartment and that is innervated by the radial nerve.The anconeus muscle is also located in this back compartment and it is a distal assistant of the triceps brachii. The flexor muscles of the front compartment exert almost the double ot the force than the extensor one, in any position, so they are stronger when pulling than when pushing.

UPPER LIMB (XIV). ARM (II)

RIGHT UPPER LIMB. ANTERIOR VIEW

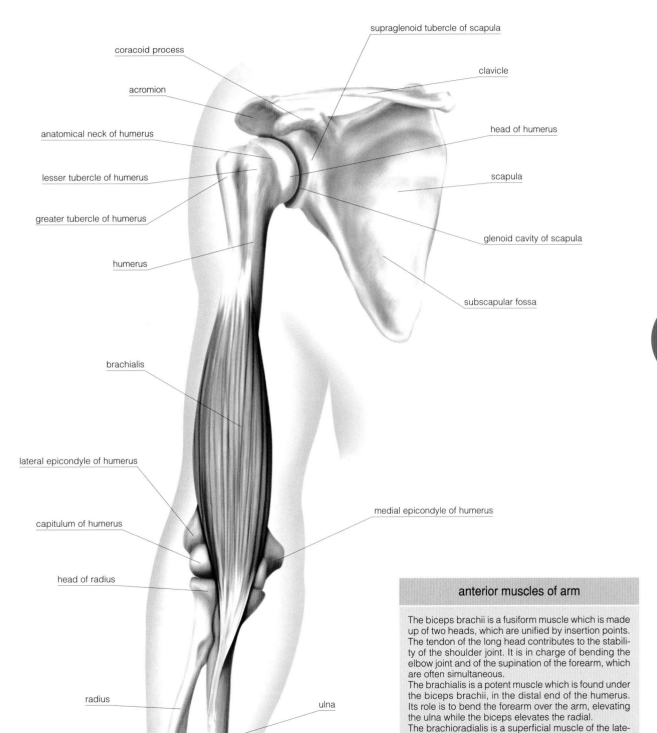

supraglenoid tubercle of scapula

coracoid process

clavicle

acromion

anatomical neck of humerus

head of humerus

lesser tubercle of humerus

greater tubercle of humerus

scapula

humerus

glenoid cavity of scapula

subscapular fossa

brachialis

lateral epicondyle of humerus

medial epicondyle of humerus

capitulum of humerus

head of radius

radius

ulna

anterior muscles of arm

The biceps brachii is a fusiform muscle which is made up of two heads, which are unified by insertion points. The tendon of the long head contributes to the stability of the shoulder joint. It is in charge of bending the elbow joint and of the supination of the forearm, which are often simultaneous.

The brachialis is a potent muscle which is found under the biceps brachii, in the distal end of the humerus. Its role is to bend the forearm over the arm, elevating the ulna while the biceps elevates the radial.

The brachioradialis is a superficial muscle of the lateral side of the forearm. It forms the lateral edge of the forearm fold. It goes from the distal end of the humerus to the distal part of the radial. It is a synergic muscle in forearm bending. The brachioradial mainly acts when the forearm is already partially folded.

UPPER LIMB (XV). ARM (III)

RIGHT UPPER LIMB. POSTERIOR VIEW

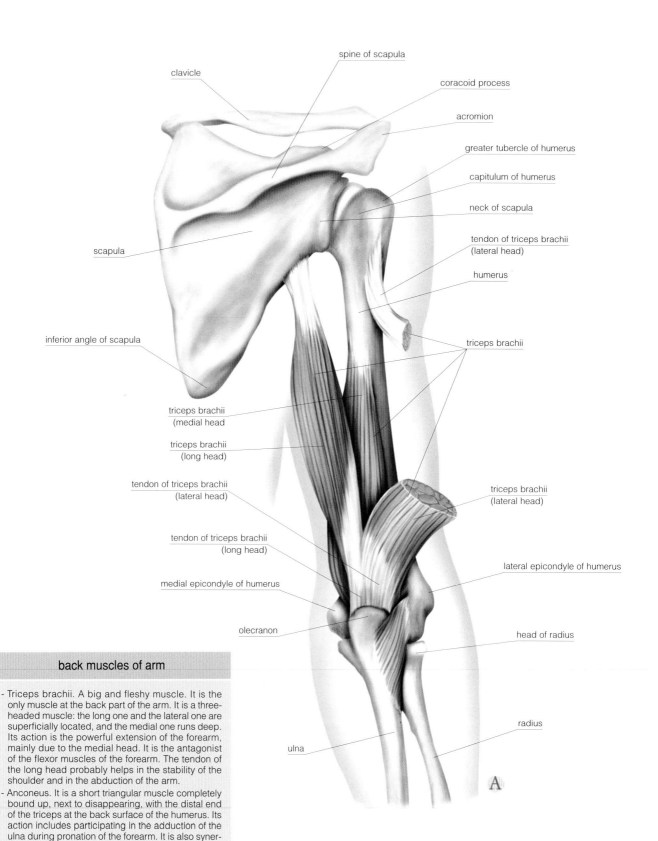

spine of scapula

clavicle

coracoid process

acromion

greater tubercle of humerus

capitulum of humerus

neck of scapula

tendon of triceps brachii
(lateral head)

humerus

scapula

triceps brachii

inferior angle of scapula

triceps brachii
(medial head)

triceps brachii
(long head)

tendon of triceps brachii
(lateral head)

triceps brachii
(lateral head)

tendon of triceps brachii
(long head)

lateral epicondyle of humerus

medial epicondyle of humerus

olecranon

head of radius

radius

ulna

A

back muscles of arm

- Triceps brachii. A big and fleshy muscle. It is the only muscle at the back part of the arm. It is a three-headed muscle: the long one and the lateral one are superficially located, and the medial one runs deep. Its action is the powerful extension of the forearm, mainly due to the medial head. It is the antagonist of the flexor muscles of the forearm. The tendon of the long head probably helps in the stability of the shoulder and in the abduction of the arm.
- Anconeus. It is a short triangular muscle completely bound up, next to disappearing, with the distal end of the triceps at the back surface of the humerus. Its action includes participating in the adduction of the ulna during pronation of the forearm. It is also synergistic of the triceps brachii during elbow extension.

UPPER LIMB (XVI). ARM (IV)

RIGHT UPPER LIMB. CROSS-SECTION. CRANIAL VIEW

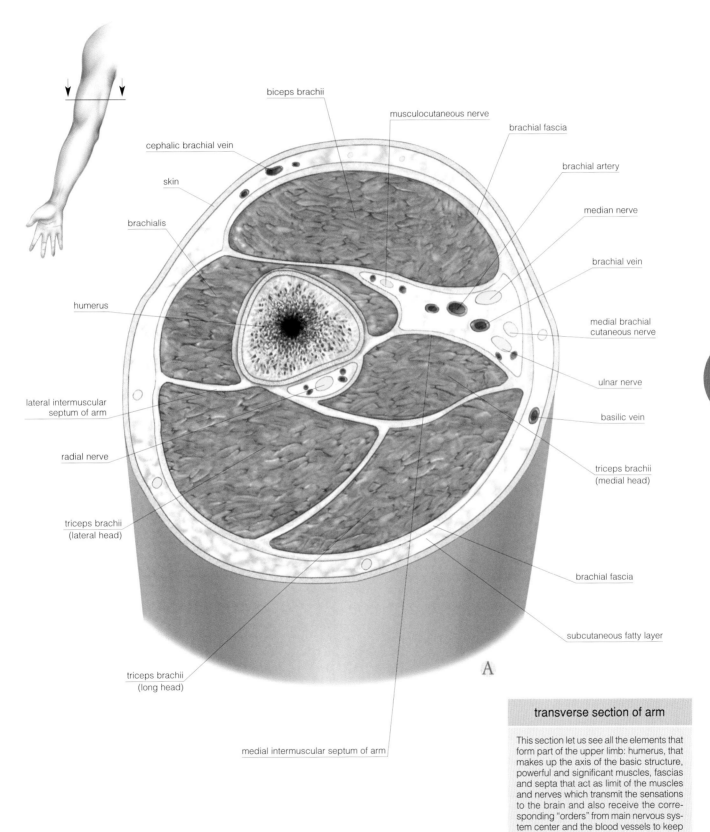

biceps brachii

musculocutaneous nerve

brachial fascia

cephalic brachial vein

brachial artery

skin

median nerve

brachialis

brachial vein

humerus

medial brachial
cutaneous nerve

ulnar nerve

lateral intermuscular
septum of arm

basilic vein

radial nerve

triceps brachii
(medial head)

triceps brachii
(lateral head)

brachial fascia

subcutaneous fatty layer

A

triceps brachii
(long head)

medial intermuscular septum of arm

107

transverse section of arm

This section let us see all the elements that form part of the upper limb: humerus, that makes up the axis of the basic structure, powerful and significant muscles, fascias and septa that act as limit of the muscles and nerves which transmit the sensations to the brain and also receive the corresponding "orders" from main nervous system center and the blood vessels to keep the limb alive and healthy.

UPPER LIMB (XVII). FOREARM (I)

RIGHT UPPER LIMB. ANTERIOR SUPERFICIAL VIEW

muscles of forearm

Having in mind its function, the muscles of the forearm may be divided into two very similar groups: the ones helping in the movement of the wrist and the ones making possible the movement of the fingers of the hand. Almost in all of them the fleshy parts make up the protuberance of the proximal part of the forearm, so they run thinner and thinner as they get near the hand to become the long tendines of the insertion. The point of insertion are firmly tied by strong ligaments (extensor retinaculum and flexor retinaculum), and they are covered by the synovial bursa of lubricated tendines that ease movements and avoid friction.

In fact, since many of the muscles of the forearm have their origin in the humerus and for that reason they cross the articulation of the elbow and the wrist, they have minimum action over the elbow. Flexion and extension processes are the most characteristic movements worked out by the articulations of the wrist and the fingers. This way wrist is able to make abduction and adduction movements.

108

humerus

lateral epicondyle of humerus

medial epicondyle of humerus

capitulum of humerus

pronator teres

palmaris longus

radius

flexor carpi radialis

flexor carpi ulnaris

flexor digitorum superficialis of hand

tendon of flexor superficialis digitorum manus

tendon of flexor carpi ulnaris

tendon of flexor carpi radialis

A

UPPER LIMB (XVIII). FOREARM (II)

RIGHT UPPER LIMB. ANTERIOR VIEW

anterior muscles of forearm

The muscles of the forearm may be divided into two main groups: front and back muscles, having in mind they are separated by aponeurotic compartments. For its part, each one of these groups may be divided into two: superficials and deep muscles. The difference of each one of the groups depends on the situation but also on the function.

The front muscles start at the humerus in a common tendon and most of them are innervated by the median nerve. The majority of these muscles are flexors of the wrist and fingers. Two muscles of this group are the pronator teres, which is superficial, and the pronator quadratus, which is deep, and they have as a function to pronating the forearm, one of the most important movements of this limb.

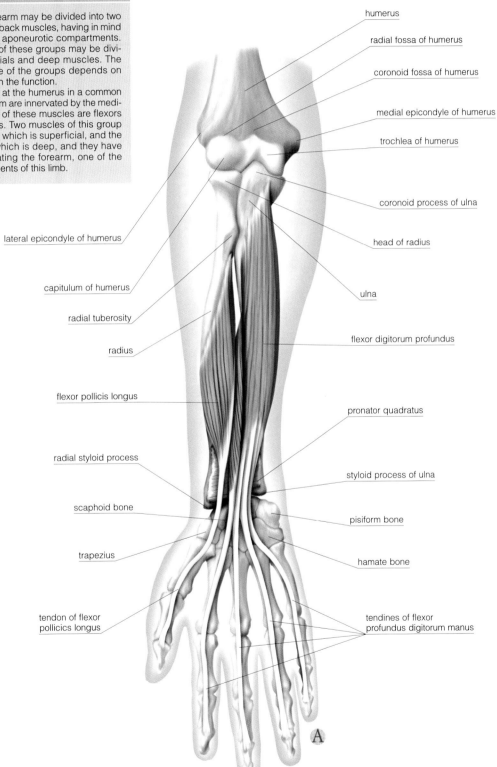

humerus

radial fossa of humerus

coronoid fossa of humerus

medial epicondyle of humerus

trochlea of humerus

coronoid process of ulna

head of radius

lateral epicondyle of humerus

capitulum of humerus

radial tuberosity

ulna

radius

flexor digitorum profundus

flexor pollicis longus

pronator quadratus

radial styloid process

styloid process of ulna

scaphoid bone

pisiform bone

trapezius

hamate bone

tendon of flexor pollicics longus

tendines of flexor profundus digitorum manus

A

109

UPPER LIMB (XIX). FOREARM (III)

RIGHT UPPER LIMB. LATERAL SUPERFICIAL VIEW

superficial muscles of forearm

- Extensor carpi radialis longus. It is located in the lateral part of the forearm and goes parallel to the brachioradialis, that may cover it. Its function is the extension and abduction of the thumb.
- Extensor carpi radialis brevis. Is a little bit shorter than the extensor carpi radialis longus, that covers it. Its function is the extension and abduction of the thumb. It works in a synergistic process with the extensor carpi radialis longus to stabilize the thumb when fingers are bent.
- Extensor digitorum. It is located in a median position in regards to the extensor carpi radialis brevis. A differentiated portion of this muscle, the extensor digiti minimi, helps when the 5th digit is extended. It is an agonist of the extension of the fingers of the hand and also of the thumb. It can also produce the abduction of all the fingers in the hand.
- Extensor carpi ulnaris. It is a long and thin superficial posterior muscle, located in a more medial position. Its function is the extension and abduction of the thumb in cooperation with the flexor carpi ulnaris.

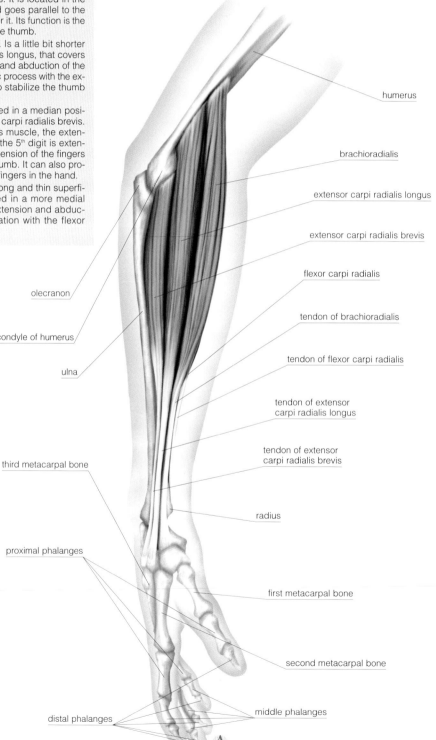

humerus

brachioradialis

extensor carpi radialis longus

extensor carpi radialis brevis

flexor carpi radialis

tendon of brachioradialis

tendon of flexor carpi radialis

tendon of extensor carpi radialis longus

tendon of extensor carpi radialis brevis

radius

first metacarpal bone

second metacarpal bone

middle phalanges

olecranon

lateral epicondyle of humerus

ulna

third metacarpal bone

proximal phalanges

distal phalanges

A

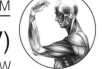

UPPER LIMB (XX). FOREARM (IV)

RIGHT UPPER LIMB. POSTERIOR VIEW

back muscles of forearm

The back muscles of the forearm are the extensors of the wrist and of the fingers of the hand, except for the supinator muscles that help the biceps brachii when the supination of the forearm takes place. Most of these muscles have their origin in the humerus from a common tendon, though their location in regards to the humerus may be different. The back muscles of the forearm are innervated by the radial nerve. While most of the movements of the hand are made by the muscles of the forearm, some little intrinsic muscles of the hand give a higher precision. They are the lumbrical muscles.

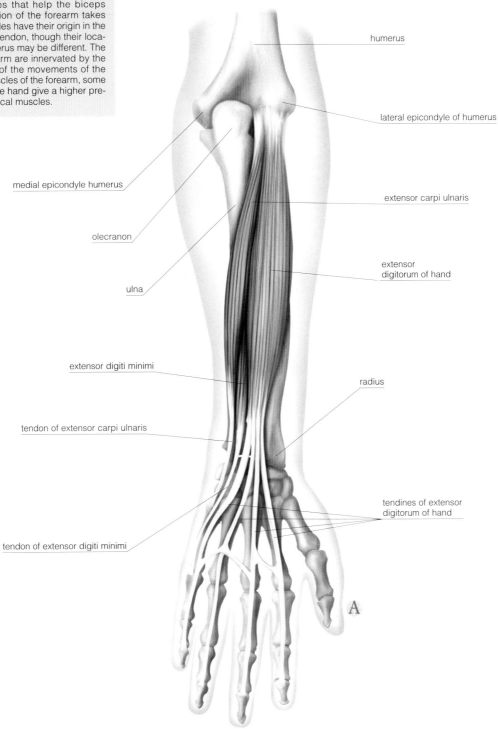

humerus

lateral epicondyle of humerus

medial epicondyle humerus

extensor carpi ulnaris

olecranon

extensor digitorum of hand

ulna

extensor digiti minimi

radius

tendon of extensor carpi ulnaris

tendines of extensor digitorum of hand

tendon of extensor digiti minimi

A

UPPER LIMB (XXI). FOREARM (V)

RIGHT UPPER LIMB. POSTERIOR DEEP VIEW

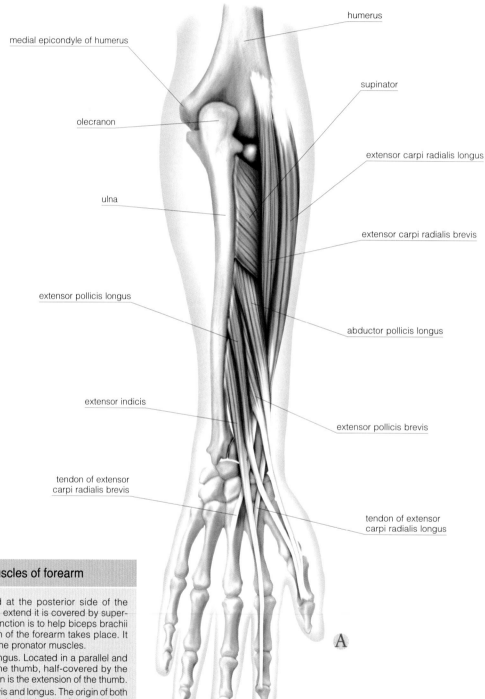

humerus

medial epicondyle of humerus

supinator

olecranon

extensor carpi radialis longus

ulna

extensor carpi radialis brevis

extensor pollicis longus

abductor pollicis longus

extensor indicis

extensor pollicis brevis

tendon of extensor carpi radialis brevis

tendon of extensor carpi radialis longus

A

deep muscles of forearm

- Supinator. Located at the posterior side of the elbow. In most of its extend it is covered by superficial muscles. Its function is to help biceps brachii when the supination of the forearm takes place. It is an antagonist of the pronator muscles.
- Abductor pollicis longus. Located in a parallel and lateral position of the thumb, half-covered by the supinator. Its function is the extension of the thumb.
- Extensor pollicis brevis and longus. The origin of both of them is similar, at the back side of the radius, in the interosseus membrane, and so it is their function, the abduction and extension of the thumb in the metacarpophalangeal joint. They are covered by the extensor carpi ulnanis.
- Extensor indicis. A very small muscle originated near the thumb, in the back part of the ulna. Its function is the extension of the pointer finger and the dorsal contraction of the hand.

UPPER LIMB (XXII). FOREARM (VI)
RIGHT UPPER LIMB. CROSS-SECTION. CAUDAL VIEW

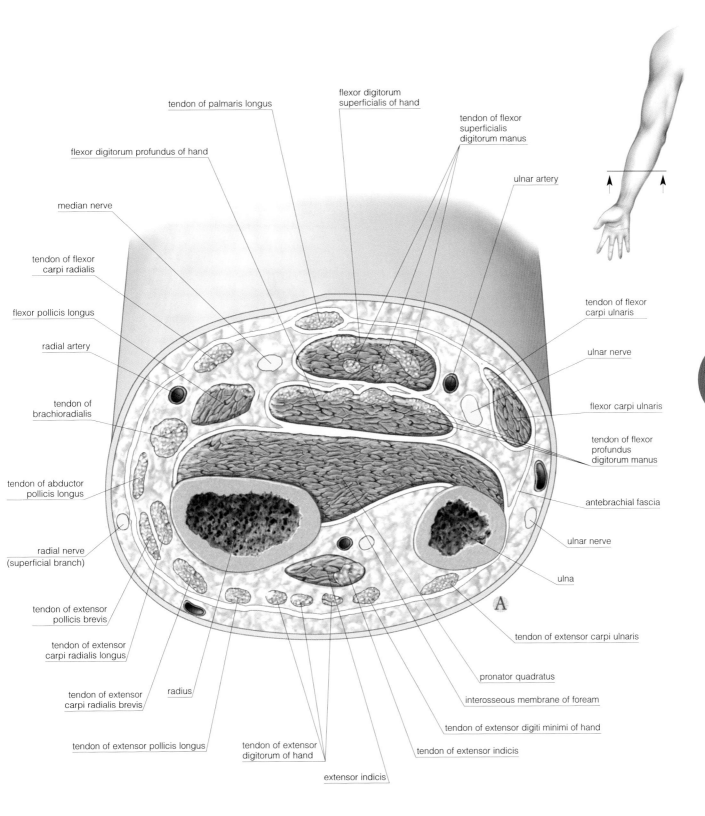

tendon of palmaris longus

flexor digitorum superficialis of hand

tendon of flexor superficialis digitorum manus

flexor digitorum profundus of hand

ulnar artery

median nerve

tendon of flexor carpi radialis

tendon of flexor carpi ulnaris

flexor pollicis longus

ulnar nerve

radial artery

tendon of flexor carpi ulnaris

tendon of brachioradialis

flexor carpi ulnaris

tendon of flexor profundus digitorum manus

tendon of abductor pollicis longus

antebrachial fascia

radial nerve (superficial branch)

ulnar nerve

tendon of extensor pollicis brevis

ulna

tendon of extensor carpi radialis longus

tendon of extensor carpi ulnaris

tendon of extensor carpi radialis brevis

radius

pronator quadratus

interosseous membrane of foream

tendon of extensor pollicis longus

tendon of extensor digitorum of hand

tendon of extensor digiti minimi of hand

tendon of extensor indicis

extensor indicis

113

UPPER LIMB (XXIII). FOREARM and HAND

RIGHT UPPER LIMB. LATERAL SUPERFICIAL VIEW

114

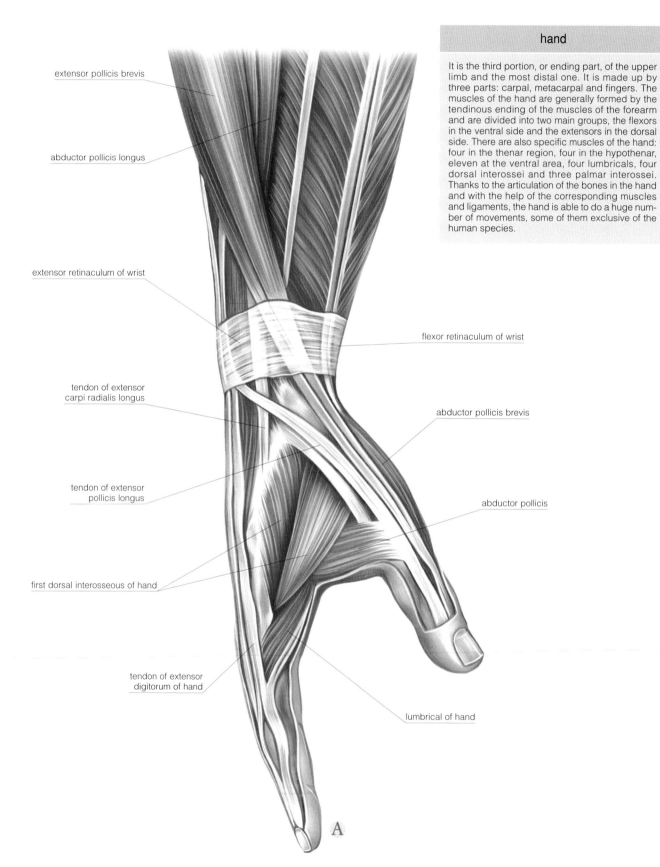

extensor pollicis brevis

abductor pollicis longus

extensor retinaculum of wrist

tendon of extensor
carpi radialis longus

tendon of extensor
pollicis longus

first dorsal interosseous of hand

tendon of extensor
digitorum of hand

flexor retinaculum of wrist

abductor pollicis brevis

abductor pollicis

lumbrical of hand

A

hand

It is the third portion, or ending part, of the upper limb and the most distal one. It is made up by three parts: carpal, metacarpal and fingers. The muscles of the hand are generally formed by the tendinous ending of the muscles of the forearm and are divided into two main groups, the flexors in the ventral side and the extensors in the dorsal side. There are also specific muscles of the hand: four in the thenar region, four in the hypothenar, eleven at the ventral area, four lumbricals, four dorsal interossei and three palmar interossei. Thanks to the articulation of the bones in the hand and with the help of the corresponding muscles and ligaments, the hand is able to do a huge number of movements, some of them exclusive of the human species.

UPPER LIMB (XXIV). HAND (I)
RIGHT UPPER LIMB. PALMAR SUPERFICIAL VIEW

thenar and hypothenar muscles

Thenar muscles form the thenar eminence, that is, the elevation of the palm that appears at the base of the thumb. Their main function is the opposition of this finger. The normal movements of the thumb are very important in regards to the activities develop by the hand. The wide range of movements of the thumb come as a result of the independence of the first metacarpal, provided with mobile articulations at both ends. To develop and control all this freedom of movements many different muscles are required:

- Extension: extensor pollicis longus, extensor pollicis brevis and abductor pollicis brevis.
- Flexion: flexor pollicis longus and flexor pollicis brevis.
- Abduction: abductor pollicis longus and abductor pollicis brevis.
- Adduction: adductor pollicis and first dorsal interossei.
- Opposition: opponens pollicis.

The first four movements take place in the carpometacarpal and metacarpophalangeal joints.

The hypothenar muscles are three and they form the hypothenar eminence, that is, the muscular eminence there is in the palm of the hand all along the ulnar border, and they move the little finger. The abductor minimi digiti is the most superficial of the three of them and its function, besides the abduction of little finger, is the flexion of the proximal phalanx of the same finger.

- Flexor digiti minimi brevis. The size of this muscle may vary. It goes along the same way the abductor minimi digiti. It also flexes the proximal phalanx of the little finger in the metacarpophalangeal joint.
- Opponens digiti minimi. Square muscle located deeper than abductor and flexor muscles. It draws 5th metacarpal anteriorly and rotates it, making deeper the palmar cavity and bringing little finger (5th digit) into opposition with thumb. As well as in the case of the opposition of the thumb (opponens pollicis), the opponens digiti minimi exclusively acts in the carpometacarpal joint.

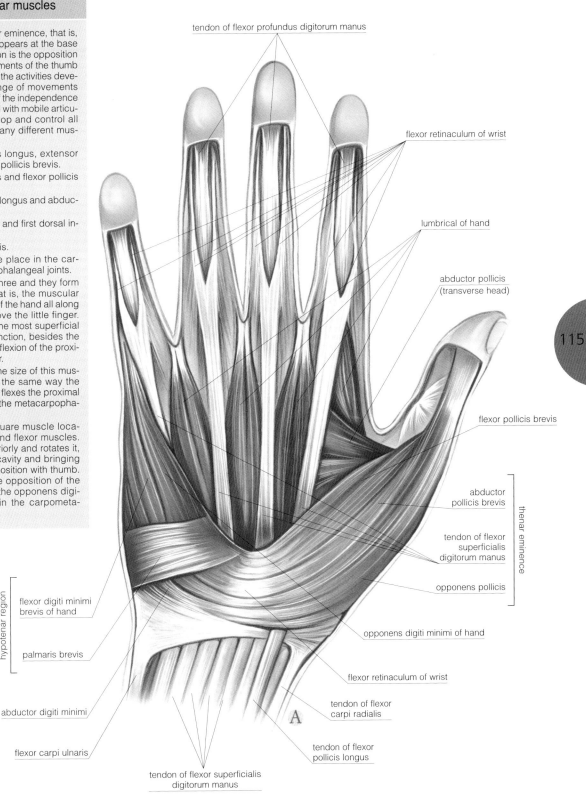

tendon of flexor profundus digitorum manus

flexor retinaculum of wrist

lumbrical of hand

abductor pollicis (transverse head)

flexor pollicis brevis

abductor pollicis brevis

tendon of flexor superficialis digitorum manus

opponens pollicis

thenar eminence

opponens digiti minimi of hand

flexor retinaculum of wrist

tendon of flexor carpi radialis

tendon of flexor pollicis longus

flexor digiti minimi brevis of hand

palmaris brevis

hypotenar region

abductor digiti minimi

flexor carpi ulnaris

tendon of flexor superficialis digitorum manus

A

115

UPPER LIMB (XXV). HAND (II)

RIGHT UPPER LIMB. PALMAR DEEP VIEW

116

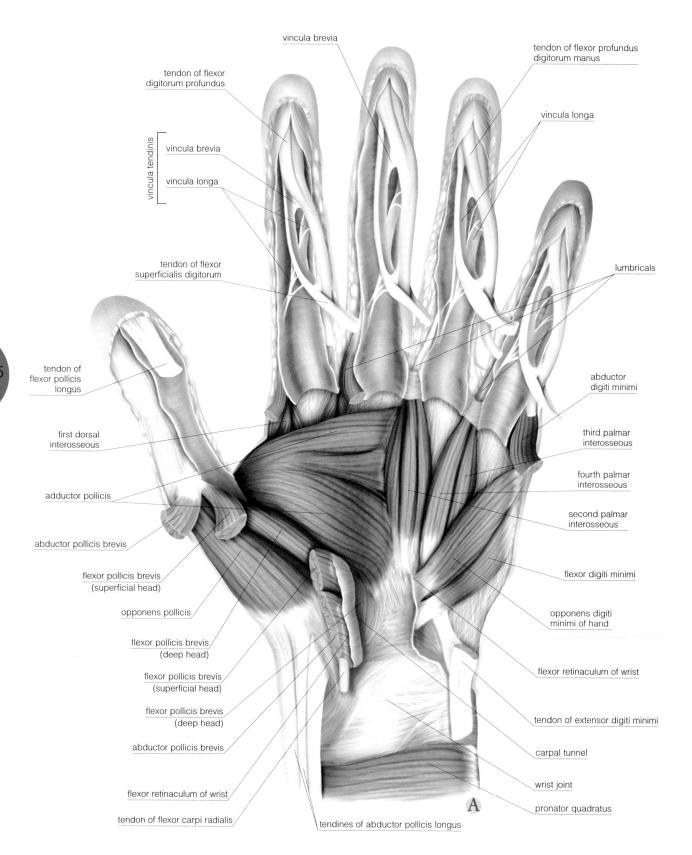

vincula brevia

tendon of flexor profundus
digitorum manus

tendon of flexor
digitorum profundus

vincula longa

vincula tendinis
vincula brevia

vincula longa

lumbricals

tendon of flexor
superficialis digitorum

abductor
digiti minimi

tendon of
flexor pollicis
longus

third palmar
interosseous

first dorsal
interosseous

fourth palmar
interosseous

adductor pollicis

second palmar
interosseous

abductor pollicis brevis

flexor digiti minimi

flexor pollicis brevis
(superficial head)

opponens pollicis

opponens digiti
minimi of hand

flexor pollicis brevis
(deep head)

flexor retinaculum of wrist

flexor pollicis brevis
(superficial head)

tendon of extensor digiti minimi

flexor pollicis brevis
(deep head)

abductor pollicis brevis

carpal tunnel

wrist joint

flexor retinaculum of wrist

A

pronator quadratus

tendon of flexor carpi radialis

tendines of abductor pollicis longus

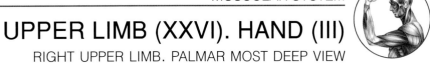

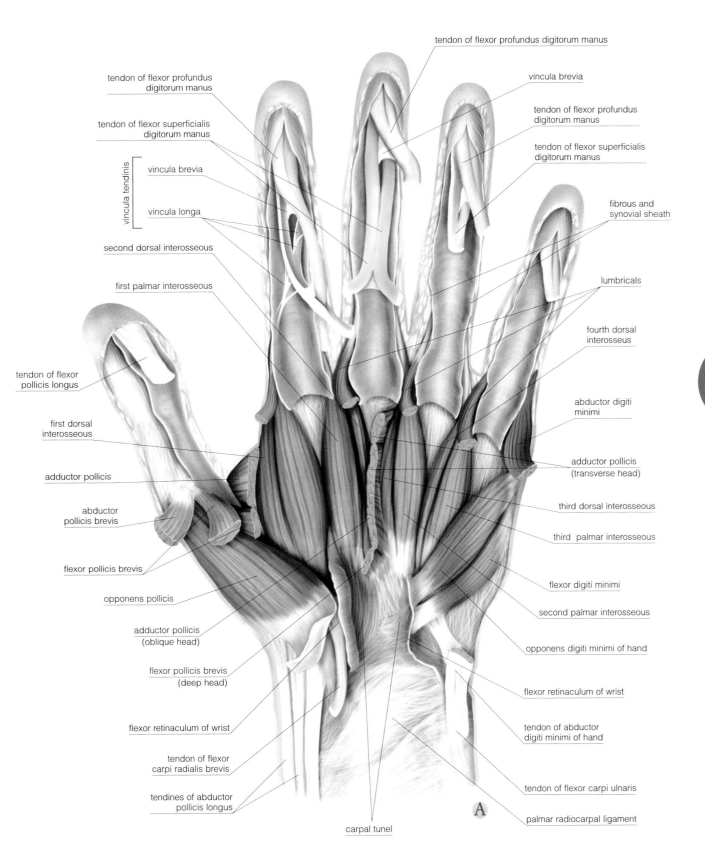

tendon of flexor profundus digitorum manus

vincula brevia

tendon of flexor profundus digitorum manus

tendon of flexor superficialis digitorum manus

fibrous and synovial sheath

tendon of flexor profundus digitorum manus

tendon of flexor superficialis digitorum manus

vincula tendinis

vincula brevia

vincula longa

second dorsal interosseous

first palmar interosseous

lumbricals

fourth dorsal interosseus

tendon of flexor pollicis longus

first dorsal interosseous

abductor digiti minimi

adductor pollicis

abductor pollicis brevis

adductor pollicis (transverse head)

third dorsal interosseous

third palmar interosseous

flexor pollicis brevis

opponens pollicis

flexor digiti minimi

second palmar interosseous

adductor pollicis (oblique head)

opponens digiti minimi of hand

flexor pollicis brevis (deep head)

flexor retinaculum of wrist

flexor retinaculum of wrist

tendon of abductor digiti minimi of hand

tendon of flexor carpi radialis brevis

tendines of abductor pollicis longus

tendon of flexor carpi ulnaris

palmar radiocarpal ligament

carpal tunel

117

UPPER LIMB (XXVII). HAND (IV)

RIGHT UPPER LIMB. DORSAL SUPERFICIAL VIEW

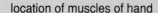

location of muscles of hand

The intrinsic muscles of the hand are located in five compartments:
- Thenar compartment: abductor pollicis brevis, flexor pollicis brevis and opponens pollicis.
- Adductor compartment: adductor pollicis.
- Hypothenar compartment: abductor mini-mi digiti, flexor digiti minimi brevis and opponens digiti minimi.
- Central compartment: short muscles of the hand, lumbricals and long flexor tendons.
- Interossei compartment (between the metacarpal bones): interossei muscles.

118

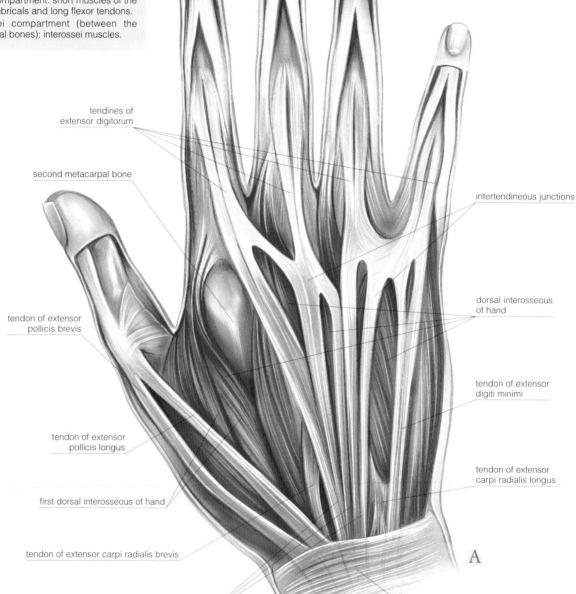

tendines of
extensor digitorum

second metacarpal bone

intertendineous junctions

tendon of extensor
pollicis brevis

dorsal interosseous
of hand

tendon of extensor
digiti minimi

tendon of extensor
pollicis longus

first dorsal interosseous of hand

tendon of extensor
carpi radialis longus

tendon of extensor carpi radialis brevis

tendines of extensor digitorum

extensor retinaculum of wrist

A

UPPER LIMB (XXVIII). HAND (V)
LEFT UPPER LIMB. DORSAL SUPERFICIAL VIEW

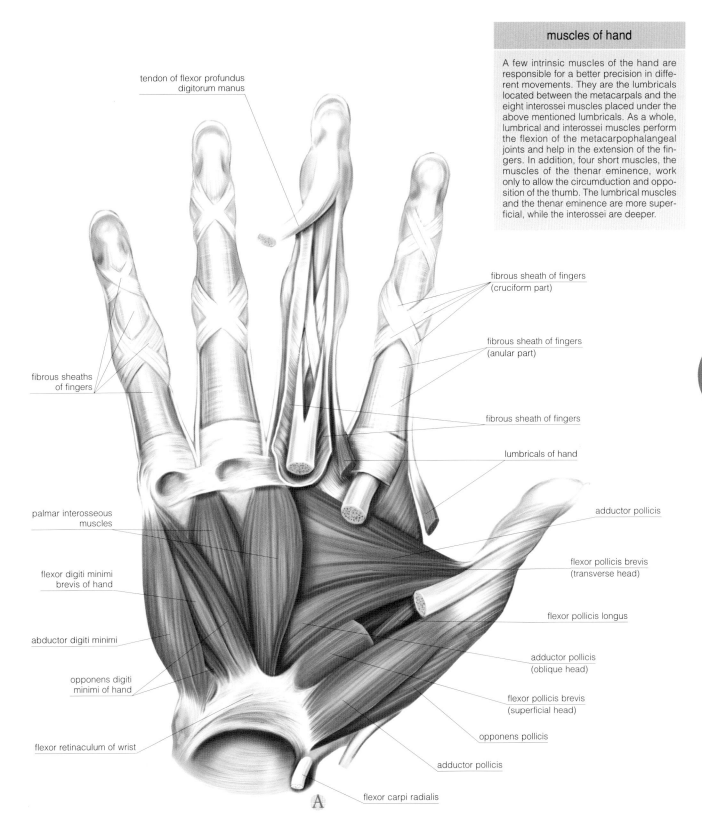

muscles of hand

A few intrinsic muscles of the hand are responsible for a better precision in different movements. They are the lumbricals located between the metacarpals and the eight interossei muscles placed under the above mentioned lumbricals. As a whole, lumbrical and interossei muscles perform the flexion of the metacarpophalangeal joints and help in the extension of the fingers. In addition, four short muscles, the muscles of the thenar eminence, work only to allow the circumduction and opposition of the thumb. The lumbrical muscles and the thenar eminence are more superficial, while the interossei are deeper.

tendon of flexor profundus digitorum manus

fibrous sheath of fingers (cruciform part)

fibrous sheath of fingers (anular part)

fibrous sheaths of fingers

fibrous sheath of fingers

lumbricals of hand

palmar interosseous muscles

adductor pollicis

flexor pollicis brevis (transverse head)

flexor digiti minimi brevis of hand

flexor pollicis longus

abductor digiti minimi

adductor pollicis (oblique head)

opponens digiti minimi of hand

flexor pollicis brevis (superficial head)

flexor retinaculum of wrist

opponens pollicis

adductor pollicis

flexor carpi radialis

A

119

UPPER LIMB (XXIX). HAND (VI)
LEFT UPPER LIMB

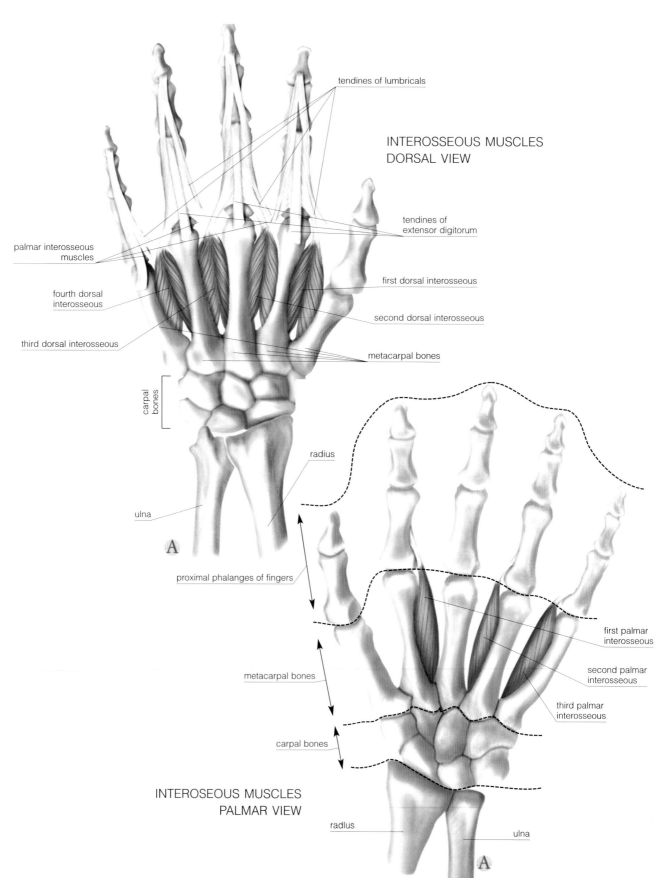

tendines of lumbricals

INTEROSSEOUS MUSCLES
DORSAL VIEW

tendines of
extensor digitorum

palmar interosseous
muscles

first dorsal interosseous

fourth dorsal
interosseous

second dorsal interosseous

third dorsal interosseous

metacarpal bones

carpal bones

radius

ulna

A

proximal phalanges of fingers

first palmar
interosseous

second palmar
interosseous

metacarpal bones

third palmar
interosseous

carpal bones

INTEROSEOUS MUSCLES
PALMAR VIEW

radlus

ulna

A

120

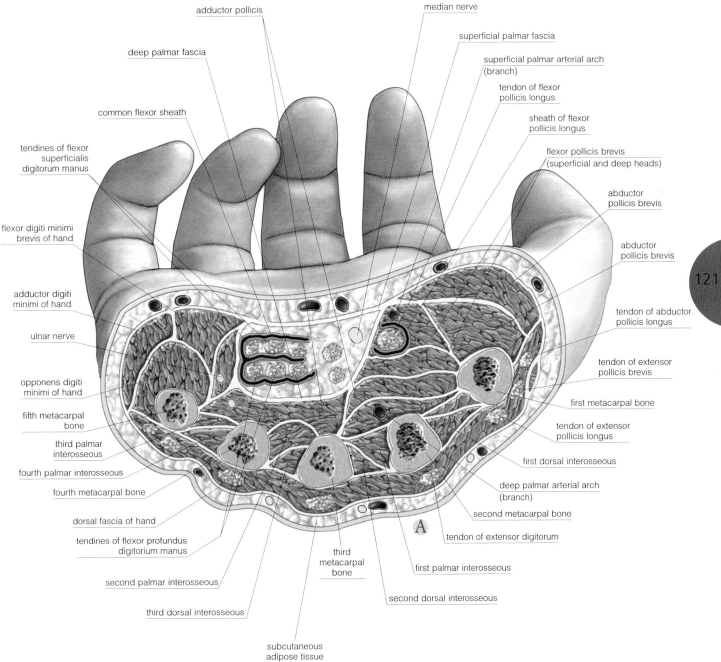

adductor pollicis

median nerve

superficial palmar fascia

deep palmar fascia

superficial palmar arterial arch
(branch)

tendon of flexor
pollicis longus

common flexor sheath

sheath of flexor
pollicis longus

tendines of flexor
superficialis
digitorum manus

flexor pollicis brevis
(superficial and deep heads)

abductor
pollicis brevis

flexor digiti minimi
brevis of hand

abductor
pollicis brevis

adductor digiti
minimi of hand

tendon of abductor
pollicis longus

ulnar nerve

tendon of extensor
pollicis brevis

opponens digiti
minimi of hand

first metacarpal bone

fifth metacarpal
bone

tendon of extensor
pollicis longus

third palmar
interosseous

first dorsal interosseous

fourth palmar interosseous

deep palmar arterial arch
(branch)

fourth metacarpal bone

second metacarpal bone

dorsal fascia of hand

tendon of extensor digitorum

tendines of flexor profundus
digitorium manus

third
metacarpal
bone

first palmar interosseous

second palmar interosseous

second dorsal interosseous

third dorsal interosseous

subcutaneous
adipose tissue

LOWER LIMB (I)

RIGHT LOWER LIMB. ANTERIOR SUPERFICIAL VIEW

lower limbs

They are two appendages starting, one each side, at the inferior and lateral zone of the abdomen. They are made up of four basic parts: thigh, which skeletal component is the femur; knee, which formation includes the osseous structure known as patella; leg, which osseous structure is made up by the tibia and the fibula; and foot, where there are bones forming the tarsus, the metatarsus and phalanges of the fingers. The osseous structure and the muscles that covers this structure, also with the various joints (the one in the hip, patella, tibiofibular articulations, tarsometatarsal joints, transverse of the tarsus, metatarsophalangeal and interphalangeal joints) are able to turn in a wide range of movements. Thanks to all of them is possible to keep the whole structure of the body upright (to keep the bipedal position) and to rove.

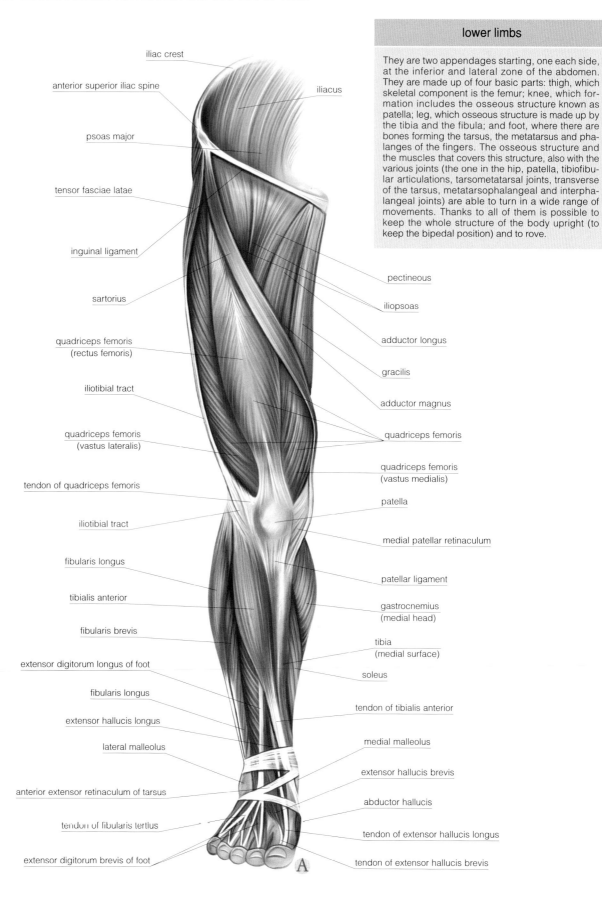

iliac crest

anterior superior iliac spine

iliacus

psoas major

tensor fasciae latae

inguinal ligament

pectineous

iliopsoas

sartorius

adductor longus

quadriceps femoris (rectus femoris)

gracilis

adductor magnus

iliotibial tract

quadriceps femoris

quadriceps femoris (vastus lateralis)

quadriceps femoris (vastus medialis)

tendon of quadriceps femoris

patella

iliotibial tract

medial patellar retinaculum

fibularis longus

patellar ligament

tibialis anterior

gastrocnemius (medial head)

fibularis brevis

tibia (medial surface)

extensor digitorum longus of foot

soleus

fibularis longus

tendon of tibialis anterior

extensor hallucis longus

lateral malleolus

medial malleolus

anterior extensor retinaculum of tarsus

extensor hallucis brevis

abductor hallucis

tendon of fibularis tertius

tendon of extensor hallucis longus

extensor digitorum brevis of foot

tendon of extensor hallucis brevis

A

122

LOWER LIMB (II)
RIGHT LOWER LIMB. ANTERIOR DEEP VIEW

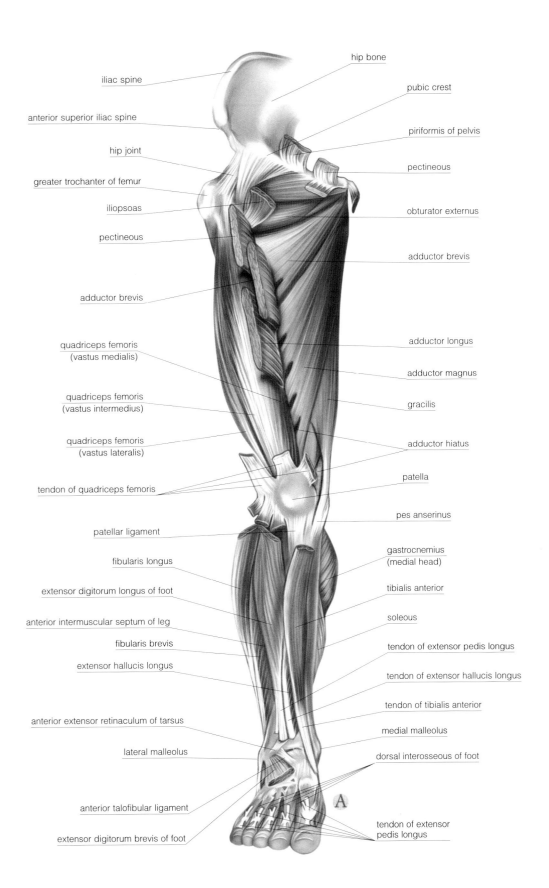

iliac spine

anterior superior iliac spine

hip joint

greater trochanter of femur

iliopsoas

pectineous

adductor brevis

quadriceps femoris
(vastus medialis)

quadriceps femoris
(vastus intermedius)

quadriceps femoris
(vastus lateralis)

tendon of quadriceps femoris

patellar ligament

fibularis longus

extensor digitorum longus of foot

anterior intermuscular septum of leg

fibularis brevis

extensor hallucis longus

anterior extensor retinaculum of tarsus

lateral malleolus

anterior talofibular ligament

extensor digitorum brevis of foot

hip bone

pubic crest

piriformis of pelvis

pectineous

obturator externus

adductor brevis

adductor longus

adductor magnus

gracilis

adductor hiatus

patella

pes anserinus

gastrocnemius
(medial head)

tibialis anterior

soleous

tendon of extensor pedis longus

tendon of extensor hallucis longus

tendon of tibialis anterior

medial malleolus

dorsal interosseous of foot

tendon of extensor
pedis longus

A

123

LOWER LIMB (III)

RIGHT LOWER LIMB. POSTERIOR SUPERFICIAL VIEW

muscles of lower limbs

The muscles of the lower limbs can be divided as hip muscles, thigh muscles, leg muscles and foot muscles. It is a group of muscles that the more proximal they are the bigger and stronger they are, because they act not only to move different articulations but to hold the weight of the lower limbs, whether they are static or in motion.

124

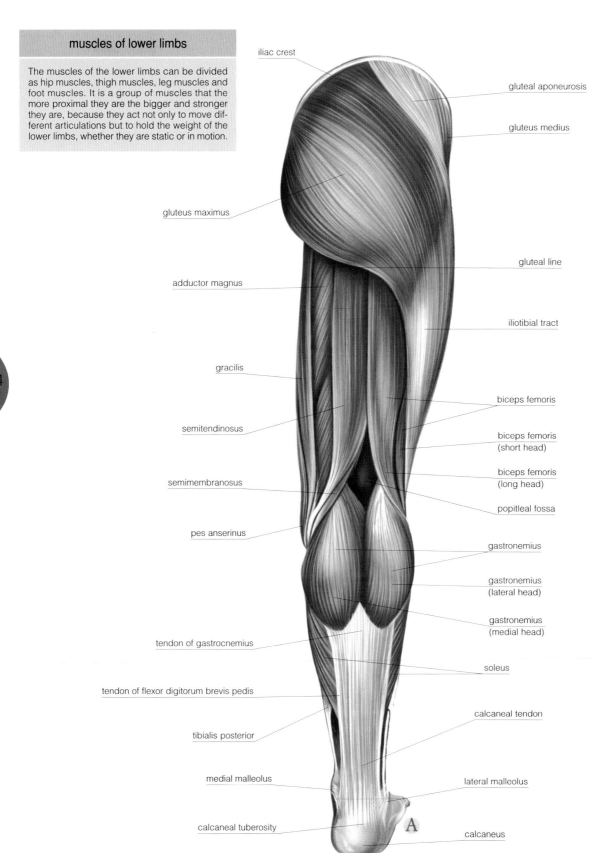

iliac crest

gluteal aponeurosis

gluteus medius

gluteus maximus

gluteal line

adductor magnus

iliotibial tract

gracilis

biceps femoris

biceps femoris
(short head)

semitendinosus

biceps femoris
(long head)

semimembranosus

popitleal fossa

pes anserinus

gastronemius

gastronemius
(lateral head)

gastronemius
(medial head)

tendon of gastrocnemius

soleus

tendon of flexor digitorum brevis pedis

calcaneal tendon

tibialis posterior

medial malleolus

lateral malleolus

calcaneal tuberosity

A

calcaneus

LOWER LIMB (IV)

RIGHT LOWER LIMB. POSTERIOR DEEP VIEW

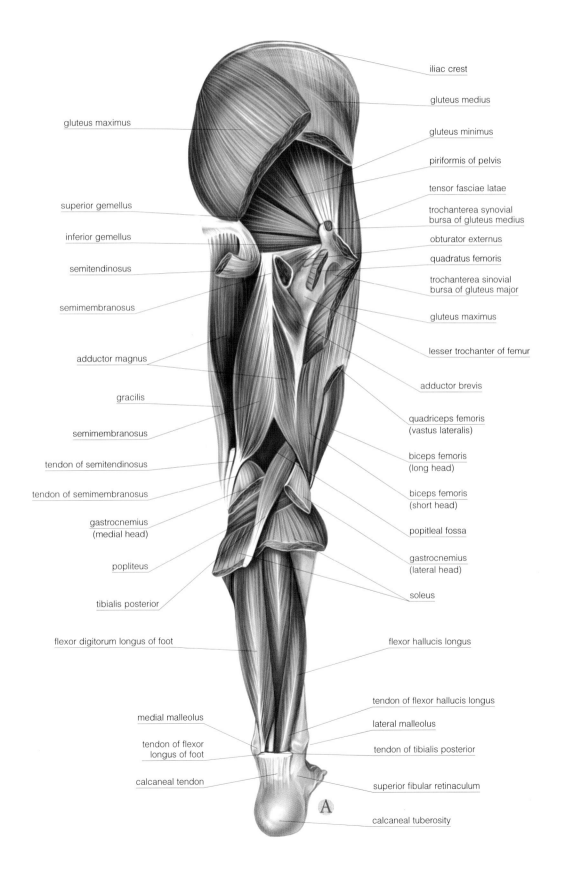

iliac crest

gluteus medius

gluteus maximus

gluteus minimus

piriformis of pelvis

tensor fasciae latae

superior gemellus

trochanterea synovial bursa of gluteus medius

inferior gemellus

obturator externus

semitendinosus

quadratus femoris

trochanterea sinovial bursa of gluteus major

semimembranosus

gluteus maximus

adductor magnus

lesser trochanter of femur

gracilis

adductor brevis

semimembranosus

quadriceps femoris (vastus lateralis)

tendon of semitendinosus

biceps femoris (long head)

tendon of semimembranosus

biceps femoris (short head)

gastrocnemius (medial head)

popitleal fossa

popliteus

gastrocnemius (lateral head)

tibialis posterior

soleus

flexor digitorum longus of foot

flexor hallucis longus

tendon of flexor hallucis longus

medial malleolus

lateral malleolus

tendon of flexor longus of foot

tendon of tibialis posterior

calcaneal tendon

superior fibular retinaculum

A

calcaneal tuberosity

125

LOWER LIMB (V)

RIGHT LOWER LIMB. LATERAL SUPERFICIAL VIEW

126

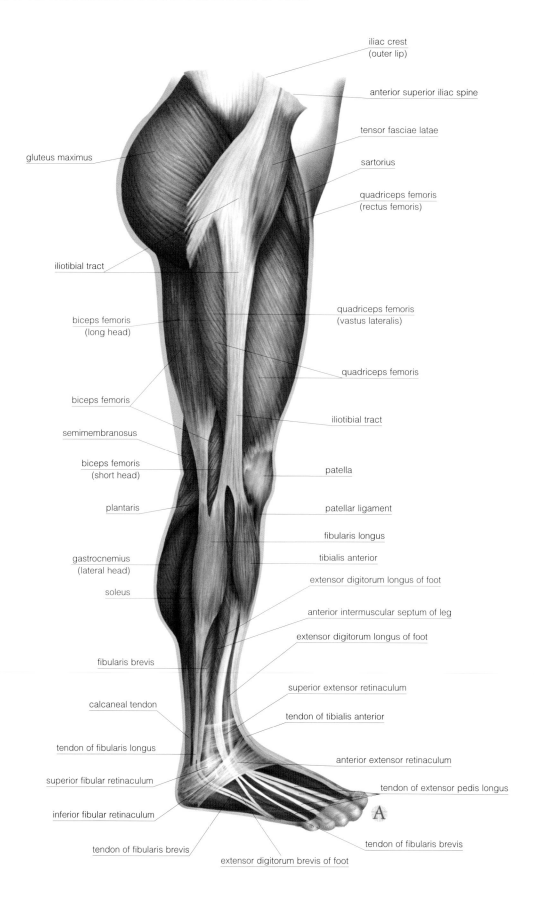

iliac crest
(outer lip)

anterior superior iliac spine

tensor fasciae latae

sartorius

quadriceps femoris
(rectus femoris)

gluteus maximus

iliotibial tract

quadriceps femoris
(vastus lateralis)

biceps femoris
(long head)

quadriceps femoris

biceps femoris

iliotibial tract

semimembranosus

biceps femoris
(short head)

patella

plantaris

patellar ligament

fibularis longus

gastrocnemius
(lateral head)

tibialis anterior

soleus

extensor digitorum longus of foot

anterior intermuscular septum of leg

extensor digitorum longus of foot

fibularis brevis

superior extensor retinaculum

calcaneal tendon

tendon of tibialis anterior

tendon of fibularis longus

anterior extensor retinaculum

superior fibular retinaculum

tendon of extensor pedis longus

inferior fibular retinaculum

A

tendon of fibularis brevis

tendon of fibularis brevis

extensor digitorum brevis of foot

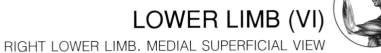

LOWER LIMB (VI)

RIGHT LOWER LIMB. MEDIAL SUPERFICIAL VIEW

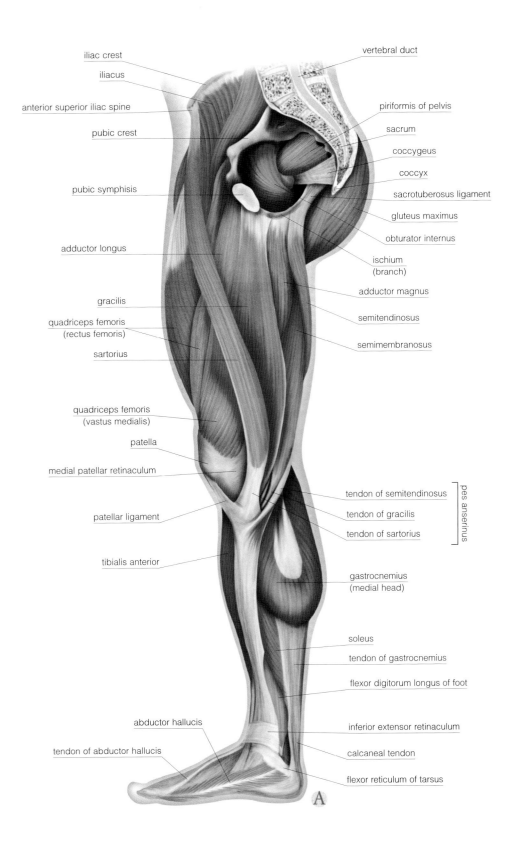

iliac crest

iliacus

anterior superior iliac spine

pubic crest

pubic symphisis

adductor longus

gracilis

quadriceps femoris
(rectus femoris)

sartorius

quadriceps femoris
(vastus medialis)

patella

medial patellar retinaculum

patellar ligament

tibialis anterior

abductor hallucis

tendon of abductor hallucis

vertebral duct

piriformis of pelvis

sacrum

coccygeus

coccyx

sacrotuberosus ligament

gluteus maximus

obturator internus

ischium
(branch)

adductor magnus

semitendinosus

semimembranosus

tendon of semitendinosus
tendon of gracilis
tendon of sartorius

pes anserinus

gastrocnemius
(medial head)

soleus

tendon of gastrocnemius

flexor digitorum longus of foot

inferior extensor retinaculum

calcaneal tendon

flexor reticulum of tarsus

A

127

128

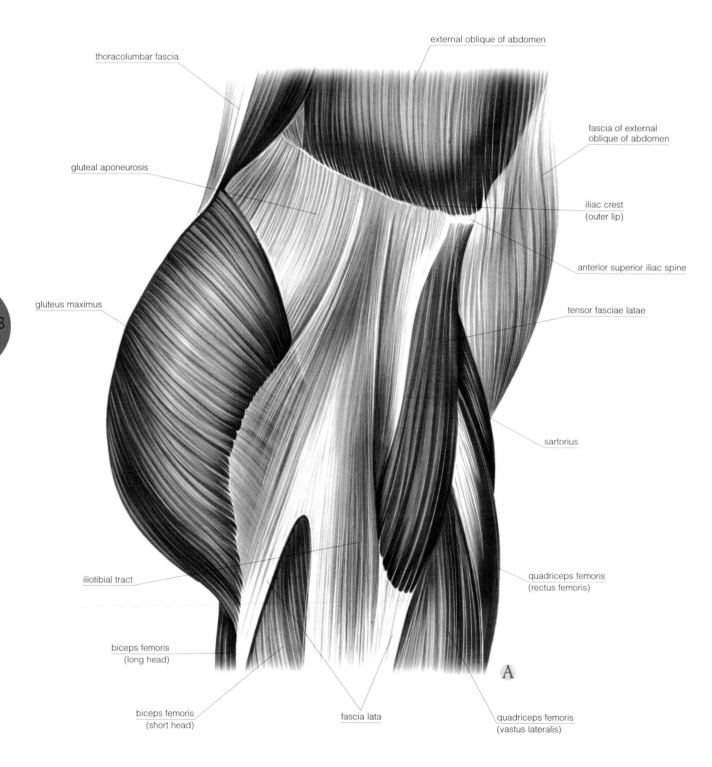

thoracolumbar fascia

external oblique of abdomen

fascia of external
oblique of abdomen

gluteal aponeurosis

iliac crest
(outer lip)

anterior superior iliac spine

gluteus maximus

tensor fasciae latae

sartorius

iliotibial tract

quadriceps femoris
(rectus femoris)

biceps femoris
(long head)

biceps femoris
(short head)

fascia lata

quadriceps femoris
(vastus lateralis)

A

LOWER LIMB (VIII). GLUTEAL REGION (II)
RIGHT LOWER LIMB. LATERAL DEEP VIEW

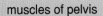

muscles of pelvis

The ones pertaining to this area are the most powerful muscles of the human body. They shape buttocks, a human species trait. Its main function is to keep trunk upright and prevent pelvis to rotate forward because of the weight of the above mentioned, which would lead to adopt a bow position, absolutely harmful to the spine.

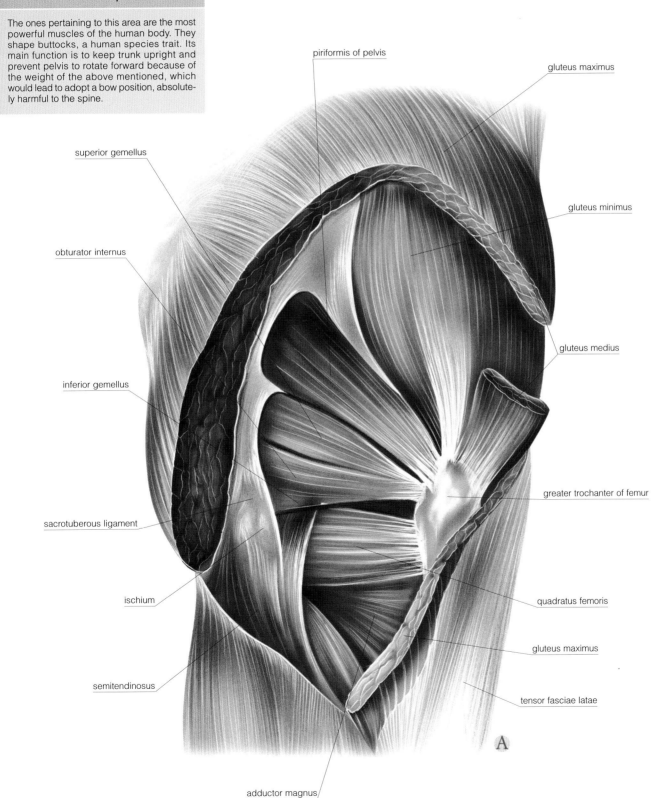

piriformis of pelvis

gluteus maximus

superior gemellus

gluteus minimus

obturator internus

gluteus medius

inferior gemellus

greater trochanter of femur

sacrotuberous ligament

quadratus femoris

ischium

gluteus maximus

semitendinosus

tensor fasciae latae

adductor magnus

A

129

LOWER LIMB (IX). THIGH (I)

RIGHT LOWER LIMB. ANTERIOR SUPERFICIAL VIEW

muscles of thigh

From the functional point of view, it is a difficult task to divide the muscles that form the fleshy chunk of the thigh into different groups. Thus, while some of them contribute with the hip joint and others do the same with the knee joint, a third group take part in both joints. Is is also difficult to classify them according to their location, because some of them, even though located in the same area, execute very different actions; nevertheless it is true that anterior muscles generally work to favor the flexion of femur in the thigh and the extension of the leg in the knee, which is the first phase of walking. On the other hand, most of the posterior muscles of thigh guarantee the extension of the same mentioned thigh and the flexion of the leg, in other words, the second phase of walking. A third group is formed by the muscles located in the median section of thigh. They produce the adduction of thigh and they do not accomplish any job in regards to the leg. Anterior, posterior and adductor muscles of thigh are separated by aponeurotic compartments. In any case, the tensor fasciae latae (femoral aponeurosis) surrounds the three groups of muscles forming a supporting group.

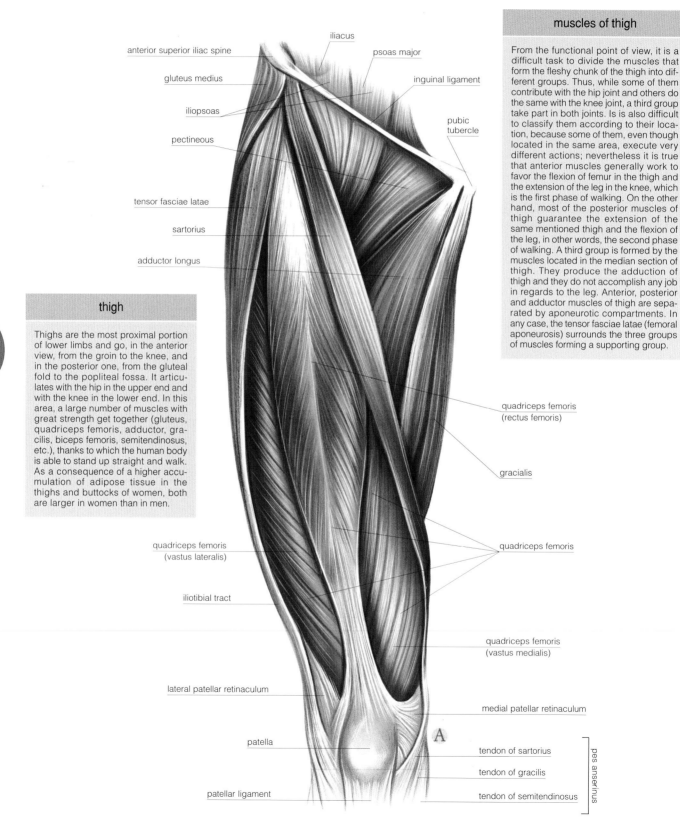

iliacus

anterior superior iliac spine

psoas major

gluteus medius

inguinal ligament

iliopsoas

pectineous

pubic tubercle

tensor fasciae latae

sartorius

adductor longus

quadriceps femoris (rectus femoris)

gracialis

quadriceps femoris

quadriceps femoris (vastus lateralis)

iliotibial tract

quadriceps femoris (vastus medialis)

lateral patellar retinaculum

medial patellar retinaculum

patella

A

tendon of sartorius

tendon of gracilis

patellar ligament

tendon of semitendinosus

pes anserinus

thigh

Thighs are the most proximal portion of lower limbs and go, in the anterior view, from the groin to the knee, and in the posterior one, from the gluteal fold to the popliteal fossa. It articulates with the hip in the upper end and with the knee in the lower end. In this area, a large number of muscles with great strength get together (gluteus, quadriceps femoris, adductor, gracilis, biceps femoris, semitendinosus, etc.), thanks to which the human body is able to stand up straight and walk. As a consequence of a higher accumulation of adipose tissue in the thighs and buttocks of women, both are larger in women than in men.

LOWER LIMB (X). THIGH (II)
RIGHT LOWER LIMB. ANTERIOR INTERMEDIATE VIEW

movements of thigh

Movements of thigh, that participate in the articulation of the hip, are produced generally by muscles originated in the pelvic girdle. The hip joint is spheroidal, which enables hip to make movements like flexion, extension, abduction adduction, circumduction and rotation. Muscles that make possible all this activity are the strongest ones of the human body. Most of the flexors of thigh ran in front of the hip joint. Among them the most important ones are the iliopsoas, the tensor fasciae latae and the quadriceps femoris. All of them are helped by the abductors from the median part of thigh and for the sartorius, a rhomboidal shape muscle. On the other hand, the iliopsoas acts as an agonist of the flexion of thigh and hip.

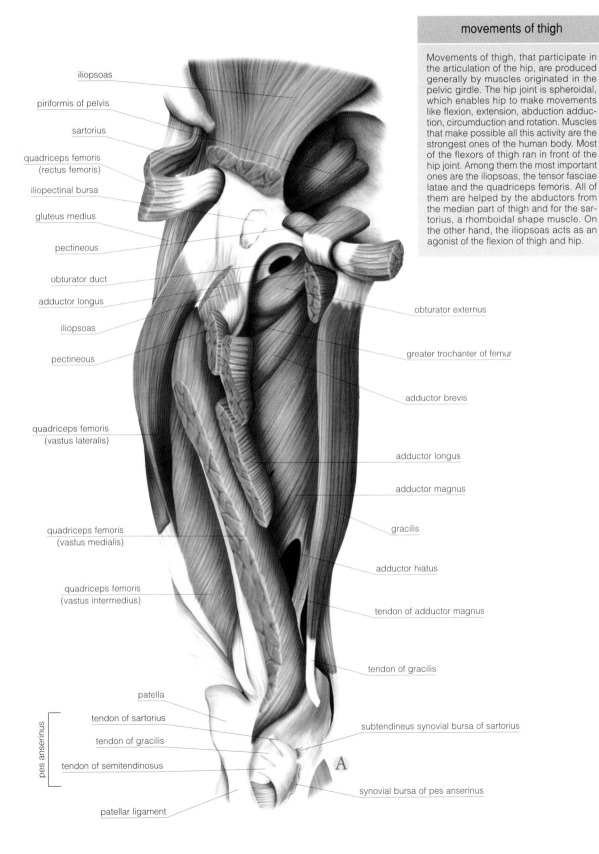

iliopsoas

piriformis of pelvis

sartorius

quadriceps femoris
(rectus femoris)

iliopectinal bursa

gluteus medius

pectineous

obturator duct

adductor longus

iliopsoas

pectineous

quadriceps femoris
(vastus lateralis)

quadriceps femoris
(vastus medialis)

quadriceps femoris
(vastus intermedius)

patella

tendon of sartorius

tendon of gracilis

tendon of semitendinosus

patellar ligament

pes anserinus

obturator externus

greater trochanter of femur

adductor brevis

adductor longus

adductor magnus

gracilis

adductor hiatus

tendon of adductor magnus

tendon of gracilis

subtendineus synovial bursa of sartorius

synovial bursa of pes anserinus

A

131

LOWER LIMB (XI). THIGH (III)

RIGHT LOWER LIMB. ANTERIOR DEEP VIEW

anterior femoral area

Anterior area of thigh is made up by the own muscles of thigh and others from the hip distally expanded so as to occupy part of the thigh. The anterior group of muscles of thigh is formed by the sartorius and the quadriceps. While in the median part of thigh it appears a gruop of adductor muscles: adductor longus, adductor brevis, adductor magnus, gracilis and pectineus.

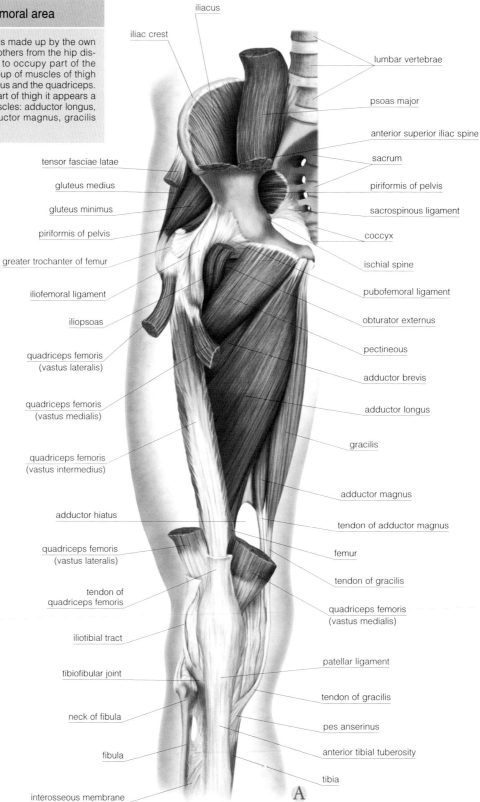

iliacus

iliac crest

lumbar vertebrae

psoas major

anterior superior iliac spine

sacrum

tensor fasciae latae

gluteus medius

piriformis of pelvis

gluteus minimus

sacrospinous ligament

piriformis of pelvis

coccyx

greater trochanter of femur

ischial spine

iliofemoral ligament

pubofemoral ligament

iliopsoas

obturator externus

quadriceps femoris
(vastus lateralis)

pectineous

adductor brevis

quadriceps femoris
(vastus medialis)

adductor longus

quadriceps femoris
(vastus intermedius)

gracilis

adductor magnus

adductor hiatus

tendon of adductor magnus

quadriceps femoris
(vastus lateralis)

femur

tendon of gracilis

tendon of
quadriceps femoris

quadriceps femoris
(vastus medialis)

iliotibial tract

patellar ligament

tibiofibular joint

tendon of gracilis

neck of fibula

pes anserinus

anterior tibial tuberosity

fibula

tibia

interosseous membrane

A

LOWER LIMB (XII). THIGH (IV)

RIGHT LOWER LIMB. POSTERIOR SUPERFICIAL VIEW

extension of thigh

The extension of thigh is possible thanks to the great back muscles. When a forced extension takes place, the gluteus maximus goes into action. Gluteus muscles are located laterally in connection with the hip joint (gluteus medius and gluteus minimus) and are responsible for the abduction of thigh and its median rotation. Six small deep muscles of the gluteal region (lateral rotators) are the antagonists of the median rotation. The adduction of thigh is the responsibility of the adductors of the median part of thigh. Abduction and adduction are extremely essential to keep the balance of the body over the limb that is standing on the floor during the course of gait.

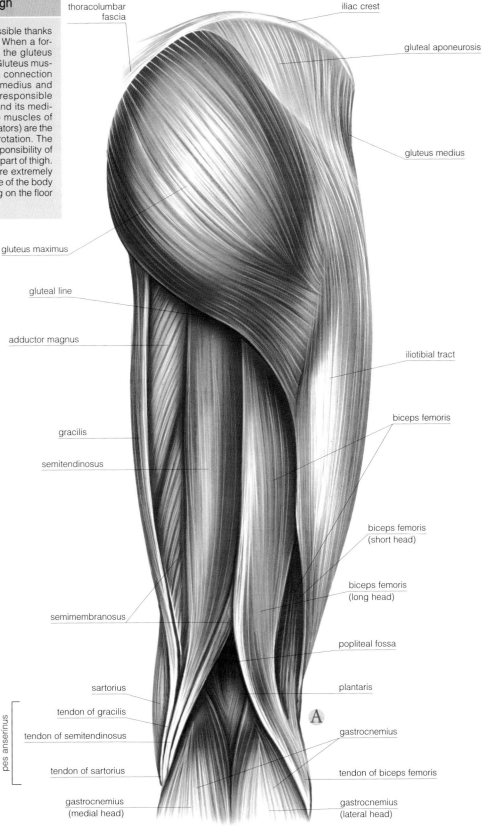

thoracolumbar fascia

iliac crest

gluteal aponeurosis

gluteus medius

gluteus maximus

gluteal line

adductor magnus

iliotibial tract

gracilis

biceps femoris

semitendinosus

biceps femoris (short head)

biceps femoris (long head)

semimembranosus

popliteal fossa

sartorius

plantaris

tendon of gracilis

A

tendon of semitendinosus

gastrocnemius

tendon of sartorius

tendon of biceps femoris

pes anserinus

gastrocnemius (medial head)

gastrocnemius (lateral head)

133

LOWER LIMB (XIII). THIGH (V)

RIGHT LOWER LIMB. POSTERIOR SUPERFICIAL VIEW

back muscles of thigh

They are originated from the tuberosity of ischium and the front branch of pubis by means of a common muscular mass. For that reason they are normally called (no doubt erroneously) ischiotibial muscles. Starting from this common mass, they extend up to their insertions whether be in the tibia (in the case of the semitendinosus and semimembranosus) or in the fibula (in the case of the biceps femoris).

134

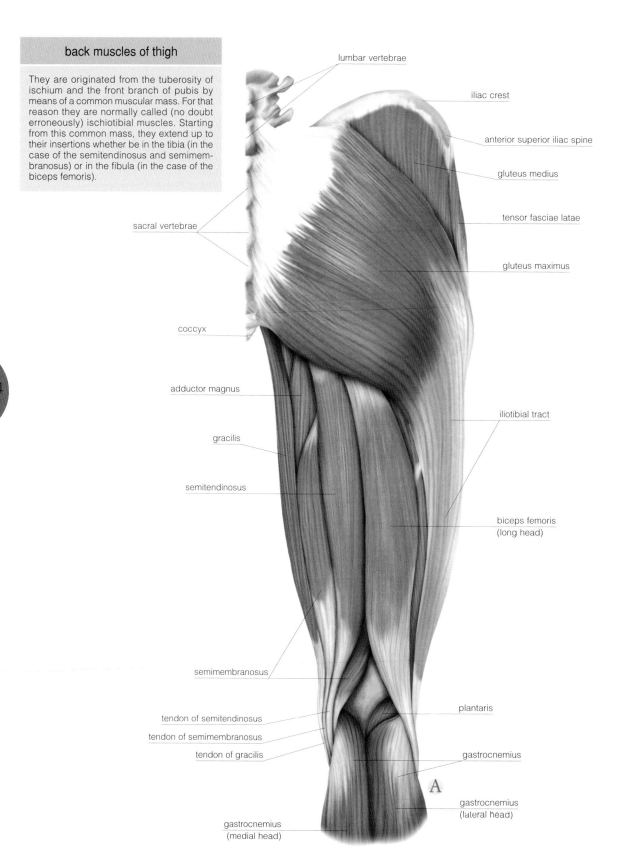

lumbar vertebrae

iliac crest

anterior superior iliac spine

gluteus medius

tensor fasciae latae

gluteus maximus

sacral vertebrae

coccyx

adductor magnus

gracilis

iliotibial tract

semitendinosus

biceps femoris
(long head)

semimembranosus

plantaris

tendon of semitendinosus

tendon of semimembranosus

tendon of gracilis

gastrocnemius

A

gastrocnemius
(lateral head)

gastrocnemius
(medial head)

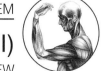

LOWER LIMB (XIV). THIGH (VI)

RIGHT LOWER LIMB. POSTERIOR DEEP VIEW

deep gluteal area

In the deep view of the gluteal area the next muscles are shown: gluteus minimus, piriformis, obturator internus, gemellus and quadratus femoris. When sectioning the long head of biceps femoris and the semitendinosus, the deep view of the back region of thigh shows a complete glimpse of the semimembranosus muscle and its characteristic membrane of origin.

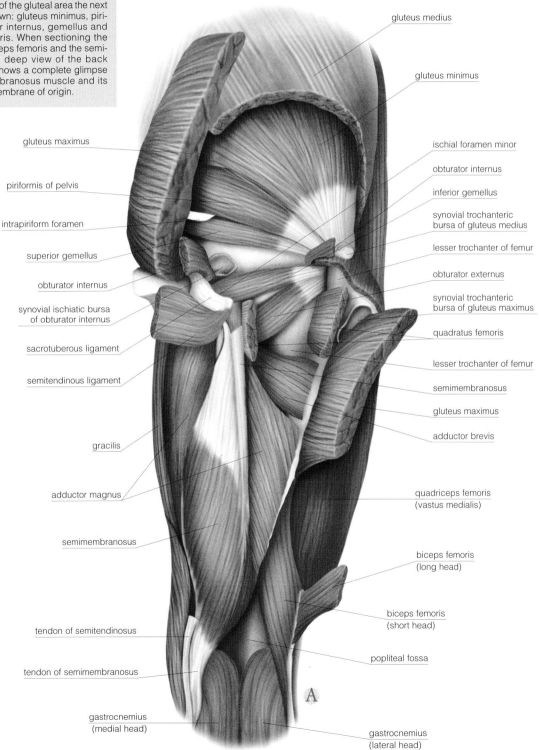

gluteus medius

gluteus minimus

gluteus maximus

piriformis of pelvis

intrapiriform foramen

superior gemellus

obturator internus

synovial ischiatic bursa of obturator internus

sacrotuberous ligament

semitendinous ligament

gracilis

adductor magnus

semimembranosus

tendon of semitendinosus

tendon of semimembranosus

gastrocnemius (medial head)

ischial foramen minor

obturator internus

inferior gemellus

synovial trochanteric bursa of gluteus medius

lesser trochanter of femur

obturator externus

synovial trochanteric bursa of gluteus maximus

quadratus femoris

lesser trochanter of femur

semimembranosus

gluteus maximus

adductor brevis

quadriceps femoris (vastus medialis)

biceps femoris (long head)

biceps femoris (short head)

popliteal fossa

gastrocnemius (lateral head)

A

LOWER LIMB (XV). THIGH (VII)

RIGHT LOWER LIMB. LATERAL SUPERFICIAL VIEW

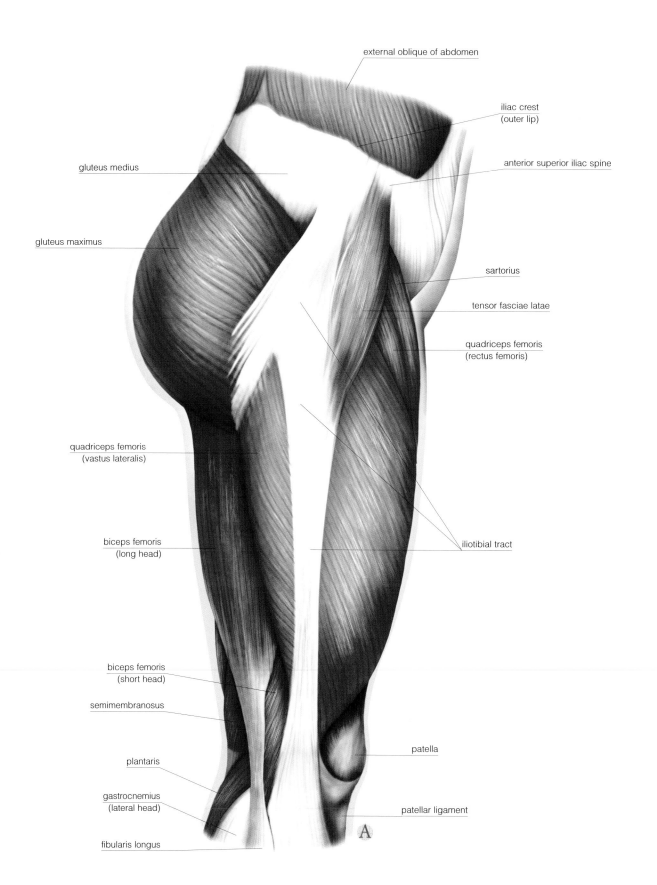

external oblique of abdomen

iliac crest
(outer lip)

anterior superior iliac spine

gluteus medius

gluteus maximus

sartorius

tensor fasciae latae

quadriceps femoris
(rectus femoris)

quadriceps femoris
(vastus lateralis)

biceps femoris
(long head)

iliotibial tract

biceps femoris
(short head)

semimembranosus

patella

plantaris

gastrocnemius
(lateral head)

patellar ligament

fibularis longus

A

LOWER LIMB (XVI). THIGH (VIII)

RIGHT LOWER LIMB. LATERAL INTERMEDIATE VIEW

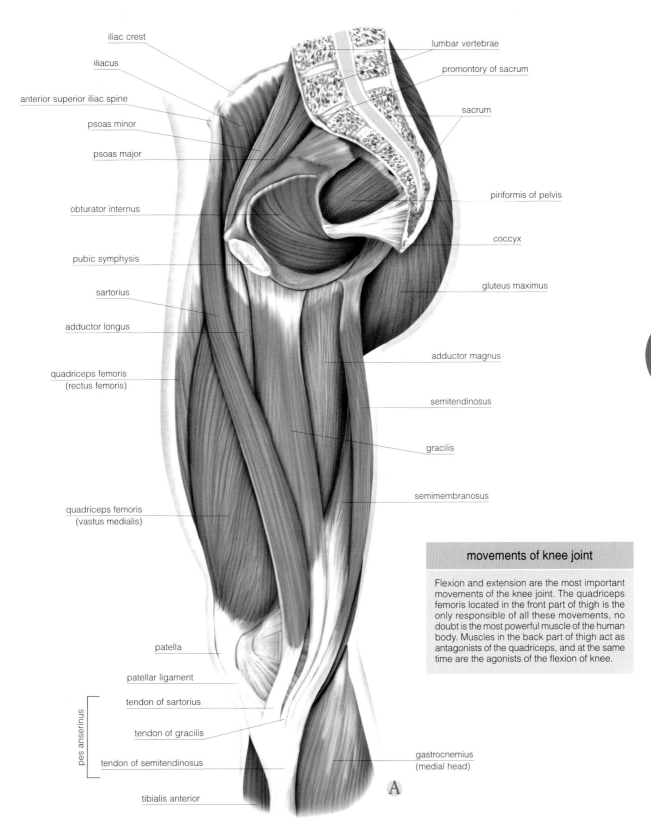

iliac crest

iliacus

anterior superior iliac spine

psoas minor

psoas major

obturator internus

pubic symphysis

sartorius

adductor longus

quadriceps femoris
(rectus femoris)

quadriceps femoris
(vastus medialis)

patella

patellar ligament

tendon of sartorius

tendon of gracilis

tendon of semitendinosus

tibialis anterior

pes anserinus

lumbar vertebrae

promontory of sacrum

sacrum

piriformis of pelvis

coccyx

gluteus maximus

adductor magnus

semitendinosus

gracilis

semimembranosus

gastrocnemius
(medial head)

movements of knee joint

Flexion and extension are the most important movements of the knee joint. The quadriceps femoris located in the front part of thigh is the only responsible of all these movements, no doubt is the most powerful muscle of the human body. Muscles in the back part of thigh act as antagonists of the quadriceps, and at the same time are the agonists of the flexion of knee.

A

137

LOWER LIMB (XVII). LEG and FOOT (I)

RIGHT LOWER LIMB. ANTERIOR SUPERFICIAL VIEW

muscles of leg

The leg contains a significant amount of muscles. Even though each one of them performs a specific function. As a rule they are intended to turn the foot and to move the fingers of the same foot, as well as to flex the leg towards the thigh. All these movements make possible the whole skeletal structure of the body stand upright and also wandering, that is, the body can go from one place to another. The front part of the leg lacks of muscles in the median area, because is occupied by the front face of the tibial structure. The front and peroneal groups of muscles are sited in the lateral part of leg. The muscles of the front group are the tibialis anterior, the extensor digitorum longus and the extensor hallucis longus. Also, its tendons pass the extensor retinaculum and go in direction to the foot.

138

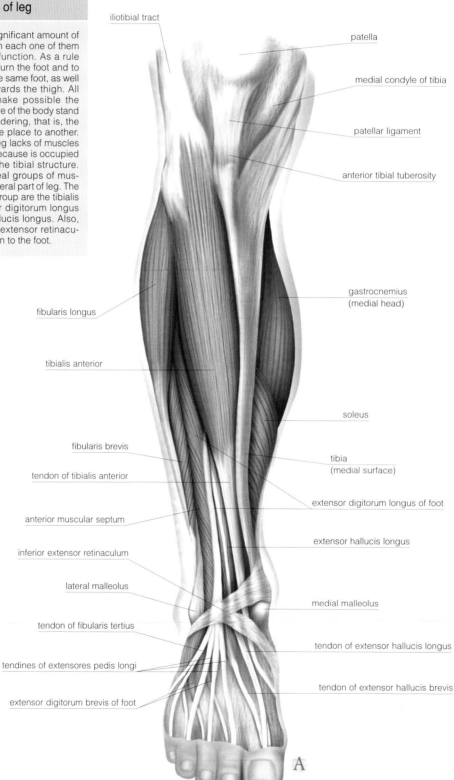

iliotibial tract

patella

medial condyle of tibia

patellar ligament

anterior tibial tuberosity

gastrocnemius (medial head)

fibularis longus

tibialis anterior

soleus

fibularis brevis

tibia (medial surface)

tendon of tibialis anterior

extensor digitorum longus of foot

anterior muscular septum

extensor hallucis longus

inferior extensor retinaculum

lateral malleolus

medial malleolus

tendon of fibularis tertius

tendon of extensor hallucis longus

tendines of extensores pedis longi

extensor digitorum brevis of foot

tendon of extensor hallucis brevis

A

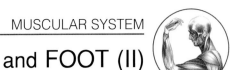

LOWER LIMB (XVIII). LEG and FOOT (II)

RIGHT LOWER LIMB. ANTERIOR SUPERFICIAL VIEW

physiology of the muscles of leg

According to the location and position, muscles of leg have the main function of making possible the movements of the ankle (dorsiflexion and plantar flexion), of the intertarsal joints (inversion and eversion of foot), and of the fingers of foot (flexion and extension). Muscles of the front group (tibialis anterior, extensor digitorum longus, extensor hallucis longus and fibularis tertius) have the function of extending the fingers and the dorsiflexion of ankle. Muscles of the lateral group (fibularis longus and fibularis brevis) take the responsibility of the plantar flexion and the eversion of the foot, while the muscles of the back group (gastrocnemius, soleus, tibialis posterior, flexor digitoum longus, flexor hallucis longus) are the main plantar flexors and flexors of the fingers.

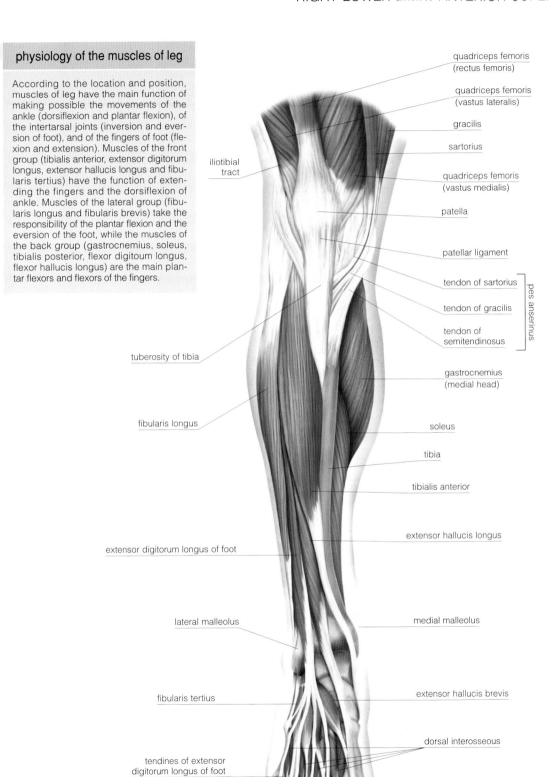

quadriceps femoris (rectus femoris)

quadriceps femoris (vastus lateralis)

gracilis

sartorius

quadriceps femoris (vastus medialis)

patella

patellar ligament

tendon of sartorius

tendon of gracilis

tendon of semitendinosus

pes anserinus

gastrocnemius (medial head)

soleus

tibia

tibialis anterior

extensor hallucis longus

medial malleolus

extensor hallucis brevis

dorsal interosseous

extensor hallucis longus

iliotibial tract

tuberosity of tibia

fibularis longus

extensor digitorum longus of foot

lateral malleolus

fibularis tertius

tendines of extensor digitorum longus of foot

A

139

LOWER LIMB (XIX). LEG and FOOT (III)

RIGHT LOWER LIMB. POSTERIOR SUPERFICIAL VIEW

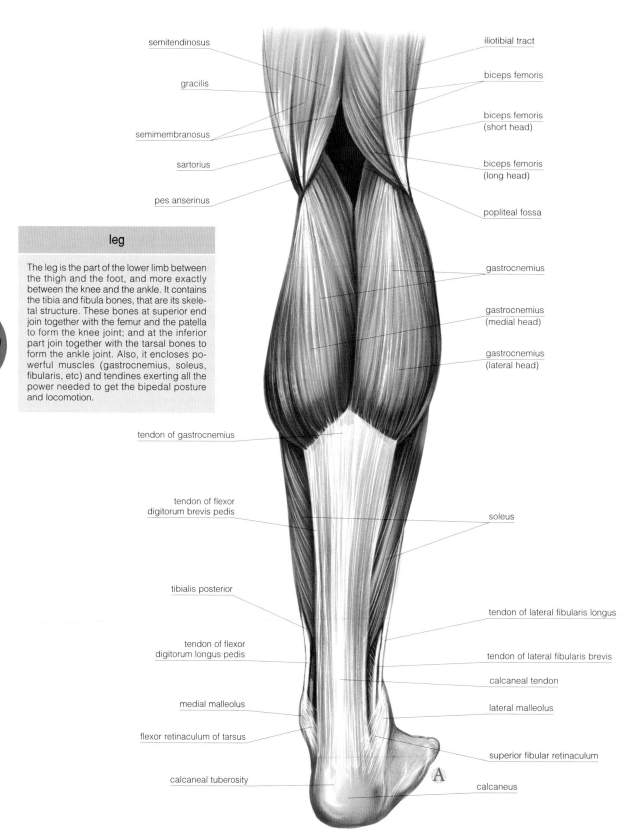

semitendinosus

gracilis

semimembranosus

sartorius

pes anserinus

iliotibial tract

biceps femoris

biceps femoris
(short head)

biceps femoris
(long head)

popliteal fossa

gastrocnemius

gastrocnemius
(medial head)

gastrocnemius
(lateral head)

leg

The leg is the part of the lower limb between the thigh and the foot, and more exactly between the knee and the ankle. It contains the tibia and fibula bones, that are its skeletal structure. These bones at superior end join together with the femur and the patella to form the knee joint; and at the inferior part join together with the tarsal bones to form the ankle joint. Also, it encloses powerful muscles (gastrocnemius, soleus, fibularis, etc) and tendines exerting all the power needed to get the bipedal posture and locomotion.

140

tendon of gastrocnemius

tendon of flexor
digitorum brevis pedis

tibialis posterior

tendon of flexor
digitorum longus pedis

medial malleolus

flexor retinaculum of tarsus

calcaneal tuberosity

soleus

tendon of lateral fibularis longus

tendon of lateral fibularis brevis

calcaneal tendon

lateral malleolus

superior fibular retinaculum

calcaneus

A

LOWER LIMB (XX). LEG and FOOT (IV)

RIGHT LOWER LIMB. POSTERIOR SUPERFICIAL VIEW

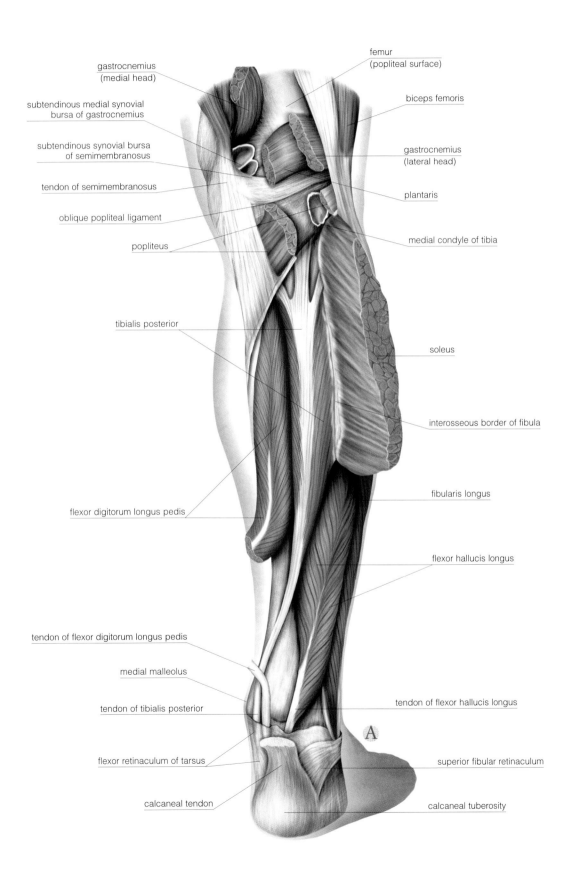

gastrocnemius
(medial head)

subtendinous medial synovial
bursa of gastrocnemius

subtendinous synovial bursa
of semimembranosus

tendon of semimembranosus

oblique popliteal ligament

popliteus

tibialis posterior

flexor digitorum longus pedis

tendon of flexor digitorum longus pedis

medial malleolus

tendon of tibialis posterior

flexor retinaculum of tarsus

calcaneal tendon

femur
(popliteal surface)

biceps femoris

gastrocnemius
(lateral head)

plantaris

medial condyle of tibia

soleus

interosseous border of fibula

fibularis longus

flexor hallucis longus

tendon of flexor hallucis longus

superior fibular retinaculum

calcaneal tuberosity

A

141

LOWER LIMB (XXI). LEG and FOOT (V)

RIGHT LOWER LIMB. POSTERIOR DEEP VIEW

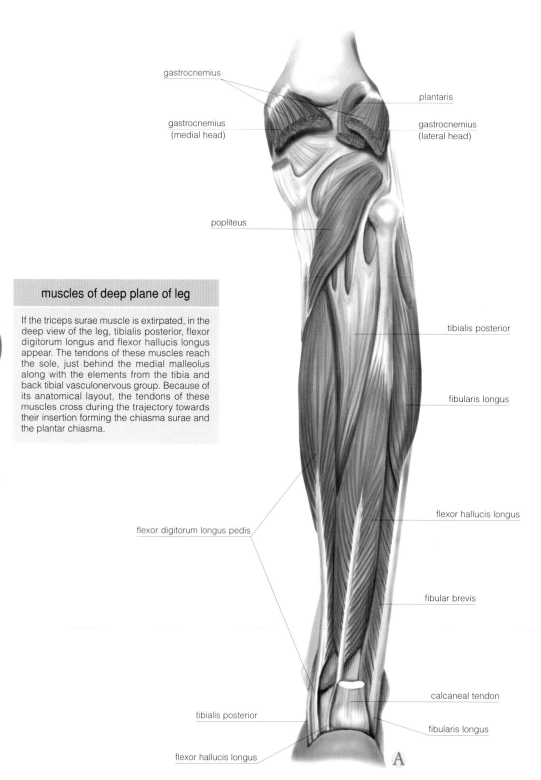

gastrocnemius

plantaris

gastrocnemius
(medial head)

gastrocnemius
(lateral head)

popliteus

tibialis posterior

fibularis longus

flexor hallucis longus

flexor digitorum longus pedis

fibular brevis

calcaneal tendon

tibialis posterior

fibularis longus

flexor hallucis longus

A

muscles of deep plane of leg

If the triceps surae muscle is extirpated, in the deep view of the leg, tibialis posterior, flexor digitorum longus and flexor hallucis longus appear. The tendons of these muscles reach the sole, just behind the medial malleolus along with the elements from the tibia and back tibial vasculonervous group. Because of its anatomical layout, the tendons of these muscles cross during the trajectory towards their insertion forming the chiasma surae and the plantar chiasma.

142

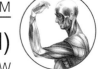

LOWER LIMB (XXII). LEG and FOOT (VI)
RIGHT LOWER LIMB. POSTERIOR DEEP VIEW

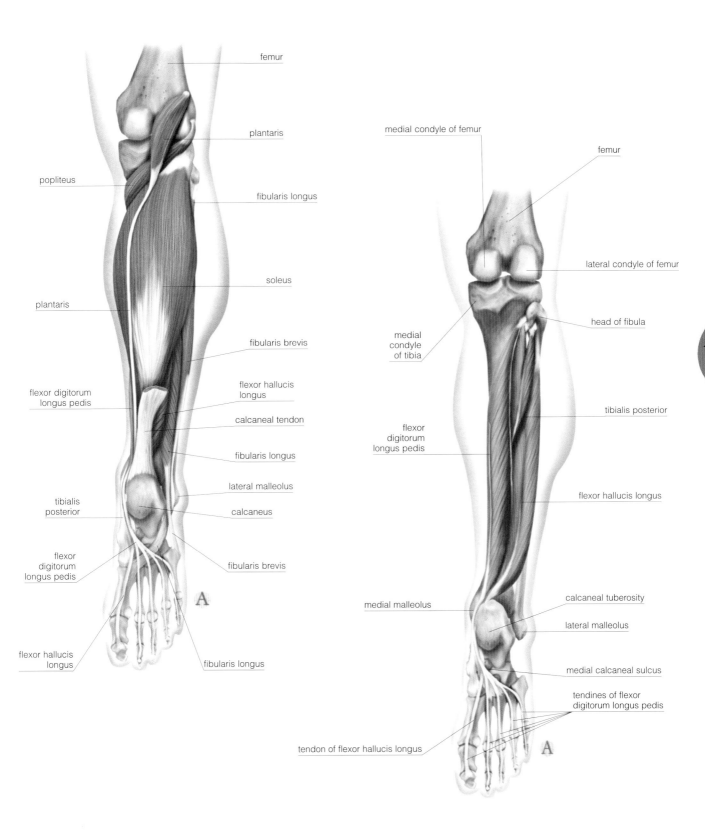

femur

plantaris

popliteus

fibularis longus

soleus

plantaris

fibularis brevis

flexor hallucis longus

flexor digitorum longus pedis

calcaneal tendon

fibularis longus

lateral malleolus

tibialis posterior

calcaneus

flexor digitorum longus pedis

fibularis brevis

flexor hallucis longus

fibularis longus

A

medial condyle of femur

femur

lateral condyle of femur

head of fibula

medial condyle of tibia

tibialis posterior

flexor digitorum longus pedis

flexor hallucis longus

medial malleolus

calcaneal tuberosity

lateral malleolus

medial calcaneal sulcus

tendines of flexor digitorum longus pedis

tendon of flexor hallucis longus

A

143

LOWER LIMB (XXIII). LEG and FOOT (VII)

LEFT LOWER LIMB. LATERAL SUPERFICIAL VIEW

fascia of leg

The deep fascia of the leg forms a sort of covering that is the continuation of the fasciae latae and brings together and holds the muscles of the leg and prevents them to swell excessively while exercising, therefore favoring the return of venous blood to the right atrium of the heart. This aponeurosis makes possible the separation of the muscles, that may be classified as anterior, posterior and lateral muscles, each one with its own vascularization and innervation. In the distal end, this aponeurosis of the leg becomes stronger in order to form the inferior extensor retinaculum, that keeps the tendons of the muscles firmly tied to the ankle, before leaving this area and going to the foot.

144

quadriceps femoris
(vastus lateralis)

biceps femoris

iliotibial tract

biceps femoris
(short head)

head of fibula

lateral muscular group of the leg

The muscles forming the lateral group of the leg are the fibularis brevis and the fibularis longus. Both get to the sole of the foot behind the lateral malleolus, passing under the inferior extensor retinaculum of the fibularis muscles. Due to this situation they are plantar flexors, different from the rest of anterior muscles that are dorsal flexors.

patella

patellar ligament

anterior tubercle of tibia

extensor digitorum
longus of foot

tibialis anterior

anterior intermuscular septum of leg

fibularis tertius

tendon of tibialis anterior

extensor hallucis longus

anterior extensor retinaculum of tarsus

tendon of fibularis tertius

extensor digitorum brevis of foot

extensor hallucis brevis

tendon of extensor pedis longus

fibularis longus

gastrocnemius
(medial head)

soleus

fibularis brevis

tendon of lateral fibularis longus

calcaneal tendon

lateral malleolus

superior fibular retinaculum

inferior fibular retinaculum

calcaneal tuberosity

calcaneus

tendon of lateral fibularis brevis

A

LOWER LIMB (XXIV). LEG and FOOT (VIII)

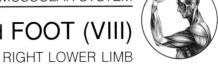

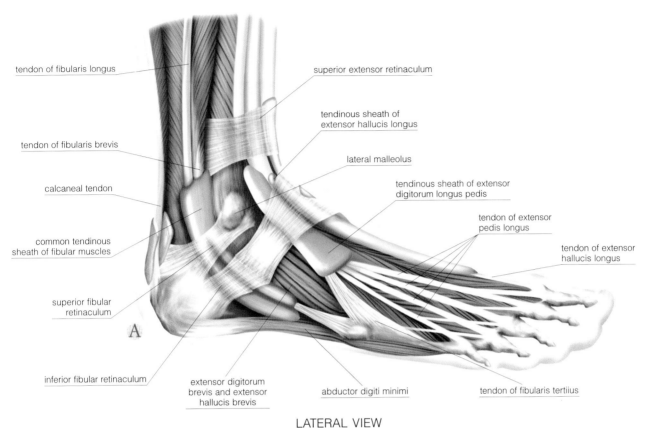

tendon of fibularis longus

superior extensor retinaculum

tendinous sheath of
extensor hallucis longus

tendon of fibularis brevis

lateral malleolus

calcaneal tendon

tendinous sheath of extensor
digitorum longus pedis

tendon of extensor
pedis longus

common tendinous
sheath of fibular muscles

tendon of extensor
hallucis longus

superior fibular
retinaculum

A

inferior fibular retinaculum

extensor digitorum
brevis and extensor
hallucis brevis

abductor digiti minimi

tendon of fibularis tertiius

145

LATERAL VIEW

superior extensor retinaculum

flexor digitorum
longus

medial malleolus

inferior extensor retinaculum

tendinous sheath
of flexor hallucis longus

tendinous sheath
of extensor hallucis longus

calcaneal tendon

flexor retinaculum
of tarsus

A

abductor hallucis

tendinous sheath of tibialis anterior

flexor digitorum brevis

tendinous sheath of flexor digitorum longus pedis

tendinous sheath of tibialis posterior

MEDIAL VIEW

LOWER LIMB (XXV). THIGH (IX)

LEFT LOWER LIMB. CROSS-SECTION. CAUDAL VIEW

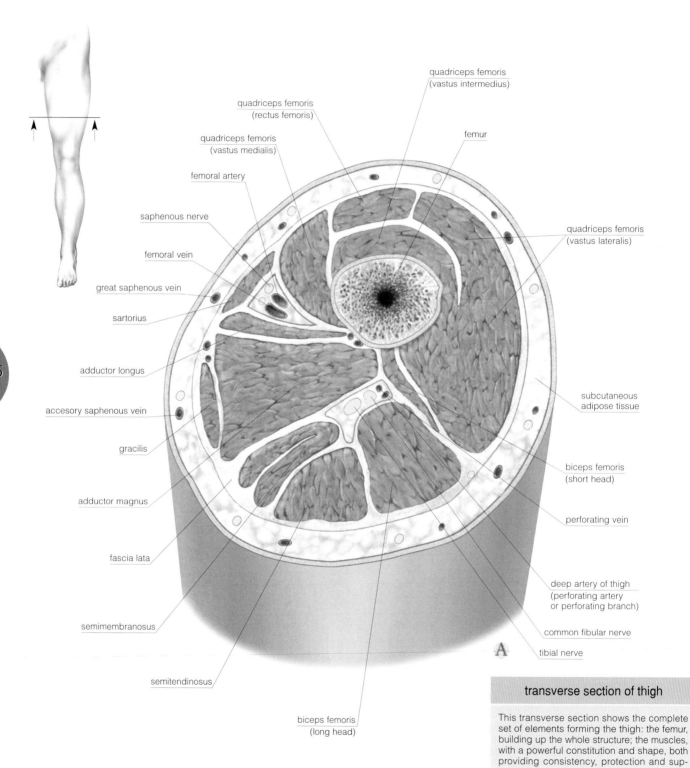

quadriceps femoris
(vastus intermedius)

quadriceps femoris
(rectus femoris)

quadriceps femoris
(vastus medialis)

femur

femoral artery

saphenous nerve

quadriceps femoris
(vastus lateralis)

femoral vein

great saphenous vein

sartorius

adductor longus

subcutaneous
adipose tissue

accesory saphenous vein

gracilis

adductor magnus

biceps femoris
(short head)

perforating vein

fascia lata

semimembranosus

deep artery of thigh
(perforating artery
or perforating branch)

common fibular nerve

A   tibial nerve

semitendinosus

biceps femoris
(long head)

146

transverse section of thigh

This transverse section shows the complete
set of elements forming the thigh: the femur,
building up the whole structure; the muscles,
with a powerful constitution and shape, both
providing consistency, protection and support; the fasciae and septa demarcating each
one of the muscle elements; the nerves, that
transmit the sensations and always act in a
two way direction; and finally, the elements
(arteries and veins) of the cardiovascular system, which keeps the lower limb purified and
with an appropriate irrigation.

LOWER LIMB (XXVI). LEG
RIGHT LOWER LIMB. CROSS-SECTION. CRANIAL VIEW

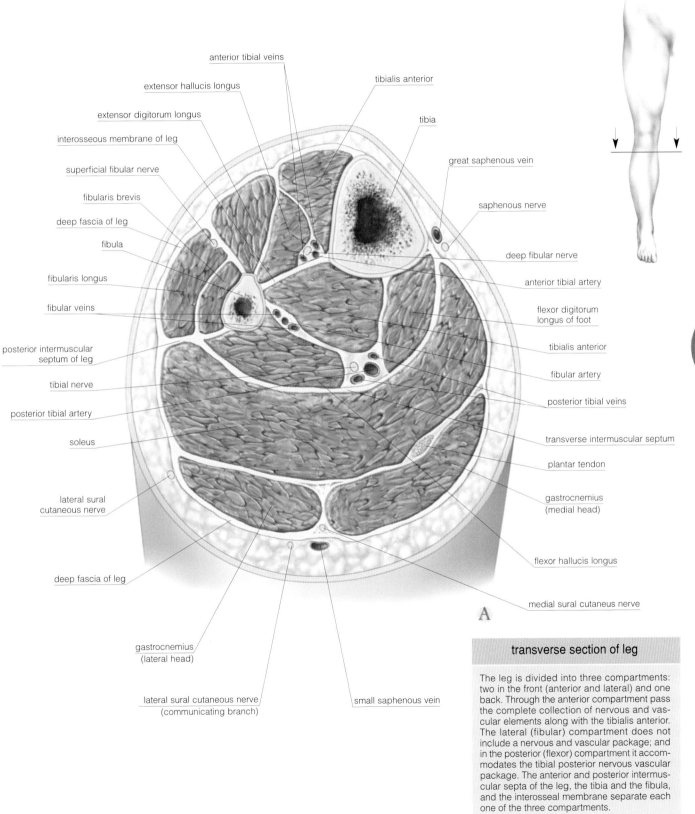

anterior tibial veins

extensor hallucis longus

extensor digitorum longus

interosseous membrane of leg

superficial fibular nerve

fibularis brevis

deep fascia of leg

fibula

fibularis longus

fibular veins

posterior intermuscular septum of leg

tibial nerve

posterior tibial artery

soleus

lateral sural cutaneous nerve

deep fascia of leg

gastrocnemius (lateral head)

lateral sural cutaneous nerve (communicating branch)

tibialis anterior

tibia

great saphenous vein

saphenous nerve

deep fibular nerve

anterior tibial artery

flexor digitorum longus of foot

tibialis anterior

fibular artery

posterior tibial veins

transverse intermuscular septum

plantar tendon

gastrocnemius (medial head)

flexor hallucis longus

medial sural cutaneus nerve

small saphenous vein

A

147

transverse section of leg

The leg is divided into three compartments: two in the front (anterior and lateral) and one back. Through the anterior compartment pass the complete collection of nervous and vascular elements along with the tibialis anterior. The lateral (fibular) compartment does not include a nervous and vascular package; and in the posterior (flexor) compartment it accommodates the tibial posterior nervous vascular package. The anterior and posterior intermuscular septa of the leg, the tibia and the fibula, and the interosseal membrane separate each one of the three compartments.

LOWER LIMB (XXVII). FOOT (I)

RIGHT LOWER LIMB. TENDINOUS SHEATHS. DORSAL VIEW

148

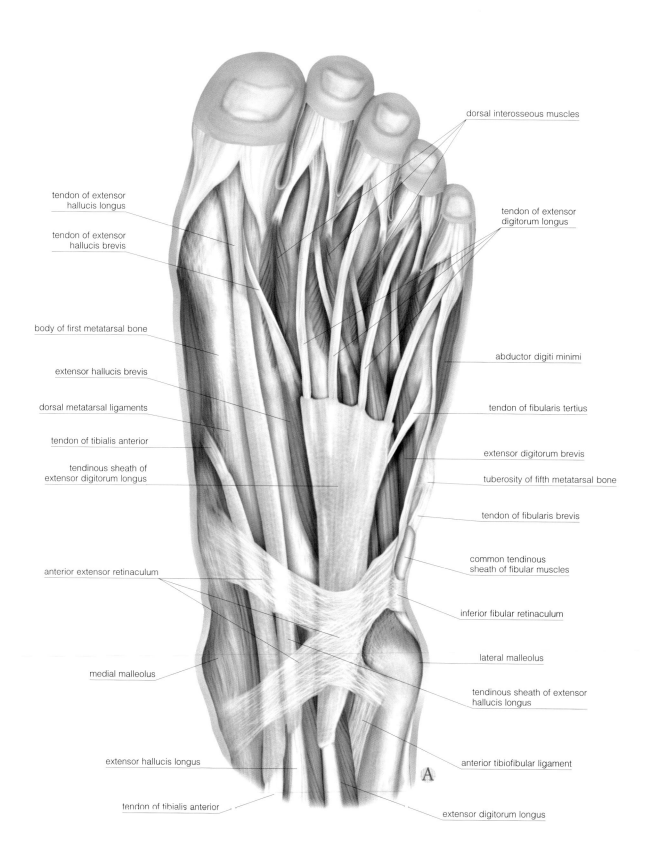

dorsal interosseous muscles

tendon of extensor
hallucis longus

tendon of extensor
hallucis brevis

tendon of extensor
digitorum longus

body of first metatarsal bone

abductor digiti minimi

extensor hallucis brevis

tendon of fibularis tertius

dorsal metatarsal ligaments

extensor digitorum brevis

tendon of tibialis anterior

tuberosity of fifth metatarsal bone

tendinous sheath of
extensor digitorum longus

tendon of fibularis brevis

common tendinous
sheath of fibular muscles

anterior extensor retinaculum

inferior fibular retinaculum

lateral malleolus

medial malleolus

tendinous sheath of extensor
hallucis longus

extensor hallucis longus

anterior tibiofibular ligament

tendon of tibialis anterior

extensor digitorum longus

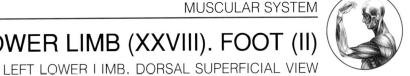

LOWER LIMB (XXVIII). FOOT (II)
LEFT LOWER LIMB. DORSAL SUPERFICIAL VIEW

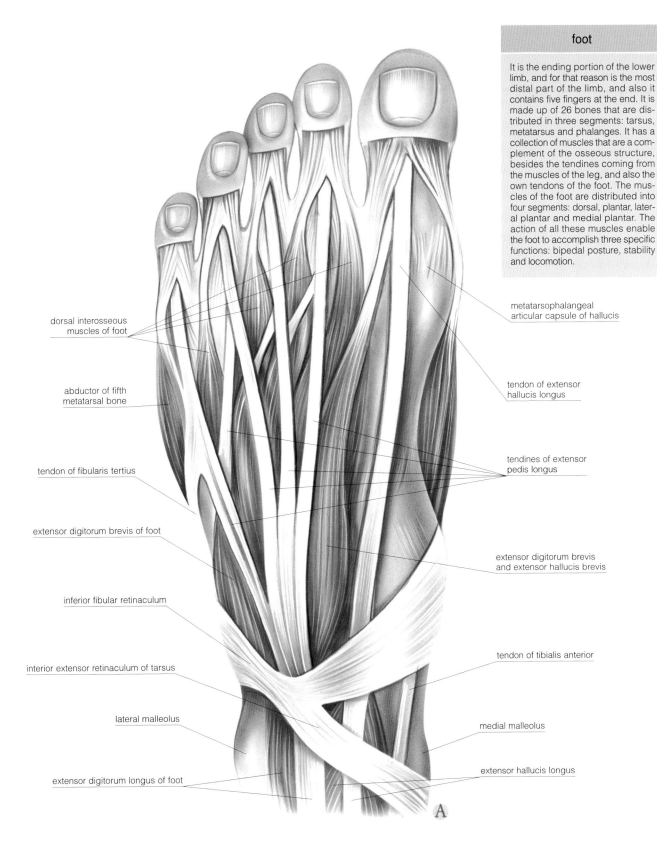

dorsal interosseous muscles of foot

abductor of fifth metatarsal bone

tendon of fibularis tertius

extensor digitorum brevis of foot

inferior fibular retinaculum

interior extensor retinaculum of tarsus

lateral malleolus

extensor digitorum longus of foot

metatarsophalangeal articular capsule of hallucis

tendon of extensor hallucis longus

tendines of extensor pedis longus

extensor digitorum brevis and extensor hallucis brevis

tendon of tibialis anterior

medial malleolus

extensor hallucis longus

A

LOWER LIMB (XXIX). FOOT (III)

RIGHT LOWER LIMB. DORSAL SUPERFICIAL VIEW

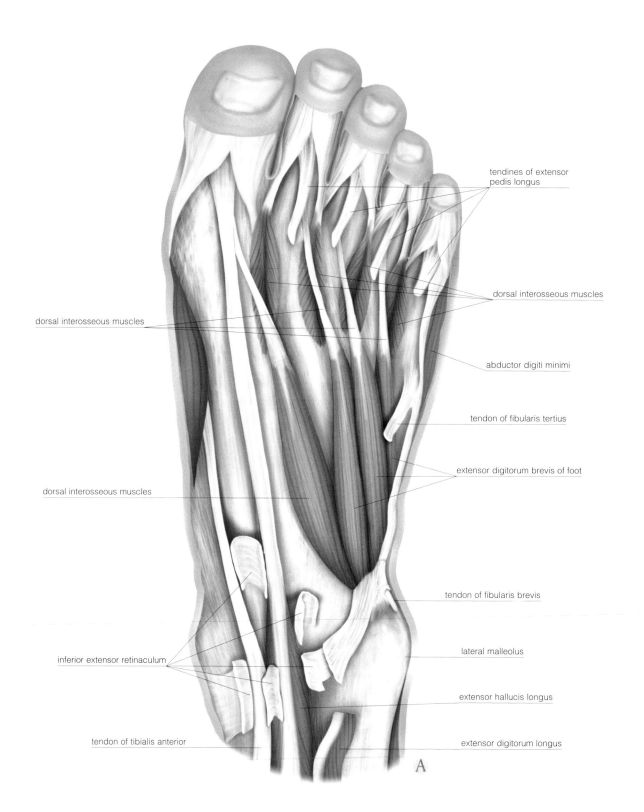

tendines of extensor pedis longus

dorsal interosseous muscles

dorsal interosseous muscles

abductor digiti minimi

tendon of fibularis tertius

extensor digitorum brevis of foot

dorsal interosseous muscles

tendon of fibularis brevis

lateral malleolus

inferior extensor retinaculum

extensor hallucis longus

tendon of tibialis anterior

extensor digitorum longus

A

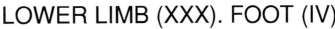
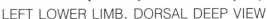

muscles of foot

The muscles of the foot form a large collection. Most of them are in the plantar area and between the metatarsal bones. They normally go along with many tendines, sometimes long-run ones and having to accomplish various functions, besides the strength that is needed. That is the reason why they provide a large mobility to the foot as well as the fingers, which eases the act of walking. Also, they are very effective in the task of keeping the stability of the complete body structure when in standing position.

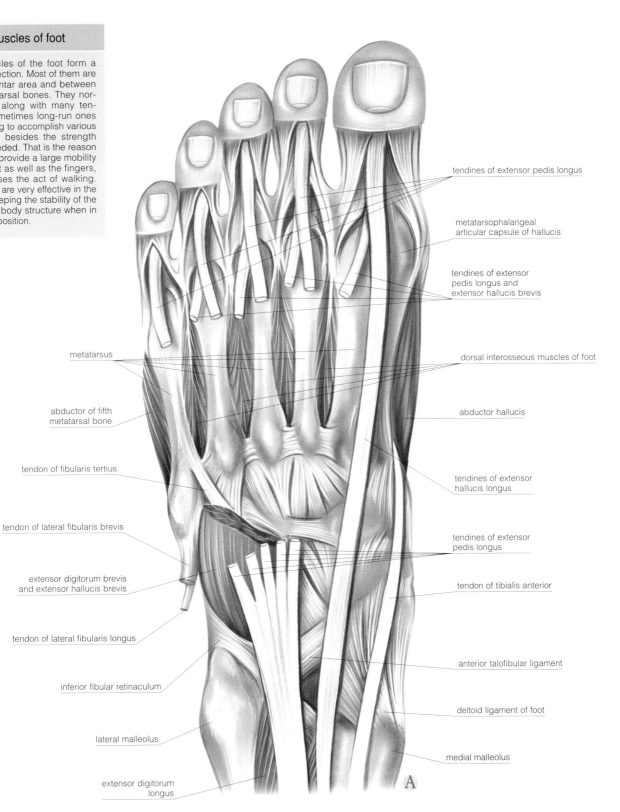

tendines of extensor pedis longus

metatarsophalangeal articular capsule of hallucis

tendines of extensor pedis longus and extensor hallucis brevis

dorsal interosseous muscles of foot

abductor hallucis

tendines of extensor hallucis longus

tendines of extensor pedis longus

tendon of tibialis anterior

anterior talofibular ligament

deltoid ligament of foot

medial malleolus

metatarsus

abductor of fifth metatarsal bone

tendon of fibularis tertius

tendon of lateral fibularis brevis

extensor digitorum brevis and extensor hallucis brevis

tendon of lateral fibularis longus

inferior fibular retinaculum

lateral malleolus

extensor digitorum longus

151

A

LOWER LIMB (XXXI). FOOT (V)

RIGHT LOWER LIMB. PLANTAR SUPERFICIAL VIEW

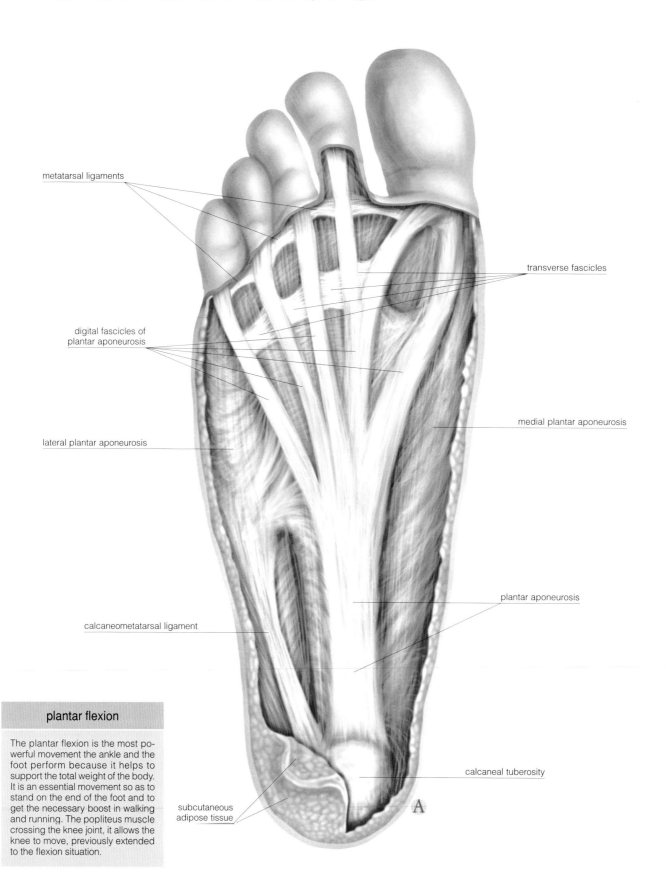

metatarsal ligaments

transverse fascicles

digital fascicles of
plantar aponeurosis

medial plantar aponeurosis

lateral plantar aponeurosis

plantar aponeurosis

calcaneometatarsal ligament

calcaneal tuberosity

subcutaneous
adipose tissue

plantar flexion

The plantar flexion is the most powerful movement the ankle and the foot perform because it helps to support the total weight of the body. It is an essential movement so as to stand on the end of the foot and to get the necessary boost in walking and running. The popliteus muscle crossing the knee joint, it allows the knee to move, previously extended to the flexion situation.

152

LOWER LIMB (XXXII). FOOT (VI)

RIGHT LOWER LIMB. PLANTAR SUPERFICIAL VIEW

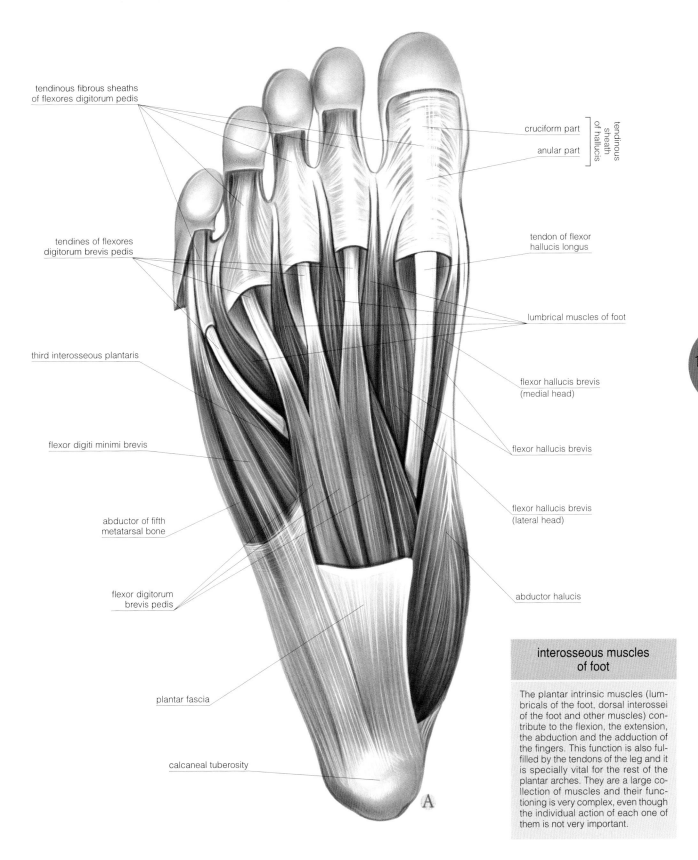

tendinous fibrous sheaths
of flexores digitorum pedis

cruciform part

anular part

tendinous sheath of hallucis

tendines of flexores
digitorum brevis pedis

tendon of flexor
hallucis longus

lumbrical muscles of foot

third interosseous plantaris

flexor hallucis brevis
(medial head)

flexor hallucis brevis

flexor digiti minimi brevis

flexor hallucis brevis
(lateral head)

abductor of fifth
metatarsal bone

flexor digitorum
brevis pedis

abductor halucis

plantar fascia

calcaneal tuberosity

A

interosseous muscles of foot

The plantar intrinsic muscles (lumbricals of the foot, dorsal interossei of the foot and other muscles) contribute to the flexion, the extension, the abduction and the adduction of the fingers. This function is also fulfilled by the tendons of the leg and it is specially vital for the rest of the plantar arches. They are a large collection of muscles and their functioning is very complex, even though the individual action of each one of them is not very important.

LOWER LIMB (XXXIII). FOOT (VII)

RIGHT LOWER LIMB. PLANTAR INTERMEDIATE VIEW

physiology of plantar muscles

During erect position, plantar muscles work together as a group to maintain the arches of the foot. Its main function is to endure the forces trying to reduce the longitudinal arch when the weight is received on the heel line, at the posterior end of the arch; this weight is transferred to the posterior plantar prominence and to the big toe. These group of muscles get mainly activated during the last phase of the movement to obtain the stability of the foot and then initiate the propulsion, just in the moment the forces try to get flat the transverse arch of the foot. They also adjust the efforts of the long muscles, thus causing pronation and supination and letting the foot adapts to an uneven surface.

154

tendon of flexor hallucis longus

tendines of flexor digitorum longus

tendines of flexor digitorum brevis

sesamoid bone

lumbricals

flexor hallucis brevis (lateral head)

flexor hallucis brevis

tendon of abductor hallucis

flexor hallucis brevis (medial head)

tendon of extensor hallucis longus

tendon of flexor digitorum longus

abductor hallucis

flexor digitorum brevis

calcaneal tuberocity

tendinous sheath of toes

plantar interosseous

flexor digiti minimi brevis of foot

fourth dorsal interosseous

abductor digiti minimi

quadratus plantae

flexor digitorum brevis

plantar aponeurosis

A

LOWER LIMB (XXXIV). FOOT (VIII)

RIGHT LOWER LIMB. PLANTAR DEEP VIEW

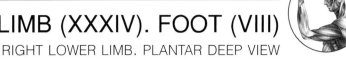

plantar muscle groups

The plantar muscles of the foot form three groups: big toe muscles, little (5th) toe muscles, which are in the lateral region of the sole; and finally the muscles of the plantar medial region. These three groups are divided by three compartments. In the plantar medial region is the flexor digitorum brevis, that corresponds to the flexor digititorum superficialis of the fingers in the forearm; the layout of the tendons is very similar in both cases.

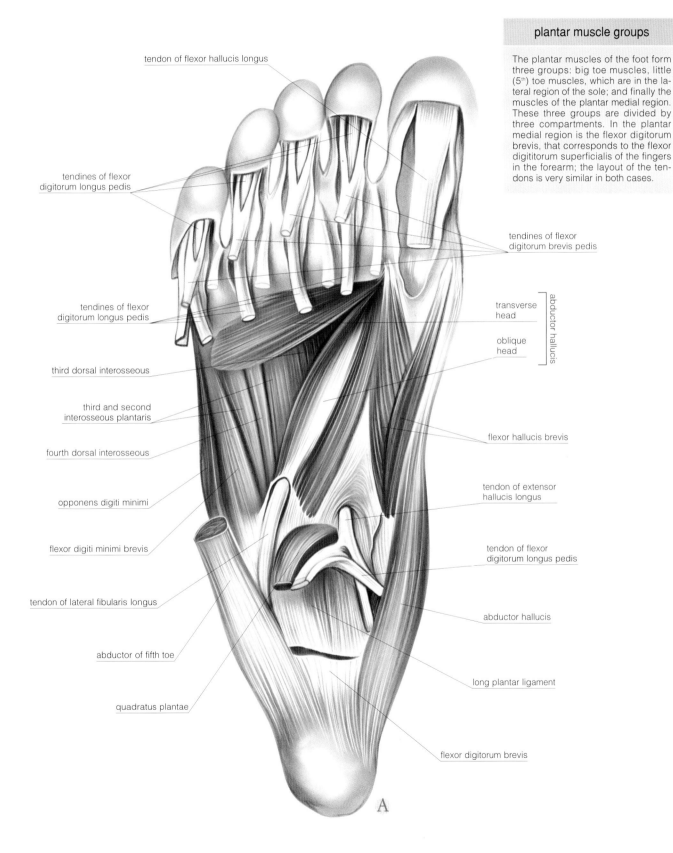

tendon of flexor hallucis longus

tendines of flexor digitorum longus pedis

tendines of flexor digitorum longus pedis

third dorsal interosseous

third and second interosseous plantaris

fourth dorsal interosseous

opponens digiti minimi

flexor digiti minimi brevis

tendon of lateral fibularis longus

abductor of fifth toe

quadratus plantae

tendines of flexor digitorum brevis pedis

transverse head

oblique head

abductor hallucis

flexor hallucis brevis

tendon of extensor hallucis longus

tendon of flexor digitorum longus pedis

abductor hallucis

long plantar ligament

flexor digitorum brevis

A

155

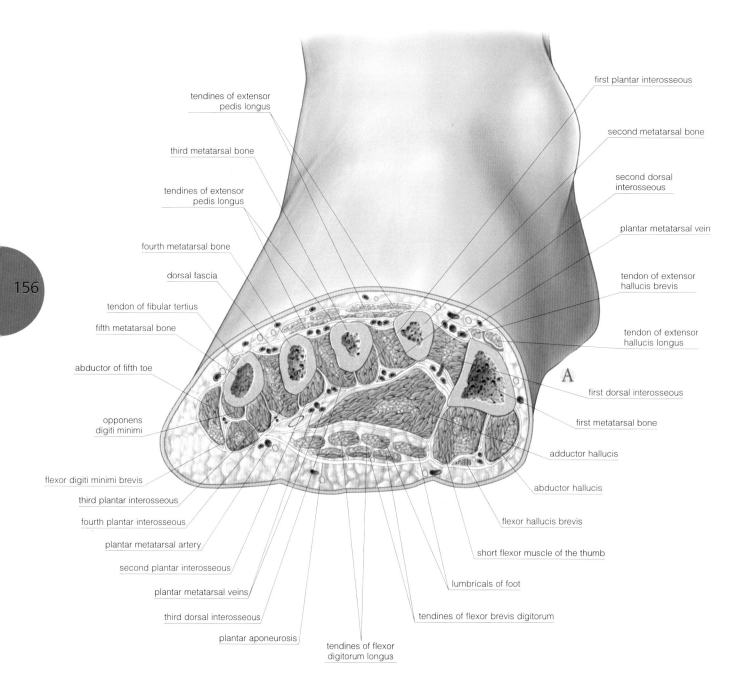

tendines of extensor pedis longus

third metatarsal bone

tendines of extensor pedis longus

fourth metatarsal bone

dorsal fascia

tendon of fibular tertius

fifth metatarsal bone

abductor of fifth toe

opponens digiti minimi

flexor digiti minimi brevis

third plantar interosseous

fourth plantar interosseous

plantar metatarsal artery

second plantar interosseous

plantar metatarsal veins

third dorsal interosseous

plantar aponeurosis

tendines of flexor digitorum longus

tendines of flexor brevis digitorum

lumbricals of foot

short flexor muscle of the thumb

flexor hallucis brevis

abductor hallucis

adductor hallucis

first metatarsal bone

first dorsal interosseous

tendon of extensor hallucis longus

tendon of extensor hallucis brevis

plantar metatarsal vein

second dorsal interosseous

second metatarsal bone

first plantar interosseous

A

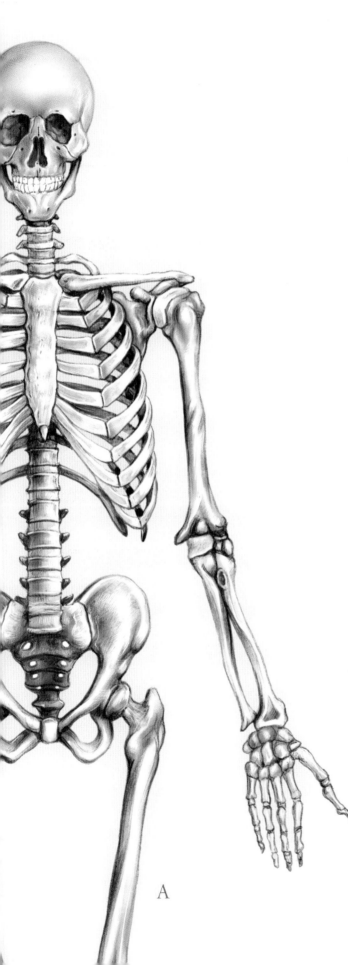

SKELETAL SYSTEM

As skeleton is known the collection of hard and resistant osseous pieces that made up the basic structure which the organism is assembled and organized over and as a consequence this organism is provided with stiffness and solidity. So, this structure is the support of muscles and mobile organs, it protects the soft parts, it holds the weight of the systems and many organs, and besides protection it makes possible, along with muscles, cartilages, ligaments and etc., the articulation of the human body as a whole and of its different parts in a wide range of movements thanks to the combined action of all these elements together.

The human body has a large amount of bones, a total 206, with very original and specific forms. Thus, there are long bones and short ones, small bones and flat ones. Each one of them has a design in accordance with the function it is appointed to.

The human skeleton may be divided into the following groups: skull, spinal column, ribs and sternum, scapula girdle, pelvic girdle and the bones of the upper and lower limbs. It is also worth considering the existence of some groups of bones arranged in a specific way in order to form cavities to protect vital organs, like the skull, where lays the brain, cerebellum, and other organs of nervous central system; or the thoracic cage, where other vital organs appear, like the heart and the lungs.

If the microscopic structure of bone tissue is examined, one can state that it mainly presents three cellular types which characterize it: osteoblasts, osteocytes, and osteoclasts. These three cellular components are in charge of creating, mineralizing and remodeling the abundant extracellular matrix which gives rigidity to this tissue. At the same time, they enable the bone to be a plastic tissue with capacity to recover. The most abundant components of this ossified or mineralized extracellular matrix will be calcium and phosphorous crystals. All of these mentioned processes would not be possible without the broad vascularization present in bones.

The bones of a newborn baby are very spongy because of the high levels of red bone marrow. But soon after it begins the ossification process which is faster in the long bones (femur, humerus, tibia, etc.). Bones play an important role during the growing process, which takes place by the effect of some hormones during childhood and adolescence. When an adult reaches 40 year age, it begins a degenerative process and the osseous mass starts a progressive phase of impoverishment that will continue up to the death of the individual. This will cause a reduction in the height of the body and it will render it more vulnerable when facing various diseases (osteoporosis, arthrosis, fractures, etc.).

A

LONG BONE (I). STRUCTURE (I)

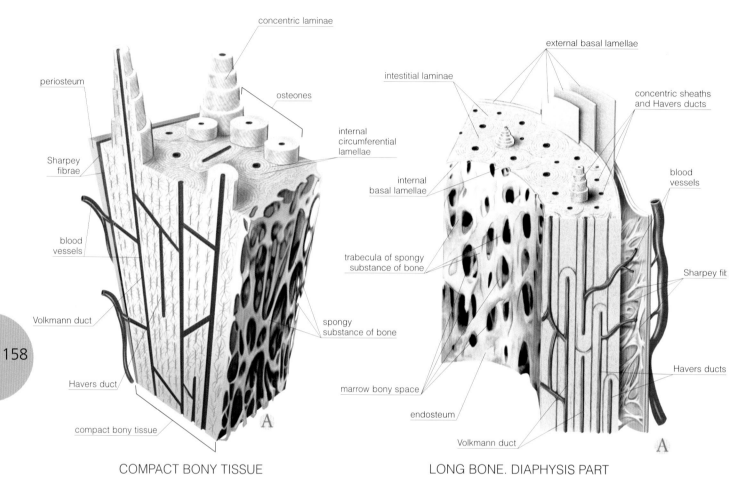

concentric laminae

external basal lamellae

intestitial laminae

periosteum

osteones

concentric sheaths
and Havers ducts

internal
circumferential
lamellae

Sharpey
fibrae

internal
basal lamellae

blood
vessels

blood
vessels

trabecula of spongy
substance of bone

Sharpey fib

Volkmann duct

spongy
substance of bone

Havers ducts

marrow bony space

endosteum

Havers duct

compact bony tissue

Volkmann duct

COMPACT BONY TISSUE

LONG BONE. DIAPHYSIS PART

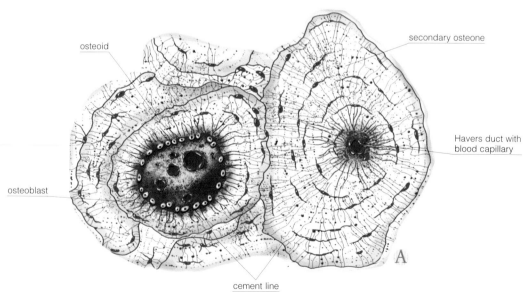

osteoid

secondary osteone

osteoblast

Havers duct with
blood capillary

cement line

DEVELOPMENT of HAVERS SYSTEM
(secondary osteone)

158

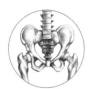

LONG BONE (II). STRUCTURE (II)

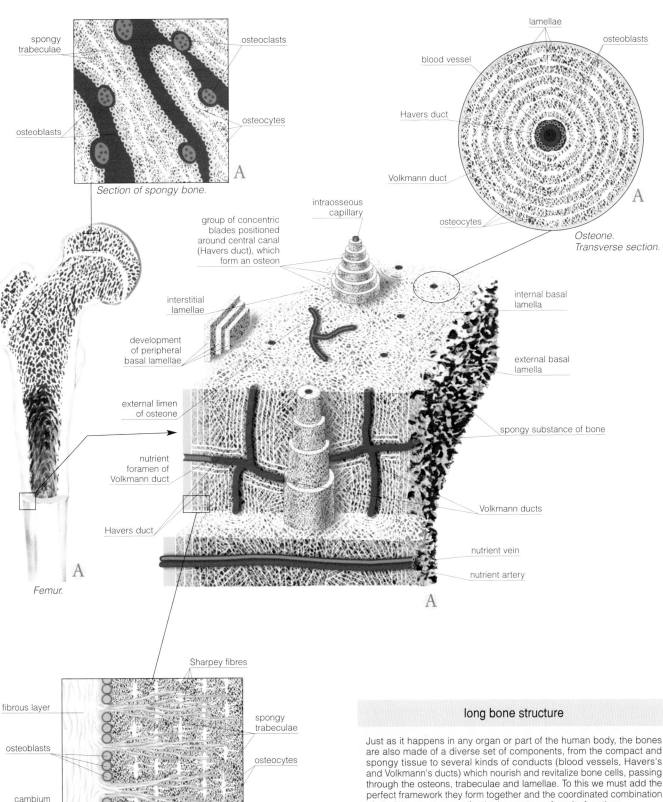

spongy trabeculae

osteoblasts

osteoclasts

osteocytes

Section of spongy bone.

lamellae

osteoblasts

blood vessel

Havers duct

Volkmann duct

osteocytes

*Osteone.
Transverse section.*

intraosseous capillary

group of concentric blades positioned around central canal (Havers duct), which form an osteon

interstitial lamellae

development of peripheral basal lamellae

external limen of osteone

nutrient foramen of Volkmann duct

Havers duct

internal basal lamella

external basal lamella

spongy substance of bone

Volkmann ducts

nutrient vein

nutrient artery

Femur.

Sharpey fibres

fibrous layer

spongy trabeculae

osteoblasts

osteocytes

cambium

periosteum   spongy substance of bone

159

long bone structure

Just as it happens in any organ or part of the human body, the bones are also made of a diverse set of components, from the compact and spongy tissue to several kinds of conducts (blood vessels, Havers's and Volkmann's ducts) which nourish and revitalize bone cells, passing through the osteons, trabeculae and lamellae. To this we must add the perfect framework they form together and the coordinated combination of all of these structures for the bones to perform its functions.

Source: Schunke, Schulte & Schumacher (2005). *General Anatomy and Musculoskeletal System.*

LONG BONE(V). PARTS and CONSTITUENTS

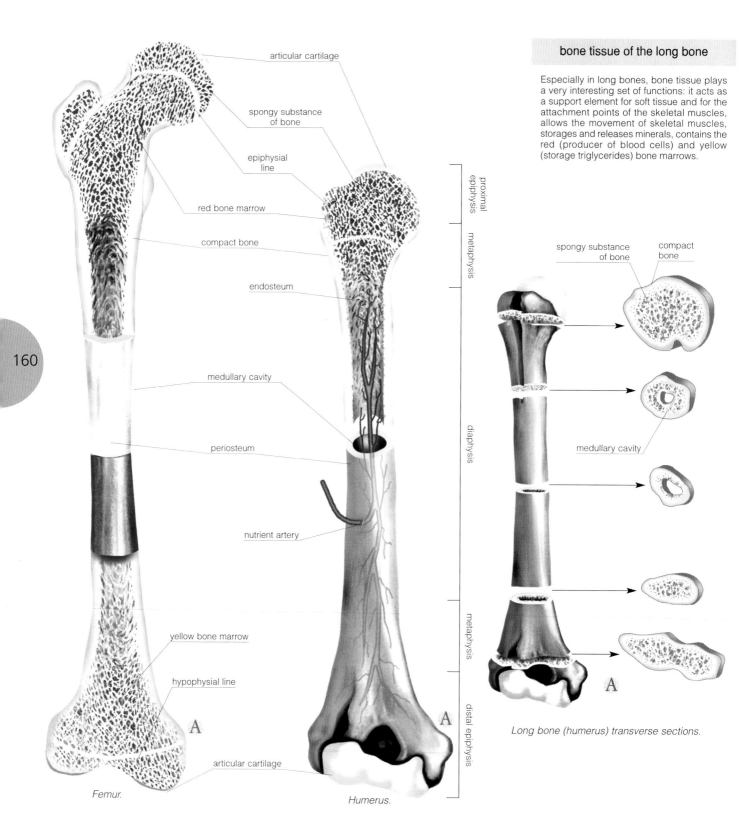

articular cartilage

spongy substance of bone

epiphysial line

red bone marrow

compact bone

endosteum

medullary cavity

periosteum

nutrient artery

yellow bone marrow

hypophysial line

articular cartilage

proximal epiphysis

metaphysis

diaphysis

metaphysis

distal epiphysis

A

Femur.

Humerus.

bone tissue of the long bone

Especially in long bones, bone tissue plays a very interesting set of functions: it acts as a support element for soft tissue and for the attachment points of the skeletal muscles, allows the movement of skeletal muscles, storages and releases minerals, contains the red (producer of blood cells) and yellow (storage triglycerides) bone marrows.

spongy substance of bone

compact bone

medullary cavity

A

Long bone (humerus) transverse sections.

BONE TYPES

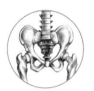

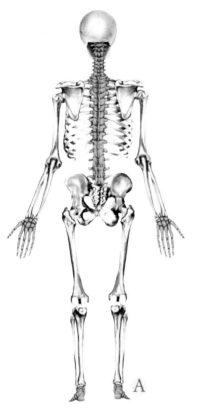

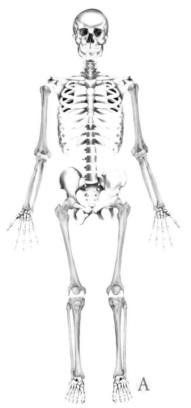

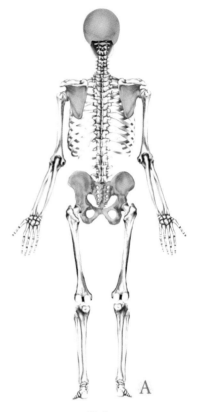

short bone

These are small bones which dimensions are practically the same. Their shape is cuboid. They are resistant and allow a great variety of mobility. Although these are not too wide, guarantee certain accuracy and safety. Short bones are the vertebrae, carpal bone (trapeze, trapezoid, scaphoid, capitation, crescent, unciform, pyramidal and pisiform) and tarsus bones (calcaneo, navicular, astragalus and cuboid) and cuneiforms.

long bone

They are the ones that length predominates over then width and thickness. They are the ones that form the skeleton of upper and lower members and allow a great variety of movements, for that reason is that their extremes (or epiphyses) show some special forms (concave or convex) which allow the bones to unite and articulate with the extremes of other neighbors bones. Among large bones are highlighted humerus, ulna and radius in the upper member, and femur, tibia and fibula in lower member.

wide bone

Wide bones are the ones that width predominates over thickness and height. Their external shape is flattened and smooth. Their common function is to form a cavity in order to be able to host and protect vital organs. Bones which form cranial cavity are flattened (frontal, occipital, temporal and parietal), where the brain is hosted, or chest cavity (ribs and sternum), where the heart is located, and also the scapula, which protects lungs.

carpal bones

calcaneum

talus

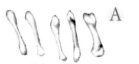

metatarsal bones

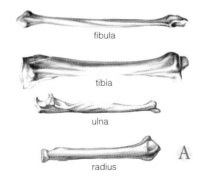

fibula

tibia

ulna

radius

hip bone

scapula

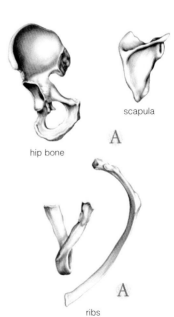

ribs

bone types

It is commonly said that the function makes the organ, this saying may be also applied to the shapes, specially in the case of bones. In the human body there are 206 bones, that may be classified according to three typologies, however there could be a lot more classifications. Each bones has specific shape and size in order to perfectly fit the function it has been appointed to. So, while femur may reach more that 50 centimeters, the little bones of the ear are just a few millimeters long. Regarding this subject, the human body has an unusual ability for adaptation; an excellent hint of this is that the evolution of the human species and the change of habits have caused the disappearance of certain bones (for examples, the ones forming the tail, that now they do not exist anymore) and the change of others (this is the case of the sacrum, that after initially being a group of five independent vertebrae has turned into a unique bone which components have ended knitted one to the other).

BONES of HEAD

162

EXTERNAL VIEW

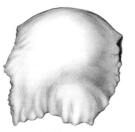

parietal bone

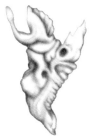

temporal bone

zygomaticus

lacrimal bone

incus   malleus   stapes   palatlne bone

concha

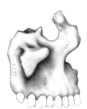

maxilla

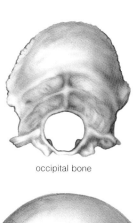

occipital bone

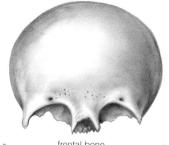

frontal bone

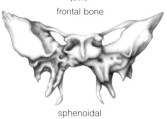

sphenoidal

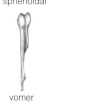

vomer

ethmoidal bone

nasal bones

hyoid bone

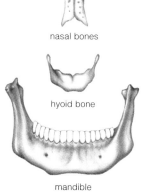

mandible

ANTERIOR VIEW

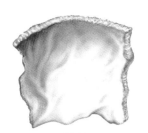

parietal bone

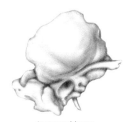

temporal bone

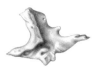

zygomaticus

lacrimal bone

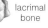

palatine bone   stapes   malleus   incus

concha

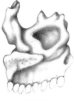

maxilla

A

BONES of TRUNK and LIMBS

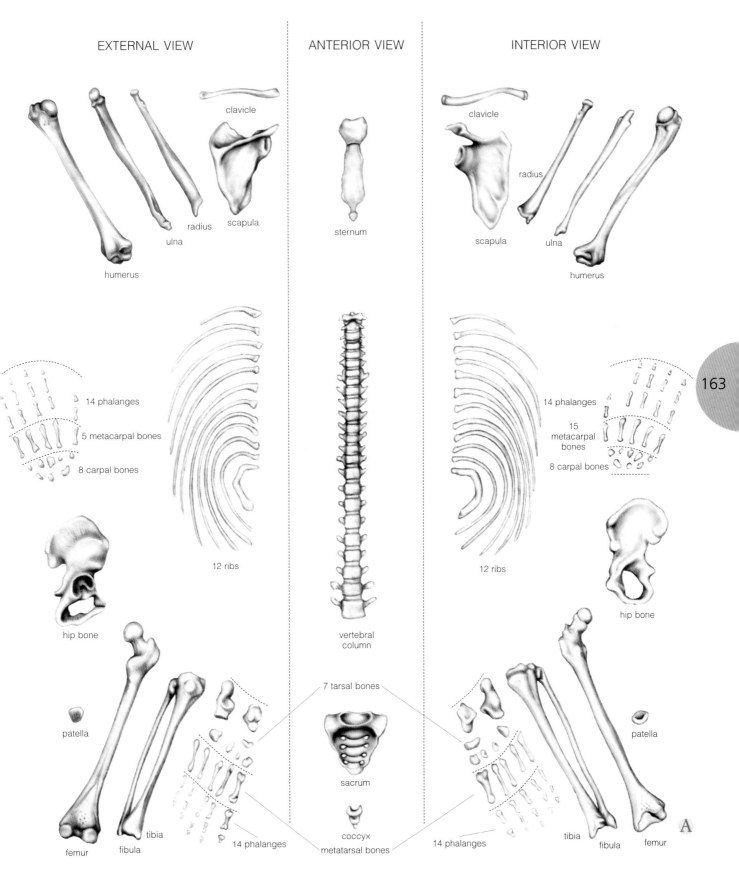

EXTERNAL VIEW

ANTERIOR VIEW

INTERIOR VIEW

clavicle

radius

ulna

scapula

humerus

sternum

clavicle

radius

scapula

ulna

humerus

14 phalanges

5 metacarpal bones

8 carpal bones

12 ribs

14 phalanges

15 metacarpal bones

8 carpal bones

12 ribs

163

hip bone

patella

femur

fibula

tibia

14 phalanges

vertebral column

7 tarsal bones

sacrum

coccyx

metatarsal bones

14 phalanges

hip bone

patella

tibia

fibula

femur

A

SKELETAL SYSTEM (I)
ANTERIOR GENERAL VIEW

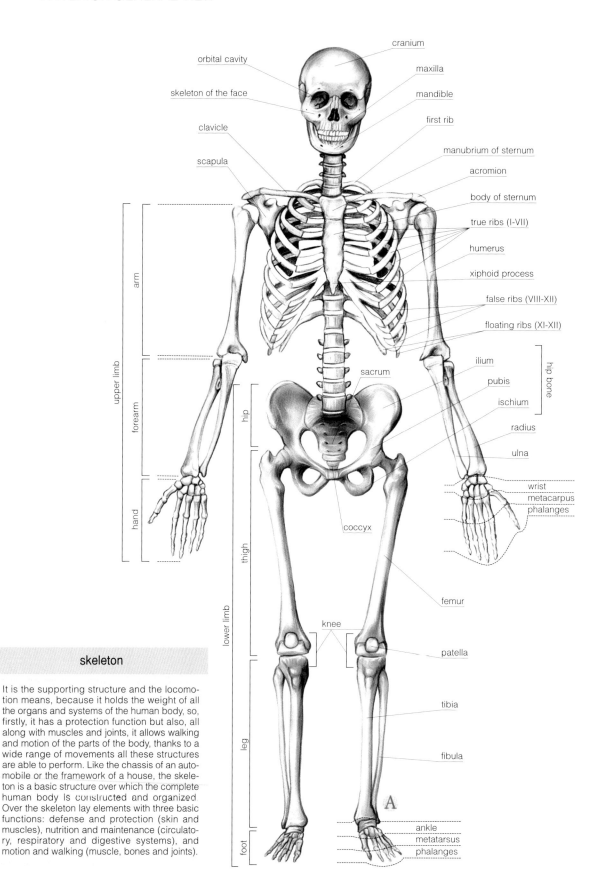

cranium

orbital cavity

maxilla

skeleton of the face

mandible

first rib

clavicle

manubrium of sternum

scapula

acromion

body of sternum

true ribs (I-VII)

arm

humerus

xiphoid process

false ribs (VIII-XII)

floating ribs (XI-XII)

upper limb

ilium

sacrum

pubis

hip bone

ischium

forearm

radius

ulna

hip

wrist

metacarpus

phalanges

hand

coccyx

thigh

femur

lower limb

knee

patella

tibia

fibula

leg

A

skeleton

ankle

metatarsus

phalanges

foot

skeleton

It is the supporting structure and the locomotion means, because it holds the weight of all the organs and systems of the human body, so, firstly, it has a protection function but also, all along with muscles and joints, it allows walking and motion of the parts of the body, thanks to a wide range of movements all these structures are able to perform. Like the chassis of an automobile or the framework of a house, the skeleton is a basic structure over which the complete human body is constructed and organized Over the skeleton lay elements with three basic functions: defense and protection (skin and muscles), nutrition and maintenance (circulatory, respiratory and digestive systems), and motion and walking (muscle, bones and joints).

164

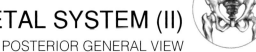

SKELETAL SYSTEM (II)
POSTERIOR GENERAL VIEW

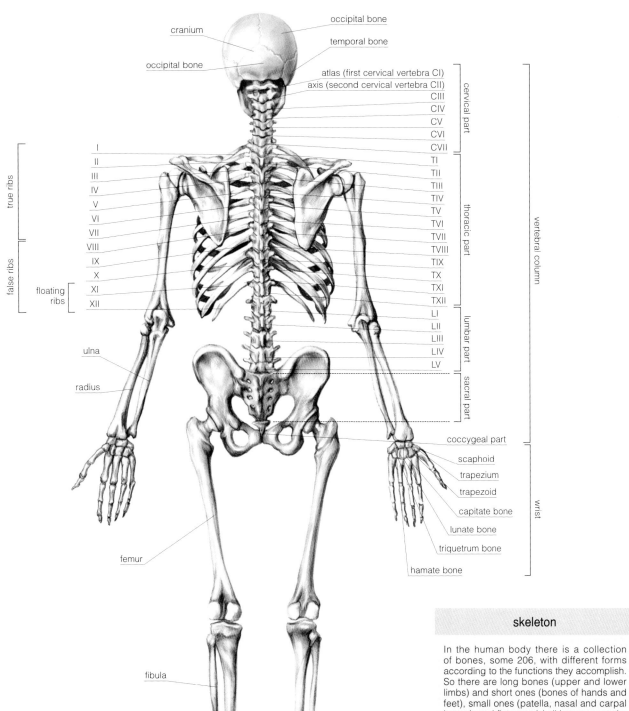

cranium

occipital bone

temporal bone

occipital bone

atlas (first cervical vertebra CI)
axis (second cervical vertebra CII)
CIII
CIV
CV
CVI
CVII

cervical part

true ribs

I
II
III
IV
V
VI
VII
VIII
IX
X
XI
XII

false ribs

floating ribs

TI
TII
TIII
TIV
TV
TVI
TVII
TVIII
TIX
TX
TXI
TXII

thoracic part

LI
LII
LIII
LIV
LV

lumbar part

sacral part

vertebral column

ulna

radius

coccygeal part

scaphoid

trapezium

trapezoid

capitate bone

lunate bone

triquetrum bone

hamate bone

wrist

femur

fibula

tibia

A

talus

calcaneus

165

skeleton

In the human body there is a collection of bones, some 206, with different forms according to the functions they accomplish. So there are long bones (upper and lower limbs) and short ones (bones of hands and feet), small ones (patella, nasal and carpal bones), and flat ones (skull bones, scapula, coccyx). Each one of them is perfectly designed accordingly to the function it fulfills. The bones of a new-born baby are very spongy because of the high levels of red bone marrow. But soon after birth it continues the ossification process which is faster in the long bones (femur, humerus, tibia, etc.). One of the signs of maturity is the presence of a secondary center of ossification in the femoral epiphysis.

CRANIUM (I)
ANTERIOR VIEW

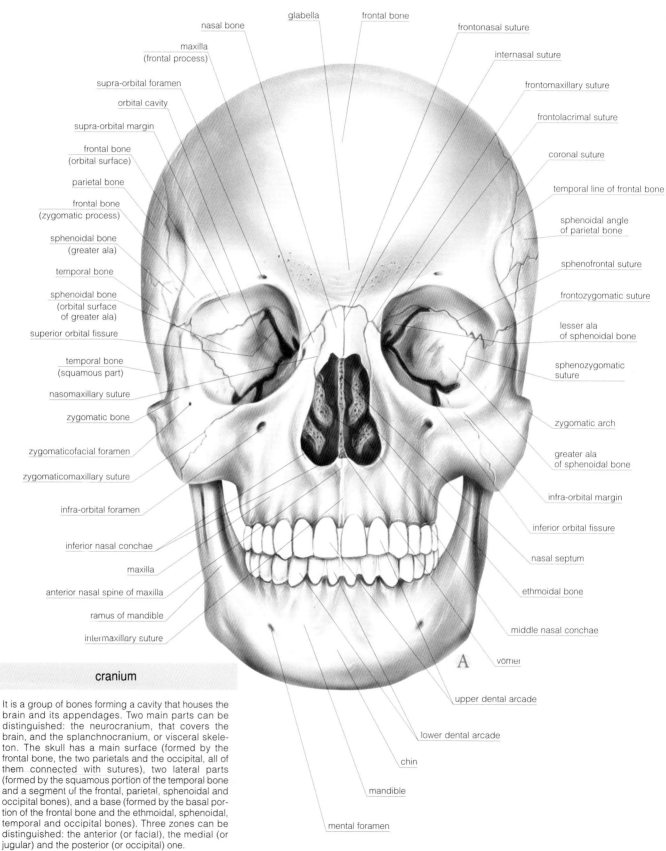

nasal bone

glabella

frontal bone

frontonasal suture

maxilla
(frontal process)

internasal suture

supra-orbital foramen

frontomaxillary suture

orbital cavity

frontolacrimal suture

supra-orbital margin

coronal suture

frontal bone
(orbital surface)

temporal line of frontal bone

parietal bone

sphenoidal angle
of parietal bone

frontal bone
(zygomatic process)

sphenoidal bone
(greater ala)

sphenofrontal suture

temporal bone

frontozygomatic suture

sphenoidal bone
(orbital surface
of greater ala)

lesser ala
of sphenoidal bone

superior orbital fissure

sphenozygomatic
suture

temporal bone
(squamous part)

nasomaxillary suture

zygomatic arch

zygomatic bone

greater ala
of sphenoidal bone

zygomaticofacial foramen

zygomaticomaxillary suture

infra-orbital margin

infra-orbital foramen

inferior orbital fissure

inferior nasal conchae

nasal septum

maxilla

ethmoidal bone

anterior nasal spine of maxilla

middle nasal conchae

ramus of mandible

intermaxillary suture

vomer

A

upper dental arcade

lower dental arcade

chin

mandible

mental foramen

166

cranium

It is a group of bones forming a cavity that houses the brain and its appendages. Two main parts can be distinguished: the neurocranium, that covers the brain, and the splanchnocranium, or visceral skeleton. The skull has a main surface (formed by the frontal bone, the two parietals and the occipital, all of them connected with sutures), two lateral parts (formed by the squamous portion of the temporal bone and a segment of the frontal, parietal, sphenoidal and occipital bones), and a base (formed by the basal portion of the frontal bone and the ethmoidal, sphenoidal, temporal and occipital bones). Three zones can be distinguished: the anterior (or facial), the medial (or jugular) and the posterior (or occipital) one.

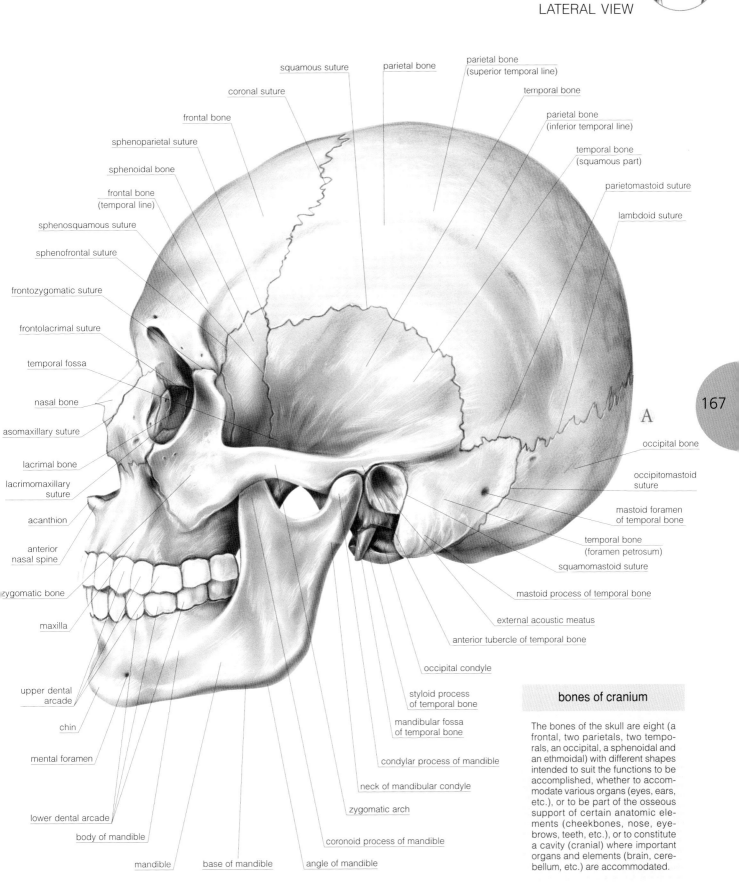

squamous suture

coronal suture

frontal bone

sphenoparietal suture

sphenoidal bone

frontal bone
(temporal line)

sphenosquamous suture

sphenofrontal suture

frontozygomatic suture

frontolacrimal suture

temporal fossa

nasal bone

asomaxillary suture

lacrimal bone

lacrimomaxillary
suture

acanthion

anterior
nasal spine

zygomatic bone

maxilla

upper dental
arcade

chin

mental foramen

lower dental arcade

body of mandible

mandible

parietal bone

parietal bone
(superior temporal line)

temporal bone

parietal bone
(inferior temporal line)

temporal bone
(squamous part)

parietomastoid suture

lambdoid suture

A

167

occipital bone

occipitomastoid
suture

mastoid foramen
of temporal bone

temporal bone
(foramen petrosum)

squamomastoid suture

mastoid process of temporal bone

external acoustic meatus

anterior tubercle of temporal bone

occipital condyle

styloid process
of temporal bone

mandibular fossa
of temporal bone

condylar process of mandible

neck of mandibular condyle

zygomatic arch

coronoid process of mandible

base of mandible

angle of mandible

bones of cranium

The bones of the skull are eight (a frontal, two parietals, two temporals, an occipital, a sphenoidal and an ethmoidal) with different shapes intended to suit the functions to be accomplished, whether to accommodate various organs (eyes, ears, etc.), or to be part of the osseous support of certain anatomic elements (cheekbones, nose, eyebrows, teeth, etc.), or to constitute a cavity (cranial) where important organs and elements (brain, cerebellum, etc.) are accommodated.

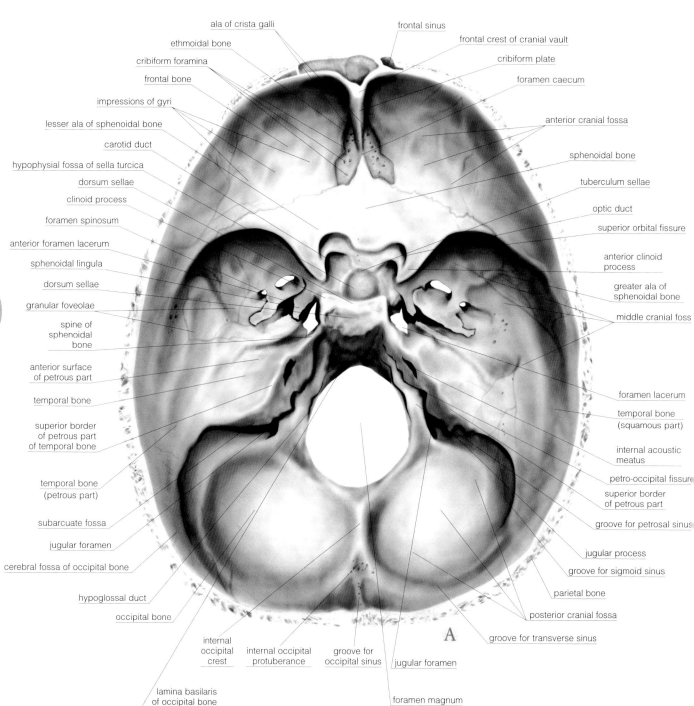

ala of crista galli
frontal sinus
ethmoidal bone
frontal crest of cranial vault
cribiform foramina
cribiform plate
frontal bone
foramen caecum
impressions of gyri
anterior cranial fossa
lesser ala of sphenoidal bone
carotid duct
sphenoidal bone
hypophysial fossa of sella turcica
tuberculum sellae
dorsum sellae
clinoid process
optic duct
foramen spinosum
superior orbital fissure
anterior foramen lacerum
anterior clinoid process
sphenoidal lingula
dorsum sellae
greater ala of sphenoidal bone
granular foveolae
middle cranial foss
spine of sphenoidal bone
anterior surface of petrous part
foramen lacerum
temporal bone
temporal bone (squamous part)
superior border of petrous part of temporal bone
internal acoustic meatus
temporal bone (petrous part)
petro-occipital fissure
superior border of petrous part
subarcuate fossa
groove for petrosal sinus
jugular foramen
jugular process
cerebral fossa of occipital bone
groove for sigmoid sinus
hypoglossal duct
parietal bone
occipital bone
posterior cranial fossa

A

internal occipital crest
internal occipital protuberance
groove for occipital sinus
jugular foramen
groove for transverse sinus

lamina basilaris of occipital bone
foramen magnum

CRANIUM (IV). BASE (II)
INFERIOR VIEW

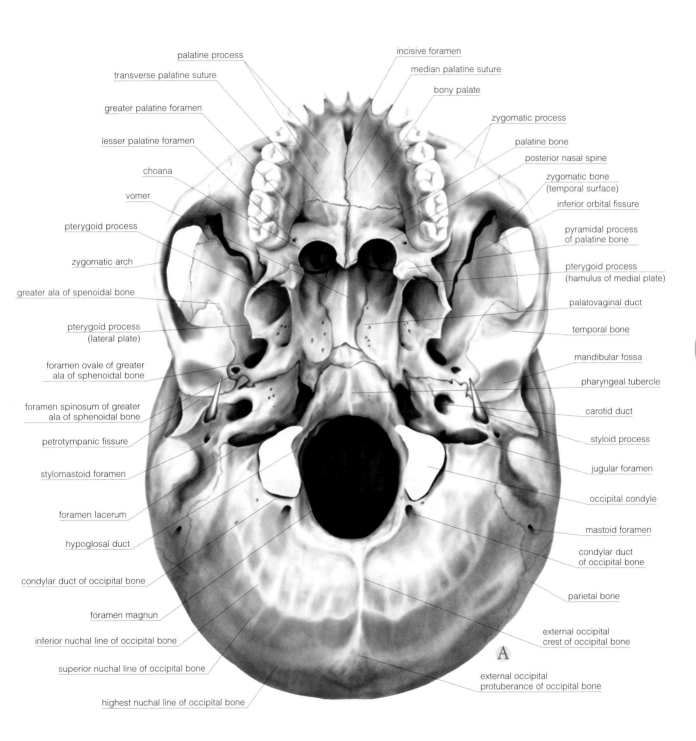

palatine process

incisive foramen

median palatine suture

transverse palatine suture

bony palate

greater palatine foramen

zygomatic process

palatine bone

lesser palatine foramen

posterior nasal spine

choana

zygomatic bone
(temporal surface)

vomer

inferior orbital fissure

pterygoid process

pyramidal process
of palatine bone

zygomatic arch

pterygoid process
(hamulus of medial plate)

greater ala of spenoidal bone

palatovaginal duct

pterygoid process
(lateral plate)

temporal bone

foramen ovale of greater
ala of sphenoidal bone

mandibular fossa

pharyngeal tubercle

foramen spinosum of greater
ala of sphenoidal bone

carotid duct

petrotympanic fissure

styloid process

stylomastoid foramen

jugular foramen

foramen lacerum

occipital condyle

hypoglosal duct

mastoid foramen

condylar duct of occipital bone

condylar duct
of occipital bone

foramen magnun

parietal bone

inferior nuchal line of occipital bone

external occipital
crest of occipital bone

superior nuchal line of occipital bone

A

highest nuchal line of occipital bone

external occipital
protuberance of occipital bone

169

CRANIUM (V). BASE (III). FORAMINA
ENDOCRANIAL VIEW

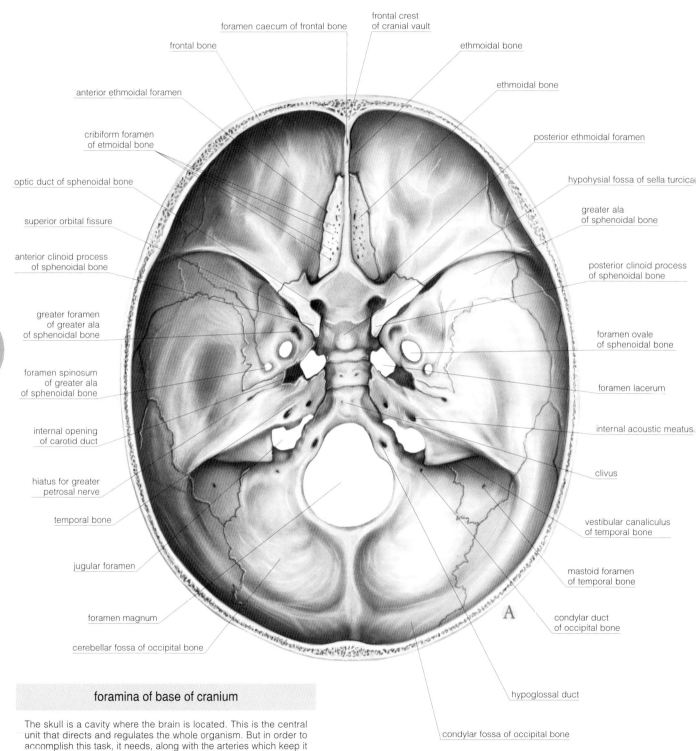

frontal crest
of cranial vault

foramen caecum of frontal bone

frontal bone

ethmoidal bone

ethmoidal bone

anterior ethmoidal foramen

posterior ethmoidal foramen

cribiform foramen
of etmoidal bone

hypohysial fossa of sella turcica

optic duct of sphenoidal bone

greater ala
of sphenoidal bone

superior orbital fissure

anterior clinoid process
of sphenoidal bone

posterior clinoid process
of sphenoidal bone

greater foramen
of greater ala
of sphenoidal bone

foramen ovale
of sphenoidal bone

foramen spinosum
of greater ala
of sphenoidal bone

foramen lacerum

internal opening
of carotid duct

internal acoustic meatus

hiatus for greater
petrosal nerve

clivus

temporal bone

vestibular canaliculus
of temporal bone

jugular foramen

mastoid foramen
of temporal bone

A

foramen magnum

condylar duct
of occipital bone

cerebellar fossa of occipital bone

hypoglossal duct

condylar fossa of occipital bone

foramina of base of cranium

The skull is a cavity where the brain is located. This is the central
unit that directs and regulates the whole organism. But in order to
accomplish this task, it needs, along with the arteries which keep it
alive and the veins that remove the waste materials, various nerves
that provide with the information needed and by this means getting
to know the impulses coming from all over the body and transmit the
orders of the timely answers. For all this, the skull is pierced by many
foramina which allow the pass of many structures, like arteries, veins
and nerves.

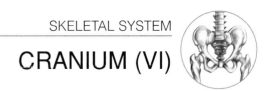

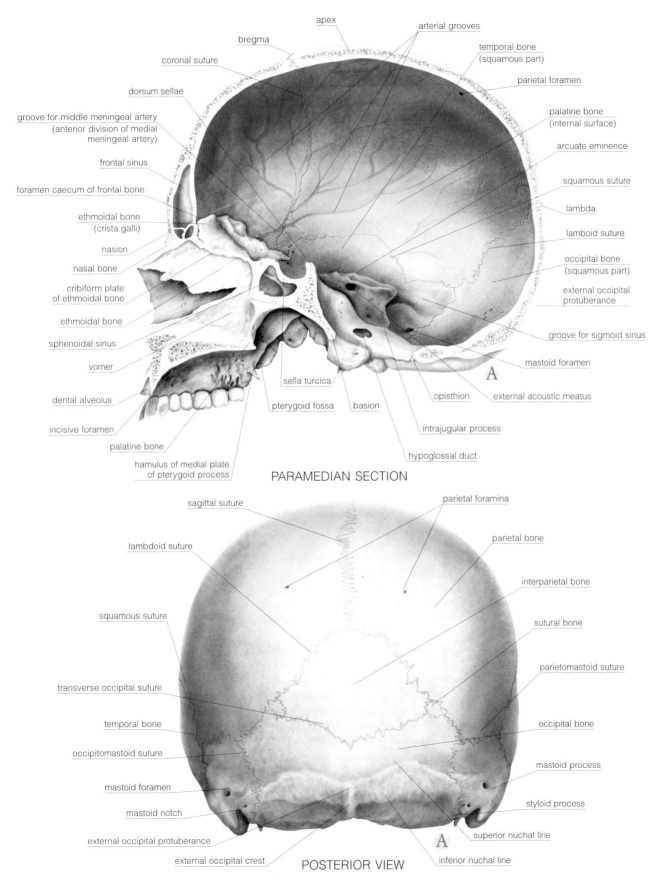

apex

bregma

arterial grooves

coronal suture

temporal bone
(squamous part)

parietal foramen

dorsum sellae

palatine bone
(internal surface)

groove for middle meningeal artery
(anterior division of medial
meningeal artery)

arcuate eminence

squamous suture

frontal sinus

lambda

foramen caecum of frontal bone

lamboid suture

ethmoidal bone
(crista galli)

occipital bone
(squamous part)

nasion

nasal bone

external occipital
protuberance

cribiform plate
of ethmoidal bone

ethmoidal bone

groove for sigmoid sinus

sphenoidal sinus

mastoid foramen

vomer

A

dental alveolus

sella turcica

opisthion

external acoustic meatus

incisive foramen

pterygoid fossa

basion

intrajugular process

palatine bone

hypoglossal duct

hamulus of medial plate
of pterygoid process

PARAMEDIAN SECTION

sagittal suture

parietal foramina

lambdoid suture

parietal bone

interparietal bone

squamous suture

sutural bone

parietomastoid suture

transverse occipital suture

temporal bone

occipital bone

occipitomastoid suture

mastoid process

mastoid foramen

styloid process

mastoid notch

external occipital protuberance

superior nuchal line

A

external occipital crest

inferior nuchal line

POSTERIOR VIEW

171

CRANIUM (VII)

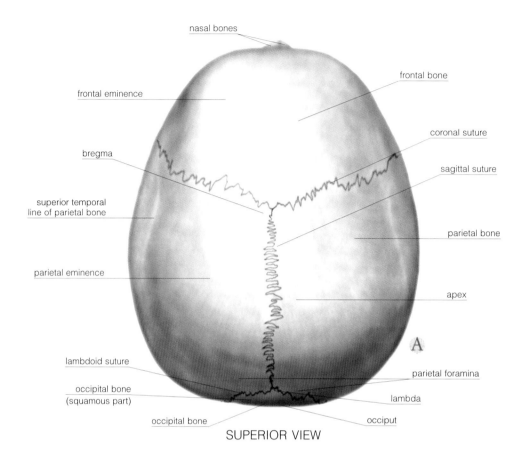

nasal bones

frontal bone

frontal eminence

coronal suture

bregma

sagittal suture

superior temporal
line of parietal bone

parietal bone

parietal eminence

apex

lambdoid suture

parietal foramina

occipital bone
(squamous part)

lambda

occipital bone

occiput

SUPERIOR VIEW

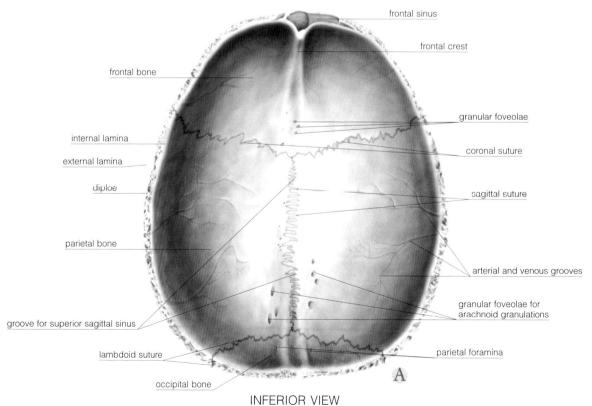

frontal sinus

frontal crest

frontal bone

granular foveolae

internal lamina

coronal suture

external lamina

diploe

sagittal suture

parietal bone

arterial and venous grooves

groove for superior sagittal sinus

granular foveolae for
arachnoid granulations

lambdoid suture

parietal foramina

occipital bone

INFERIOR VIEW

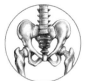

CRANIUM (VIII). FRONTAL BONE

frontal bone

It is an unpaired and flat bone that shapes the forehead and works as the osseous base of the anterior part of the brain. It is primitively formed by two halves with a separation line that is sometimes perceptible, even in adult individuals. It has a primary ossification point on about the 50th day of the life of the embryo and another six complementary points. The anterior part is a convex surface corresponding to the forehead. At the back it forms a cavity, the cranial cavity, that figures the fossae that accommodates the frontal lobes. At the back and sideways is linked with the parietal and sphenoidal bones, and at the inferior part with the zygomatic, maxilla, nasal and ethmoid bones, all of them forming the roof of the orbital cavity.

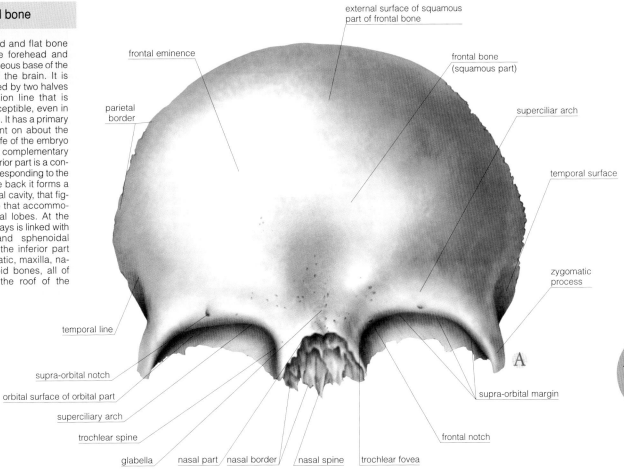

external surface of squamous part of frontal bone

frontal bone (squamous part)

frontal eminence

superciliar arch

parietal border

temporal surface

zygomatic process

temporal line

supra-orbital notch

orbital surface of orbital part

superciliary arch

trochlear spine

glabella

nasal part / nasal border / nasal spine

trochlear fovea

frontal notch

supra-orbital margin

ANTERIOR VIEW

173

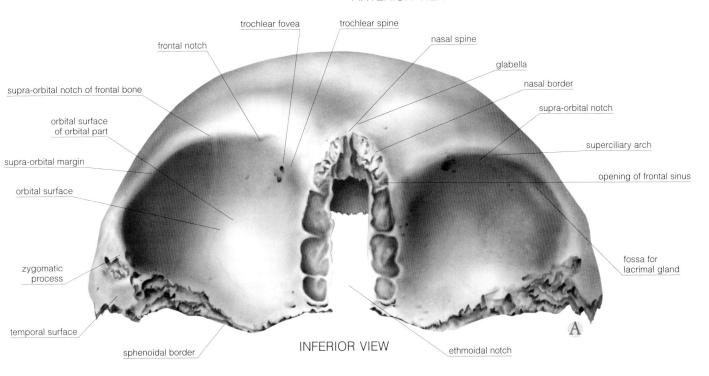

trochlear fovea

trochlear spine

nasal spine

frontal notch

glabella

nasal border

supra-orbital notch of frontal bone

supra-orbital notch

orbital surface of orbital part

superciliary arch

supra-orbital margin

opening of frontal sinus

orbital surface

zygomatic process

fossa for lacrimal gland

temporal surface

sphenoidal border

ethmoidal notch

INFERIOR VIEW

CRANIUM (IX). PARIETAL BONE

parietal bone

The parietal bones are two flat and symmetric bones of intramembranous origin and square-shape, closing the cranial cavity both sides. At the superior border, they join between them by means of the interparietal or saggittal suture. Anteriorly they join with the frontal bone, posteriorly they do with the occipital bone, and inferiorly with temporal and sphenoidal bones. Its external surface is rounded and it has an eminence, while its interior surface has a peculiar morphology known as figleaf, that is the consequence of the numerous furrows due to the ramifications of the middle meningeal artery.

sagittal border

sternal surface

parietal tuber

parietal foramen

occipital angle

frontal angle

frontal border

superior temporal line

inferior temporal line

occipital border

LEFT PARIETAL BONE LATERAL VIEW

mastoid angle

squamosal border

sphenoidal angle

A

174

sagittal border

internal surface

parietal foramen

groove for superior sagittal sinus

occipital angle

frontal angle

frontal border

occipital border

RIGHT PARIETAL BONE MEDIAL VIEW

groove for sigmoid sinus

groove for middle meningeal artery (anterior division of medial meningeal artery)

sphenoidal angle

squamosal border

mastoid angle

groove for middle meningeal artery (posterior division of medial meningeal artery)

A

CRANIUM (X). OCCIPITAL BONE

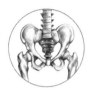

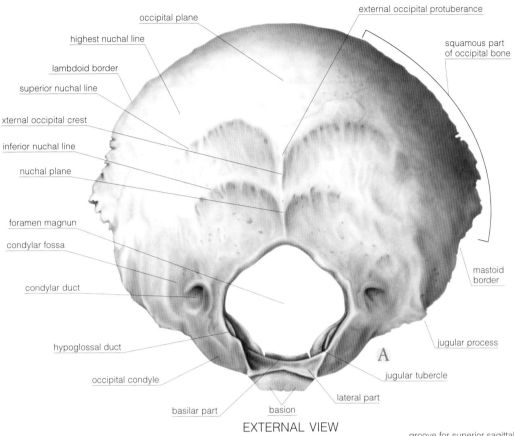

external occipital protuberance

occipital plane

highest nuchal line

lambdoid border

superior nuchal line

xternal occipital crest

inferior nuchal line

nuchal plane

foramen magnun

condylar fossa

condylar duct

hypoglossal duct

occipital condyle

basilar part

basion

squamous part
of occipital bone

mastoid
border

jugular process

jugular tubercle

lateral part

A

EXTERNAL VIEW

occipital bone

It is a flat and unpaired bone, with an irregular diamond shape, located at the back and lower part of the cranium, in a medial position, behind the sphenoidal bone and just above the atlas vertebra. It has two surfaces, one posterior-inferior and the other one anterior-superior, four borders and four angles. It is the posterior and inferior part of the cranium and it contains the occipital lobes of the brain and the cerebellum. It is pierced by the foramen magnum which is flanked by the condyles that articulate with the atlas. It is the joining point between the atlas vertebra and the spinal column and where the spinal cord gets out of the cranium. Some prevertebrae muscles get inserted in its jugular process and its basilar part. Also, it articulates with sphenoidal, parietal and temporal bones. From the second to the third month of intrauterine life, it has five main points of ossification: one at the basilar apophysis, two at the condylar regions and two in the squamous portion. It also has various secondary points.

175

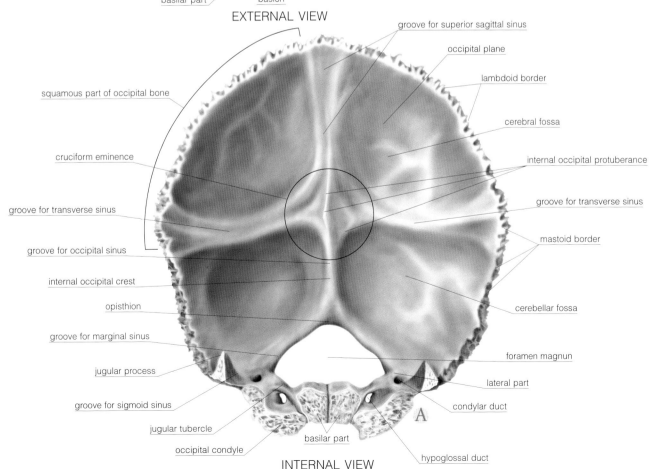

groove for superior sagittal sinus

occipital plane

lambdoid border

cerebral fossa

squamous part of occipital bone

internal occipital protuberance

cruciform eminence

groove for transverse sinus

groove for transverse sinus

mastoid border

groove for occipital sinus

internal occipital crest

opisthion

cerebellar fossa

groove for marginal sinus

jugular process

foramen magnun

lateral part

groove for sigmoid sinus

condylar duct

jugular tubercle

occipital condyle

basilar part

hypoglossal duct

A

INTERNAL VIEW

CRANIUM (XI). TEMPORAL BONE (I)

RIGHT TEMPORAL BONE. INFERIOR VIEW

temporal bone

It is an unpaired and complex bone that makes part of the cranial border and the floor of the cranium. It closes the lateral area of the cranium and protects the organs of the ear and of the balance. It is linked at the back with the occipital, at the top with the parietal, and at the front with the sphenoidal and the mandible. From an anatomic point of view, it can be divided in four portions: mastoid and petrous portions that make part of the auditive organ), squamous (that makes part of the cranial vault), and the tympanic part. It has also four main ossification points: one for the squama, other for petrous part, a third one for the tympanic ring, and finally the styloid process. It has also various secondary points.

- sphenoidal border
- articular tubercle
- musculotubaric duct
- apex of petrous part
- zygomatic process
- internal opening of carotid duct
- mandibular fossa
- petrotympanic fissure
- styloid process
- sheath of stiloid process
- external acoustic meatus
- duct of facial nerve
- external opening of carotid duct
- mastoid process
- intrajugular process
- petrosal fossula
- occipital groove
- jugular fossa
- tympanic part
- mastoid notch
- occipital border
- mastoid foramen

A

176

CRANIUM (XII). TEMPORAL BONE (II)

RIGHT TEMPORAL BONE

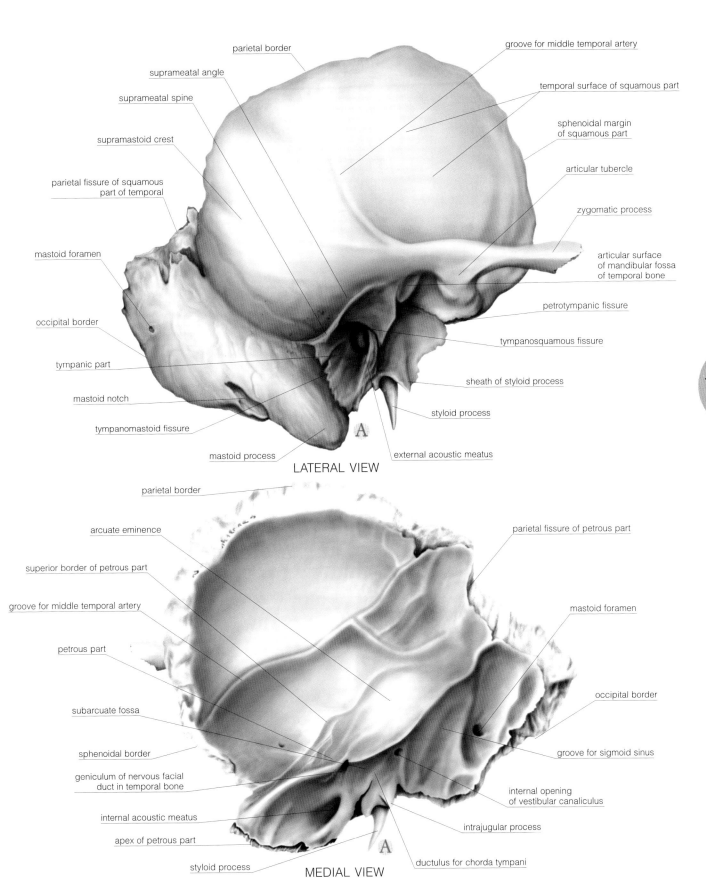

parietal border

suprameatal angle

suprameatal spine

supramastoid crest

parietal fissure of squamous part of temporal

mastoid foramen

occipital border

tympanic part

mastoid notch

tympanomastoid fissure

mastoid process

groove for middle temporal artery

temporal surface of squamous part

sphenoidal margin of squamous part

articular tubercle

zygomatic process

articular surface of mandibular fossa of temporal bone

petrotympanic fissure

tympanosquamous fissure

sheath of styloid process

styloid process

external acoustic meatus

A

LATERAL VIEW

177

parietal border

arcuate eminence

superior border of petrous part

groove for middle temporal artery

petrous part

subarcuate fossa

sphenoidal border

geniculum of nervous facial duct in temporal bone

internal acoustic meatus

apex of petrous part

styloid process

parietal fissure of petrous part

mastoid foramen

occipital border

groove for sigmoid sinus

internal opening of vestibular canaliculus

intrajugular process

ductulus for chorda tympani

A

MEDIAL VIEW

CRANIUM (XIII). TEMPORAL BONE (III)

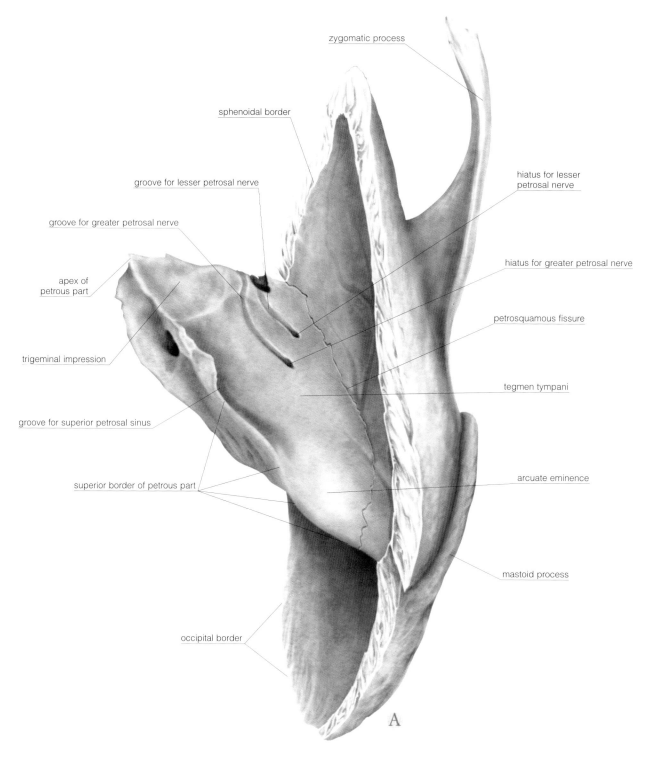

zygomatic process

sphenoidal border

groove for lesser petrosal nerve

groove for greater petrosal nerve

apex of
petrous part

trigeminal impression

groove for superior petrosal sinus

superior border of petrous part

occipital border

hiatus for lesser
petrosal nerve

hiatus for greater petrosal nerve

petrosquamous fissure

tegmen tympani

arcuate eminence

mastoid process

A

SUPERIOR VIEW

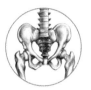

CRANIUM (XIV). ETHMOIDAL BONE

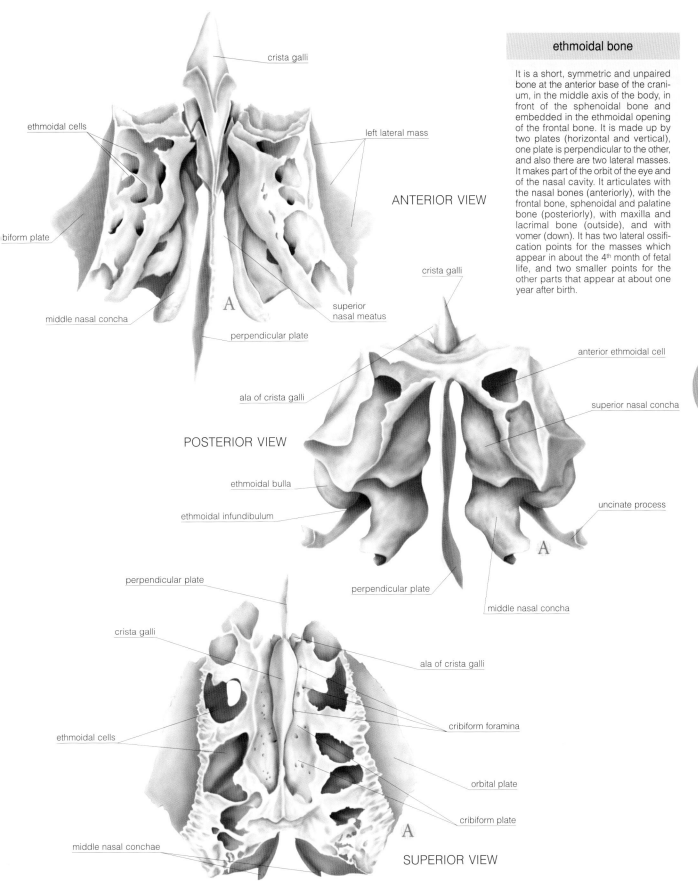

crista galli

ethmoidal cells

left lateral mass

ANTERIOR VIEW

biform plate

middle nasal concha

superior
nasal meatus

perpendicular plate

ethmoidal bone

It is a short, symmetric and unpaired bone at the anterior base of the cranium, in the middle axis of the body, in front of the sphenoidal bone and embedded in the ethmoidal opening of the frontal bone. It is made up by two plates (horizontal and vertical), one plate is perpendicular to the other, and also there are two lateral masses. It makes part of the orbit of the eye and of the nasal cavity. It articulates with the nasal bones (anteriorly), with the frontal bone, sphenoidal and palatine bone (posteriorly), with maxilla and lacrimal bone (outside), and with vomer (down). It has two lateral ossification points for the masses which appear in about the 4th month of fetal life, and two smaller points for the other parts that appear at about one year after birth.

179

crista galli

anterior ethmoidal cell

superior nasal concha

ala of crista galli

POSTERIOR VIEW

ethmoidal bulla

ethmoidal infundibulum

uncinate process

perpendicular plate

middle nasal concha

perpendicular plate

crista galli

ala of crista galli

cribiform foramina

ethmoidal cells

orbital plate

cribiform plate

middle nasal conchae

SUPERIOR VIEW

CRANIUM (XV). SPHENOIDAL BONE (I)

sphenoidal bone

Short and unpaired bone with a form evoking an extended-wing bat. It is located in the median and inferior zone of the cranium. It articulates with parietal and ethmoidal bones (anteriorly), with the occipital (posteriorly), with parietal and temporal bones (both sides), with zygomatic (anteriorly and outside), and with palatine and vomer bones (down). It may be divided into three sections; central one (body of sphenoidal bone), anterior (alae of sphenoidal), and the external one (pterygoid processes of the sphenoides). The anterior part contains four points of ossification and the posterior one eight points. These points appear from the 3rd to 7th month of foetal life.

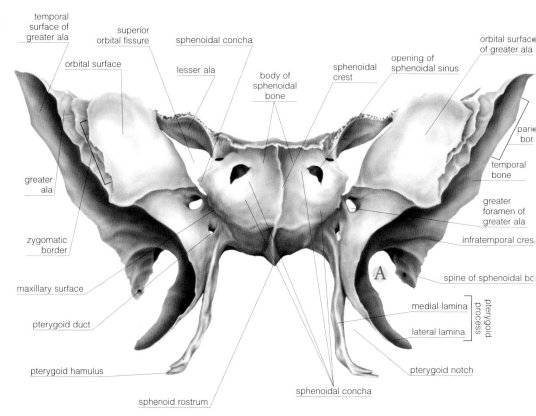

temporal surface of greater ala
superior orbital fissure
sphenoidal concha
orbital surface of greater ala
orbital surface
lesser ala
body of sphenoidal bone
sphenoidal crest
opening of sphenoidal sinus
parietal bone
greater ala
temporal bone
greater foramen of greater ala
zygomatic border
infratemporal crest
maxillary surface
spine of sphenoidal bone
medial lamina
lateral lamina
pterygoid process
pterygoid duct
pterygoid hamulus
pterygoid notch
sphenoidal concha
sphenoid rostrum

ANTERIOR VIEW

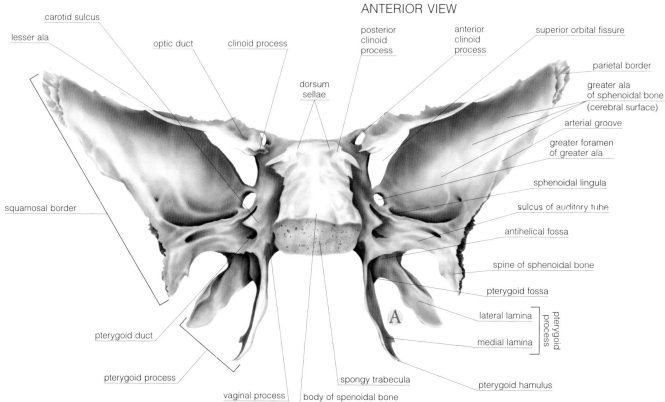

carotid sulcus
lesser ala
optic duct
clinoid process
posterior clinoid process
anterior clinoid process
superior orbital fissure
parietal border
greater ala of sphenoidal bone (cerebral surface)
dorsum sellae
arterial groove
greater foramen of greater ala
sphenoidal lingula
sulcus of auditory tube
squamosal border
antihelical fossa
spine of sphenoidal bone
pterygoid fossa
lateral lamina
medial lamina
pterygoid process
pterygoid duct
pterygoid process
vaginal process
spongy trabecula
body of spenoidal bone
pterygoid hamulus

POSTERIOR VIEW

CRANIUM (XVI). SPHENOIDAL BONE (II)

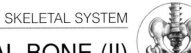

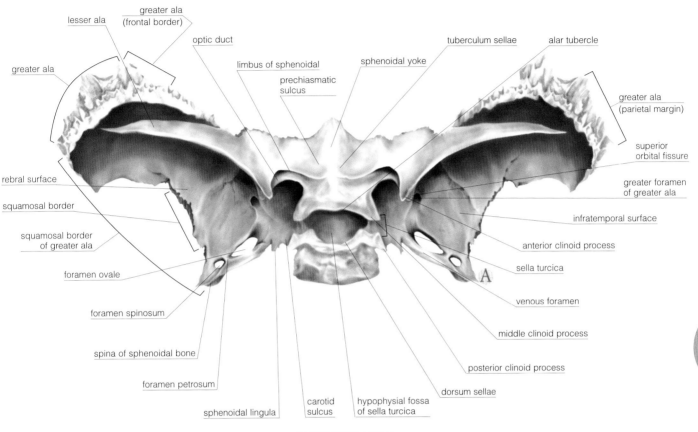

lesser ala

greater ala
(frontal border)

greater ala

optic duct

limbus of sphenoidal

prechiasmatic
sulcus

sphenoidal yoke

tuberculum sellae

alar tubercle

greater ala
(parietal margin)

superior
orbital fissure

rebral surface

squamosal border

squamosal border
of greater ala

foramen ovale

foramen spinosum

spina of sphenoidal bone

foramen petrosum

sphenoidal lingula

carotid
sulcus

hypophysial fossa
of sella turcica

dorsum sellae

posterior clinoid process

middle clinoid process

venous foramen

sella turcica

anterior clinoid process

infratemporal surface

greater foramen
of greater ala

A

SUPERIOR VIEW

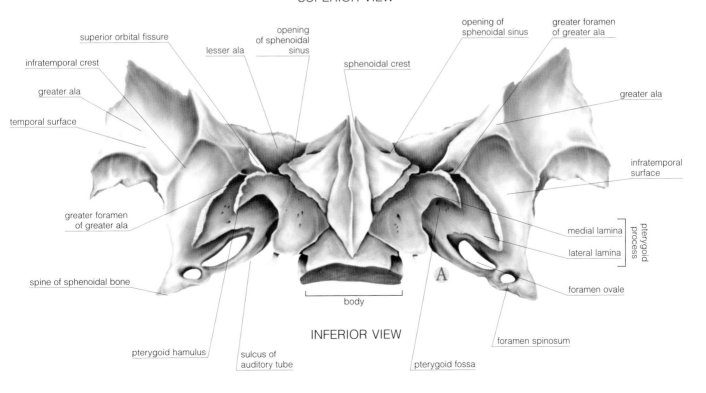

superior orbital fissure

infratemporal crest

greater ala

temporal surface

lesser ala

opening
of sphenoidal
sinus

sphenoidal crest

opening of
sphenoidal sinus

greater foramen
of greater ala

greater ala

infratemporal
surface

greater foramen
of greater ala

spine of sphenoidal bone

pterygoid hamulus

sulcus of
auditory tube

body

medial lamina

lateral lamina

pterygoid
process

foramen ovale

A

foramen spinosum

pterygoid fossa

INFERIOR VIEW

181

CRANIUM (XVII). MAXILLA

RIGHT MAXILLA

maxilla

It is a short and even bone, with irregular square form and two surfaces, internal and external; it also has four borders and four angles. This structure works together with its similar counterpart and meet at the anterior-inferior part of the face to form the upper jaw. Besides the upper jaw, it assist in the forming of the orbit of the eye, the nasal antrum and the palate. All this turns the maxilla into the center of the structure of the face which all the facial bones are linked with. It is located below the frontal and ethmoidal bones, and it articulates with them and with the zygomatic, lacrimale, nasale and vomer bones. At the inferior border, it has some cavities, the alveoli, that house the dental pieces of the jaw. It has five primary points of ossification (zygomatic, orbital, nasal, palatine and premaxillary) appearing in about the second month of the life of the embryo.

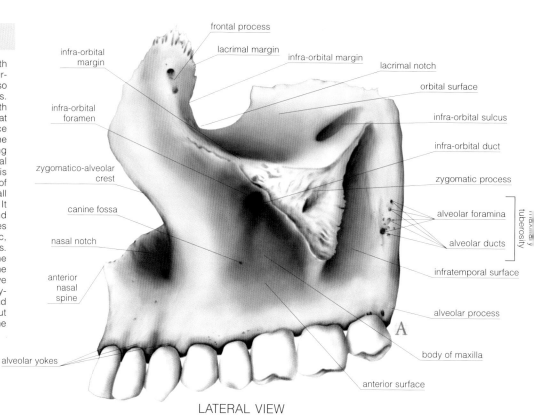

LATERAL VIEW

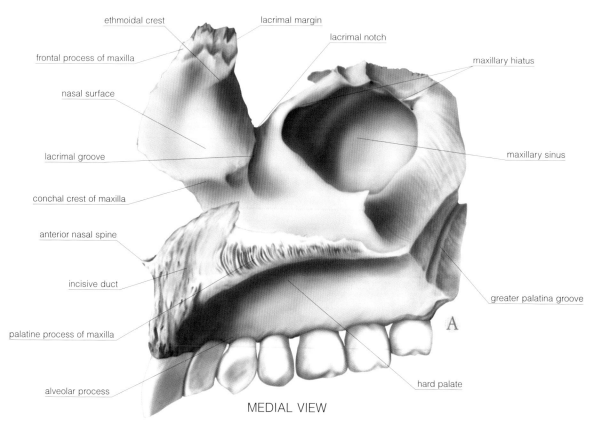

MEDIAL VIEW

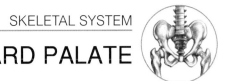

CRANIUM (XVIII). HARD PALATE

hard palate

It is the anterior part of the palate and its structure is formed by the union of the palatine apophyses of the maxilla and the inferior surface of the horizontal plate of both palatine bones. For that reason is also called bony palate, and it it forms the anterior part of the oral cavity. It is covered, in the superior surface by the mucosa of the nasal cavity and the surface that makes the roof of the mouth is covered by the mucoperiostium.

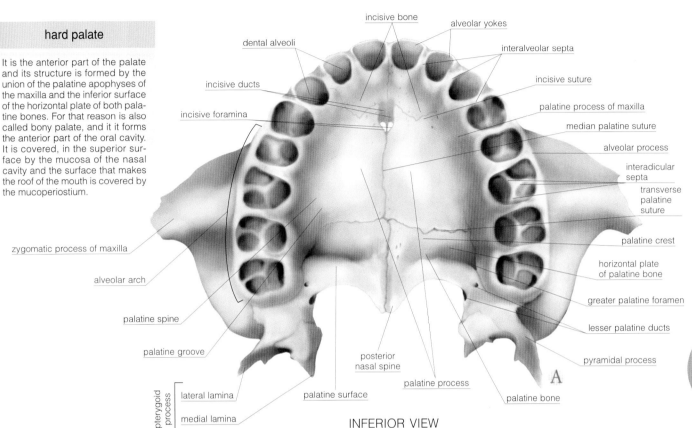

incisive bone
alveolar yokes
dental alveoli
interalveolar septa
incisive ducts
incisive suture
incisive foramina
palatine process of maxilla
median palatine suture
alveolar process
interadicular septa
transverse palatine suture
zygomatic process of maxilla
palatine crest
alveolar arch
horizontal plate of palatine bone
greater palatine foramen
palatine spine
lesser palatine ducts
palatine groove
pyramidal process
posterior nasal spine
palatine process
palatine bone
lateral lamina
medial lamina
pterygoid process
palatine surface

INFERIOR VIEW

183

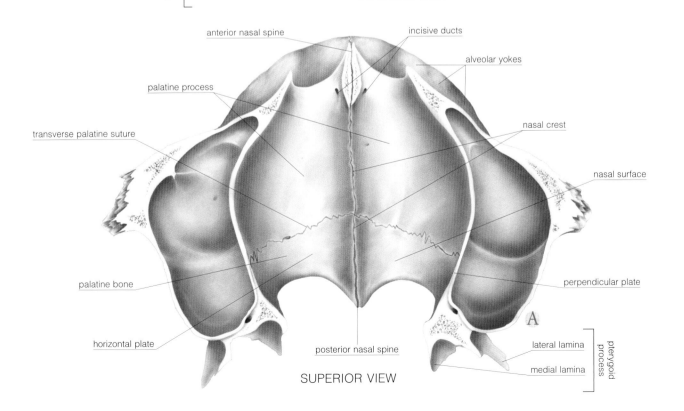

anterior nasal spine
incisive ducts
alveolar yokes
palatine process
transverse palatine suture
nasal crest
nasal surface
palatine bone
perpendicular plate
horizontal plate
lateral lamina
medial lamina
pterygoid process
posterior nasal spine

SUPERIOR VIEW

CRANIUM (XIX). ZYGOMATIC BONE

zygomatic bone

It is a short, paired and square-shape bone, with two surfaces, external and internal. It also has four borders and four angles. It gives form to the osseous support of the lateral areas of the face known as cheekbones. It is located on both sides of the face, below the frontal bone, between the maxilla and the all the bones forming the temporal fossa, which it articulates with. Thus, it is medially linked with the maxilla, it is superiorly linked with the frontal bone, and it is posteriorly united with the great wings of the sphenoidal and the zygomatic process of the temporal bone. The face muscles are inserted on the anterior surface of this bone and the masticatory muscles are inserted on the posterior surface. The superior borders of this bone form the floor and the external wall of the orbital cavity and the lateral ends of the zygomatic bone made up the zygomatic arch. It has two points of ossification by the second month of intra-uterine life.

184

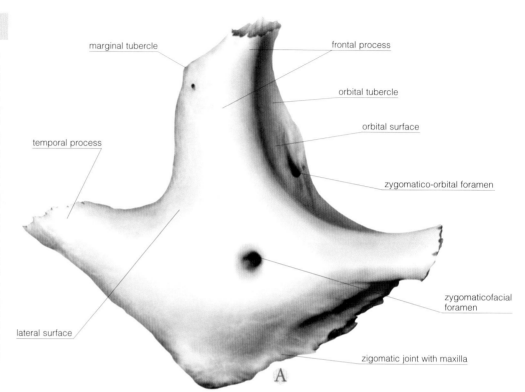

marginal tubercle
frontal process
orbital tubercle
orbital surface
zygomatico-orbital foramen
temporal process
zygomaticofacial foramen
lateral surface
zygomatic joint with maxilla

A

LATERAL VIEW

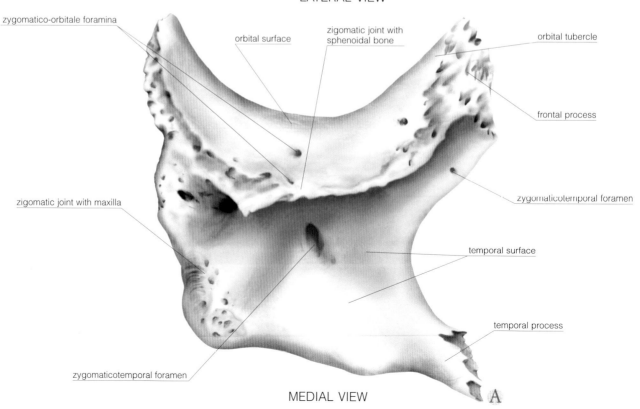

zygomatico-orbitale foramina
orbital surface
zygomatic joint with sphenoidal bone
orbital tubercle
frontal process
zygomaticotemporal foramen
zigomatic joint with maxilla
temporal surface
temporal process
zygomaticotemporal foramen

MEDIAL VIEW

A

CRANIUM (XX). PALATINE BONE

RIGHT PALATINE BONE

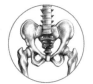

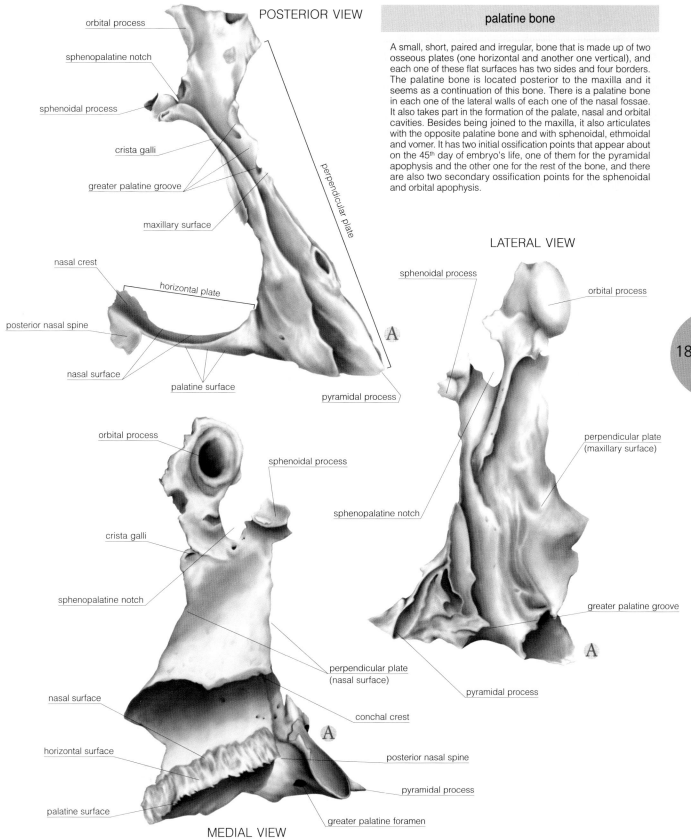

POSTERIOR VIEW

orbital process

sphenopalatine notch

sphenoidal process

crista galli

greater palatine groove

maxillary surface

perpendicular plate

nasal crest

horizontal plate

posterior nasal spine

nasal surface

palatine surface

A

palatine bone

A small, short, paired and irregular, bone that is made up of two osseous plates (one horizontal and another one vertical), and each one of these flat surfaces has two sides and four borders. The palatine bone is located posterior to the maxilla and it seems as a continuation of this bone. There is a palatine bone in each one of the lateral walls of each one of the nasal fossae. It also takes part in the formation of the palate, nasal and orbital cavities. Besides being joined to the maxilla, it also articulates with the opposite palatine bone and with sphenoidal, ethmoidal and vomer. It has two initial ossification points that appear about on the 45th day of embryo's life, one of them for the pyramidal apophysis and the other one for the rest of the bone, and there are also two secondary ossification points for the sphenoidal and orbital apophysis.

LATERAL VIEW

sphenoidal process

orbital process

pyramidal process

185

perpendicular plate
(maxillary surface)

sphenopalatine notch

greater palatine groove

A

orbital process

sphenoidal process

crista galli

sphenopalatine notch

perpendicular plate
(nasal surface)

nasal surface

conchal crest

horizontal surface

A

posterior nasal spine

pyramidal process

palatine surface

greater palatine foramen

MEDIAL VIEW

CRANIUM (XXI). CAVITIES

orbital cavity

The orbital cavities are two and they are placed interiorly on both sides of the nasal fossae and exteriorly the limit with the temporal and pterygomaxillare regions. They are intended to house inside the eyeballs and pertaining muscles, nerves and blood vessels. Also, they are quadrangular and pyramidal shaped even though with rounded borders. Among others, they are formed by the following bones: frontal, zygomatic, maxilla, nasal, sphenoidal, palatine and lacrimal. Anteriorly, they communicate with the exterior and posteriorly they get in contact with the cranial cavity, nasal fossae and the pterygomaxillary region.

186

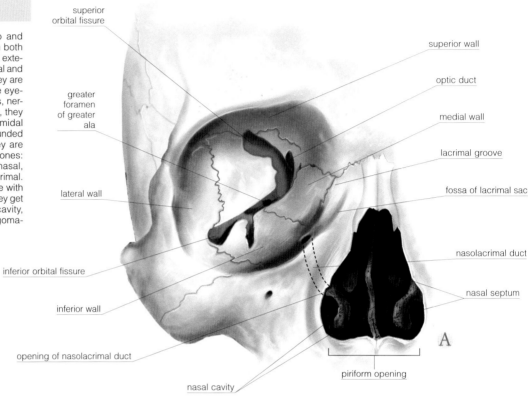

superior orbital fissure

greater foramen of greater ala

lateral wall

inferior orbital fissure

inferior wall

opening of nasolacrimal duct

nasal cavity

superior wall

optic duct

medial wall

lacrimal groove

fossa of lacrimal sac

nasolacrimal duct

nasal septum

piriform opening

A

ORBITAL CAVITY. RIGHT PART

nasal cavity

The nasal cavities are two and are basal to the cranium and the roof of the mouth. Anteriorly, they open through the nose, and posteriorly the open to the nasopharyngeal passage. Laterally the are confined by the maxilla, palatine bone, inferior nasal conchae, and lacrimal; medially they are limited by ethmoid and vomer and have direct communication with the exterior through the nostrils. The nasal cavity is divided into left and right airways and they are separated by the nasal septum. The floor of the nasal cavities is the hard palate that separates it from the oral cavity. The lateral walls contain nasal conchae and meatus. In the nasal fossae it begins the inhalation and ends the exhalation of the respiratory cycle.

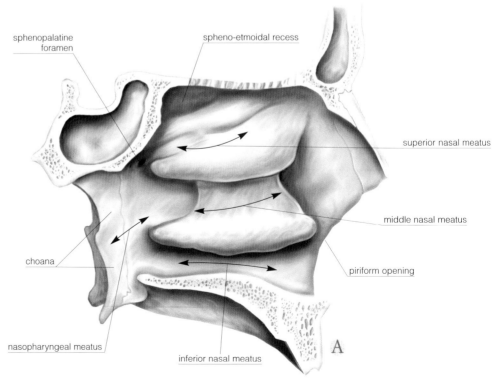

sphenopalatine foramen

spheno-etmoidal recess

superior nasal meatus

middle nasal meatus

piriform opening

choana

nasopharyngeal meatus

inferior nasal meatus

A

NASAL CAVITY. LATERAL WALL

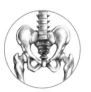

CRANIUM (XXII). VOMER, LACRIMAL and NASAL BONES

vomer

The only bone located in the midsaggital line of the face is the posterior-inferior support to the septum that splits the nasal fossae into two. It is a square-shaped, thin and transparent plate. It articulates with sphenoidal (at its posterior-superior border), the perpendicular wall of the ethmoidal bone (at its superior-anterior border) and the palatine and maxilla bones (at its inferior border) and when fresh it articulates with the cartilage of the septum. The posterior-superior border remains loose.

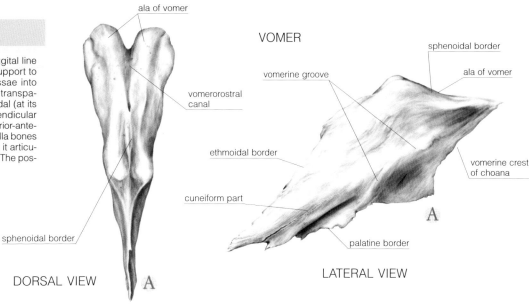

VOMER

ala of vomer

vomerorostral canal

sphenoidal border

DORSAL VIEW

sphenoidal border

ala of vomer

vomerine groove

ethmoidal border

cuneiform part

vomerine crest of choana

palatine border

LATERAL VIEW

lacrimal bone

Lacrimal bones are two tiny and compact square-shaped plates, with two surfaces and four borders, they are situated at the front part of the medial wall of the orbit, which is also formed by the following bones: maxilla, frontal and ethmoidal; all of them are articulated between them. Moreover, they take part in the formation of the nasolacrimal duct. It presents one point of ossification during the third month of intra-uterine life.

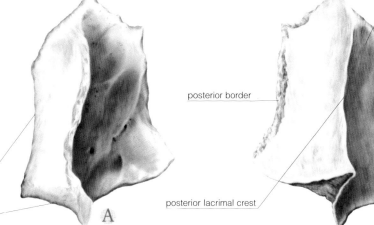

LACRIMAL BONE

lacrimal surface

posterior border

anterior border

anterior border

inferior border

posterior lacrimal crest

MEDIAL SURFACE

LATERAL SURFACE

187

nasal bone

The nasal bones are two small flat bones; they are also short and with two surfaces, anterior and posterior, and four borders. They are located at the upper part of the anterior surface of the nasal fossae and form the osseous support of the base of the nose. They articulate between them at the medial border, in the upper area, above the nostrils. They also articulate with the frontal bone and inferiorly with the upward apophysis of the maxilla, and with the ethmoidal bone. It presents one point of ossification during the third month of the intra-uterine life.

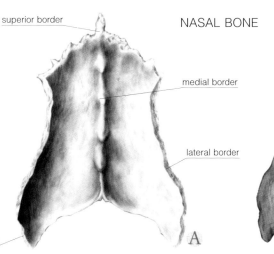
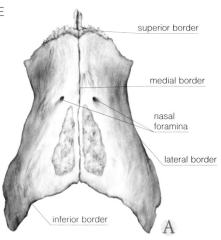

NASAL BONE

superior border

medial border

lateral border

inferior border

POSTERIOR VIEW

superior border

medial border

nasal foramina

lateral border

inferior border

ANTERIOR BORDER

CRANIUM (XXIII). MANDIBLE (I)

mandible

It is a flat and robust bone, horseshoe-shaped, formed by a body with two surfaces, anterior and posterior, two borders and two lateral ends or rami. It is located in the inferior part of the face and forms the skeleton of the inferior maxillary. In its superior border it has a chain of alveoli where all the dental pieces of the lower jaw are implanted. It has a central portion, or chin, which has other two portions, left and right, they are the two horizontal portions of the mandible that become vertical and from that point they are known as mandibular ramus; they articulate with the temporal bone. This articulation enables the mandible to exert a great force and do all the necessary movements during the masticatory process of food once it has been introduced into the mouth during one of the first phases of digestion. It also articulates with the maxilla. Many of the masticatory muscles are inserted in the mandible. Initially is a double bone and each one of the two halves comes from various ossification points. Which are perceptible from the 90th day of the mental level.

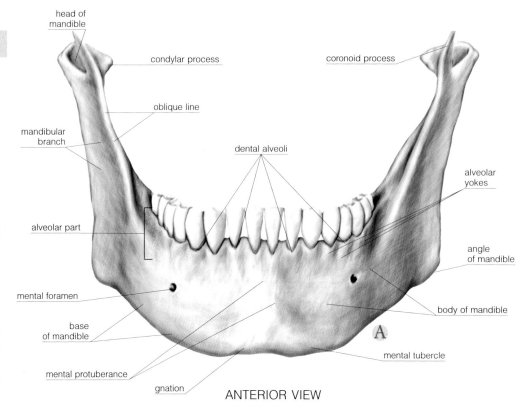

ANTERIOR VIEW

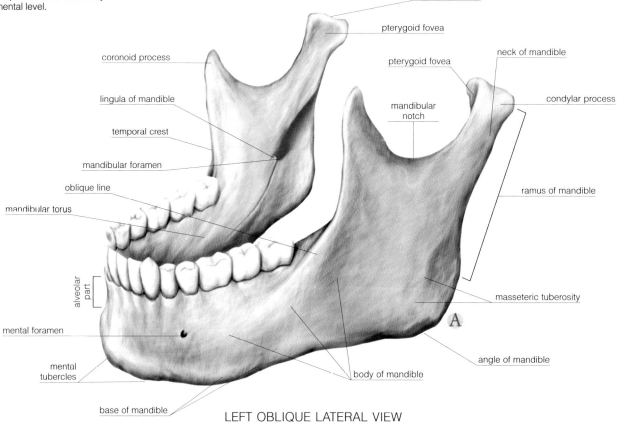

LEFT OBLIQUE LATERAL VIEW

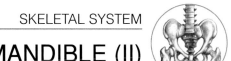

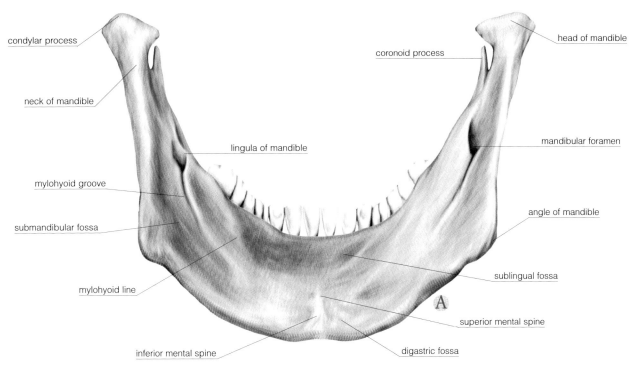

condylar process

neck of mandible

lingula of mandible

mylohyoid groove

submandibular fossa

mylohyoid line

inferior mental spine

head of mandible

coronoid process

mandibular foramen

angle of mandible

sublingual fossa

superior mental spine

digastric fossa

A

POSTERIOR VIEW

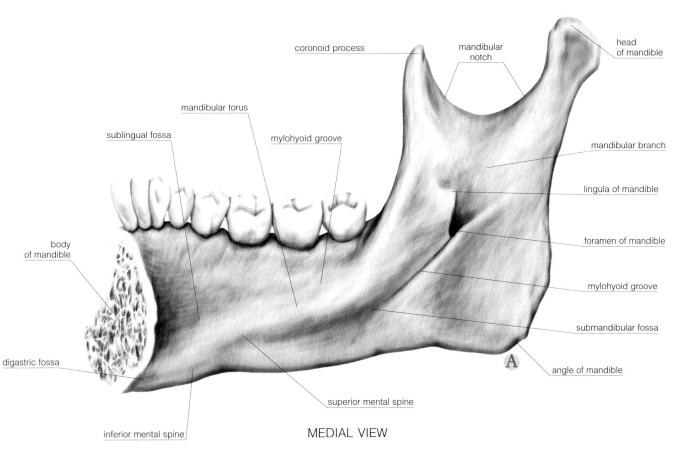

coronoid process

mandibular notch

head of mandible

mandibular torus

sublingual fossa

mylohyoid groove

mandibular branch

lingula of mandible

foramen of mandible

mylohyoid groove

submandibular fossa

body of mandible

digastric fossa

angle of mandible

A

superior mental spine

inferior mental spine

MEDIAL VIEW

CRANIUM (XXV). SECTIONS

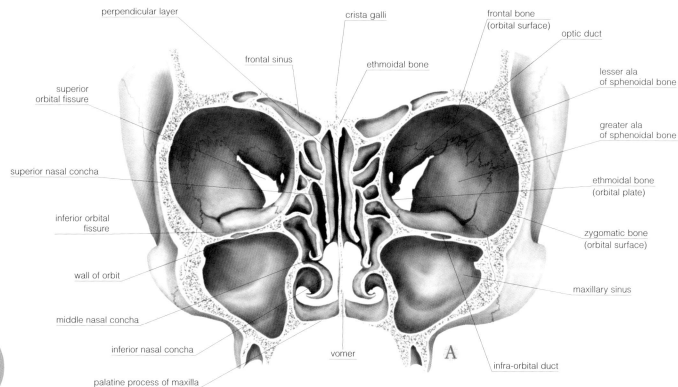

perpendicular layer

frontal sinus

crista galli

ethmoidal bone

frontal bone (orbital surface)

optic duct

lesser ala of sphenoidal bone

superior orbital fissure

superior nasal concha

greater ala of sphenoidal bone

ethmoidal bone (orbital plate)

inferior orbital fissure

zygomatic bone (orbital surface)

wall of orbit

maxillary sinus

middle nasal concha

inferior nasal concha

vomer

infra-orbital duct

palatine process of maxilla

190

ORBITAL CAVITY and ADJACENT STRUCTURES
CORONAL SECTION. ANTERIOR VIEW

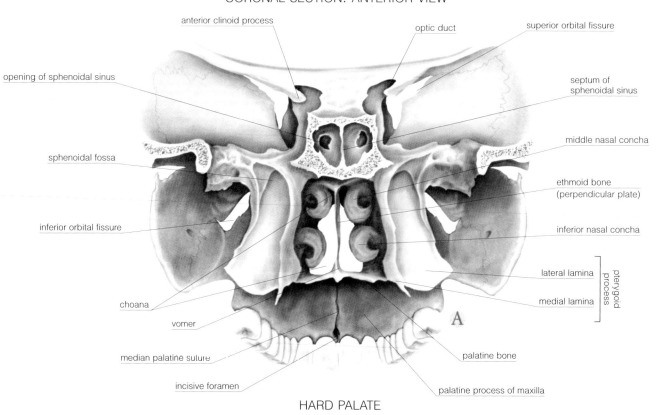

anterior clinoid process

optic duct

superior orbital fissure

opening of sphenoidal sinus

septum of sphenoidal sinus

middle nasal concha

sphenoidal fossa

ethmoid bone (perpendicular plate)

inferior orbital fissure

inferior nasal concha

lateral lamina

medial lamina

pterygoid process

choana

vomer

median palatine suture

palatine bone

incisive foramen

palatine process of maxilla

HARD PALATE
POSTERIOR OBLIQUE VIEW

HEAD and NECK (I)
GENERAL LATERAL VIEW

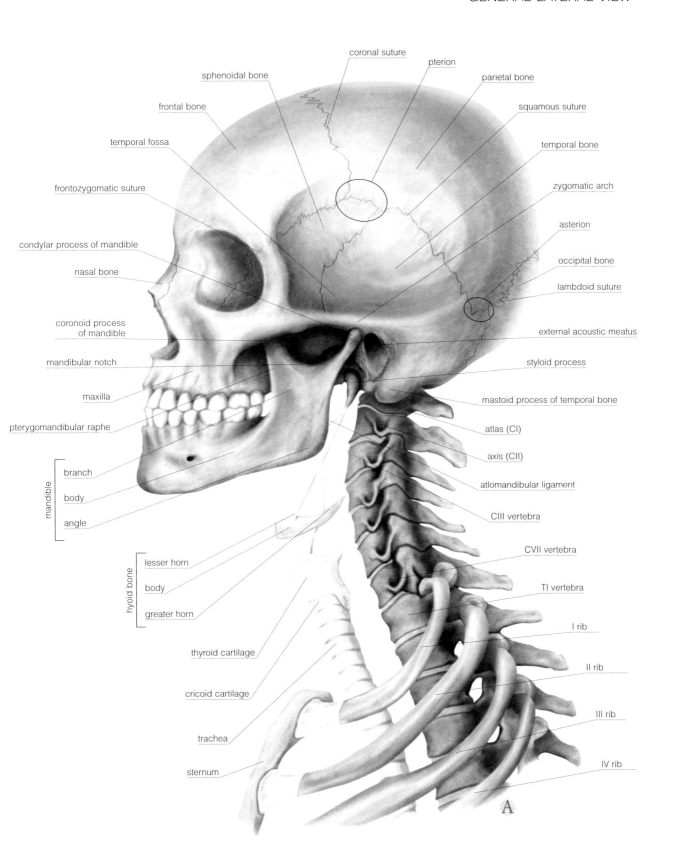

coronal suture

pterion

sphenoidal bone

parietal bone

frontal bone

squamous suture

temporal fossa

temporal bone

frontozygomatic suture

zygomatic arch

asterion

condylar process of mandible

occipital bone

nasal bone

lambdoid suture

coronoid process of mandible

external acoustic meatus

mandibular notch

styloid process

maxilla

mastoid process of temporal bone

pterygomandibular raphe

atlas (CI)

axis (CII)

branch

atlomandibular ligament

mandible

body

CIII vertebra

angle

CVII vertebra

lesser horn

TI vertebra

hyoid bone

body

I rib

greater horn

thyroid cartilage

II rib

cricoid cartilage

III rib

trachea

IV rib

sternum

A

HEAD and NECK (II)

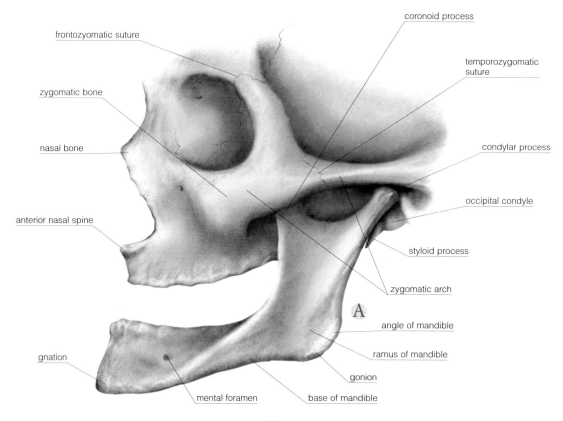

frontozyomatic suture

zygomatic bone

nasal bone

anterior nasal spine

gnation

mental foramen

coronoid process

temporozygomatic suture

condylar process

occipital condyle

styloid process

zygomatic arch

angle of mandible

ramus of mandible

gonion

base of mandible

MANDIBLE of AGED

hyoid bone

It is a short, unpaired, thin and symmetric bone, with the form of a U. It has a main body, two surfaces, two borders, two ends and four lateral extensions (greater and lesser horns). It is placed at the anterior part of the neck, below the mandible, above the thyroid cartilage, above the larynx, below the tongue, which skeleton is the hyoid bone. On this bone get inserted a huge numbers of muscles of the tongue, and also do the muscles of the pharynx and of the floor of the mouth. It presents six points of primary ossification, two for the body, two for the greater cornu (2), appearing at the end of the intra-uterine life, and two for the lesser horns, that appear at the end of the adolescence.

HYOID BONE

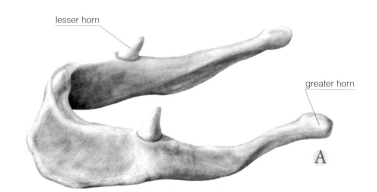

lesser horn

greater horn

LEFT LATERAL VIEW

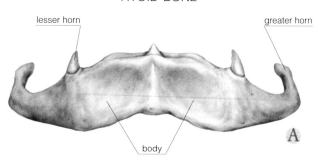

lesser horn

greater horn

body

ANTERIOR VIEW

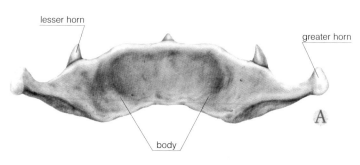

lesser horn

greater horn

body

POSTERIOR VIEW

VERTEBRAL COLUMN (I)
GENERAL VIEWS

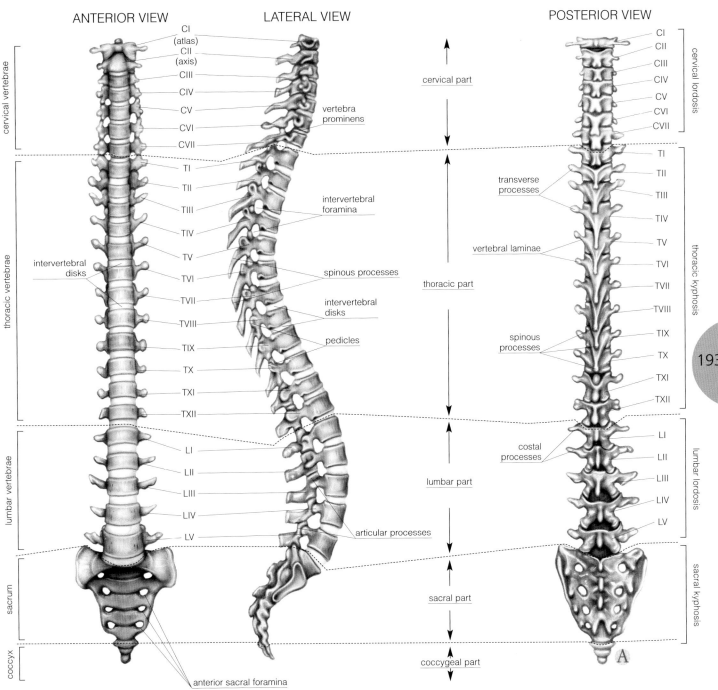

ANTERIOR VIEW

LATERAL VIEW

POSTERIOR VIEW

CI
(atlas)
CII
(axis)
CIII
CIV
CV
CVI
CVII

cervical vertebrae

vertebra prominens

cervical part

CI
CII
CIII
CIV
CV
CVI
CVII

cervical lordosis

TI
TII
TIII
TIV
TV
TVI
TVII
TVIII
TIX
TX
TXI
TXII

thoracic vertebrae

intervertebral disks

intervertebral foramina

spinous processes

intervertebral disks

pedicles

thoracic part

transverse processes

vertebral laminae

spinous processes

TI
TII
TIII
TIV
TV
TVI
TVII
TVIII
TIX
TX
TXI
TXII

thoracic kyphosis

193

LI
LII
LIII
LIV
LV

lumbar vertebrae

articular processes

lumbar part

costal processes

LI
LII
LIII
LIV
LV

lumbar lordosis

sacrum

anterior sacral foramina

sacral part

sacral kyphosis

coccyx

coccygeal part

A

vertebral column

A set of 24 bones, or vertebrae, arranged one in top of the other in a column fashion and located in the medial section of the trunk. It is the support structure of the dorsal portion of the skeleton. Its spiny apophyses are easily felt through the skin.
It is divided into 5 portions:
- cervical or superior (CI-CVII vertebrae).
- thoracic (TI-TXII vertebrae).
- lumbar (LI-LV vertebrae).

- sacrum (SI-SV vertebrae, fused).
- coccygeal (4 vertebrae, fused).
The increase in volume and weight of the mother's abdomen during pregnancy due to fetal growth, placenta and amniotic fluid, among others, forces the anterior part of the body to demand a stronger support from the spine in order to maintain balance. As a consequence, lumbar vertebrae support more weight and thus the spine curves more, a usually painful condition known as lordosis.

VERTEBRAL COLUMN (II). CERVICAL PART (I)

cervical part

It is the upper portion of the spine column and it is formed by seven overlapped vertebrae that build up the skeleton of the neck. The first and second from these vertebrae, the atlas and the axis, have special peculiarities due to the fact that they make up the union between the neck and the head. The other five of them are very similar. In the cervical vertebrae, the cervical muscles of the prevertebral region are inserted through tendinous extensions.

ATLAS (or CI VERTEBRA)

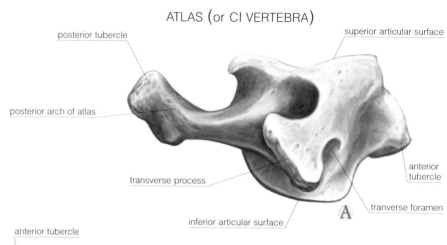

posterior tubercle

superior articular surface

posterior arch of atlas

transverse process

anterior tubercle

inferior articular surface

tranverse foramen

RIGHT LATERAL VIEW

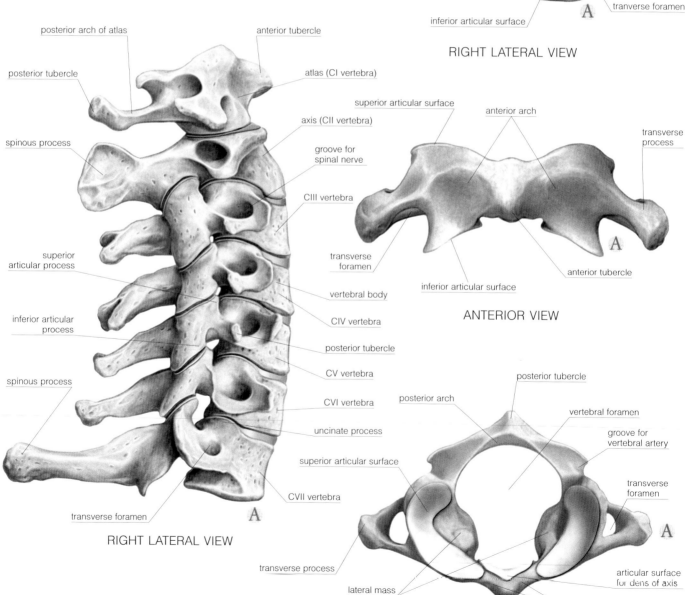

posterior arch of atlas

anterior tubercle

posterior tubercle

atlas (CI vertebra)

spinous process

axis (CII vertebra)

superior articular surface

anterior arch

transverse process

groove for spinal nerve

CIII vertebra

superior articular process

transverse foramen

inferior articular surface

anterior tubercle

inferior articular process

vertebral body

CIV vertebra

spinous process

posterior tubercle

CV vertebra

CVI vertebra

uncinate process

superior articular surface

CVII vertebra

transverse foramen

RIGHT LATERAL VIEW

ANTERIOR VIEW

posterior tubercle

posterior arch

vertebral foramen

groove for vertebral artery

transverse foramen

transverse process

articular surface for dens of axis

lateral mass

anterior arch

anterior tubercle

SUPERIOR VIEW

VERTEBRAL COLUMN (III). CERVICAL PART (II)

AXIS (or CII VERTEBRA)

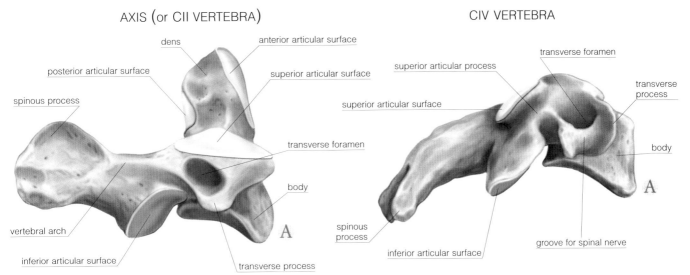

RIGHT LATERAL VIEW

CIV VERTEBRA

RIGHT LATERAL VIEW

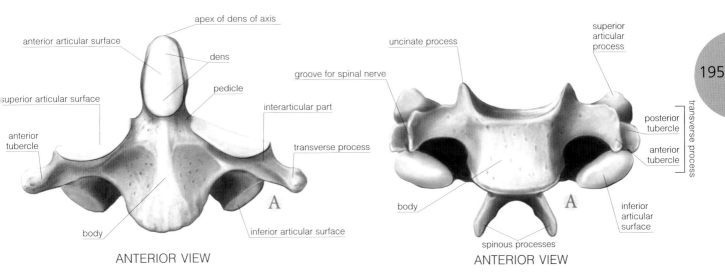

ANTERIOR VIEW

ANTERIOR VIEW

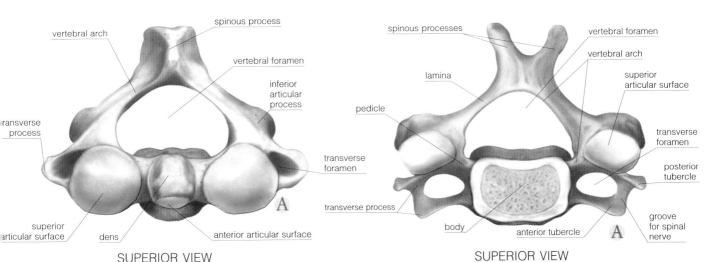

SUPERIOR VIEW

SUPERIOR VIEW

VERTEBRAL COLUMN (IV). THORACIC PART

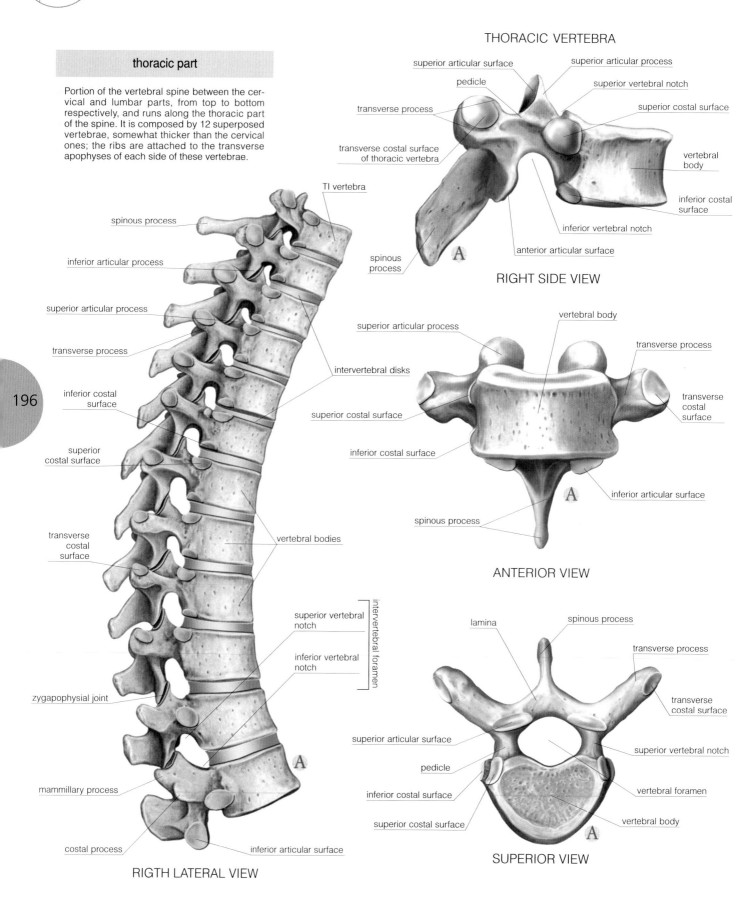

thoracic part

Portion of the vertebral spine between the cervical and lumbar parts, from top to bottom respectively, and runs along the thoracic part of the spine. It is composed by 12 superposed vertebrae, somewhat thicker than the cervical ones; the ribs are attached to the transverse apophyses of each side of these vertebrae.

THORACIC VERTEBRA

superior articular surface
superior articular process
pedicle
superior vertebral notch
transverse process
superior costal surface
transverse costal surface of thoracic vertebra
vertebral body
inferior costal surface
spinous process
inferior vertebral notch
anterior articular surface

RIGHT SIDE VIEW

superior articular process
vertebral body
transverse process
intervertebral disks
transverse costal surface
superior costal surface
inferior costal surface
inferior articular surface
spinous process

ANTERIOR VIEW

TI vertebra
spinous process
inferior articular process
superior articular process
transverse process
inferior costal surface
superior costal surface
transverse costal surface
vertebral bodies
superior vertebral notch
inferior vertebral notch
intervertebral foramen
zygapophysial joint
mammillary process
costal process
inferior articular surface

RIGTH LATERAL VIEW

lamina
spinous process
transverse process
transverse costal surface
superior articular surface
pedicle
superior vertebral notch
inferior costal surface
vertebral foramen
superior costal surface
vertebral body

SUPERIOR VIEW

196

VERTEBRAL COLUMN (V). LUMBAR PART

lumbar part

Refers to part of the vertebral column, which is a continuation of the thoracic part. It covers the back, from the abdominal region to the sacrum. It is made up of five very wide and thick vertebrae which overlap and which are sustained in the sacrum. The first lumbar vertebrae act as insertion to the sinewy extensions emitted by the diaphragm in their posterior part, and will unite the vertebral body and to their transverse processes.

LUMBAR VERTEBRA

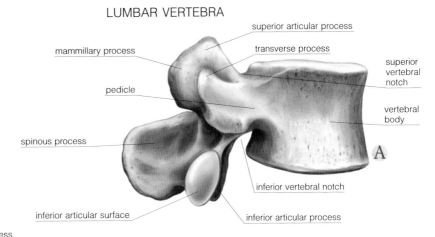

superior articular process
mammillary process
transverse process
superior vertebral notch
pedicle
vertebral body
spinous process
inferior vertebral notch
inferior articular surface
inferior articular process

RIGHT LATERAL VIEW

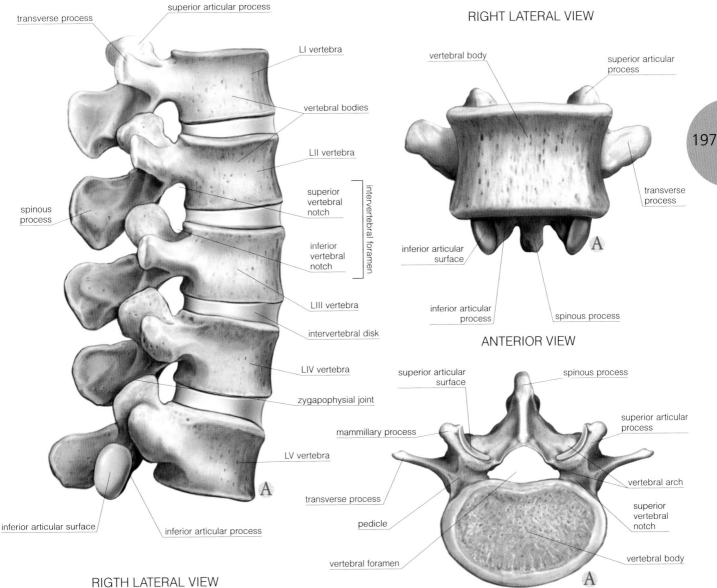

transverse process
superior articular process
LI vertebra
vertebral bodies
LII vertebra
superior vertebral notch
intervertebral foramen
spinous process
inferior vertebral notch
LIII vertebra
intervertebral disk
LIV vertebra
zygapophysial joint
LV vertebra
inferior articular surface
inferior articular process

RIGTH LATERAL VIEW

vertebral body
superior articular process
inferior articular surface
inferior articular process
spinous process
transverse process

ANTERIOR VIEW

superior articular surface
spinous process
mammillary process
superior articular process
transverse process
vertebral arch
pedicle
superior vertebral notch
vertebral foramen
vertebral body

SUPERIOR VIEW

197

VERTEBRAL COLUMN (VI). SACRUM (I)

sacrum

Triangular-shaped osseous structure made up of five vertebrae which are all welded in a unique bone that is housed by the two hip bones. It is the base of the vertebral column and its inferior part connects with the coccyx. The sacrum actively participates in various movements of the trunk: inclination, extension, both forward and backward. It articulates with the last lumbar vertebra (LV) above (lumbosacral joint), with the coccyx below (sacrococcygeal joint), and with the illium part of the hip bones (sacro-illiac joint) on either side, and consequently all together with the other two portions of the hip bone, ischium and pubis, it forms the pelvic cavity.

promontory
base of sacrum
superior articular process
ala of sacrum
lateral part
transverse ridges
anterior sacral foramina
sacrococcygeal joint
apex of sacrum
coccygeal cornu
lateral part
coccyx

ANTERIOR VIEW

superior articular process
base of sacrum
promontory
articular surface
anterior surface
sacral cornu
coccyx
sacral tuberosity
middle sacral crest
dorsal surface
lateral sacral crest
coccygeal cornu

LEFT LATERAL VIEW

coccygeal cornu

COCCYX

ANTERIOR VIEW

coccygeal cornu

POSTERIOR VIEW

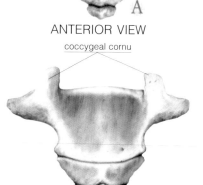

coccyx

Small and unpaired bone, central and symmetric, it is the ending portion of the vertebral column. It articulates with the lower part of the sacrum above and it is formed by three to five primitive bones, almost atrophied ones (residual vertebrae), that are joined one to the other and become the lower final segment of the vertebral column. It is triangular-shape, with one base, one vertex, two surfaces and two borders. In spite of being covered by a very strong group of muscles, its hard consistency can be perceptible at the intergluteal area.

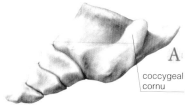

coccygeal cornu

LEFT LATERAL VIEW

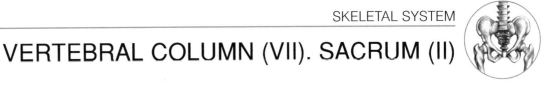

VERTEBRAL COLUMN (VII). SACRUM (II)

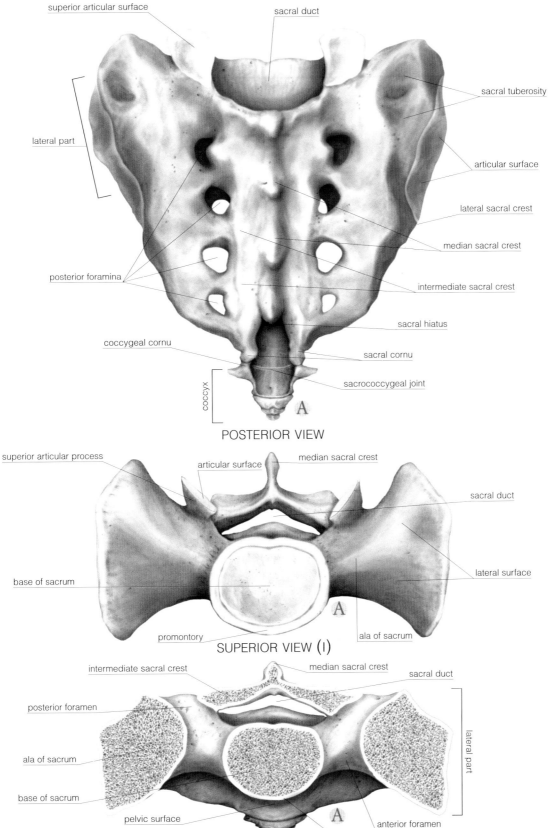

superior articular surface

sacral duct

sacral tuberosity

lateral part

articular surface

lateral sacral crest

median sacral crest

posterior foramina

intermediate sacral crest

sacral hiatus

coccygeal cornu

sacral cornu

coccyx

sacrococcygeal joint

199

POSTERIOR VIEW

superior articular process

articular surface

median sacral crest

sacral duct

base of sacrum

lateral surface

promontory

ala of sacrum

SUPERIOR VIEW (I)

intermediate sacral crest

median sacral crest

sacral duct

posterior foramen

ala of sacrum

base of sacrum

lateral part

pelvic surface

anterior foramen

coccyx

promontory of sacrum

SUPERIOR VIEW (II)

TRUNK (I)
ANTERIOR VIEW

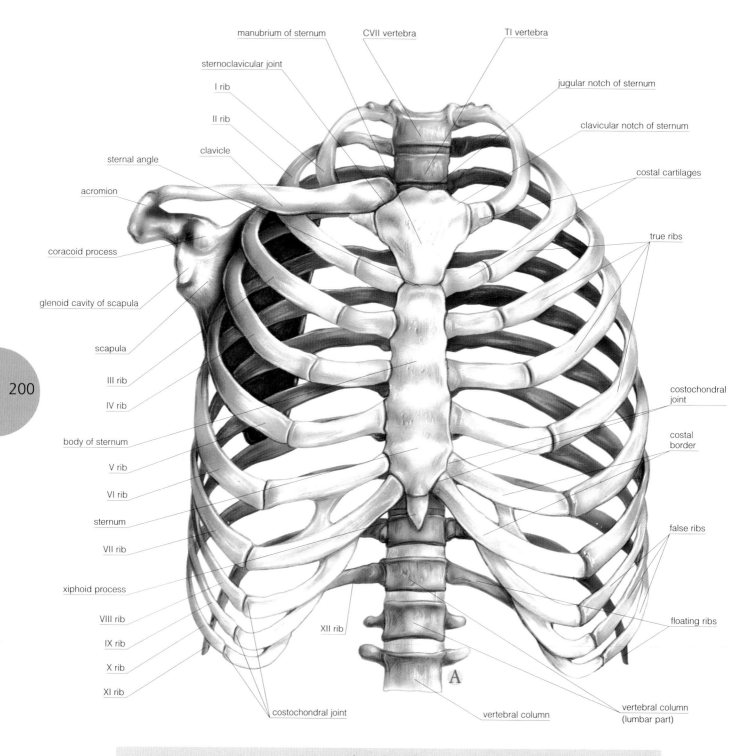

manubrium of sternum

CVII vertebra

TI vertebra

sternoclavicular joint

I rib

II rib

jugular notch of sternum

clavicular notch of sternum

sternal angle

clavicle

acromion

costal cartilages

coracoid process

true ribs

glenoid cavity of scapula

scapula

III rib

IV rib

costochondral joint

body of sternum

costal border

V rib

VI rib

sternum

false ribs

VII rib

xiphoid process

VIII rib

floating ribs

XII rib

IX rib

X rib

XI rib

A

costochondral joint

vertebral column

vertebral column (lumbar part)

thoracic cavity

It is a collection of bones and soft tissues that covers the thorax. This structure is formed by twelve pairs of ribs (seven of them true and other five of them false) that limit the thorax all the way round; the thoracic segment of the vertebral column, which vertebrae are linked to the above mentioned ribs at the back; and finally, the sternum where the ribs end at the front of the thorax. All these elements form a kind of cage sited be- tween the neck and the diaphragm that houses very important organs like the heart or the lungs. The thoracic cage is like a protector shield to all these organs. In order to favor breathing movements, the thoracic cavity is able to expand and contract itself with the help of the respiratory muscles, thus, it enables the lungs to take as much air as possible (during inhalation) or to expel it to the exterior (during exhalation).

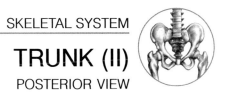

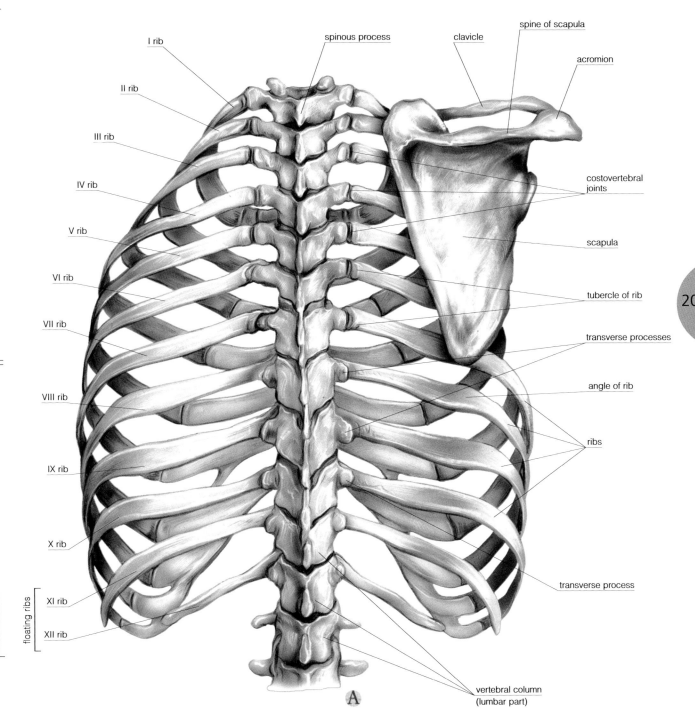

true ribs (I-VII)

false ribs (VIII-XII)

floating ribs

I rib

II rib

III rib

IV rib

V rib

VI rib

VII rib

VIII rib

IX rib

X rib

XI rib

XII rib

spinous process

clavicle

spine of scapula

acromion

costovertebral joints

scapula

tubercle of rib

transverse processes

angle of rib

ribs

transverse process

vertebral column (lumbar part)

A

201

TRUNK (III)

LATERAL VIEW

rib

The ribs are a series of flat and curved bones forming the skeleton structure of the thorax. The distribution, form and structure of ribs can be perceived through the walls of the thoracic cavity. The ribs start at the spine of the thoracic wall and end at the sternum, namely, posteriorly they find support on the vertebral column and anteriorly on the sternum and this way they form a cavity, a kind of cage (thoracic cavity), where many important organs are housed, mainly the lungs and the heart. There are twelve ribs. Anatomically, going forward from the back, the rib has an enlarged end (head) that articulates with the corresponding vertebra; then, it has a narrow area (neck); also, a prominence (tubercle) which articulates with the transverse process of the corresponding vertebra; and, finally, a flat part (body). Some of the ribs are fixed at both ends and with the form and distribution just mentioned; but there is another group of ribs below in which the ribs are joined between them or free. Some ribs are true ribs (the ones directly joined with the sternum), some others are false ribs (the ones that reached the sternum through a common costal cartilage), and a third group of ribs, known as floating, due to the fact that they do no have any anterior point of fixation. Many muscles of the abdominal wall and also of the diaphragm are inserted in the ribs.

202

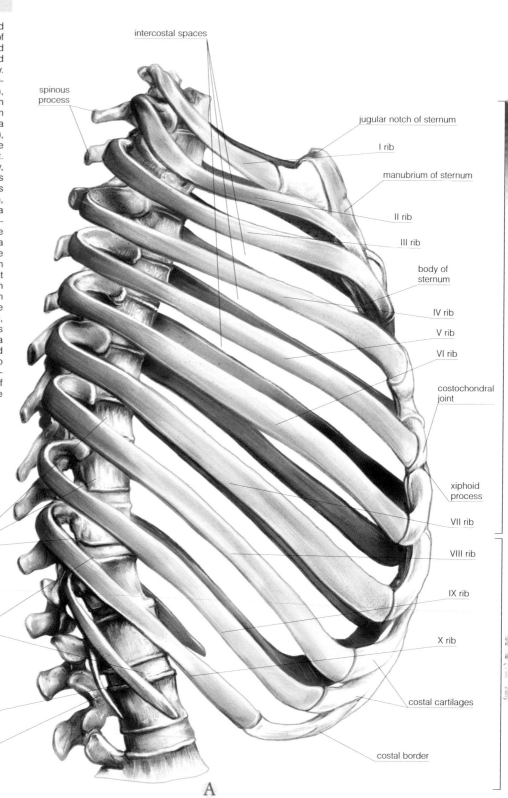

intercostal spaces

spinous process

jugular notch of sternum

I rib

manubrium of sternum

II rib

III rib

body of sternum

IV rib

V rib

VI rib

costochondral joint

xiphoid process

VII rib

VIII rib

vertebral bodies

IX rib

X rib

intervertebral disks

costal cartilages

XI rib

true ribs

XII rib

costal border

A

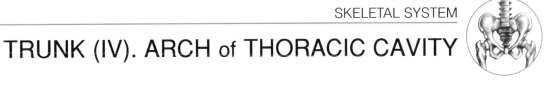

TRUNK (IV). ARCH of THORACIC CAVITY

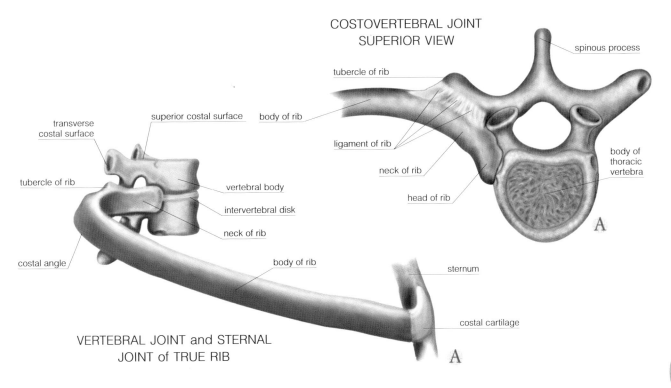

COSTOVERTEBRAL JOINT
SUPERIOR VIEW

spinous process

tubercle of rib

body of rib

transverse
costal surface

superior costal surface

ligament of rib

tubercle of rib

vertebral body

neck of rib

intervertebral disk

body of
thoracic
vertebra

neck of rib

head of rib

costal angle

body of rib

sternum

A

costal cartilage

VERTEBRAL JOINT and STERNAL
JOINT of TRUE RIB

A

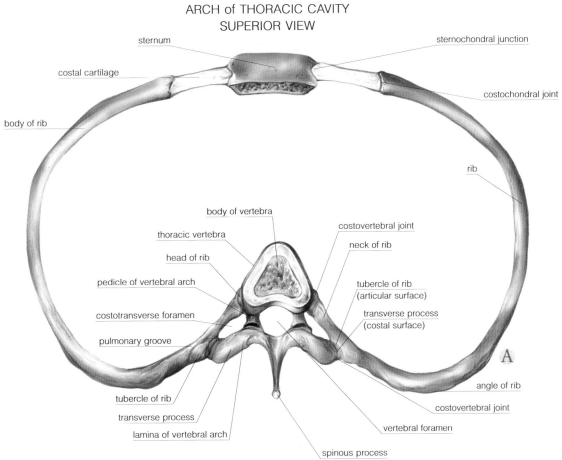

ARCH of THORACIC CAVITY
SUPERIOR VIEW

sternum

sternochondral junction

costal cartilage

costochondral joint

body of rib

rib

body of vertebra

costovertebral joint

thoracic vertebra

neck of rib

head of rib

tubercle of rib
(articular surface)

pedicle of vertebral arch

transverse process
(costal surface)

costotransverse foramen

pulmonary groove

A

tubercle of rib

angle of rib

transverse process

costovertebral joint

lamina of vertebral arch

vertebral foramen

spinous process

UPPER LIMB (I). SHOULDER and ARM

LEFT UPPER LIMB

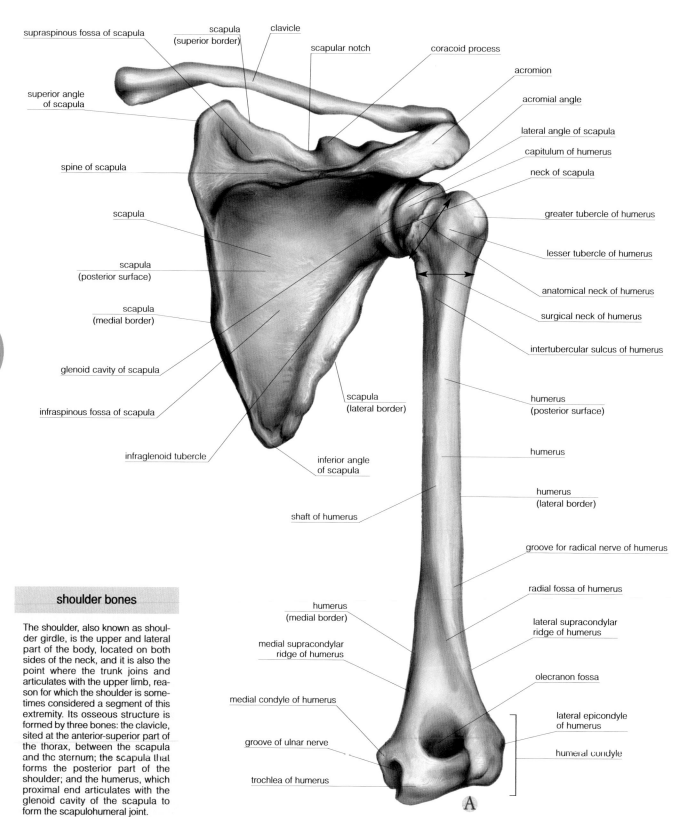

supraspinous fossa of scapula

scapula
(superior border)

clavicle

scapular notch

coracoid process

acromion

superior angle
of scapula

acromial angle

lateral angle of scapula

capitulum of humerus

neck of scapula

spine of scapula

greater tubercle of humerus

scapula

lesser tubercle of humerus

scapula
(posterior surface)

anatomical neck of humerus

surgical neck of humerus

scapula
(medial border)

intertubercular sulcus of humerus

glenoid cavity of scapula

humerus
(posterior surface)

infraspinous fossa of scapula

scapula
(lateral border)

humerus

infraglenoid tubercle

humerus
(lateral border)

inferior angle
of scapula

groove for radical nerve of humerus

shaft of humerus

radial fossa of humerus

humerus
(medial border)

lateral supracondylar
ridge of humerus

medial supracondylar
ridge of humerus

olecranon fossa

medial condyle of humerus

lateral epicondyle
of humerus

groove of ulnar nerve

humeral condyle

trochlea of humerus

Ⓐ

204

shoulder bones

The shoulder, also known as shoulder girdle, is the upper and lateral part of the body, located on both sides of the neck, and it is also the point where the trunk joins and articulates with the upper limb, reason for which the shoulder is sometimes considered a segment of this extremity. Its osseous structure is formed by three bones: the clavicle, sited at the anterior-superior part of the thorax, between the scapula and the sternum; the scapula that forms the posterior part of the shoulder; and the humerus, which proximal end articulates with the glenoid cavity of the scapula to form the scapulohumeral joint.

UPPER LIMB (II). SCAPULA

RIGHT UPPER LIMB

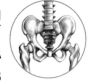

scapula

Flat bone with triangular shape located just above the costal group that can be felt through the skin, under the muscles of the shoulder, on both sides of the back, just above the costal group. It make part of the posterior segment of the shoulder. It is confined to the superior area of the posterior wall of the thoracic cavity and it articulates with the humerus and the clavicle. Its dorsal surface is convexed and is horizontally crossed by the spine of the scapula.

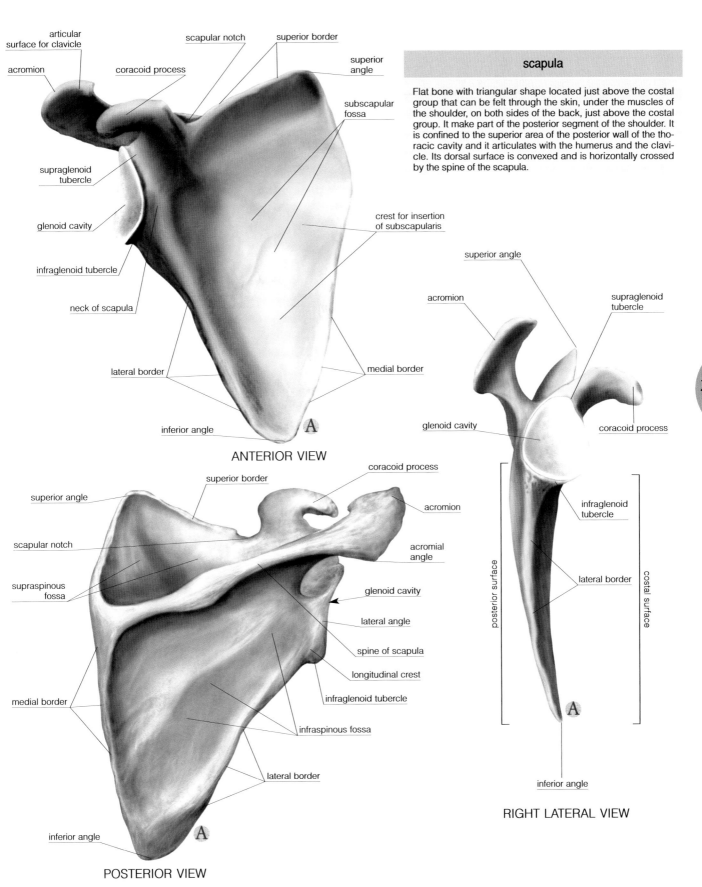

ANTERIOR VIEW

RIGHT LATERAL VIEW

POSTERIOR VIEW

UPPER LIMB (III). HUMERUS

humerus

Paired, long, thick and symmetric bone that is the skeleton of the arm, portion of the upper limb that this bone runs all along through the central part. It has a central and cylindrical part and two enlarged bodies at both ends. At its proximal end, or head, it articulates with the scapula to form the glenohumeral joint; and at its distal end it articulates with the ulna and the radius to form the elbow joint. Muscles of the shoulder, thorax and upper limb are inserted on this bone.

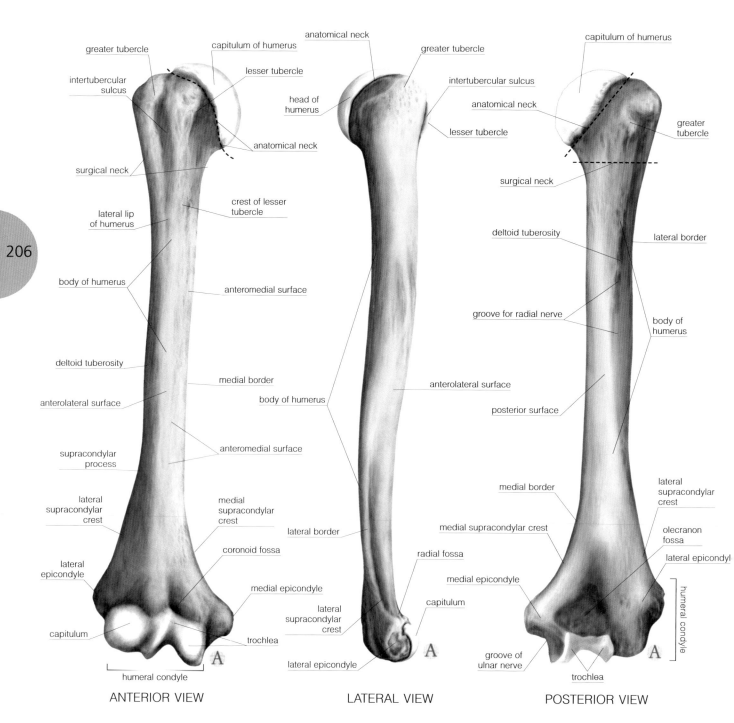

greater tubercle
capitulum of humerus
anatomical neck
intertubercular sulcus
lesser tubercle
head of humerus
anatomical neck
surgical neck
lateral lip of humerus
crest of lesser tubercle
body of humerus
anteromedial surface
deltoid tuberosity
medial border
anterolateral surface
body of humerus
supracondylar process
anteromedial surface
lateral supracondylar crest
medial supracondylar crest
lateral border
coronoid fossa
radial fossa
lateral epicondyle
medial epicondyle
lateral supracondylar crest
capitulum
trochlea
capitulum
lateral epicondyle
humeral condyle

ANTERIOR VIEW

LATERAL VIEW

greater tubercle
capitulum of humerus
intertubercular sulcus
anatomical neck
lesser tubercle
greater tubercle
surgical neck
deltoid tuberosity
lateral border
groove for radial nerve
body of humerus
anterolateral surface
posterior surface
medial border
lateral supracondylar crest
medial supracondylar crest
olecranon fossa
medial epicondyle
lateral epicondyl
groove of ulnar nerve
trochlea
humeral condyle

POSTERIOR VIEW

UPPER LIMB (IV). FOREARM
RIGHT UPPER LIMB. ANTERIOR VIEW

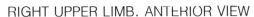

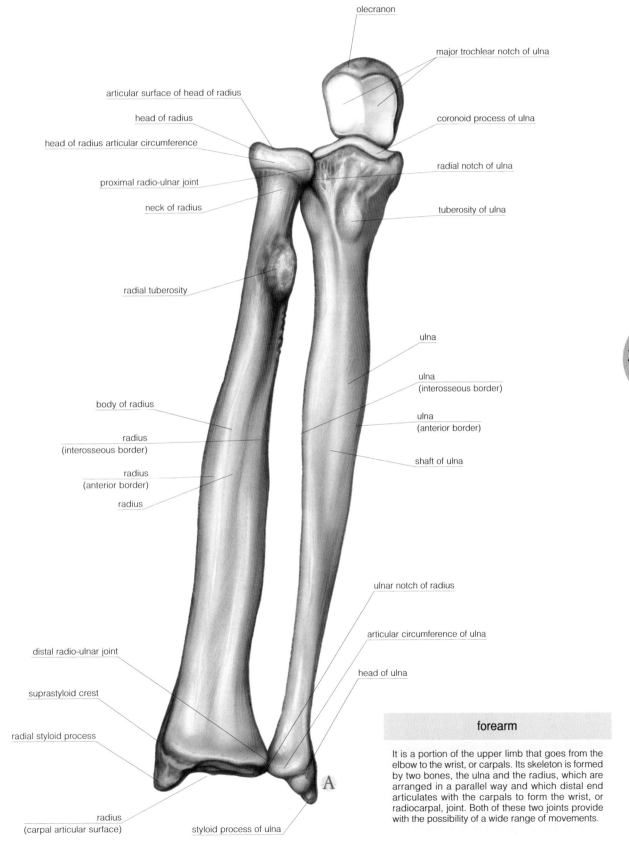

olecranon

major trochlear notch of ulna

articular surface of head of radius

coronoid process of ulna

head of radius

head of radius articular circumference

radial notch of ulna

proximal radio-ulnar joint

neck of radius

tuberosity of ulna

radial tuberosity

ulna

ulna
(interosseous border)

body of radius

ulna
(anterior border)

radius
(interosseous border)

shaft of ulna

radius
(anterior border)

radius

ulnar notch of radius

articular circumference of ulna

distal radio-ulnar joint

head of ulna

suprastyloid crest

radial styloid process

A

radius
(carpal articular surface)

styloid process of ulna

forearm

It is a portion of the upper limb that goes from the elbow to the wrist, or carpals. Its skeleton is formed by two bones, the ulna and the radius, which are arranged in a parallel way and which distal end articulates with the carpals to form the wrist, or radiocarpal, joint. Both of these two joints provide with the possibility of a wide range of movements.

UPPER LIMB (V). ULNA

LEFT UPPER LIMB

ulna

It is a long bone sited in the medial part of the forearm and along with the radius they form the skeleton of the above mentioned forearm that is able to move thanks to action of these two bones. This is the reason why it plays an essential role in all the movements of rotation of the arm and of the forearm. It is made up by a diaphysis (or central body) and two epiphysis (or ends).

At its proximal end, that is very voluminous, we can find the olecranon process, the coronoid process and the greater and lesser sigmoid cavities. It articulates with the trochlea of the humerus and the head of the radius to form the elbow joint. At its distal end, head of the ulna, which presents the styloid process, it articulates with the tarsal bones to form the wrist joint.

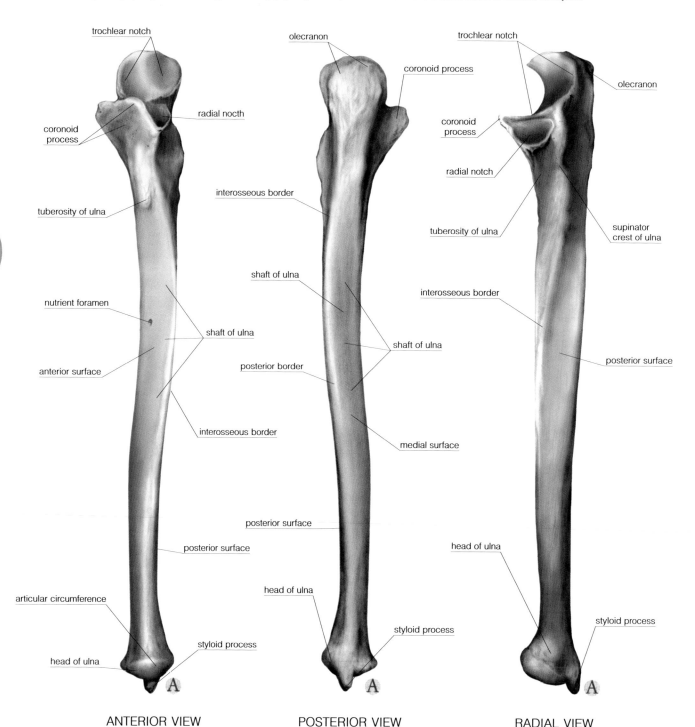

ANTERIOR VIEW

POSTERIOR VIEW

RADIAL VIEW

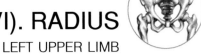

radius

Long, paired and symmetric bone, situated in the lateral part of the forearm. Together with the ulna it forms the skeleton of the forearm, which both cause to move, and so they do with the hand. It has a an almost cylindrical central body, called diaphysis, and two bulging extremities (ends), one superior and another inferior. Downwards from the superior end there is a head, a neck and the bicipital tuberosity. The head of the radius it articulates with the lateral epicondyle of the humerus through its shallow cap, or articular surface of head of radius, and with the radial notch (lesser sigmoid cavity) of the ulna, through its circumferential articular surface. Its inferior end (or epiphysis) has an inferior articular surface divided into two semi-surfaces: a most external one that articulates with the scaphoid bone and an internal one that articulates with the lunate bone of the carpals. On the internal part of this articular surface is the radial notch intended to articulate with the head of the ulna.

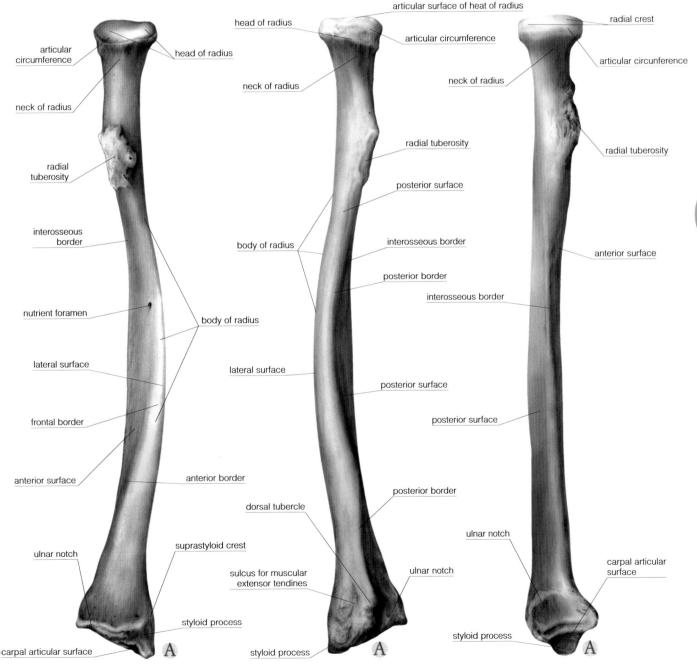

ANTERIOR VIEW

POSTERIOR VIEW

ULNAR VIEW

UPPER LIMB (VII). WRIST and METACARPUS (I)

LEFT UPPER LIMB. DORSAL VIEW

wrist

It is the region between the forearm and the palm of the hand. It is a structure made up for eight small bones, cuboid-shaped, arranged in two rows. The superior (proximal) row includes the scaphoid, lunate, triquetral and pisiform which have a proximal articulation with the inferior epiphysis of the ulna and the radius. The ones of the inferior (distal) row are the trapezium, trapezoid, capitate and hamate and they articulate with the five bones of the metacarpus so as to form the carpometacarpal joint.

metacarpus

It is the portion of the hand between the wrist and the fingers. It is an osseous structure formed by five cylindrical bones making up the palm of the hand and the first segment of the five fingers. Each one of these bones, (known as metacarpals) belongs to each one of the fingers and they are basically a cylindrical central body with two bulging ends (head and base). They decisively participate in the movements of the hand. Proximally they articulate with the carpal bones to form the carpometacarpal joint, and distally they do with the proximal phalanges of the corresponding fingers to form the metacarpophalangeal joints.

210

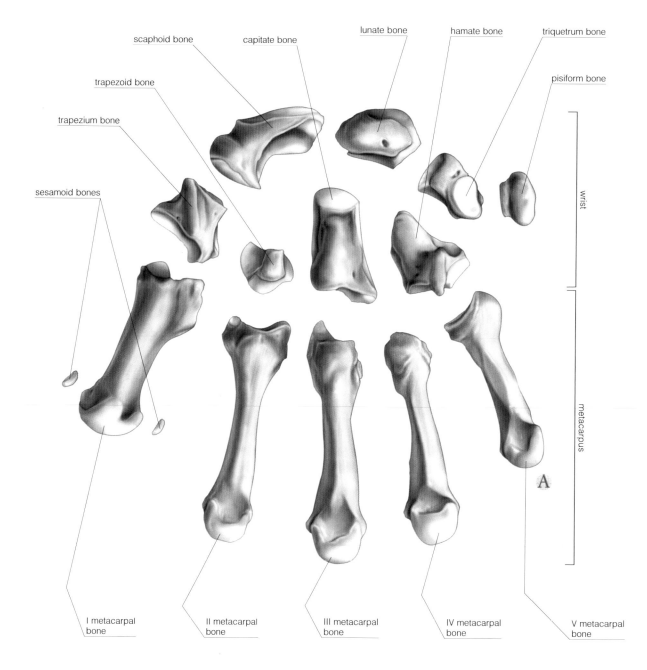

scaphoid bone

capitate bone

lunate bone

hamate bone

triquetrum bone

trapezoid bone

pisiform bone

trapezium bone

sesamoid bones

wrist

metacarpus

A

I metacarpal bone

II metacarpal bone

III metacarpal bone

IV metacarpal bone

V metacarpal bone

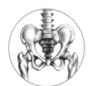

UPPER LIMB (VIII). WRIST and METACARPUS (II)

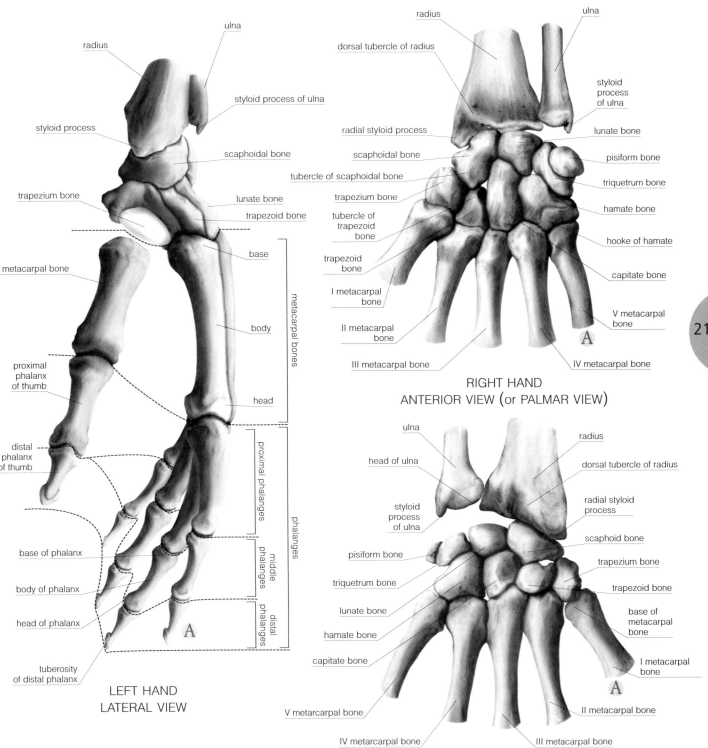

radius

ulna

dorsal tubercle of radius

styloid process of ulna

styloid process

scaphoidal bone

radial styloid process

lunate bone

trapezium bone

scaphoidal bone

pisiform bone

tubercle of scaphoidal bone

lunate bone

triquetrum bone

trapezoid bone

trapezium bone

hamate bone

base

tubercle of trapezoid bone

hooke of hamate

metacarpal bone

trapezoid bone

metacarpal bones

capitate bone

body

I metacarpal bone

proximal phalanx of thumb

II metacarpal bone

V metacarpal bone

head

III metacarpal bone

IV metacarpal bone

distal phalanx of thumb

**RIGHT HAND
ANTERIOR VIEW (or PALMAR VIEW)**

proximal phalanges

ulna

radius

base of phalanx

head of ulna

dorsal tubercle of radius

phalanges

middle phalanges

styloid process of ulna

radial styloid process

body of phalanx

pisiform bone

scaphoid bone

distal phalanges

triquetrum bone

trapezium bone

head of phalanx

lunate bone

trapezoid bone

hamate bone

base of metacarpal bone

tuberosity of distal phalanx

capitate bone

I metacarpal bone

**LEFT HAND
LATERAL VIEW**

V metacarpal bone

II metacarpal bone

IV metacarpal bone

III metacarpal bone

**RIGHT HAND
POSTERIOR VIEW (or DORSAL VIEW)**

UPPER LIMB (IX). HAND (I)

RIGHT UPPER LIMB. PALMAR VIEW

hand

It is the third or ending segment of the upper limb and also the most distal one. Three sections form the hand: carpus, metacarpus and fingers. The skeleton of the hand is figured by a series of bones with very important duties, like gestures, gripping objects, etc. This group of bones may be divided into two: carpal bones (scaphoid, lunate, triquetral, pisiform, trapezium, trapezoid, capitate and hamate) and the fingers. The last ones are made up of three groups of phalanges (proximal, medial and distal), except the thumb, which only has two of them (proximal and distal). Some groups of these bones combine one to the others to body various joints: radiocarpal joint (the distal end of the radius with the bones of the proximal row of the carpus); metacarpophalangeal joints (the bones of the carpus with the fingers); intercarpal (the proximal row of the carpal bones with the distal row of the same bones); carpometacarpal of the thumb (the trapezium with the proximal end of the first metacarpal bone); carpometacarpal of the other four fingers (bones of the distal row of the carpus with the proximal end of 2nd to 5th metacarpals) and interpahlangeal of the hand (the articular capsules of the phalanges one to the other).

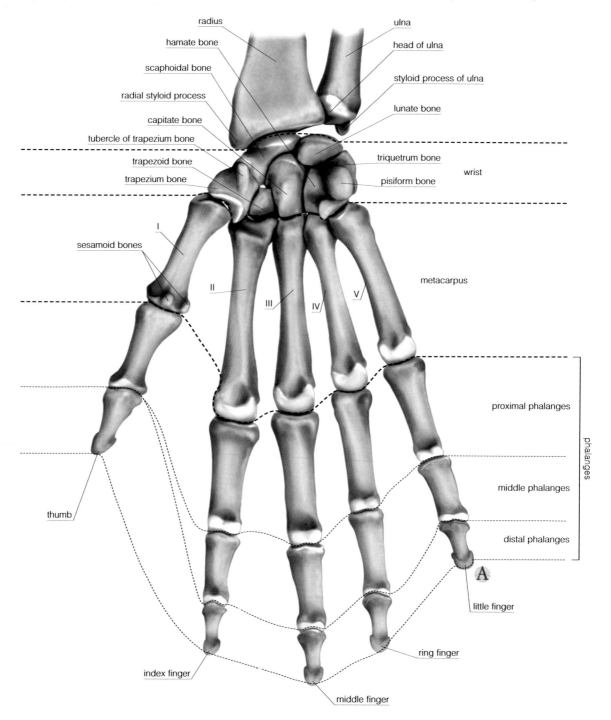

UPPER LIMB (X). HAND (II)

RIGHT UPPER LIMB. DORSAL VIEW

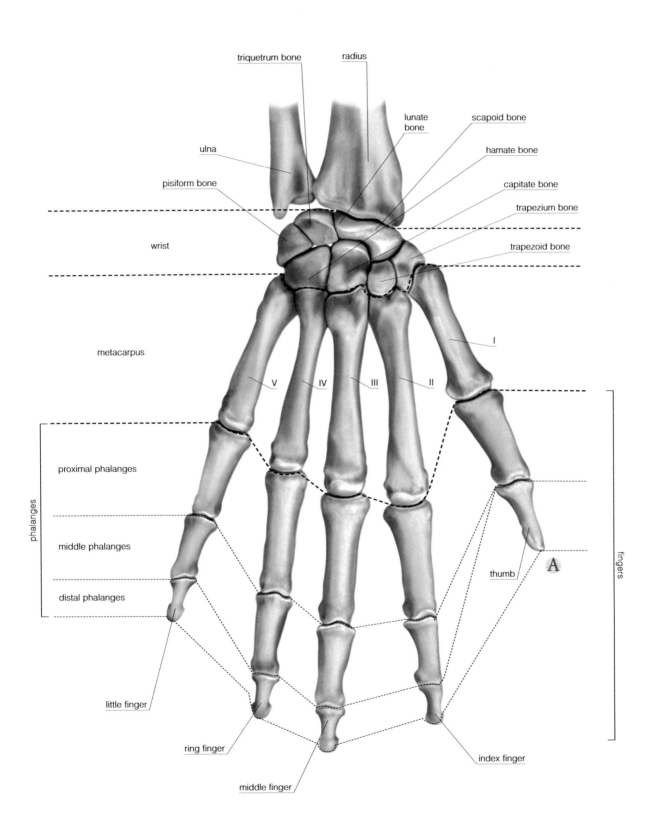

triquetrum bone

radius

lunate bone

scapoid bone

ulna

hamate bone

pisiform bone

capitate bone

trapezium bone

wrist

trapezoid bone

metacarpus

I

213

V   IV   III   II

proximal phalanges

phalanges

middle phalanges

distal phalanges

thumb

A

fingers

little finger

ring finger

index finger

middle finger

PELVIS (I)
ANTERIOR VIEW

pelvis

Osseous ring of the homonymous region of the body that is located in the inferior part of the trunk. It is formed by two hip bones and the most inferior pieces of the vertebral column: the sacrum and the coccyx. As a whole it has the shape of a truncated cone with the basis upside down, and it constitutes the pelvic cavity. It houses inside some viscus of the digestive, urinary and genital systems. The superior strait, from the base of sacrum to the superior border of the pubic symphysis, divides the pelvis into two parts: superior (grater or false pelvis) and inferior (lesser or true pelvis). The diameters of pelvis varies according to sexual differences. Thus, in women horizontal diameters predominate, which means pelvis is wider, an essential characteristic having in mind the space needed during childbirth. In a newborn the pelvis is not completely developed.

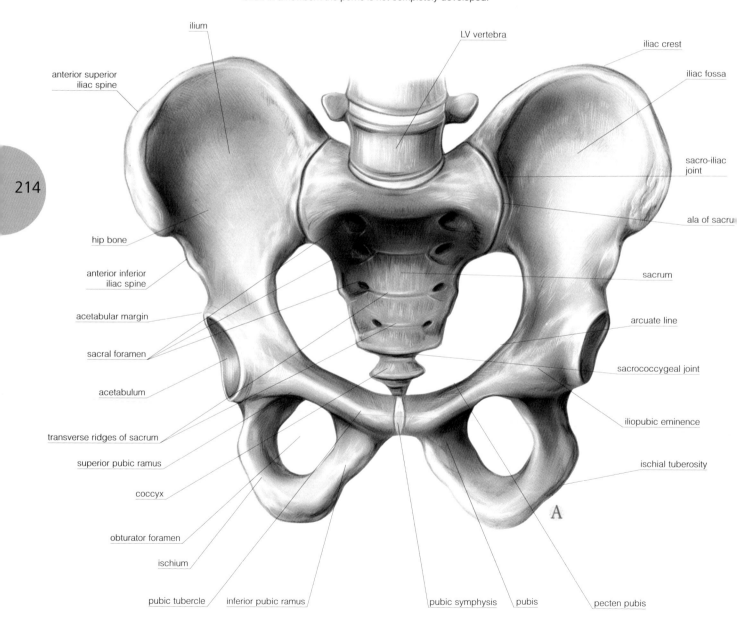

ilium

LV vertebra

iliac crest

anterior superior iliac spine

iliac fossa

sacro-iliac joint

ala of sacru

hip bone

sacrum

anterior inferior iliac spine

acetabular margin

arcuate line

sacral foramen

sacrococcygeal joint

acetabulum

iliopubic eminence

transverse ridges of sacrum

ischial tuberosity

superior pubic ramus

coccyx

A

obturator foramen

ischium

pubic tubercle   inferior pubic ramus

pubic symphysis   pubis   pecten pubis

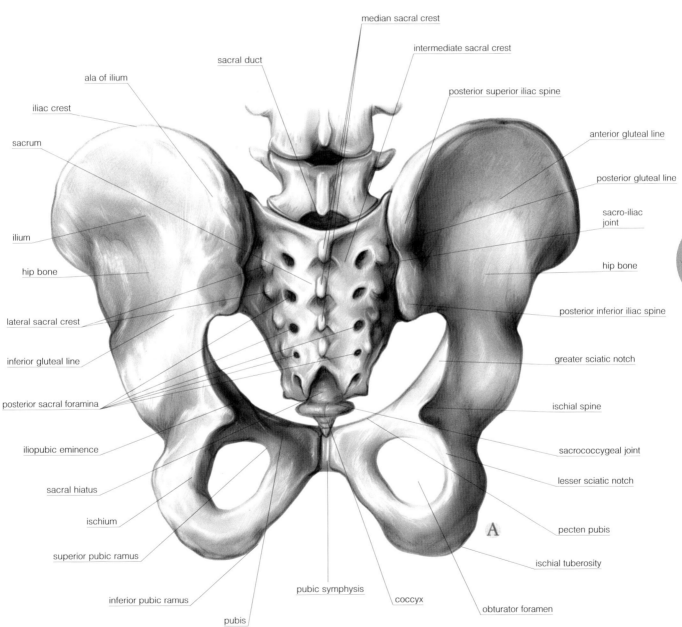

median sacral crest

intermediate sacral crest

sacral duct

posterior superior iliac spine

ala of ilium

iliac crest

anterior gluteal line

sacrum

posterior gluteal line

sacro-iliac joint

ilium

hip bone

hip bone

posterior inferior iliac spine

lateral sacral crest

inferior gluteal line

greater sciatic notch

posterior sacral foramina

ischial spine

sacrococcygeal joint

iliopubic eminence

lesser sciatic notch

sacral hiatus

ischium

A

pecten pubis

superior pubic ramus

ischial tuberosity

inferior pubic ramus

pubic symphysis

coccyx

obturator foramen

pubis

PELVIS (III). DIFFERENCES BETWEEN SEXES

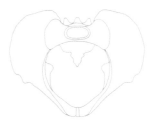

superior diameter limits
- lumbosacral and sacro-iliac joints
- arcuate line
- iliopectinal eminence
- superior border of pubis

male pelvis

The male pelvis is more oblique and narrower than in women. The dorsal surface of the sacrum is more salient in the case of women. The superior strait is less oval and smaller than in women, even though the vertical measurements are larger in the case of men.

216

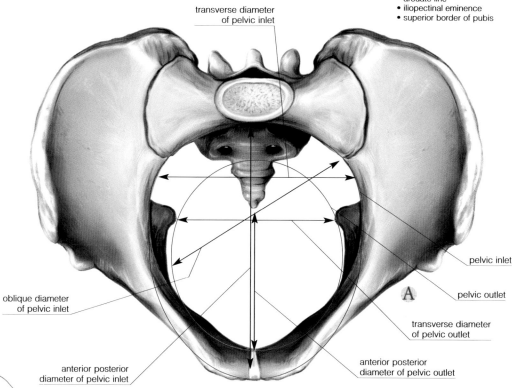

transverse diameter of pelvic inlet

oblique diameter of pelvic inlet

anterior posterior diameter of pelvic inlet

pelvic inlet

pelvic outlet

transverse diameter of pelvic outlet

anterior posterior diameter of pelvic outlet

A

MALE PELVIS. SUPERIOR VIEW

inferior diameter limits
- inferior border of symphysis
- inferior borders of ischiopubic branches
- sacrosciatic ligaments
- coccyx

female pelvis

The female pelvis is larger and broader than in men. The superior strait transversally figures an anterior segment and a posterior one, both rounded. The transversal measurements are inferior than in the case of the male pelvis. It also has a slope in regards to the vertebral column and the external surface of the sacrum is less prominent than in the case of men.

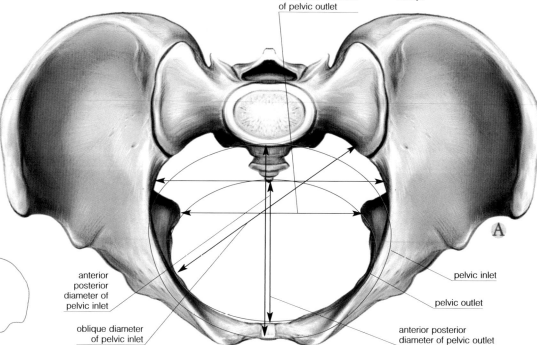

transverse diameter of pelvic outlet

anterior posterior diameter of pelvic inlet

oblique diameter of pelvic inlet

pelvic inlet

pelvic outlet

anterior posterior diameter of pelvic outlet

A

FEMALE PELVIS. SUPERIOR VIEW

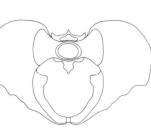

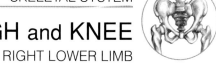

LOWER LIMB (I) THIGH and KNEE

RIGHT LOWER LIMB

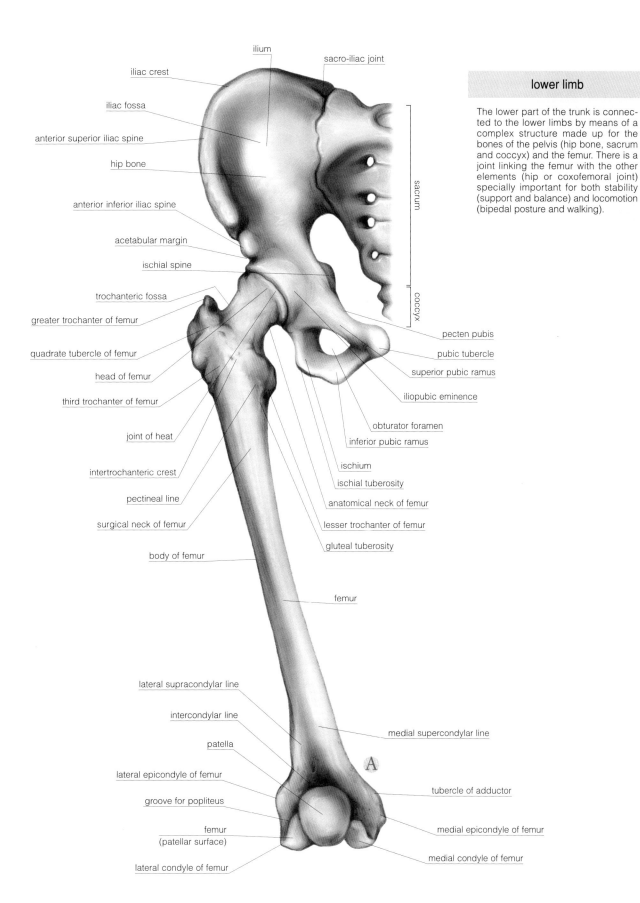

lower limb

The lower part of the trunk is connected to the lower limbs by means of a complex structure made up for the bones of the pelvis (hip bone, sacrum and coccyx) and the femur. There is a joint linking the femur with the other elements (hip or coxofemoral joint) specially important for both stability (support and balance) and locomotion (bipedal posture and walking).

217

ilium

sacro-iliac joint

iliac crest

iliac fossa

anterior superior iliac spine

hip bone

anterior inferior iliac spine

acetabular margin

ischial spine

trochanteric fossa

greater trochanter of femur

quadrate tubercle of femur

head of femur

third trochanter of femur

joint of heat

intertrochanteric crest

pectineal line

surgical neck of femur

body of femur

sacrum

coccyx

pecten pubis

pubic tubercle

superior pubic ramus

iliopubic eminence

obturator foramen

inferior pubic ramus

ischium

ischial tuberosity

anatomical neck of femur

lesser trochanter of femur

gluteal tuberosity

femur

lateral supracondylar line

intercondylar line

patella

lateral epicondyle of femur

groove for popliteus

femur
(patellar surface)

lateral condyle of femur

medial supercondylar line

tubercle of adductor

medial epicondyle of femur

medial condyle of femur

LOWER LIMB (II). HIP BONE (I)

RIGHT LOWER LIMB. LATERAL VIEW

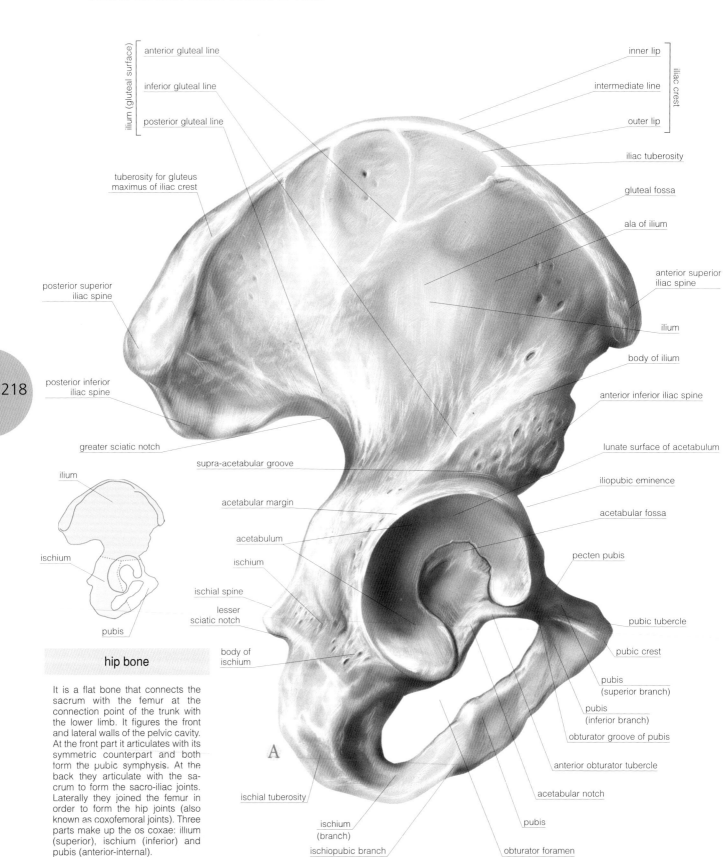

ilium (gluteal surface)

anterior gluteal line

inferior gluteal line

posterior gluteal line

inner lip

intermediate line

outer lip

iliac crest

iliac tuberosity

tuberosity for gluteus maximus of iliac crest

gluteal fossa

ala of ilium

posterior superior iliac spine

anterior superior iliac spine

ilium

body of ilium

posterior inferior iliac spine

anterior inferior iliac spine

greater sciatic notch

lunate surface of acetabulum

supra-acetabular groove

iliopubic eminence

acetabular margin

acetabular fossa

acetabulum

pecten pubis

ischium

ischial spine

lesser sciatic notch

pubic tubercle

pubic crest

body of ischium

pubis (superior branch)

pubis (inferior branch)

obturator groove of pubis

anterior obturator tubercle

acetabular notch

ischial tuberosity

ischium (branch)

pubis

ischiopubic branch

obturator foramen

A

ilium

ischium

pubis

hip bone

It is a flat bone that connects the sacrum with the femur at the connection point of the trunk with the lower limb. It figures the front and lateral walls of the pelvic cavity. At the front part it articulates with its symmetric counterpart and both form the pubic symphysis. At the back they articulate with the sacrum to form the sacro-iliac joints. Laterally they joined the femur in order to form the hip joints (also known as coxofemoral joints). Three parts make up the os coxae: ilium (superior), ischium (inferior) and pubis (anterior-internal).

218

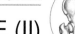

LOWER LIMB (III). HIP BONE (II)

RIGHT INFERIOR LIMB. MEDIAL VIEW

hip bone

This bone presents important prominences: the iliac crest, that is the superior border, located between two osseous prominences (anterior-superior and posterior-inferior iliac spines and the ischial spine); the arcuate line, that divides the internal surface of the bone; the acetabular fossa (acetabulum or cotyloid cavity), which figures the hip joint; and the obturator foramen that works as an essential way for vital structures of this region.

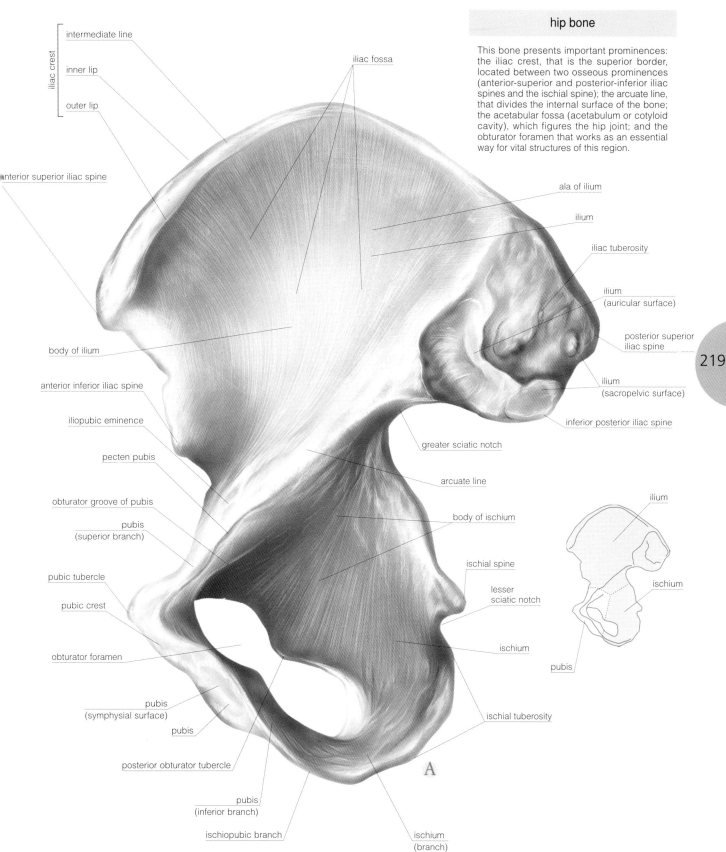

iliac crest
- intermediate line
- inner lip
- outer lip

iliac fossa

anterior superior iliac spine

ala of ilium

ilium

iliac tuberosity

ilium (auricular surface)

posterior superior iliac spine

body of ilium

ilium (sacropelvic surface)

anterior inferior iliac spine

inferior posterior iliac spine

iliopubic eminence

greater sciatic notch

pecten pubis

arcuate line

obturator groove of pubis

body of ischium

pubis (superior branch)

pubic tubercle

ischial spine

pubic crest

lesser sciatic notch

obturator foramen

ischium

pubis (symphysial surface)

pubis

posterior obturator tubercle

ischial tuberosity

pubis (inferior branch)

ischiopubic branch

ischium (branch)

ilium

ischium

pubis

A

219

LOWER LIMB (IV). FEMUR (I)

RIGHT LOWER LIMB

femur

A thick bone that makes part of the lower limb (it figures the skeleton of the thigh) which the torso is linked to. It is both the longest and strongest bone of the human body and runs from the pelvis to the knee. It is made up for a more or less cylindrical central shaft and two bulging ends, one superior (proximal), which articulates with the acetabulum of the hip bone in order to form the hip joint, and another one inferior (distal), which articulates with the tibia and fibula so as to form the knee joint. It is the point of insertion of the locomotion muscles of the lower limb.

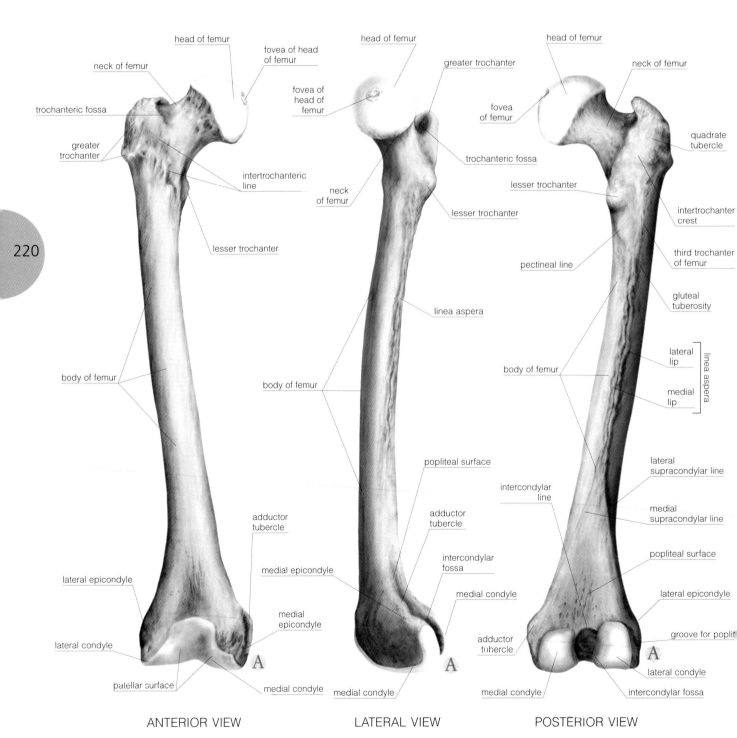

ANTERIOR VIEW

- head of femur
- fovea of head of femur
- neck of femur
- trochanteric fossa
- greater trochanter
- intertrochanteric line
- lesser trochanter
- body of femur
- adductor tubercle
- medial epicondyle
- lateral epicondyle
- medial epicondyle
- lateral condyle
- patellar surface
- medial condyle

LATERAL VIEW

- head of femur
- greater trochanter
- fovea of head of femur
- trochanteric fossa
- neck of femur
- lesser trochanter
- linea aspera
- body of femur
- popliteal surface
- adductor tubercle
- intercondylar fossa
- medial condyle
- medial epicondyle

POSTERIOR VIEW

- head of femur
- neck of femur
- fovea of femur
- quadrate tubercle
- lesser trochanter
- intertrochanter crest
- pectineal line
- third trochanter of femur
- gluteal tuberosity
- lateral lip
- body of femur
- medial lip
- linea aspera
- lateral supracondylar line
- intercondylar line
- medial supracondylar line
- popliteal surface
- lateral epicondyle
- groove for poplit
- adductor tubercle
- lateral condyle
- medial condyle
- intercondylar fossa

LOWER LIMB (V). FEMUR (II)

RIGHT LOWER LIMB

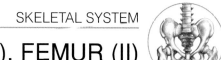

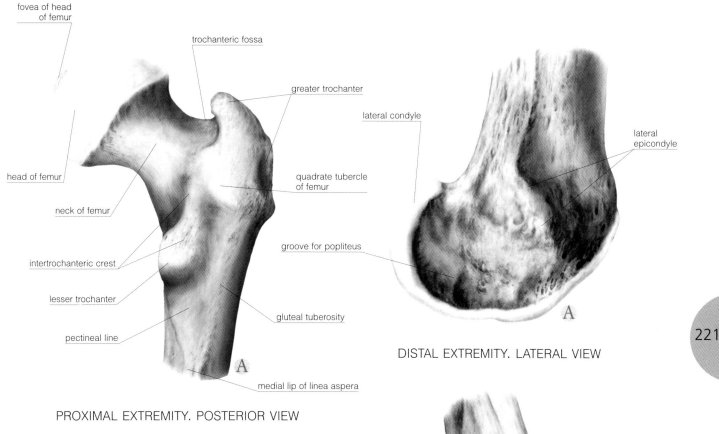

fovea of head of femur

trochanteric fossa

greater trochanter

lateral condyle

lateral epicondyle

head of femur

quadrate tubercle of femur

neck of femur

groove for popliteus

intertrochanteric crest

lesser trochanter

gluteal tuberosity

pectineal line

A

DISTAL EXTREMITY. LATERAL VIEW

medial lip of linea aspera

PROXIMAL EXTREMITY. POSTERIOR VIEW

221

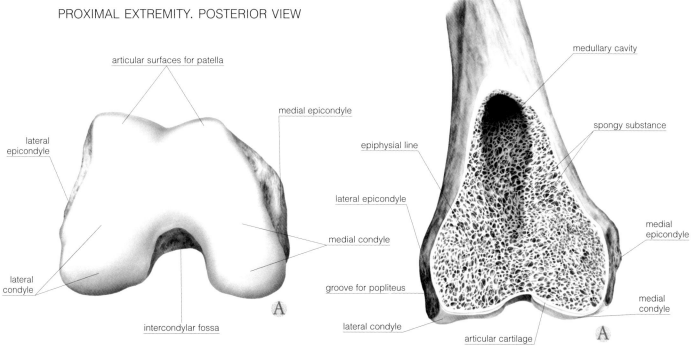

articular surfaces for patella

medial epicondyle

lateral epicondyle

epiphysial line

medullary cavity

spongy substance

lateral epicondyle

lateral condyle

medial condyle

groove for popliteus

medial epicondyle

lateral condyle

intercondylar fossa

lateral condyle

articular cartilage

medial condyle

A

A

DISTAL EXTREMITY. DISTAL VIEW

FRONTAL SECTION. ANTERIOR VIEW

LOWER LIMB (VI). KNEE

RIGHT LOWER LIMB

knee

Medial anatomic region of the lower limb, the knee is the connecting point between the thigh and the leg. It has an amazing flexion capability due to presence of two articulations: femorotibial and femoropatellar joints. The articular surfaces are formed by the distal end of the femur (trochlea femoris and femoral condyles), by the proximal end of the tibia (glenoid cavities), and by the back surface of the patella (external and internal articular surfaces). The soft parts of the knee are the internal and external menisci, the articular capsule, the medial and lateral collateral ligaments, the cruciate ligaments, the arcuate and oblique popliteal ones, the patellar ligament, the surrounding muscles and aponeurosis, as well as the infrapatellar fat pad. It is a very vital region that allows the body to keep an upright position and to walk.

patella

Flat and slightly rounded bone located in the anterior region of the knee. Its anterior surface is convex, and is covered by the prepatellar bursae, and its posterior surface is concave, with two small surfaces that fit the femoral condyles and participate in the knee joint. In the patella the quadriceps muscles get inserted (from above) and the patellar ligament (from below).

222

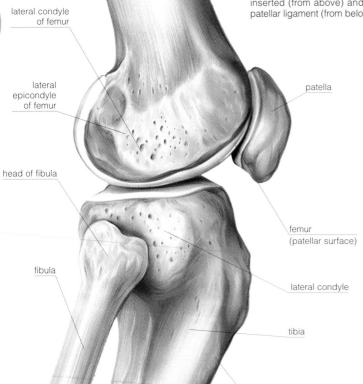

LATERAL VIEW

femur

lateral condyle of femur

lateral epicondyle of femur

head of fibula

fibula

patella

femur (patellar surface)

lateral condyle

tibia

anterior tubercle

A

PATELLA

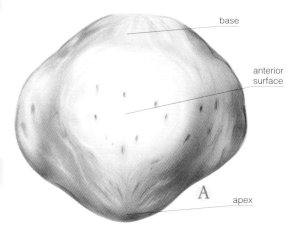

base

anterior surface

apex

A

ANTERIOR VIEW

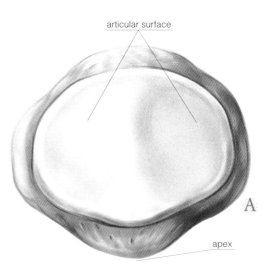

articular surface

apex

A

POSTERIOR VIEW

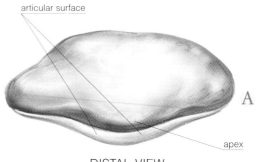

articular surface

apex

A

DISTAL VIEW

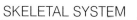

LOWER LIMB (VII). LEG
RIGHT LOWER LIMB. ANTERIOR VIEW

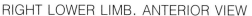

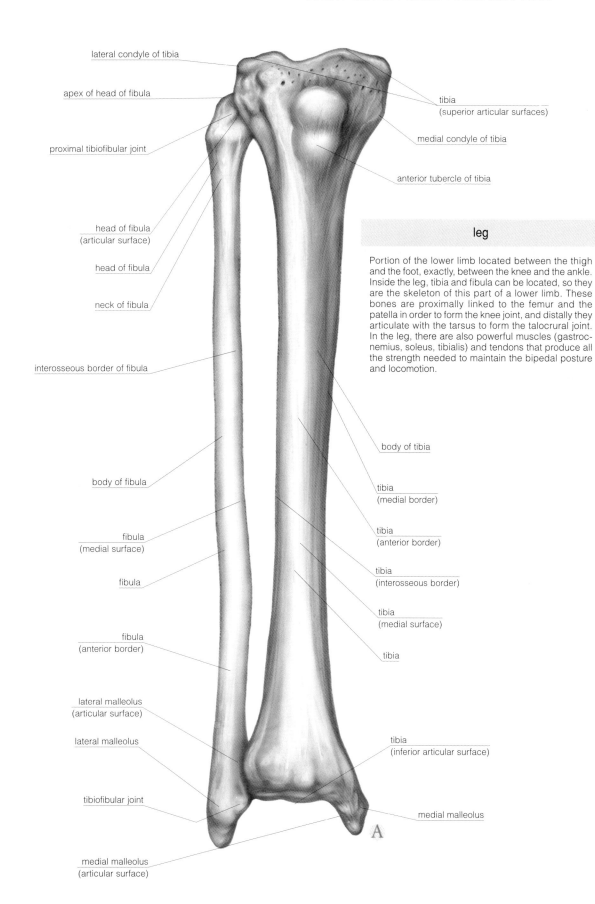

lateral condyle of tibia

apex of head of fibula

proximal tibiofibular joint

head of fibula
(articular surface)

head of fibula

neck of fibula

interosseous border of fibula

body of fibula

fibula
(medial surface)

fibula

fibula
(anterior border)

lateral malleolus
(articular surface)

lateral malleolus

tibiofibular joint

medial malleolus
(articular surface)

tibia
(superior articular surfaces)

medial condyle of tibia

anterior tubercle of tibia

leg

Portion of the lower limb located between the thigh and the foot, exactly, between the knee and the ankle. Inside the leg, tibia and fibula can be located, so they are the skeleton of this part of a lower limb. These bones are proximally linked to the femur and the patella in order to form the knee joint, and distally they articulate with the tarsus to form the talocrural joint. In the leg, there are also powerful muscles (gastrocnemius, soleus, tibialis) and tendons that produce all the strength needed to maintain the bipedal posture and locomotion.

223

body of tibia

tibia
(medial border)

tibia
(anterior border)

tibia
(interosseous border)

tibia
(medial surface)

tibia

tibia
(inferior articular surface)

medial malleolus

A

LOWER LIMB (VIII). TIBIA

RIGHT LOWER LIMB

tibia

It is a long, thick, paired and asymmetric bone sited in the lower limb, on the anterior-internal part of the leg, medial in regards to the fibula. Both, tibia an fibula, figure the skeleton of the leg, below the femur and above the tarsus. It consists of a body, also known as diaphysis, and two ends, also known as epiphysis, one superior and another inferior. The superior epiphysis presents two, internal and external, horizontal articular surfaces, which are slightly concave, and which are also known as glenoid cavities of the tibia; they both articulate with the femoral condyles. Both glenoid cavities rest on two voluminous masses, tuberosities of the tibia; all together they form the tibial plateau. The internal tuberosity presents an articular semi-surface intended to articulate with a similar semi-surface at the head of the fibula. The inferior epiphysis presents an interior surface that articulates with the talus, it also presents a differentiable internal aspect in the form of a voluminous apophysis known as medial malleolus, and a lateral concave surface intended to fit with the inferior end of the fibula.

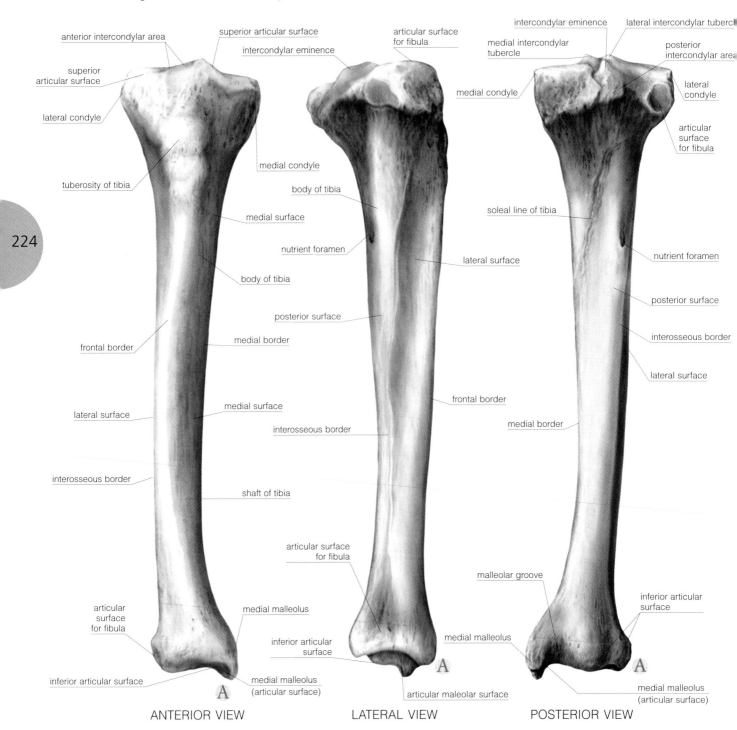

anterior intercondylar area

superior articular surface

lateral condyle

tuberosity of tibia

frontal border

lateral surface

interosseous border

articular surface for fibula

inferior articular surface

superior articular surface

intercondylar eminence

medial condyle

body of tibia

medial surface

nutrient foramen

body of tibia

posterior surface

medial border

medial surface

interosseous border

shaft of tibia

articular surface for fibula

medial malleolus

inferior articular surface

medial malleolus (articular surface)

ANTERIOR VIEW

articular surface for fibula

medial condyle

lateral surface

frontal border

articular surface for fibula

inferior articular surface

medial malleolus

articular maleolar surface

LATERAL VIEW

intercondylar eminence

medial intercondylar tubercle

medial condyle

lateral intercondylar tubercl

posterior intercondylar area

lateral condyle

articular surface for fibula

soleal line of tibia

nutrient foramen

posterior surface

interosseous border

lateral surface

medial border

malleolar groove

inferior articular surface

medial malleolus

medial malleolus (articular surface)

POSTERIOR VIEW

LOWER LIMB (IX). TIBIA and FIBULA

fibula

It is one of the longest and thinnest bones of the human body located at the lateral part of the leg. Together with the tibia if figures the skeleton of the leg. It extends downwards from the knee to the ankle. It consists of a long body and two bulging ends; one superior (proximal) that articulates with the superior end of the tibia, and another inferior (distal) that articulates with inferior end of the tibia; they both form the tibiofibular syndesmosis. It participates in the knee joint (proximally) and in the ankle joint (distally). Its distal ends it also articulates with the talus bone. The fibula represents above all a muscular insertion zone, since the function of supporting the lower limb is carried out by the tibia.

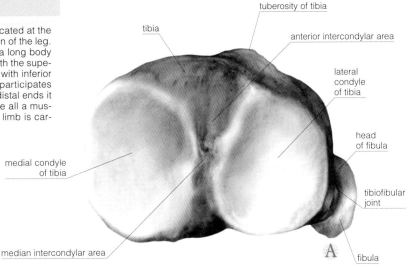

TIBIA and FIBULA. PROXIMAL VIEW

225

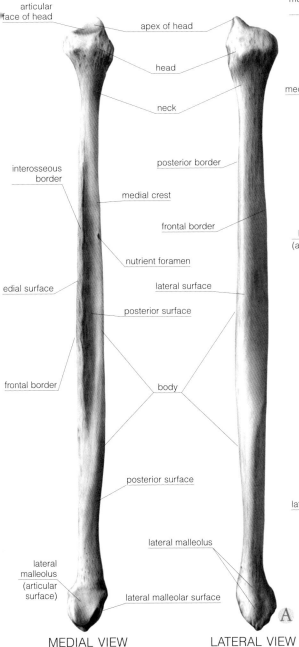

MEDIAL VIEW   LATERAL VIEW

FIBULA

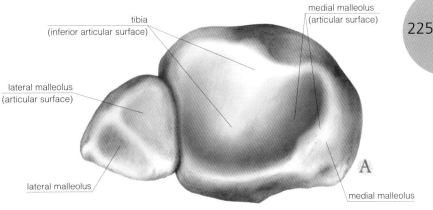

TIBIA and FIBULA. DISTAL VIEW

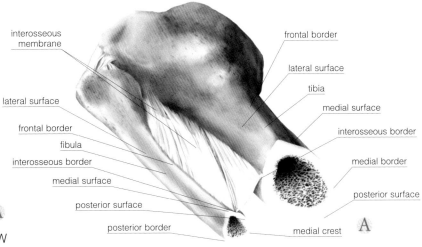

TIBIA and FIBULA. DISTAL VIEW

LOWER LIMB (X). FOOT (I)

RIGHT LOWER LIMB. DORSAL VIEW

226

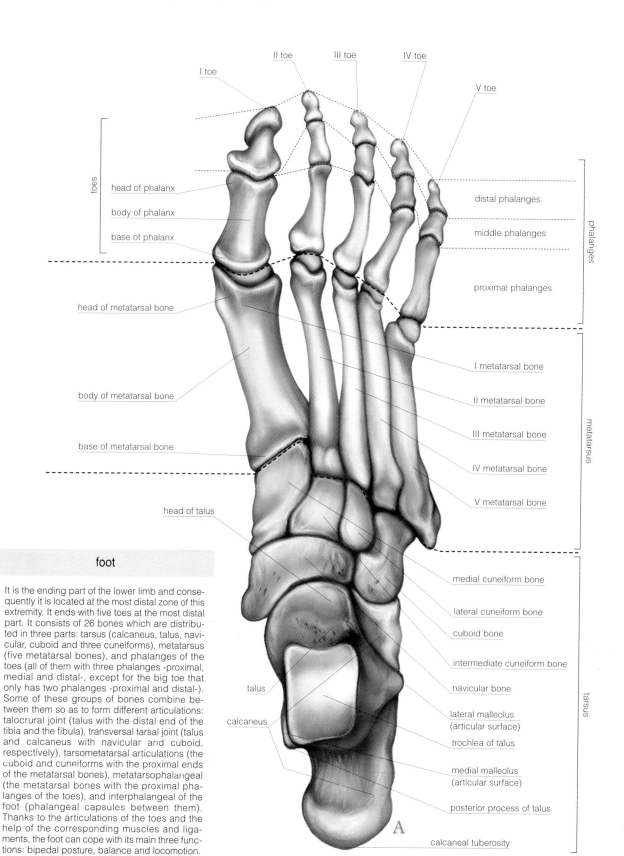

toes

I toe
II toe
III toe
IV toe
V toe

head of phalanx
body of phalanx
base of phalanx

distal phalanges
middle phalanges
proximal phalanges

phalanges

head of metatarsal bone

I metatarsal bone
II metatarsal bone
III metatarsal bone
IV metatarsal bone
V metatarsal bone

metatarsus

body of metatarsal bone

base of metatarsal bone

head of talus

medial cuneiform bone
lateral cuneiform bone
cuboid bone
intermediate cuneiform bone
navicular bone

talus
calcaneus

lateral malleolus
(articular surface)
trochlea of talus
medial malleolus
(articular surface)
posterior process of talus

tarsus

calcaneal tuberosity

A

foot

It is the ending part of the lower limb and consequently it is located at the most distal zone of this extremity. It ends with five toes at the most distal part. It consists of 26 bones which are distributed in three parts: tarsus (calcaneus, talus, navicular, cuboid and three cuneiforms), metatarsus (five metatarsal bones), and phalanges of the toes (all of them with three phalanges -proximal, medial and distal-, except for the big toe that only has two phalanges -proximal and distal-). Some of these groups of bones combine between them so as to form different articulations: talocrural joint (talus with the distal end of the tibia and the fibula), transversal tarsal joint (talus and calcaneus with navicular and cuboid, respectively), tarsometatarsal articulations (the cuboid and cuneiforms with the proximal ends of the metatarsal bones), metatarsophalangeal (the metatarsal bones with the proximal phalanges of the toes), and interphalangeal of the foot (phalangeal capsules between them). Thanks to the articulations of the toes and the help of the corresponding muscles and ligaments, the foot can cope with its main three functions: bipedal posture, balance and locomotion.

LOWER LIMB (XI). FOOT (II)

RIGHT LOWER LIMB. PLANTAR VIEW

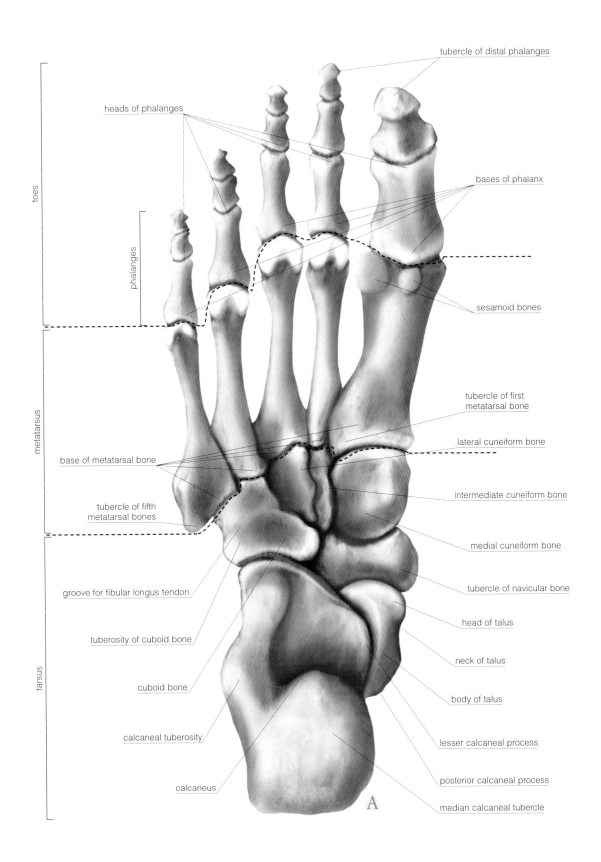

tubercle of distal phalanges

heads of phalanges

bases of phalanx

sesamoid bones

tubercle of first metatarsal bone

lateral cuneiform bone

intermediate cuneiform bone

base of metatarsal bone

medial cuneiform bone

tubercle of fifth metatarsal bones

tubercle of navicular bone

groove for fibular longus tendon

head of talus

tuberosity of cuboid bone

neck of talus

cuboid bone

body of talus

calcaneal tuberosity

lesser calcaneal process

calcaneus

posterior calcaneal process

median calcaneal tubercle

toes

phalanges

metatarsus

tarsus

A

227

LOWER LIMB (XII). FOOT (III)

RIGHT LOWER LIMB. LATERAL VIEWS

the toes

The toes are each one of the five appendages the distal extremity of the lower limb ends up. They are formed by 14 bones, known as phalanges. In all the five toes there are three phalanges (proximal, medial and distal), except for the big toe which only has two (proximal and distal). Nevertheless, they have a similar structure, the toes are not as developed as the fingers of the hands, and however they have mobility, this mobility is less than in the case of the one of the fingers of the hands.

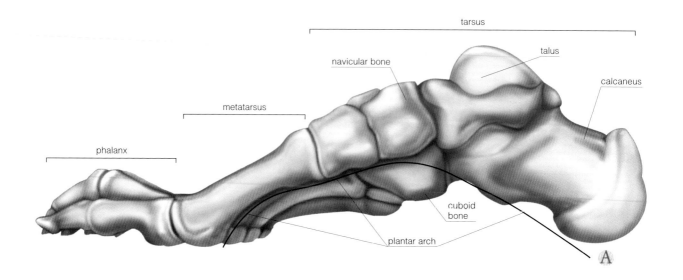

posterior process of talus

talus

neck of talus

calcaneus

cuboid bone

navicular bone

lateral

intermediate

medial

cuneiform bones

proximal phalanges

middle phalanges

distal phalanges

calcaneal tuberosity

medial process of calcaneal tuberosity

tuberosity of fifth metatarsal bone

lateral process of calcaneal tuberosity

I metatarsal bone

II metatarsal bone

III metatarsal bone

IV metatarsal bone

V metatarsal bone

A

tarsus

navicular bone

talus

calcaneus

metatarsus

phalanx

cuboid bone

plantar arch

A

LOWER LIMB (XIII). FOOT (IV). TALUS

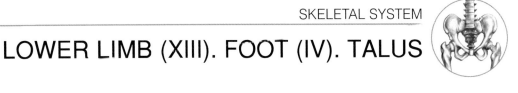

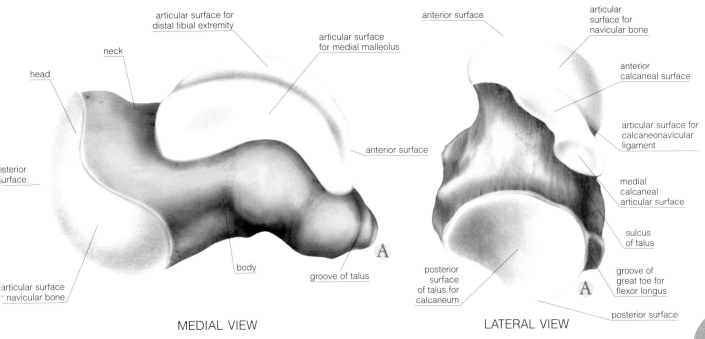

MEDIAL VIEW

- articular surface for distal tibial extremity
- neck
- head
- articular surface for medial malleolus
- posterior surface
- anterior surface
- body
- groove of talus
- articular surface for navicular bone

LATERAL VIEW

- anterior surface
- articular surface for navicular bone
- anterior calcaneal surface
- articular surface for calcaneonavicular ligament
- medial calcaneal articular surface
- sulcus of talus
- groove of great toe for flexor longus
- posterior surface
- posterior surface of talus for calcaneum

229

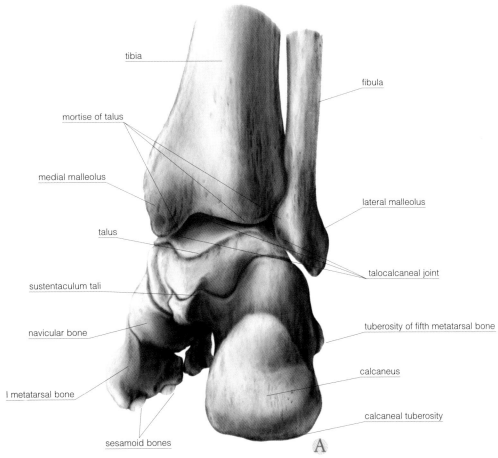

POSTERIOR VIEW

- tibia
- fibula
- mortise of talus
- medial malleolus
- talus
- lateral malleolus
- talocalcaneal joint
- sustentaculum tali
- navicular bone
- tuberosity of fifth metatarsal bone
- I metatarsal bone
- calcaneus
- calcaneal tuberosity
- sesamoid bones

LOWER LIMB (XIV). FOOT (V). TARSUS and METATARSU

RIGHT LOWER LIMB. DORSAL VIEW

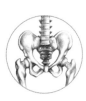

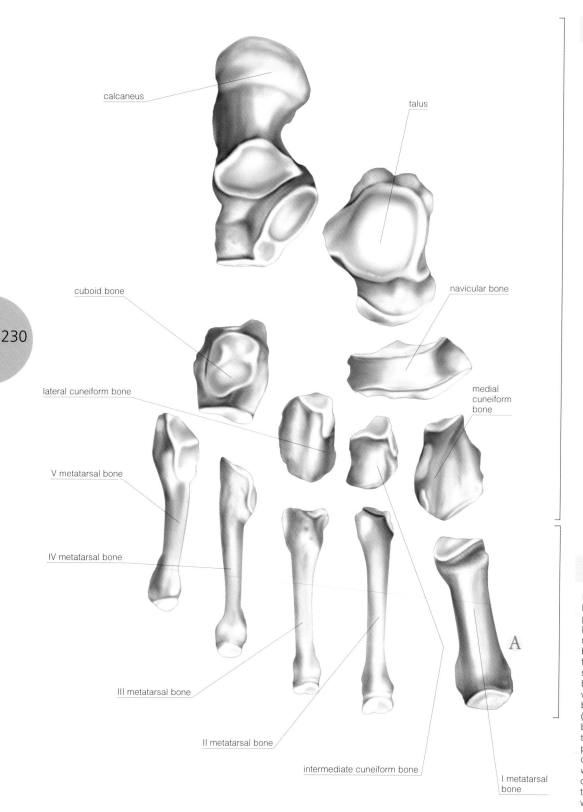

calcaneus

talus

cuboid bone

navicular bone

lateral cuneiform bone

medial cuneiform bone

V metatarsal bone

IV metatarsal bone

III metatarsal bone

II metatarsal bone

intermediate cuneiform bone

I metatarsal bone

A

230

tarsus

It is the back portion of the foot that includes the ankle and the segment of the articulation of the foot and the leg. The skeleton of the tarsus is figured by a collection of seven short bones which are arranged in two rows: in the first one (proximal) the talus and the calcaneus can be distinguished; in the second one (distal), the navicular, the cuboid and three cuneiforms appear. Different combinations of the tarsal bones give rise to different articulations: talocrural joint (talus with the distal end of the tibia and the fibula), transversal tarsal joint (talus and calcaneus with navicular and cuboid, respectively), and the tarsometatarsal articulations (the cuboid and cuneiforms with the proximal ends of the metatarsal bones).

metatarsus

It is the segment of the foot between the tarsus and the phalanges of the toes. The skeleton of the metatarsus is formed by a group of five long bones, called metatarsals, that form the plantar arch and consist of a cylindrical central body and two bulging ends which articulates with other bones: Thus, the proximal end (posterior) is linked to the bones of the tarsus and the distal end (anterior) is linked to the phalanges of the corresponding toe. They also articulate with the cuboid and the three cuneiforms in order to form the tarsometatarsal articulations with very little mobility.

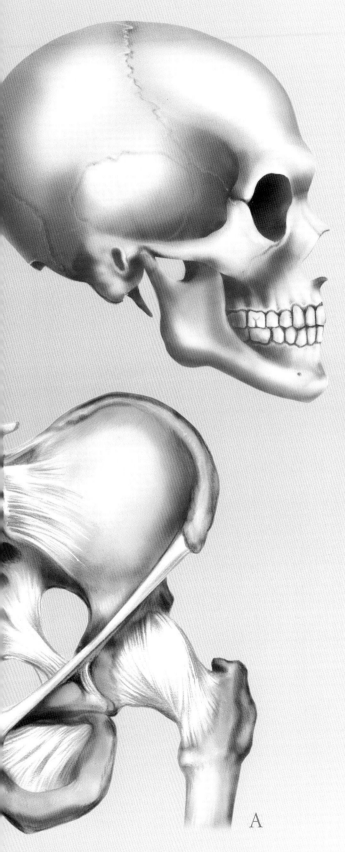

JOINTS

An articulation or joint is the area of join that exist between two contiguous bones and that plays a decisive role in the growth of the individual. But, if it's talked from a physiological point of view, the articulation is a very important structure of the locomotive apparatus. Thus joined with the bones and the muscles and activated conveniently by the nerves, contributes in a determinate way that different body parts and bone surfaces are able to move coordinately and that all the body not only dispose of a wide and varied mobility (adduction, abduction, tension, extension, pronation, supination, circumduction, etc), but also itself, as a whole be able to move and relate with its environment.

Articulations are formed by a group of components that make possible the correct development of its function. The bone articulations consist of articular surfaces -or parts of the bones that contact-, the articular cartilages -that cover the articular surfaces and avoid its outwear-, the articular ligaments -that present diversity of forms, either intra or extra articulated, to be able to guarantee the contact between articular surfaces-, the articular capsule, or synovial -that limited the articulation and besides through the synovial liquid, lubricates, such articulation and facilitates the articulated mechanic- and, in some cases, other gristly formations, like the meniscus of the knee, or the inter vertebral discs, etc. -that are interposed between the surfaces of certain articulations-. Between the articulated surfaces and the articulated capsule there is an space -articulated cavity-, that is occupied by the synovial liquid.

According to the grade and type of movement to be developed, the articulations are classified in:

- Synarthrosis: They lack of cartilages, synovial capsule and ligaments, their articulated surfaces are dented and irregular and they are immobile (cranium articulations). Is the growth of the bone or the existence of a resistant cartilage or connective fibrous tissue that maintain the bones together.

- Amphiarthrosis (or symphysis): Its capsule and ligaments are rigid and its articulated surfaces are flat (articulations of vertebral bodies and sacro-iliac). Holds strongly the bones and allows a scarce mobility.

- Synovial (or diarthrosis): Are equipped with an external layer
of fibrous cartilage, resistant ligaments, articulated cavity internally covered, smooth and lubricated by synovial liquid cartilages.
Its articulated surfaces are perfectly molded and allow wide movements, of glide of an articulated surface over other (articulations of the hip, the knee or the elbow).

Besides constituting elements of fixation and subjection of bones, articulations give the body a wide varied freedom of movements.

A

JOINTS (I)
ANTERIOR GENERAL VIEW

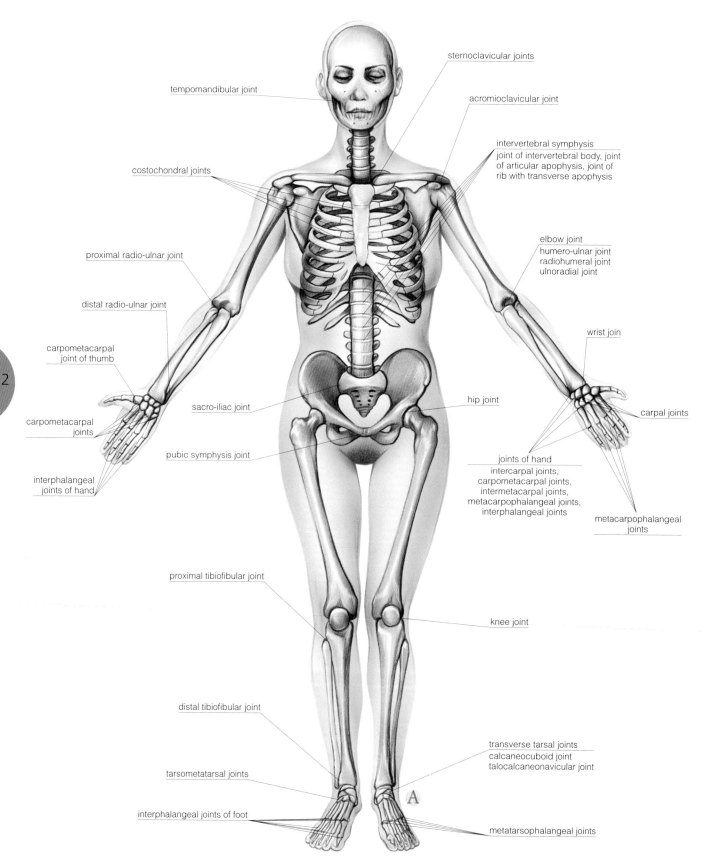

tempomandibular joint

sternoclavicular joints

acromioclavicular joint

intervertebral symphysis
joint of intervertebral body, joint
of articular apophysis, joint of
rib with transverse apophysis

costochondral joints

proximal radio-ulnar joint

elbow joint
humero-ulnar joint
radiohumeral joint
ulnoradial joint

distal radio-ulnar joint

wrist join

carpometacarpal
joint of thumb

232

hip joint

carpal joints

sacro-iliac joint

carpometacarpal
joints

joints of hand
intercarpal joints,
carpometacarpal joints,
intermetacarpal joints,
metacarpophalangeal joints,
interphalangeal joints

pubic symphysis joint

interphalangeal
joints of hand

metacarpophalangeal
joints

proximal tibiofibular joint

knee joint

distal tibiofibular joint

transverse tarsal joints
calcaneocuboid joint
talocalcaneonavicular joint

tarsometatarsal joints

A

interphalangeal joints of foot

metatarsophalangeal joints

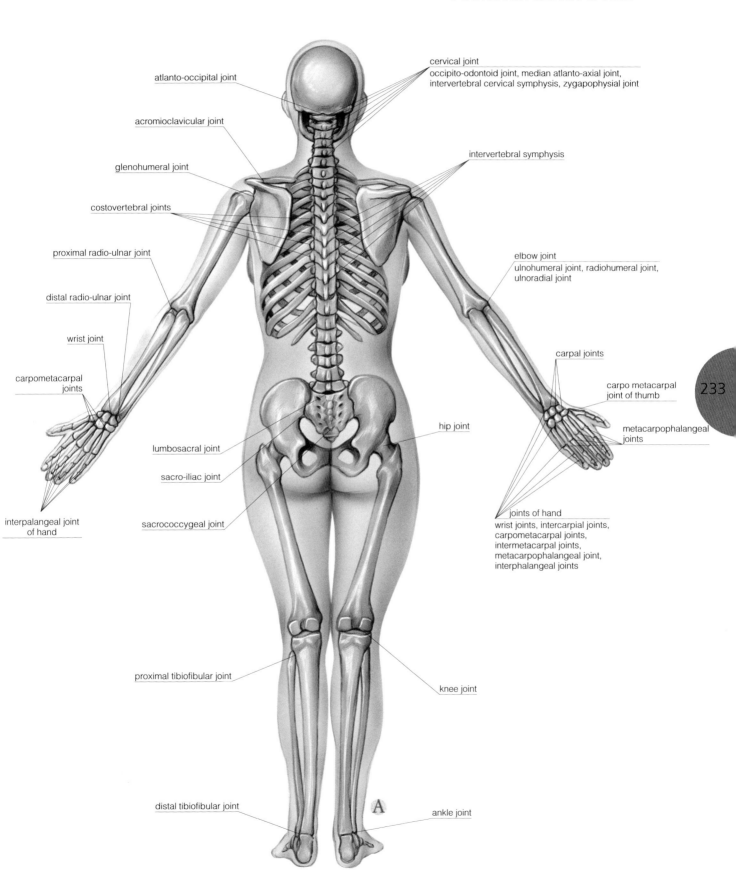

atlanto-occipital joint

acromioclavicular joint

glenohumeral joint

costovertebral joints

proximal radio-ulnar joint

distal radio-ulnar joint

wrist joint

carpometacarpal joints

interpalangeal joint of hand

lumbosacral joint

sacro-iliac joint

sacrococcygeal joint

cervical joint
occipito-odontoid joint, median atlanto-axial joint, intervertebral cervical symphysis, zygapophysial joint

intervertebral symphysis

elbow joint
ulnohumeral joint, radiohumeral joint, ulnoradial joint

carpal joints

carpo metacarpal joint of thumb

233

metacarpophalangeal joints

hip joint

joints of hand
wrist joints, intercarpial joints, carpometacarpal joints, intermetacarpal joints, metacarpophalangeal joint, interphalangeal joints

proximal tibiofibular joint

knee joint

distal tibiofibular joint

A

ankle joint

HEAD and NECK (I). NUCHAL JOINT

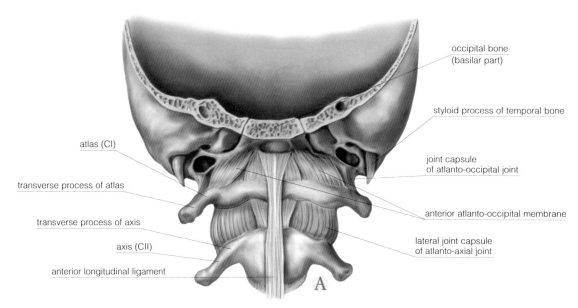

occipital bone
(basilar part)

styloid process of temporal bone

atlas (CI)

joint capsule
of atlanto-occipital joint

transverse process of atlas

transverse process of axis

anterior atlanto-occipital membrane

axis (CII)

lateral joint capsule
of atlanto-axial joint

anterior longitudinal ligament

A

ANTERIOR VIEW

234

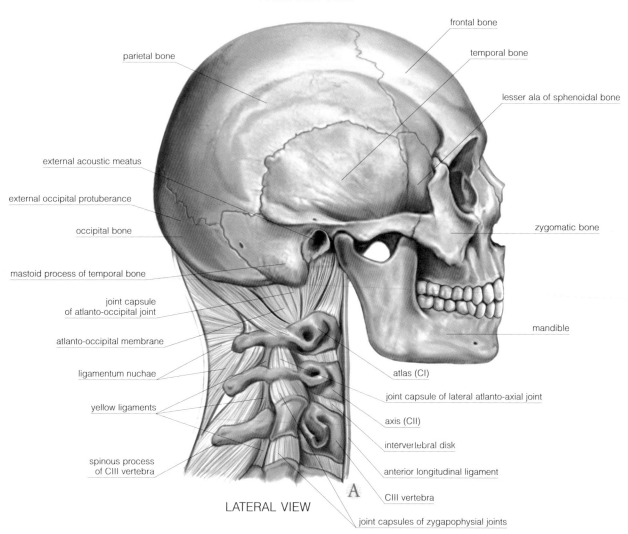

frontal bone

parietal bone

temporal bone

lesser ala of sphenoidal bone

external acoustic meatus

external occipital protuberance

occipital bone

zygomatic bone

mastoid process of temporal bone

joint capsule
of atlanto-occipital joint

atlanto-occipital membrane

ligamentum nuchae

mandible

yellow ligaments

atlas (CI)

joint capsule of lateral atlanto-axial joint

axis (CII)

intervertebral disk

spinous process
of CIII vertebra

anterior longitudinal ligament

A

CIII vertebra

LATERAL VIEW

joint capsules of zygapophysial joints

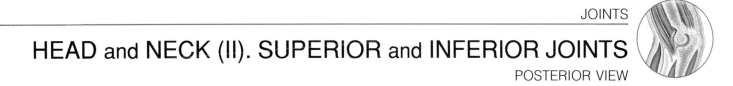

HEAD and NECK (II). SUPERIOR and INFERIOR JOINTS
POSTERIOR VIEW

cervical joints

It includes three joints: occipito-atloydea (condylea, that joins the occipital bone with the atlas and allows movements of flexion, extension and certain laterality), atlo-axoidea (trochoidea that joins the two first cervical vertebres, atlas and axis, and allows movements of rotation), cervical intervertebral (that allow to increase the movements of the previous ones) and zygapophysials (joints between the articular apophysis of vertebres, or zigapophysis).

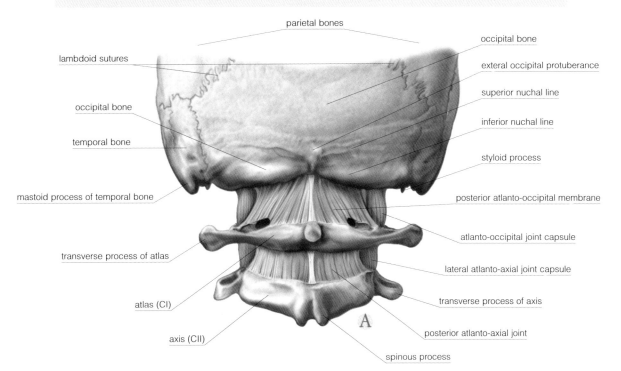

parietal bones

occipital bone

lambdoid sutures

exteral occipital protuberance

superior nuchal line

occipital bone

inferior nuchal line

temporal bone

styloid process

mastoid process of temporal bone

posterior atlanto-occipital membrane

atlanto-occipital joint capsule

transverse process of atlas

lateral atlanto-axial joint capsule

transverse process of axis

atlas (CI)

posterior atlanto-axial joint

axis (CII)

spinous process

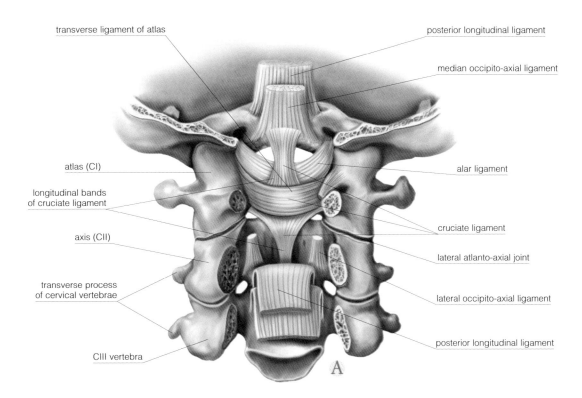

transverse ligament of atlas

posterior longitudinal ligament

median occipito-axial ligament

atlas (CI)

alar ligament

longitudinal bands
of cruciate ligament

axis (CII)

cruciate ligament

lateral atlanto-axial joint

transverse process
of cervical vertebrae

lateral occipito-axial ligament

CIII vertebra

posterior longitudinal ligament

235

HEAD and NECK (III). TEMPOROMANDIBULAR JOINT

temporomandibular joint

Is a bicondylar joint. Union of the rounded eminence, or condyle, of the jaw that is hosted in the glenoid cavity with the temporal condyle, that slides over that when the mouth is opened (that's why is considered bicondylia).This joint contains an interarticular meniscus that interposed between the two condyles and facilitates its encase. It allows several movements of the jaw that includes all that are necessary for the mastication: ascent and descent, projection towards and backwards and laterality.

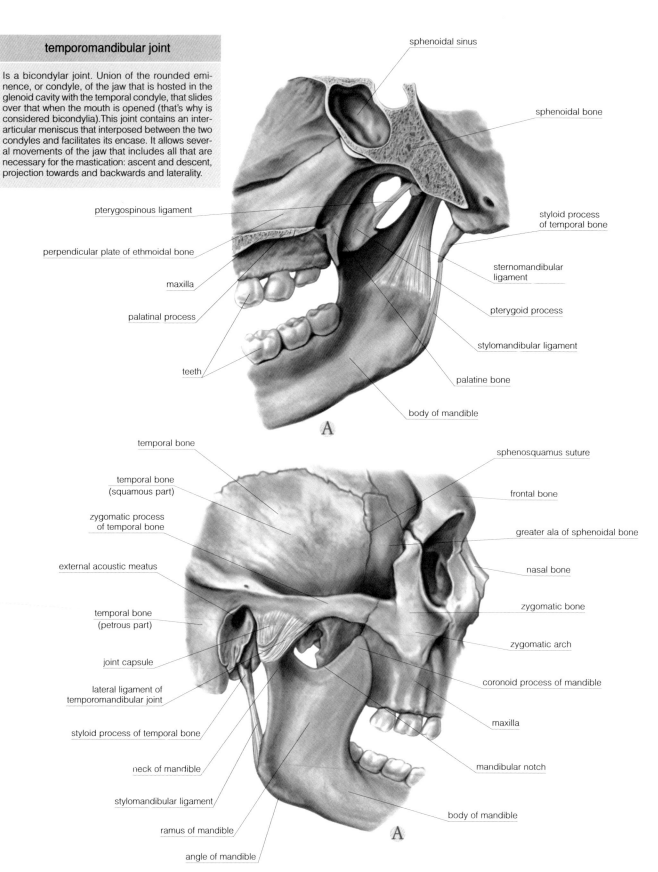

sphenoidal sinus

sphenoidal bone

pterygospinous ligament

perpendicular plate of ethmoidal bone

maxilla

palatinal process

teeth

styloid process of temporal bone

sternomandibular ligament

pterygoid process

stylomandibular ligament

palatine bone

body of mandible

A

temporal bone

temporal bone (squamous part)

zygomatic process of temporal bone

external acoustic meatus

temporal bone (petrous part)

joint capsule

lateral ligament of temporomandibular joint

styloid process of temporal bone

neck of mandible

stylomandibular ligament

ramus of mandible

angle of mandible

sphenosquamus suture

frontal bone

greater ala of sphenoidal bone

nasal bone

zygomatic bone

zygomatic arch

coronoid process of mandible

maxilla

mandibular notch

body of mandible

A

236

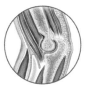

TRUNK. VERTEBRAL JOINTS

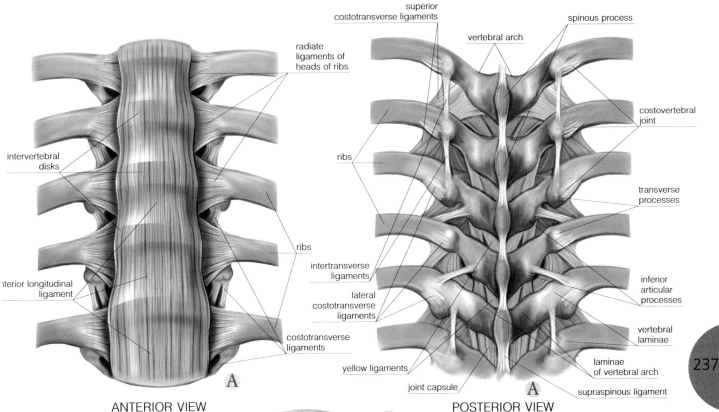

radiate
ligaments of
heads of ribs

intervertebral
disks

anterior longitudinal
ligament

ribs

costotransverse
ligaments

ANTERIOR VIEW

superior
costotransverse ligaments

vertebral arch

spinous process

costovertebral
joint

ribs

transverse
processes

intertransverse
ligaments

lateral
costotransverse
ligaments

inferior
articular
processes

vertebral
laminae

yellow ligaments

laminae
of vertebral arch

joint capsule

supraspinous ligament

POSTERIOR VIEW

237

intervertebral joints

In the conjunct of the vertebral column are distinguished various types of joints: Those of vertebral bodies between them, that are joints from the type of artrodies, and those that articulate the ribs with the transverse apophysis, that are also artrodies. The intervertebral joints are those found between the vertebras and there are of different types: zygapophysials, lumbosacrals, sacrococcigeous, and atlanto-axials laterals and medial. These joints allows movements of flexion, extension, lateralization and rotation.

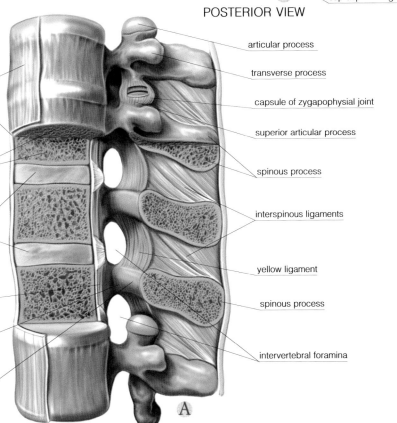

anterior
longitudinal
ligament

vertebral
body of
lumbar
vertebra

intervertebral
disks

posterior longitudinal ligament

pedicle of vertebra

lamina of vertebral arch

articular process

transverse process

capsule of zygapophysial joint

superior articular process

spinous process

interspinous ligaments

yellow ligament

spinous process

intervertebral foramina

**INTERVERTEBRAL JOINTS
LATERAL VIEW**

UPPER LIMB (I). SHOULDER (I)

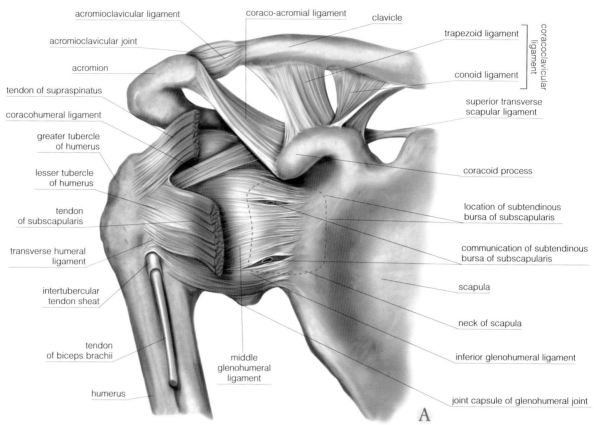

acromioclavicular ligament

coraco-acromial ligament

clavicle

trapezoid ligament

coracoclavicular ligament

acromioclavicular joint

conoid ligament

acromion

superior transverse scapular ligament

tendon of supraspinatus

coracohumeral ligament

coracoid process

greater tubercle of humerus

lesser tubercle of humerus

location of subtendinous bursa of subscapularis

tendon of subscapularis

communication of subtendinous bursa of subscapularis

transverse humeral ligament

scapula

intertubercular tendon sheat

neck of scapula

tendon of biceps brachii

inferior glenohumeral ligament

humerus

middle glenohumeral ligament

joint capsule of glenohumeral joint

A

RIGHT SIDE. ANTERIOR VIEW

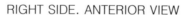

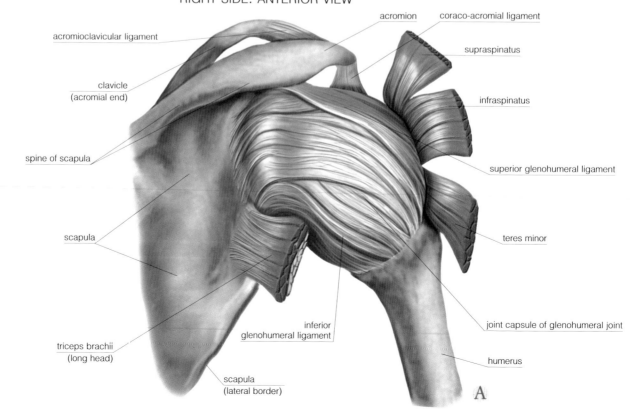

acromion

coraco-acromial ligament

acromioclavicular ligament

supraspinatus

clavicle (acromial end)

infraspinatus

spine of scapula

superior glenohumeral ligament

scapula

teres minor

triceps brachii (long head)

inferior glenohumeral ligament

joint capsule of glenohumeral joint

humerus

scapula (lateral border)

A

RIGHT SIDE. POSTERIOR VIEW

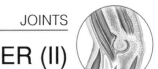

UPPER LIMB (II). SHOULDER (II)

glenohumeral joint

Is the type of the enarthrosis. Join the articular surfaces of the humerus head and the glenoid cavity of the scapula. Is surrounded by a series of serous bags that act as a padding allows movements of adduction, rotation, projection forward and backwards and of circumduction.

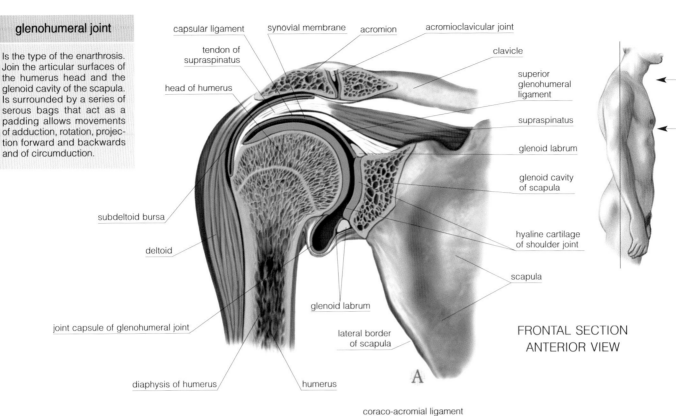

capsular ligament
synovial membrane
acromion
acromioclavicular joint
clavicle
tendon of supraspinatus
superior glenohumeral ligament
head of humerus
supraspinatus
glenoid labrum
glenoid cavity of scapula
subdeltoid bursa
deltoid
hyaline cartilage of shoulder joint
scapula
joint capsule of glenohumeral joint
glenoid labrum
lateral border of scapula
diaphysis of humerus
humerus

FRONTAL SECTION
ANTERIOR VIEW

A

239

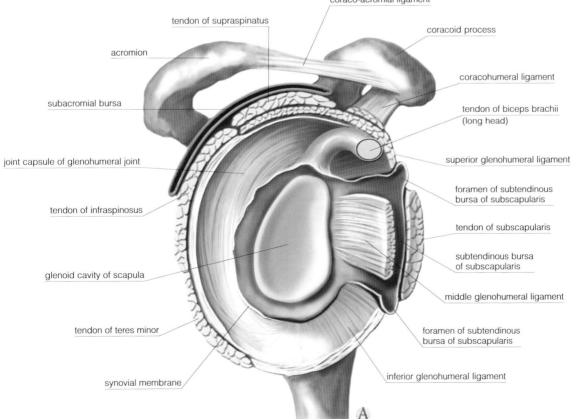

coraco-acromial ligament
tendon of supraspinatus
coracoid process
acromion
coracohumeral ligament
subacromial bursa
tendon of biceps brachii (long head)
joint capsule of glenohumeral joint
superior glenohumeral ligament
foramen of subtendinous bursa of subscapularis
tendon of infraspinosus
tendon of subscapularis
subtendinous bursa of subscapularis
glenoid cavity of scapula
middle glenohumeral ligament
tendon of teres minor
foramen of subtendinous bursa of subscapularis
synovial membrane
inferior glenohumeral ligament

A

RIGHT SIDE. LATERAL VIEW

240

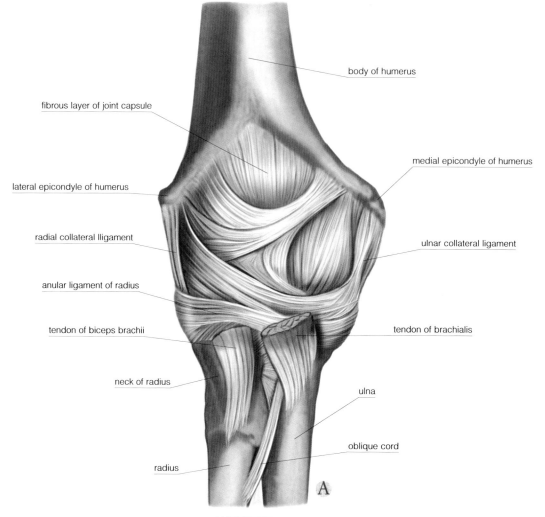

body of humerus

fibrous layer of joint capsule

medial epicondyle of humerus

lateral epicondyle of humerus

radial collateral lligament

ulnar collateral ligament

anular ligament of radius

tendon of biceps brachii

tendon of brachialis

neck of radius

ulna

radius

oblique cord

A

ANTERIOR VIEW

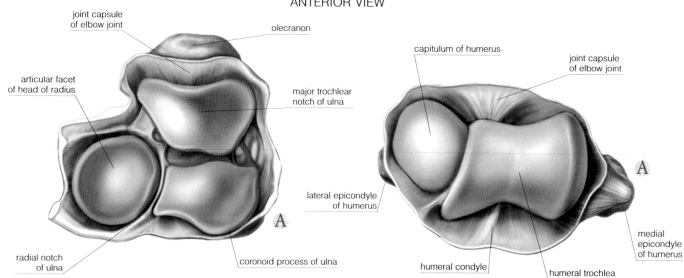

joint capsule
of elbow joint

olecranon

capitulum of humerus

joint capsule
of elbow joint

articular facet
of head of radius

major trochlear
notch of ulna

lateral epicondyle
of humerus

medial
epicondyle
of humerus

radial notch
of ulna

coronoid process of ulna

humeral condyle

humeral trochlea

PROXIMAL RADIO-ULNAR ARTICULAR SURFACE
POSTERIOR VIEW

ARTICUI AR SUPERFICIE of HUMERUS

UPPER LIMB (IV). ELBOW (II)

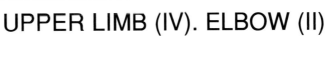

elbow joint

Includes three joints that are covered by an articular unique capsule: the ulnohumeral, or cubitohumeral or humero-ulnar or (trochlear) formed by the sigmoid cavity major than the ulna and the trochea humeral, the radiohumeral (enarthrosis), constituted by the glenoid cavity and lateral condyle of the humerus, and the ulnoradial, or cubitoradial superior (trochoid), or join of the proximal extremes of the ulna and the radius. Allows movements of flexion and extension of the forearm over the arm and the rotation of radius around the ulna which allows the hand to move in supination (towards) and pronation (backwards).

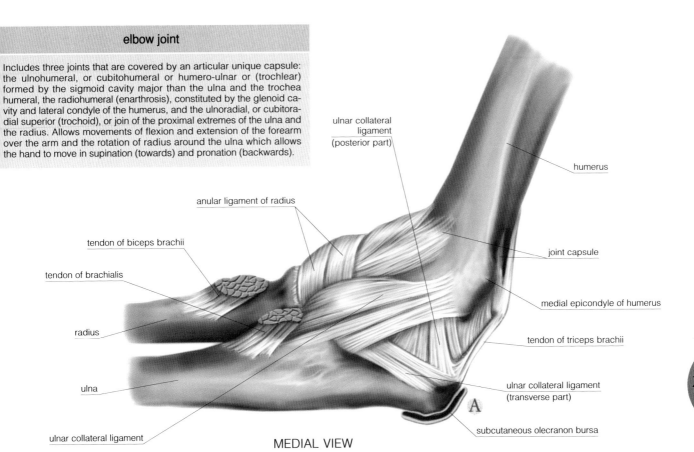

- ulnar collateral ligament (posterior part)
- humerus
- anular ligament of radius
- tendon of biceps brachii
- tendon of brachialis
- joint capsule
- medial epicondyle of humerus
- radius
- tendon of triceps brachii
- ulna
- ulnar collateral ligament (transverse part)
- subcutaneous olecranon bursa
- ulnar collateral ligament

MEDIAL VIEW

241

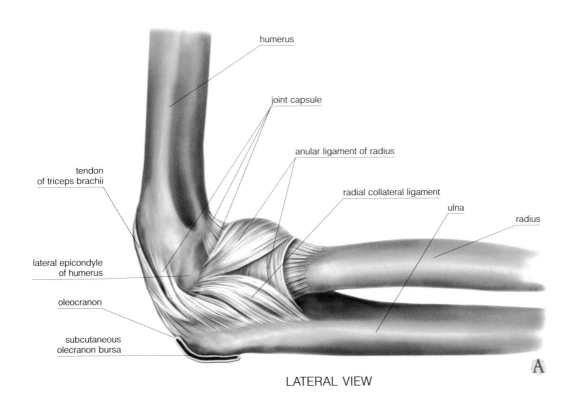

- humerus
- joint capsule
- anular ligament of radius
- tendon of triceps brachii
- radial collateral ligament
- ulna
- radius
- lateral epicondyle of humerus
- oleocranon
- subcutaneous olecranon bursa

LATERAL VIEW

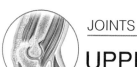

UPPER LIMB (V). ELBOW (III)

RIGHT ELBOW. FRONTAL SECTION

242

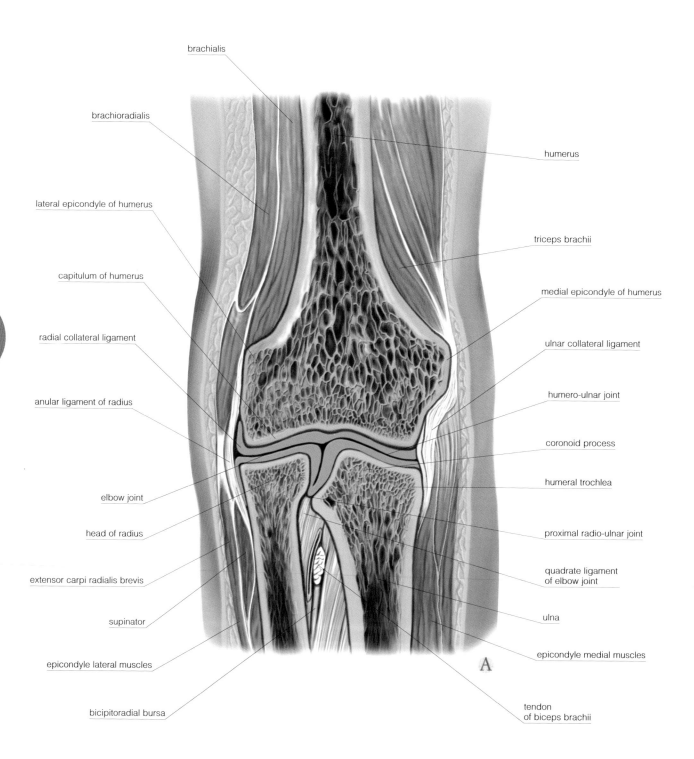

brachialis

brachioradialis

lateral epicondyle of humerus

capitulum of humerus

radial collateral ligament

anular ligament of radius

elbow joint

head of radius

extensor carpi radialis brevis

supinator

epicondyle lateral muscles

bicipitoradial bursa

humerus

triceps brachii

medial epicondyle of humerus

ulnar collateral ligament

humero-ulnar joint

coronoid process

humeral trochlea

proximal radio-ulnar joint

quadrate ligament
of elbow joint

ulna

epicondyle medial muscles

tendon
of biceps brachii

A

UPPER LIMB (VI). ELBOW (IV)
LEFT ELBOW. LATERAL SECTION

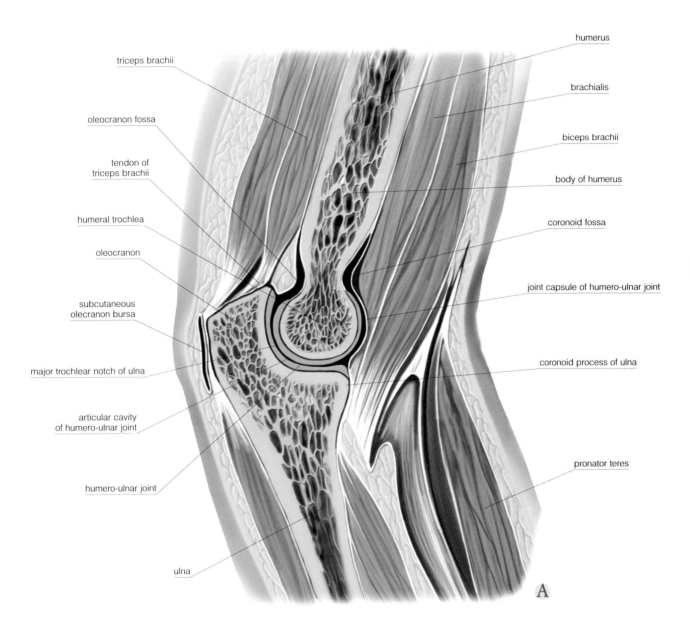

triceps brachii

oleocranon fossa

tendon of
triceps brachii

humeral trochlea

oleocranon

subcutaneous
olecranon bursa

major trochlear notch of ulna

articular cavity
of humero-ulnar joint

humero-ulnar joint

ulna

humerus

brachialis

biceps brachii

body of humerus

coronoid fossa

joint capsule of humero-ulnar joint

coronoid process of ulna

pronator teres

A

243

UPPER LIMB (VII). HAND (I)

RIGHT HAND. PALMAR VIEW

hand joints

Comprises the wrist, inter-carpal, carpometacarpal, intermetacarpal, metacar-pophalangeal and inter-phalangeal joints. Because of these joints, the hand can carry out a great number of varied movements, some of which are exclusive to the human species.

244

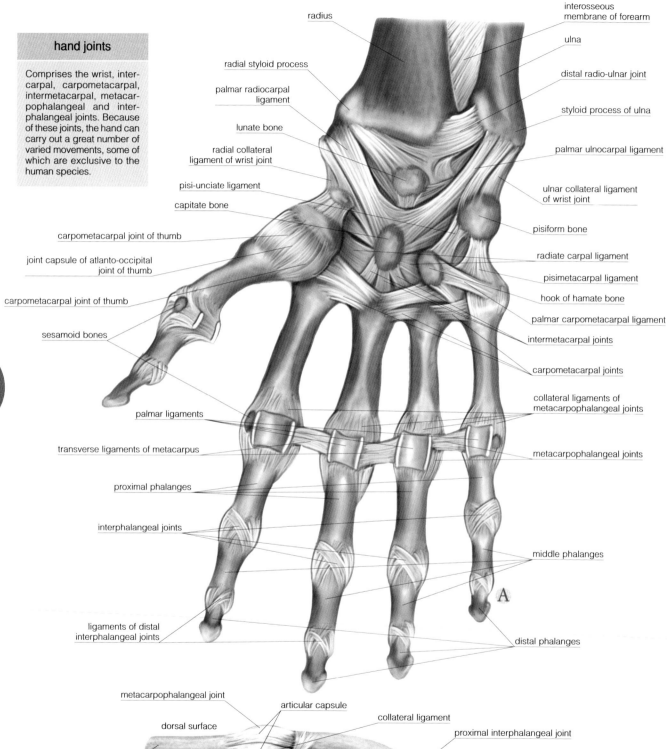

radius
interosseous membrane of forearm
ulna
radial styloid process
distal radio-ulnar joint
palmar radiocarpal ligament
styloid process of ulna
lunate bone
palmar ulnocarpal ligament
radial collateral ligament of wrist joint
ulnar collateral ligament of wrist joint
pisi-unciate ligament
capitate bone
pisiform bone
carpometacarpal joint of thumb
radiate carpal ligament
joint capsule of atlanto-occipital joint of thumb
pisimetacarpal ligament
hook of hamate bone
carpometacarpal joint of thumb
palmar carpometacarpal ligament
sesamoid bones
intermetacarpal joints
carpometacarpal joints
collateral ligaments of metacarpophalangeal joints
palmar ligaments
transverse ligaments of metacarpus
metacarpophalangeal joints
proximal phalanges
interphalangeal joints
middle phalanges
A
ligaments of distal interphalangeal joints
distal phalanges

metacarpophalangeal joint
articular capsule
collateral ligament
dorsal surface
proximal interphalangeal joint
metcarpal bone
distal interphalangeal joint
palmar surface
palmar ligaments
A
proximal phalanx   middle phalanx   distal phalanx
phalanges

JOINTS of THREE-PHALANGEAL FINGER. LATERAL VIEW

UPPER LIMB (VIII). HAND (II)
RIGHT HAND. DORSAL VIEW

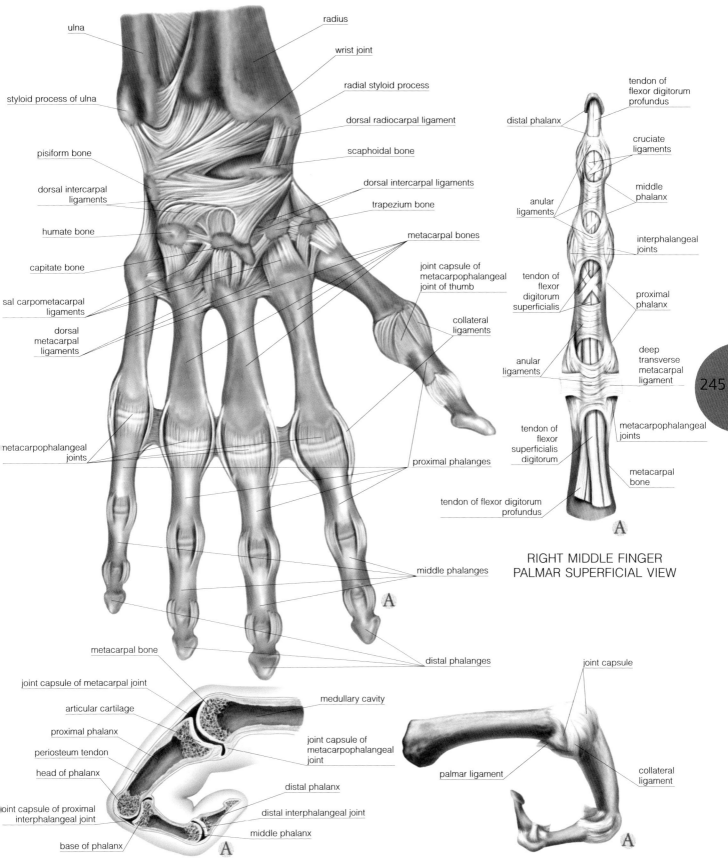

ulna

radius

wrist joint

styloid process of ulna

radial styloid process

dorsal radiocarpal ligament

scaphoidal bone

pisiform bone

dorsal intercarpal ligaments

dorsal intercarpal ligaments

trapezium bone

humate bone

capitate bone

metacarpal bones

joint capsule of metacarpophalangeal joint of thumb

sal carpometacarpal ligaments

collateral ligaments

dorsal metacarpal ligaments

metacarpophalangeal joints

proximal phalanges

middle phalanges

A

distal phalanges

tendon of flexor digitorum profundus

distal phalanx

cruciate ligaments

anular ligaments

middle phalanx

interphalangeal joints

tendon of flexor digitorum superficialis

proximal phalanx

anular ligaments

deep transverse metacarpal ligament

245

tendon of flexor superficialis digitorum

metacarpophalangeal joints

metacarpal bone

tendon of flexor digitorum profundus

A

RIGHT MIDDLE FINGER PALMAR SUPERFICIAL VIEW

metacarpal bone

joint capsule of metacarpal joint

articular cartilage

medullary cavity

proximal phalanx

joint capsule of metacarpophalangeal joint

periosteum tendon

head of phalanx

distal phalanx

joint capsule of proximal interphalangeal joint

distal interphalangeal joint

middle phalanx

base of phalanx

A

joint capsule

palmar ligament

collateral ligament

A

THREE-PHALANGEAL FINGER. SAGITAL SECTION. LATERAL VIEW

MEDIAL FLEXION of FINGER

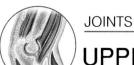

UPPER LIMB (IX). WRIST

RIGHT HAND

wrist joint

Is condyle and is formed by the union of the inferior extremity of the radius with the bones of the first row of the wrist: scaphoid, semi-lunar and pyramidal. Consist of an articular capsule that covers it and is reinforced by several liga-ments. Allows movements of fle-xion, extension, adduction and circumduction, sum of all the pre-vious movements.

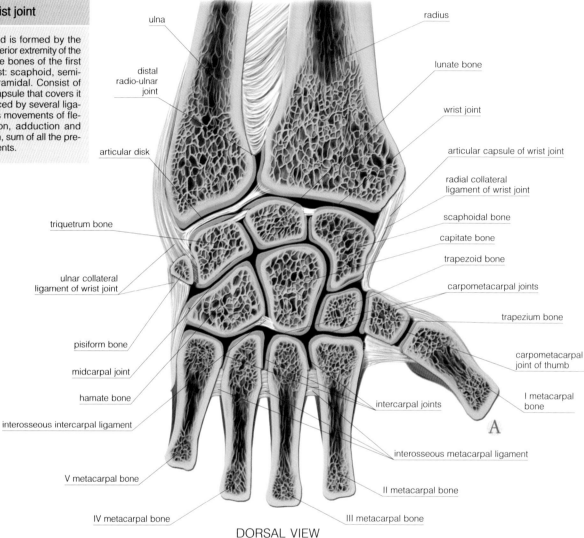

ulna
distal radio-ulnar joint
articular disk
triquetrum bone
ulnar collateral ligament of wrist joint
pisiform bone
midcarpal joint
hamate bone
interosseous intercarpal ligament
V metacarpal bone
IV metacarpal bone

radius
lunate bone
wrist joint
articular capsule of wrist joint
radial collateral ligament of wrist joint
scaphoidal bone
capitate bone
trapezoid bone
carpometacarpal joints
trapezium bone
carpometacarpal joint of thumb
I metacarpal bone
intercarpal joints
interosseous metacarpal ligament
II metacarpal bone
III metacarpal bone

A

DORSAL VIEW

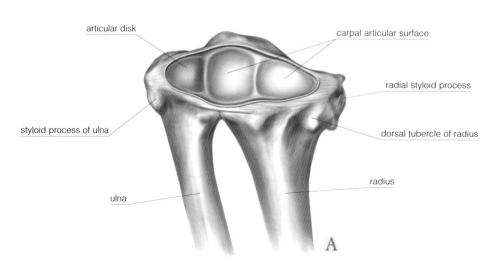

articular disk
styloid process of ulna
ulna

carpal articular surface
radial styloid process
dorsal tubercle of radius
radius

A

ANTERIOR VIEW

246

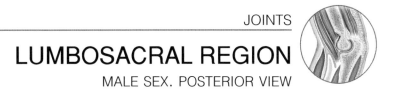

LUMBOSACRAL REGION
MALE SEX. POSTERIOR VIEW

lumbosacral joint

Joint between the sacrum and the lumbar vertebras that allows movements of inclination and extension of the thorax, forwards and backwards. The vertebras LV and SI articulate in the anterior intervertebral joint formed by the IV disk between their bodies and at two zygapophysial joints of these vertebras. The articular surfaces of the SI vertebra are faced in posterior medial sense and make contact with the inferior articular surface of the LV vertebra in anterior lateral sense, which avoids that the lumbar vertebra slides away anterior, towards down due to the inclination that the sacrum forms.

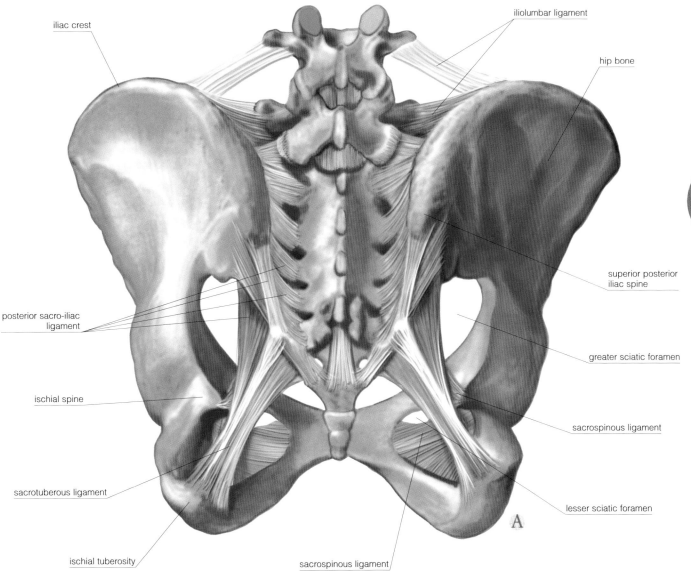

iliac crest

iliolumbar ligament

hip bone

247

superior posterior
iliac spine

posterior sacro-iliac
ligament

greater sciatic foramen

ischial spine

sacrospinous ligament

sacrotuberous ligament

lesser sciatic foramen

ischial tuberosity

sacrospinous ligament

A

LOWER LIMB (I). HIP (I)

RIGHT SIDE

hip joint

It is spheroid joint. Joins the head of the thigh bone with the acetabulum of the pelvic bone, enlarged by a fibrous ring, which is called the acetabular labrum. It consists of a joint capsule which completely covers the joint and the reinforcement ligaments. It allows bending, extension, adduction, and rotation movements.

248

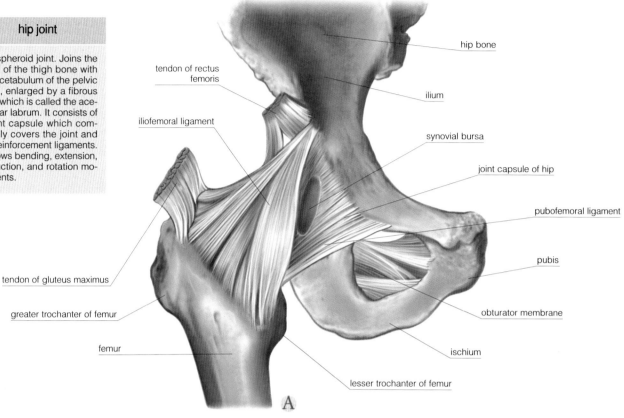

tendon of rectus femoris

iliofemoral ligament

tendon of gluteus maximus

greater trochanter of femur

femur

hip bone

ilium

synovial bursa

joint capsule of hip

pubofemoral ligament

pubis

obturator membrane

ischium

lesser trochanter of femur

A

ANTERIOR VIEW

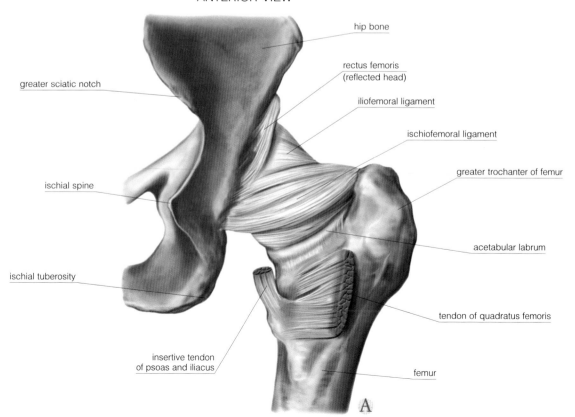

greater sciatic notch

ischial spine

ischial tuberosity

insertive tendon of psoas and iliacus

hip bone

rectus femoris (reflected head)

iliofemoral ligament

ischiofemoral ligament

greater trochanter of femur

acetabular labrum

tendon of quadratus femoris

femur

A

POSTERIOR VIEW

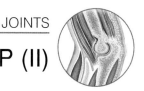

LOWER LIMB (II). HIP (II)

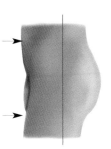

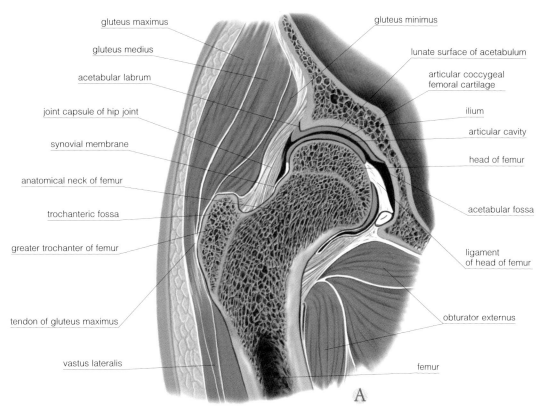

gluteus maximus

gluteus medius

acetabular labrum

joint capsule of hip joint

synovial membrane

anatomical neck of femur

trochanteric fossa

greater trochanter of femur

tendon of gluteus maximus

vastus lateralis

gluteus minimus

lunate surface of acetabulum

articular coccygeal femoral cartilage

ilium

articular cavity

head of femur

acetabular fossa

ligament of head of femur

obturator externus

femur

ANTERIOR VIEW

249

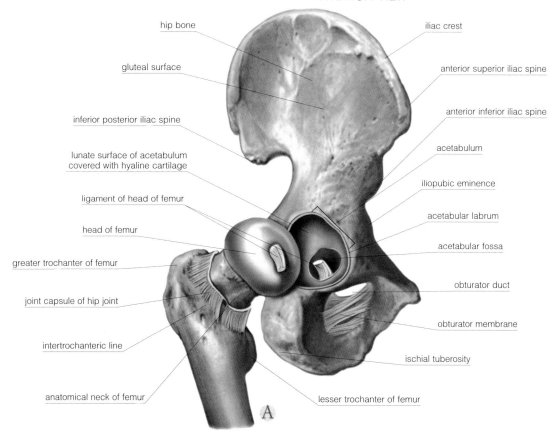

hip bone

gluteal surface

inferior posterior iliac spine

lunate surface of acetabulum covered with hyaline cartilage

ligament of head of femur

head of femur

greater trochanter of femur

joint capsule of hip joint

intertrochanteric line

anatomical neck of femur

iliac crest

anterior superior iliac spine

anterior inferior iliac spine

acetabulum

iliopubic eminence

acetabular labrum

acetabular fossa

obturator duct

obturator membrane

ischial tuberosity

lesser trochanter of femur

OPEN JOINT. LATERAL VIEW

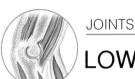

LOWER LIMB (III). KNEE (I)

knee joint

It is trochlear. It corresponds to the joining of the facet joint of the distal ending of the thigh bone, the proximal surface of the tibia, and the fact joint of the patella, interposed by two intra-articular meniscuses. It consists of a capsule which covers the entire joint and of reinforcement ligaments, in addition to crossed and intra-articular ligaments. It allows flexion, extension, and internal and external rotation movements. When the joint is flexed, it also allows light lateral inclination movement.

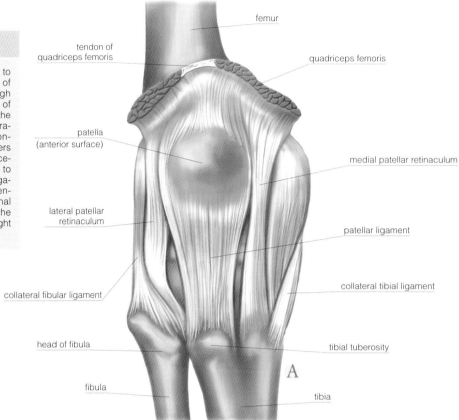

- femur
- tendon of quadriceps femoris
- quadriceps femoris
- patella (anterior surface)
- medial patellar retinaculum
- lateral patellar retinaculum
- patellar ligament
- collateral tibial ligament
- collateral fibular ligament
- head of fibula
- tibial tuberosity
- fibula
- tibia

ANTERIOR VIEW

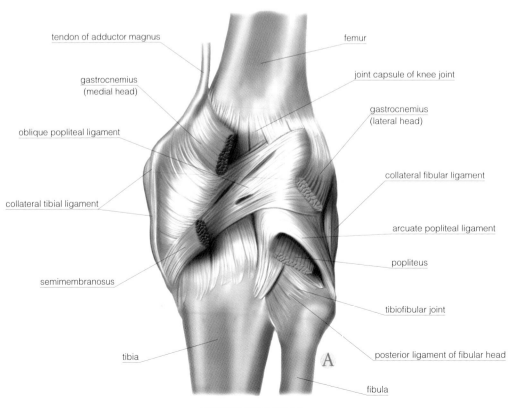

- tendon of adductor magnus
- femur
- gastrocnemius (medial head)
- joint capsule of knee joint
- gastrocnemius (lateral head)
- oblique popliteal ligament
- collateral fibular ligament
- collateral tibial ligament
- arcuate popliteal ligament
- popliteus
- semimembranosus
- tibiofibular joint
- tibia
- posterior ligament of fibular head
- fibula

POSTERIOR VIEW

250

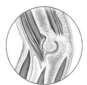

LOWER LIMB (IV). KNEE (II)

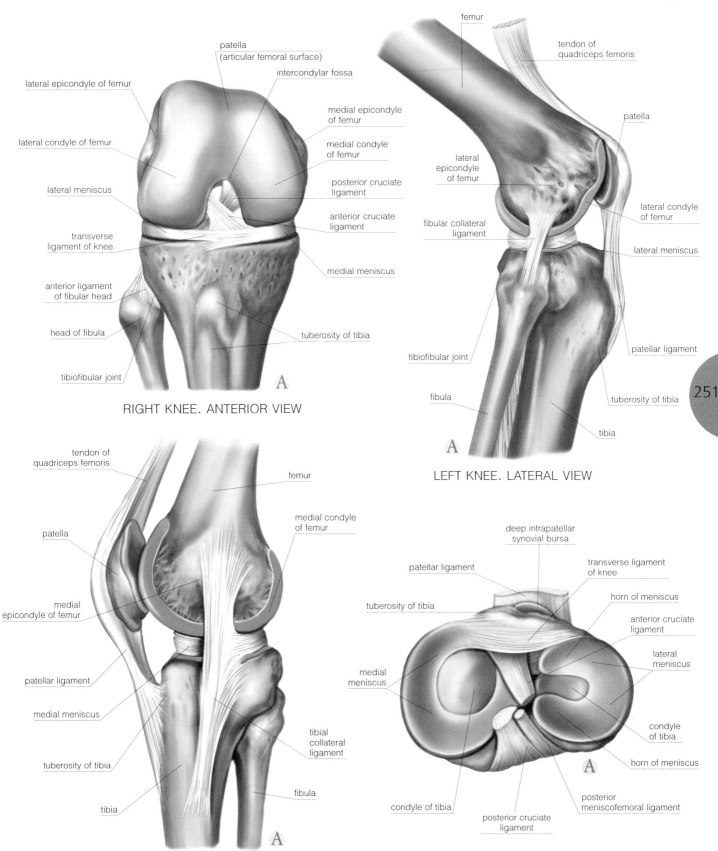

patella
(articular femoral surface)

intercondylar fossa

lateral epicondyle of femur

medial epicondyle
of femur

lateral condyle of femur

medial condyle
of femur

lateral meniscus

posterior cruciate
ligament

anterior cruciate
ligament

transverse
ligament of knee

medial meniscus

anterior ligament
of fibular head

head of fibula

tuberosity of tibia

tibiofibular joint

RIGHT KNEE. ANTERIOR VIEW

femur

tendon of
quadriceps femoris

patella

lateral
epicondyle
of femur

lateral condyle
of femur

fibular collateral
ligament

lateral meniscus

tibiofibular joint

patellar ligament

fibula

tuberosity of tibia

tibia

251

LEFT KNEE. LATERAL VIEW

tendon of
quadriceps femoris

femur

medial condyle
of femur

patella

medial
epicondyle of femur

patellar ligament

medial meniscus

tibial
collateral
ligament

tuberosity of tibia

fibula

tibia

RIGHT KNEE. MEDIAL VIEW

deep intrapatellar
synovial bursa

transverse ligament
of knee

patellar ligament

horn of meniscus

tuberosity of tibia

anterior cruciate
ligament

lateral
meniscus

medial
meniscus

condyle
of tibia

horn of meniscus

condyle of tibia

posterior
meniscofemoral ligament

posterior cruciate
ligament

TIBIAL ARTICULAR SURFACE

LOWER LIMB (V). KNEE (III)

RIGHT KNEE. LATERAL VIEW

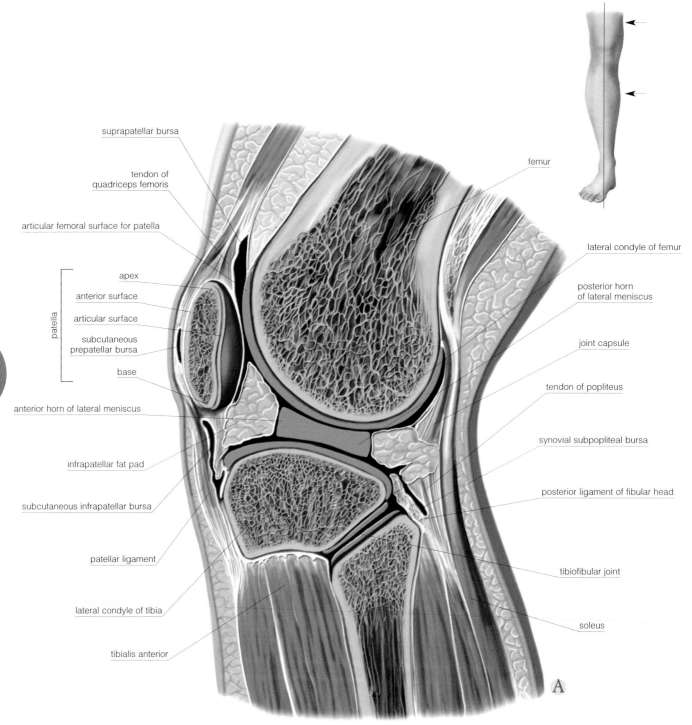

suprapatellar bursa

tendon of
quadriceps femoris

articular femoral surface for patella

apex

anterior surface

articular surface

subcutaneous
prepatellar bursa

base

patella

anterior horn of lateral meniscus

infrapatellar fat pad

subcutaneous infrapatellar bursa

patellar ligament

lateral condyle of tibia

tibialis anterior

femur

lateral condyle of femur

posterior horn
of lateral meniscus

joint capsule

tendon of popliteus

synovial subpopliteal bursa

posterior ligament of fibular head

tibiofibular joint

soleus

252

A

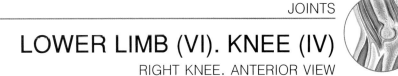

LOWER LIMB (VI). KNEE (IV)
RIGHT KNEE. ANTERIOR VIEW

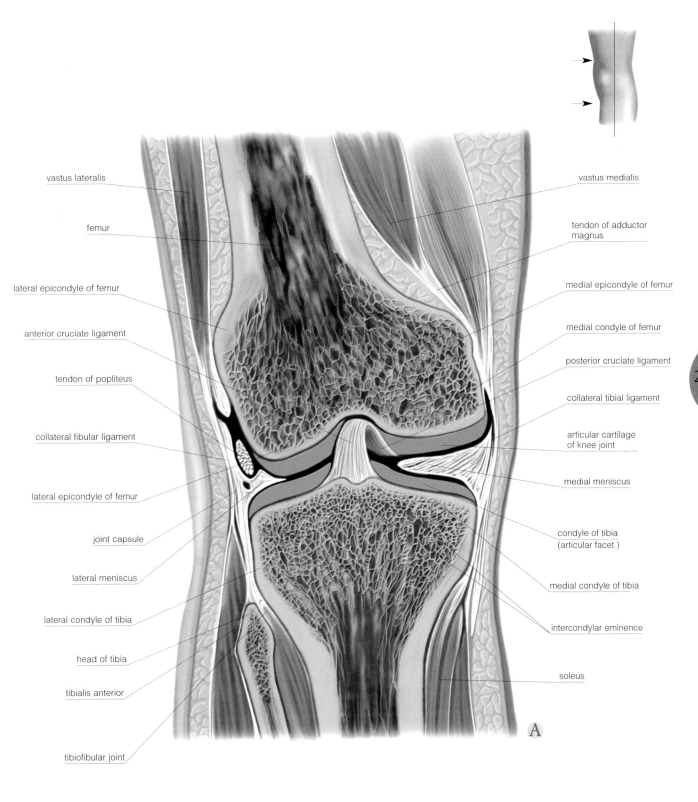

vastus lateralis

femur

lateral epicondyle of femur

anterior cruciate ligament

tendon of popliteus

collateral fibular ligament

lateral epicondyle of femur

joint capsule

lateral meniscus

lateral condyle of tibia

head of tibia

tibialis anterior

tibiofibular joint

vastus medialis

tendon of adductor magnus

medial epicondyle of femur

medial condyle of femur

posterior cruciate ligament

collateral tibial ligament

articular cartilage of knee joint

medial meniscus

condyle of tibia (articular facet)

medial condyle of tibia

intercondylar eminence

soleus

253

LOWER LIMB (VII). ANKLE
RIGHT LEG. FRONTAL SECTION. POSTERIOR VIEW

ankle joint

Is the trochlear joint. Joins the leg with the foot and articulates the inferior articular surface of the tibia and the malleolar articular surface of the fibula and the medial, lateral and superior malleolar surfaces of the talus. Is endowed of an articular capsule, that covers it and of rainforced ligaments. On either side of the ankle appear two prominences, or malleolus, lateral and medial, that correspond to the distal portions of the tibia and the fibula. Allows movements of flexion and extension, abduction, adduction and rotation.

interosseous membrane of leg

tibia

tibiofibular joint

epiphysial line

medial malleolus

ankle joint

talus of trochlea (superior surface)

body of talus

flexor retinaculum of tarsus

medial collateral ligament of ankle joint

tendon of tibialis posterior

posterior tibialis sheath

tendon of flexor digitorum longus

flexor digitorum longus sheath

tendon of flexor hallucis longus

flexor hallucis longus sheat

subtalar joint

quadratus plantae

abductor hallucis

lateral plantar nerves

flexor hallucis brevis

fibula

epiphysial line

lateral malleolus

posterior tibiofibular ligament

collateral ligament

subtalar joint

calcaneus

superior fibularis retinaculum

tendon of lateral fibularis brevis

common tendinous sheath of fibular muscles

tendon of fibularis longus

inferior fibular retinaculum

abductor digiti minimi

plantar aponeurosis

A

254

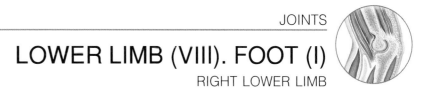

LOWER LIMB (VIII). FOOT (I)
RIGHT LOWER LIMB

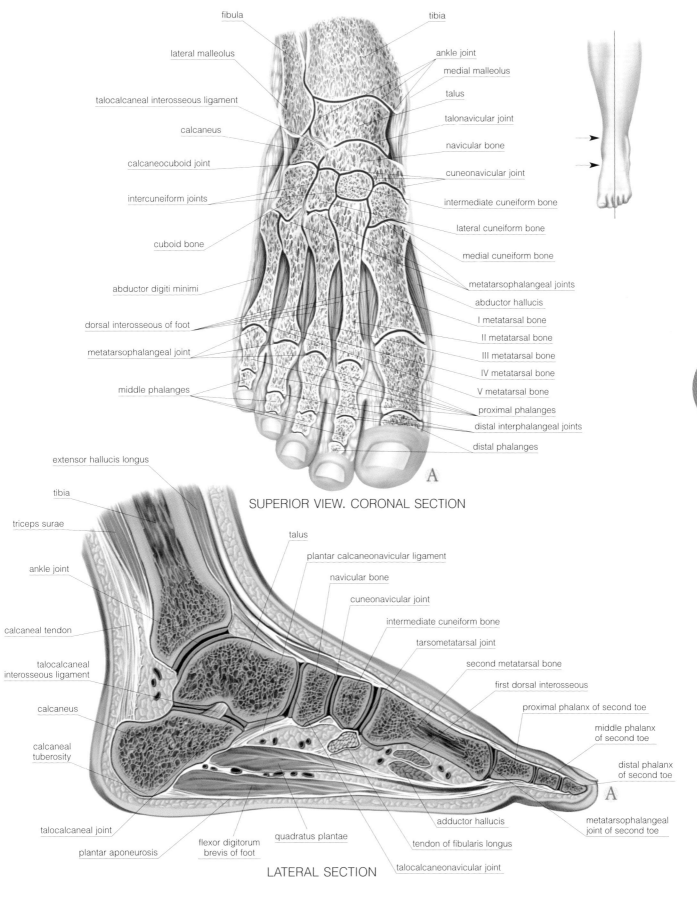

fibula

tibia

lateral malleolus

ankle joint

medial malleolus

talocalcaneal interosseous ligament

talus

calcaneus

talonavicular joint

calcaneocuboid joint

navicular bone

cuneonavicular joint

intercuneiform joints

intermediate cuneiform bone

lateral cuneiform bone

cuboid bone

medial cuneiform bone

abductor digiti minimi

metatarsophalangeal joints

abductor hallucis

dorsal interosseous of foot

I metatarsal bone

II metatarsal bone

metatarsophalangeal joint

III metatarsal bone

IV metatarsal bone

middle phalanges

V metatarsal bone

proximal phalanges

distal interphalangeal joints

distal phalanges

A

SUPERIOR VIEW. CORONAL SECTION

extensor hallucis longus

talus

tibia

plantar calcaneonavicular ligament

triceps surae

navicular bone

ankle joint

cuneonavicular joint

intermediate cuneiform bone

tarsometatarsal joint

calcaneal tendon

second metatarsal bone

talocalcaneal
interosseous ligament

first dorsal interosseous

calcaneus

proximal phalanx of second toe

middle phalanx
of second toe

calcaneal
tuberosity

distal phalanx
of second toe

A

talocalcaneal joint

adductor hallucis

metatarsophalangeal
joint of second toe

plantar aponeurosis

flexor digitorum
brevis of foot

quadratus plantae

tendon of fibularis longus

talocalcaneonavicular joint

LATERAL SECTION

255

256

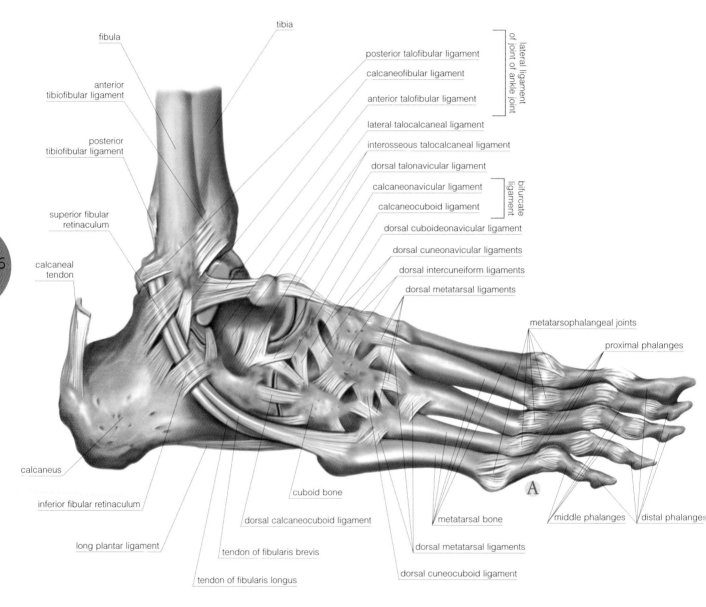

fibula

tibia

anterior
tibiofibular ligament

posterior
tibiofibular ligament

superior fibular
retinaculum

calcaneal
tendon

calcaneus

inferior fibular retinaculum

long plantar ligament

tendon of fibularis brevis

tendon of fibularis longus

posterior talofibular ligament

calcaneofibular ligament

anterior talofibular ligament

lateral talocalcaneal ligament

interosseous talocalcaneal ligament

dorsal talonavicular ligament

calcaneonavicular ligament

calcaneocuboid ligament

dorsal cuboideonavicular ligament

dorsal cuneonavicular ligaments

dorsal intercuneiform ligaments

dorsal metatarsal ligaments

lateral ligament
of joint of ankle joint

bifurcate
ligament

metatarsophalangeal joints

proximal phalanges

cuboid bone

dorsal calcaneocuboid ligament

metatarsal bone

middle phalanges

distal phalanges

dorsal metatarsal ligaments

dorsal cuneocuboid ligament

A

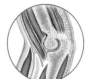

LOWER LIMB (X). FOOT (III)

RIGHT FOOT. MEDIAL VIEW

joints of foot

Involves a set of joints among them the following:
- Intertarsian: Joints that are found among the different bones of the tarsus.
- Tarsometatarsal: Union of the proximal extremes of the five metatarsal bones with the cuboid bone and the three cuneiform bones that are reinforced by interosseous, dorsal and plantar ligaments. Allows a very few movements.
- Metatarsophalangeal: Joins the distal extremes of the metacarpal bones with the proximal extremes of the proximal phalanges of the correspon-

ding toes of the foot. These unions are reinforced by lateral ligaments and by a transverse ligament that extends plantally from the first metatarsal bone until the fifth. Allows movements of flexion, extension, lateral inclination and rotation.
- Interphalangeal of the foot: Are cylindrical and articulate the phalanges of the foot between them through one each articular capsules and are reinforced by two lateral and medial ligaments. Allow flexion and extension movements.

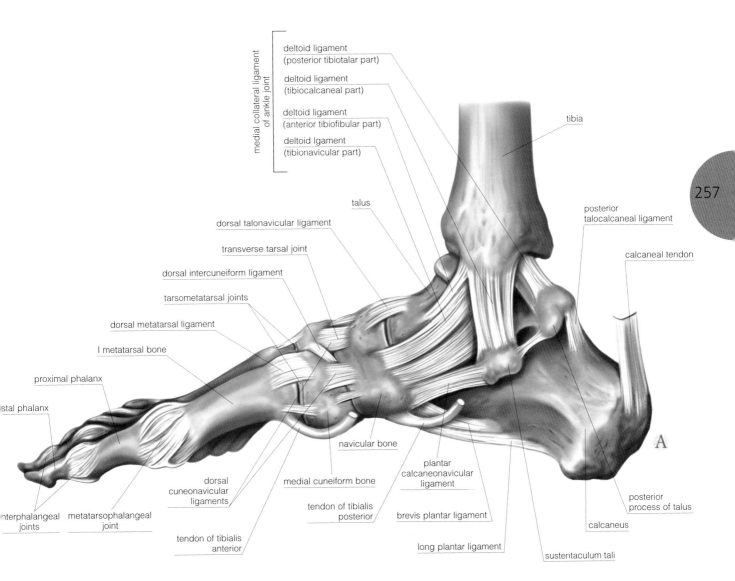

257

LOWER LIMB (XI). FOOT (IV)
RIGHT FOOT. DORSAL VIEW

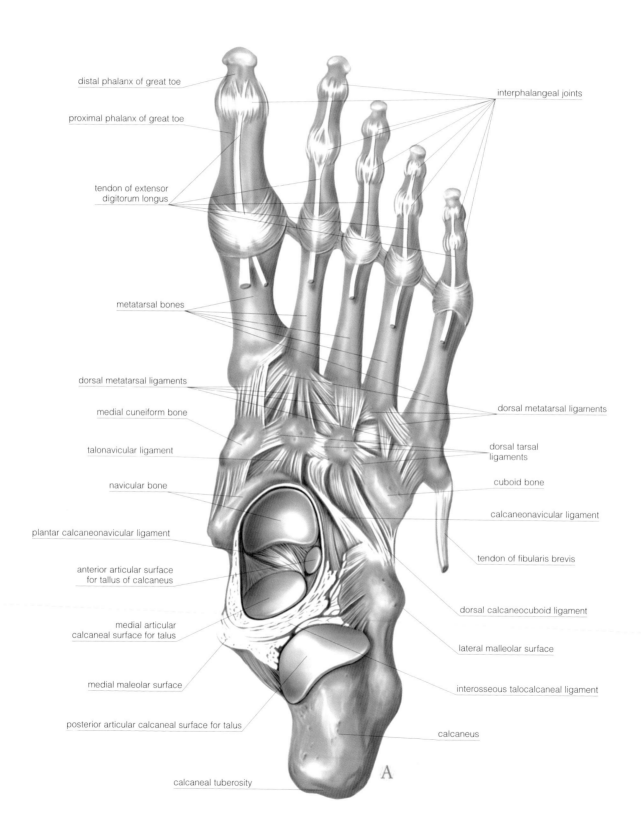

distal phalanx of great toe

proximal phalanx of great toe

tendon of extensor
digitorum longus

metatarsal bones

dorsal metatarsal ligaments

medial cuneiform bone

talonavicular ligament

navicular bone

plantar calcaneonavicular ligament

anterior articular surface
for tallus of calcaneus

medial articular
calcaneal surface for talus

medial maleolar surface

posterior articular calcaneal surface for talus

calcaneal tuberosity

interphalangeal joints

dorsal metatarsal ligaments

dorsal tarsal
ligaments

cuboid bone

calcaneonavicular ligament

tendon of fibularis brevis

dorsal calcaneocuboid ligament

lateral malleolar surface

interosseous talocalcaneal ligament

calcaneus

A

258

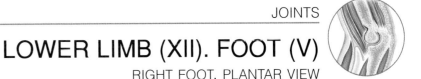

LOWER LIMB (XII). FOOT (V)
RIGHT FOOT. PLANTAR VIEW

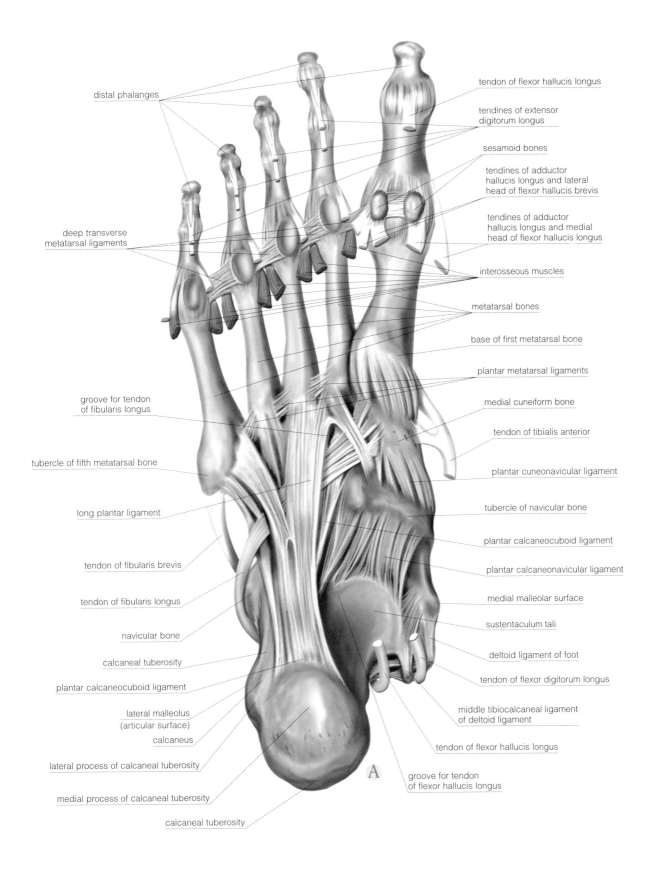

distal phalanges

tendon of flexor hallucis longus

tendines of extensor digitorum longus

sesamoid bones

tendines of adductor hallucis longus and lateral head of flexor hallucis brevis

tendines of adductor hallucis longus and medial head of flexor hallucis longus

deep transverse metatarsal ligaments

interosseous muscles

metatarsal bones

base of first metatarsal bone

plantar metatarsal ligaments

groove for tendon of fibularis longus

medial cuneiform bone

tendon of tibialis anterior

tubercle of fifth metatarsal bone

plantar cuneonavicular ligament

long plantar ligament

tubercle of navicular bone

plantar calcaneocuboid ligament

tendon of fibularis brevis

plantar calcaneonavicular ligament

tendon of fibularis longus

medial malleolar surface

navicular bone

sustentaculum tali

calcaneal tuberosity

deltoid ligament of foot

plantar calcaneocuboid ligament

tendon of flexor digitorum longus

lateral malleolus (articular surface)

middle tibiocalcaneal ligament of deltoid ligament

calcaneus

lateral process of calcaneal tuberosity

tendon of flexor hallucis longus

medial process of calcaneal tuberosity

groove for tendon of flexor hallucis longus

calcaneal tuberosity

A

259

LOWER LIMB (XIII). FOOT (VI)
RIGHT FOOT. PLANTAR VIEW

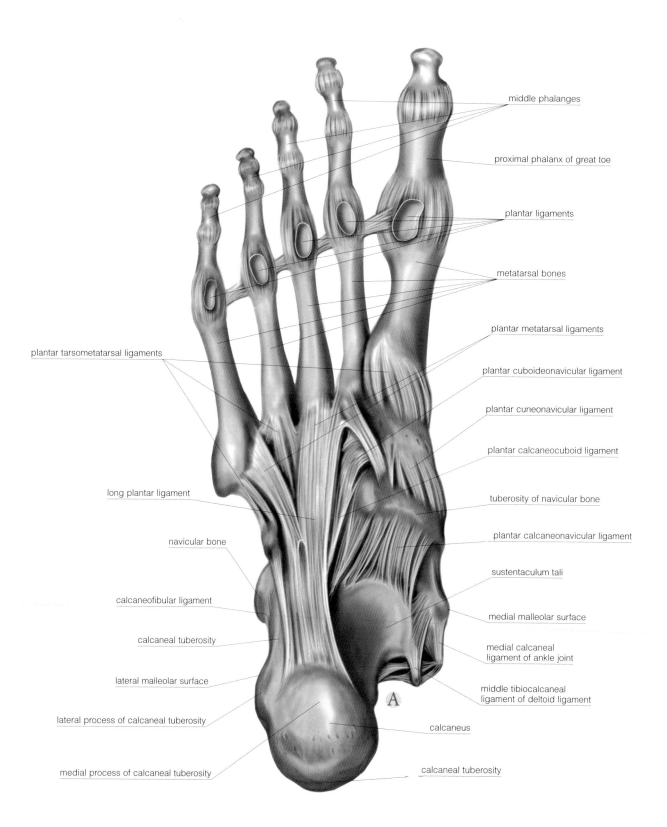

middle phalanges

proximal phalanx of great toe

plantar ligaments

metatarsal bones

plantar metatarsal ligaments

plantar cuboideonavicular ligament

plantar cuneonavicular ligament

plantar calcaneocuboid ligament

tuberosity of navicular bone

plantar calcaneonavicular ligament

sustentaculum tali

medial malleolar surface

medial calcaneal
ligament of ankle joint

middle tibiocalcaneal
ligament of deltoid ligament

calcaneus

calcaneal tuberosity

plantar tarsometatarsal ligaments

long plantar ligament

navicular bone

calcaneofibular ligament

calcaneal tuberosity

lateral malleolar surface

lateral process of calcaneal tuberosity

medial process of calcaneal tuberosity

A

CARDIOVASCULAR SYSTEM

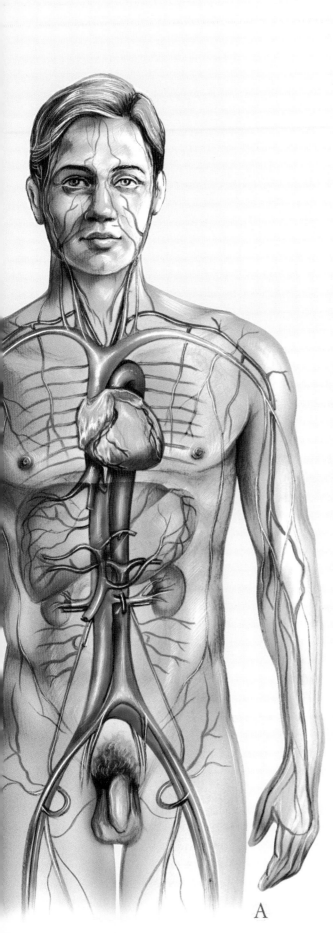

A

The cardiovascular apparatus is the conduction net that transports the oxygenated blood to any part of the body to provide the cells those nutritive elements that contains. In its return journey, this net carries the discard products, which form the venous blood, with the purpose of being eliminated. Therefore, the function of this apparatus is eminently nutritive.

The human body is formed by millions of cells that as all living being, need different substances to survive, substances that receive through the blood. The cardiovascular apparatus has a double function: That such blood is in perfect conditions and keep permanently activated its circulation, to be able to reach all the cells of the body. This route it's complemented with the return journey, in which the blood picks the residual substances from the cellular metabolism, inconvenient for the organism, to be expelled and after restart the circuit.

To be able to develop this process, the cardiovascular apparatus disposes of two big elements: The heart and the vascular net.

The heart acts as a propulsive pump which heartbeats don't stop for a single moment. Is the truly engine of all the vascular circuit. On one hand receives the oxygenated blood that comes from the lungs and impulses to all the body, through a strong contraction called systole. On the other hand thanks to the diastole or relaxation of the cardiac muscle, the blood coming from all the body provided for the veins, it's picked up and through new contractions, it's sent to the lungs to eliminate there, the carbon dioxide contained and to be charged of oxygen and then return to the heart to be distributed again through the net.

The vascular net has, therefore, two directions: one of departure (arterial) and other of arrival (venous).

The arterial blood is in charge that, the oxygenated blood reaches all the organism. Begins in the heart, from the aorta artery, it ramifies in arteries, these divide in arterioles and from them come out a multitude of arterial capillaries that, after a certain journey become venous capillaries. All these vases are of caliber progressively smaller.

The venous blood picks the inconvenient substances up to be able to be eliminated. It begins from the venous capillaries in which have derived the arterial capillaries; the venous capillaries end up in the venues, of a bigger caliber, those do that in the veins, of a even bigger caliber, and these pour out in the venae cavae, of even much more capacity, in which through them the blood reaches the heart.

Parallel to the venous net, there is the lymphatic net, that is in charge of pick the lymph up, yellow alkaline liquid that comes from the insular liquids and that contains mainly lymphocytes and monocots and that is poured out, to the venous net.

To the journey that follows the blood from the heart to the cells and from them to the heart it's denominated major circulation, or systemic. And to the sanguineous journey of the heart to the lungs and vice-versa is called minor circulation or pulmonary.

HEART (I)
ANTERIOR VIEW

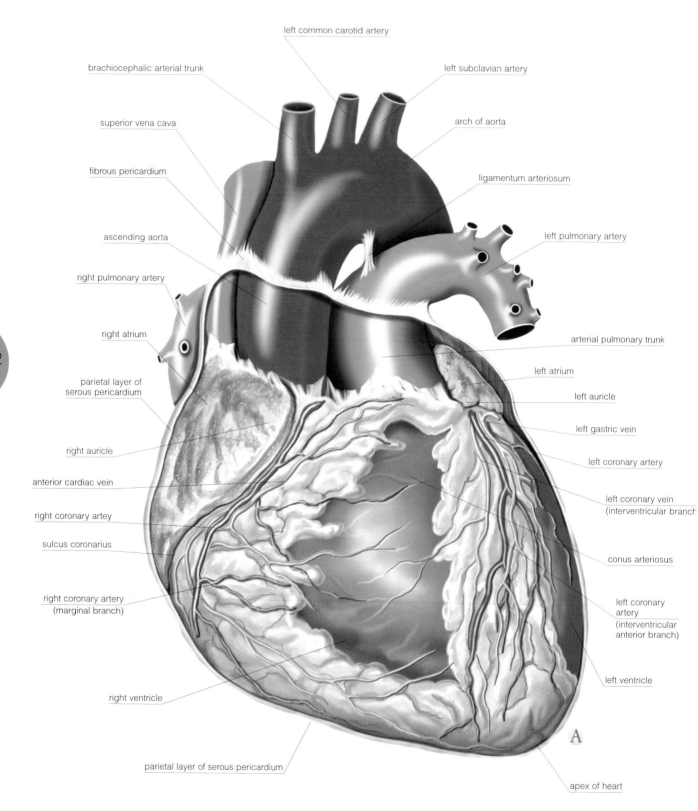

left common carotid artery

brachiocephalic arterial trunk

left subclavian artery

superior vena cava

arch of aorta

fibrous pericardium

ligamentum arteriosum

ascending aorta

left pulmonary artery

right pulmonary artery

arterial pulmonary trunk

right atrium

left atrium

parietal layer of
serous pericardium

left auricle

left gastric vein

right auricle

left coronary artery

anterior cardiac vein

left coronary vein
(interventricular branch)

right coronary artey

sulcus coronarius

conus arteriosus

right coronary artery
(marginal branch)

left coronary
artery
(interventricular
anterior branch)

left ventricle

right ventricle

parietal layer of serous pericardium

A

apex of heart

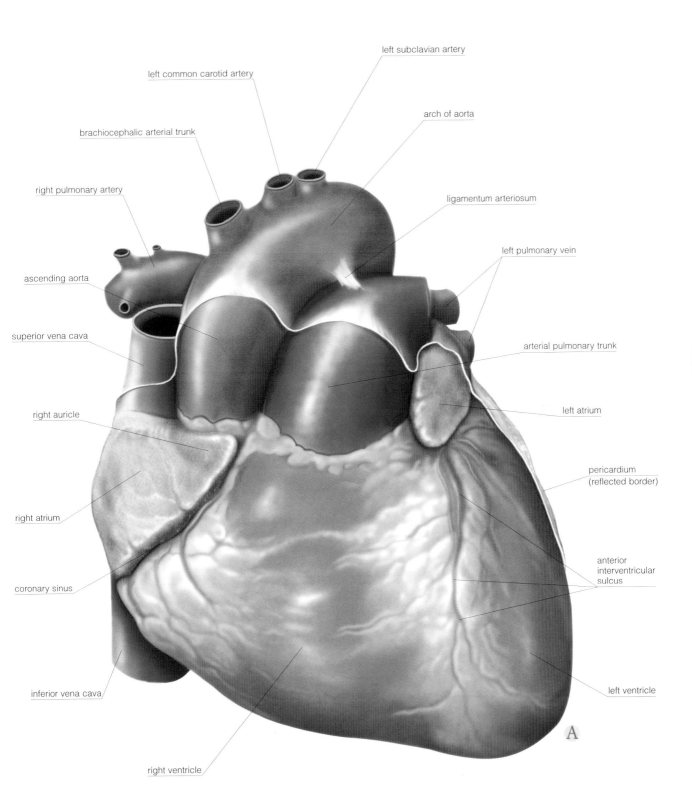

left common carotid artery

left subclavian artery

arch of aorta

brachiocephalic arterial trunk

right pulmonary artery

ligamentum arteriosum

left pulmonary vein

ascending aorta

superior vena cava

arterial pulmonary trunk

right auricle

left atrium

right atrium

pericardium (reflected border)

coronary sinus

anterior interventricular sulcus

inferior vena cava

left ventricle

right ventricle

A

HEART (III)
POSTERIOR VIEW

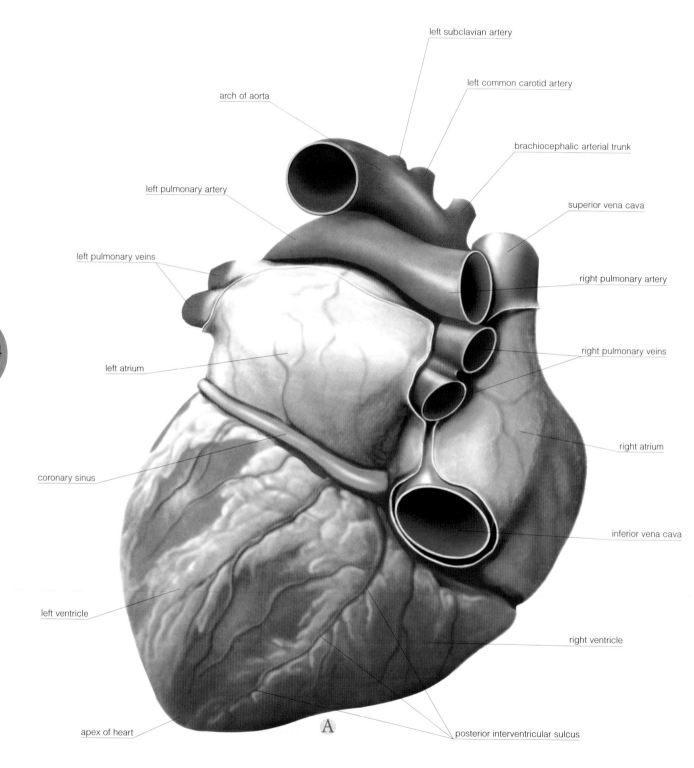

left subclavian artery

left common carotid artery

arch of aorta

brachiocephalic arterial trunk

left pulmonary artery

superior vena cava

left pulmonary veins

right pulmonary artery

left atrium

right pulmonary veins

right atrium

coronary sinus

inferior vena cava

left ventricle

right ventricle

apex of heart

posterior interventricular sulcus

264

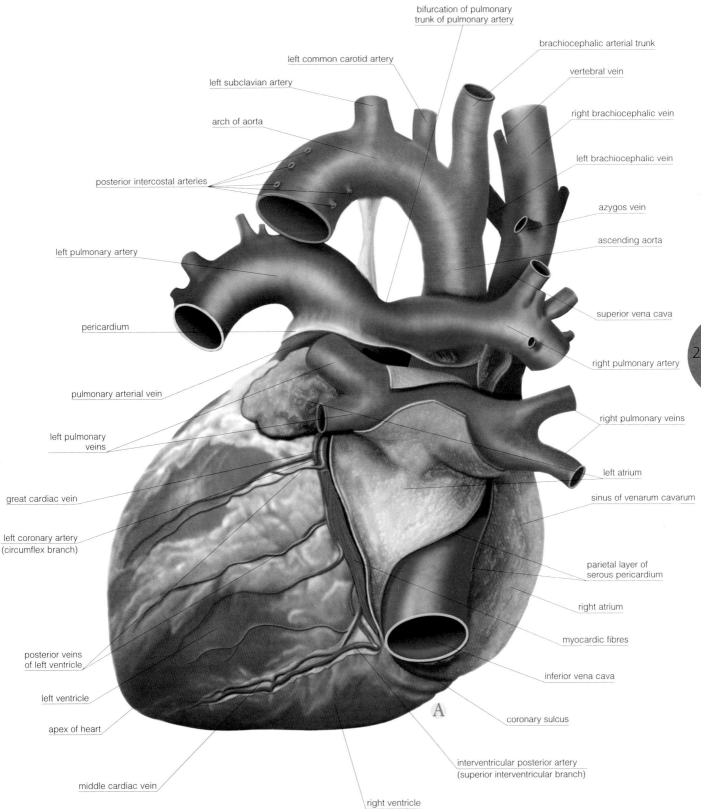

bifurcation of pulmonary
trunk of pulmonary artery

brachiocephalic arterial trunk

left common carotid artery

vertebral vein

left subclavian artery

right brachiocephalic vein

arch of aorta

left brachiocephalic vein

posterior intercostal arteries

azygos vein

ascending aorta

left pulmonary artery

pericardium

superior vena cava

pulmonary arterial vein

right pulmonary artery

right pulmonary veins

left pulmonary
veins

left atrium

great cardiac vein

sinus of venarum cavarum

left coronary artery
(circumflex branch)

parietal layer of
serous pericardium

right atrium

myocardic fibres

posterior veins
of left ventricle

inferior vena cava

left ventricle

apex of heart

coronary sulcus

middle cardiac vein

interventricular posterior artery
(superior interventricular branch)

right ventricle

A

HEART (V). RIGHT VENTRICLE
ANTERIOR VIEW

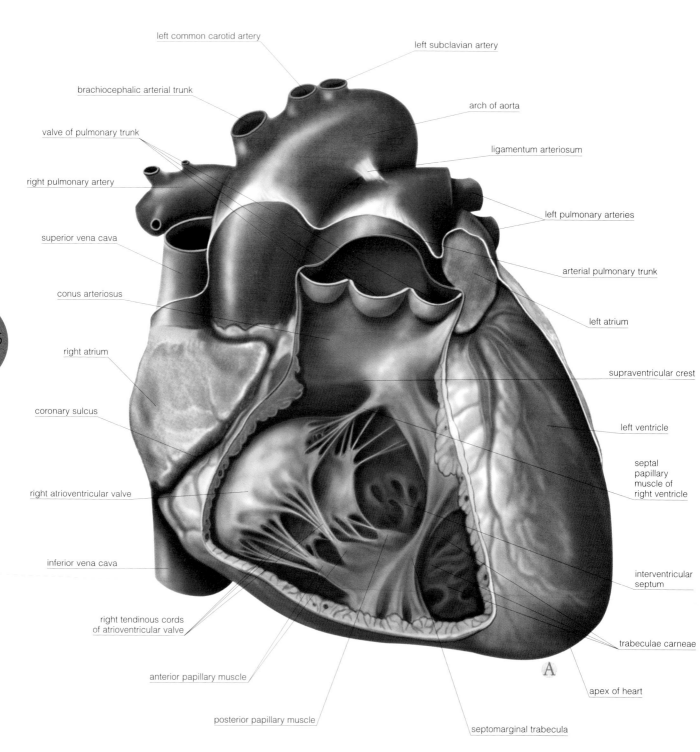

left common carotid artery

left subclavian artery

brachiocephalic arterial trunk

arch of aorta

valve of pulmonary trunk

ligamentum arteriosum

right pulmonary artery

left pulmonary arteries

superior vena cava

arterial pulmonary trunk

conus arteriosus

left atrium

266

right atrium

supraventricular crest

coronary sulcus

left ventricle

septal
papillary
muscle of
right ventricle

right atrioventricular valve

inferior vena cava

interventricular
septum

right tendinous cords
of atrioventricular valve

trabeculae carneae

A

anterior papillary muscle

apex of heart

posterior papillary muscle

septomarginal trabecula

HEART (VI). RIGHTS ATRIUM and VENTRICLE

ANTERIOR VIEW

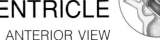

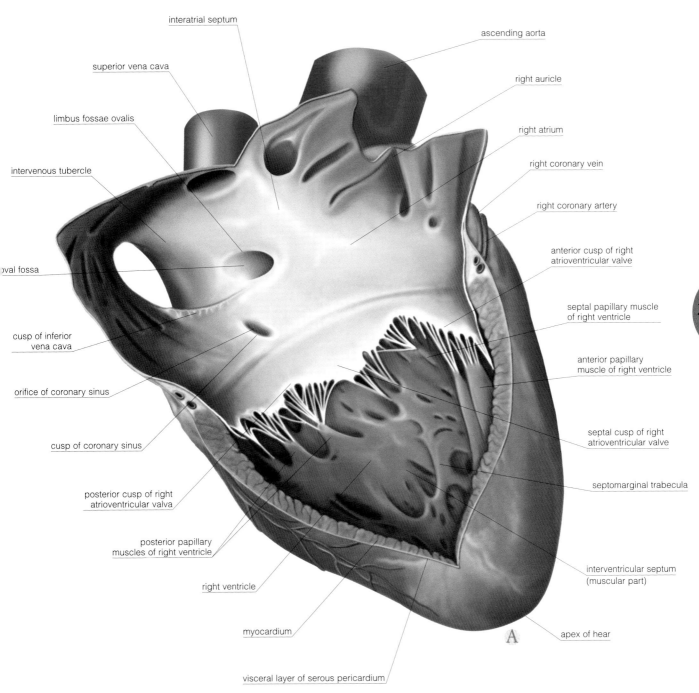

interatrial septum

ascending aorta

superior vena cava

right auricle

limbus fossae ovalis

right atrium

intervenous tubercle

right coronary vein

right coronary artery

oval fossa

anterior cusp of right
atrioventricular valve

septal papillary muscle
of right ventricle

267

cusp of inferior
vena cava

anterior papillary
muscle of right ventricle

orifice of coronary sinus

septal cusp of right
atrioventricular valve

cusp of coronary sinus

septomarginal trabecula

posterior cusp of right
atrioventricular valva

interventricular septum
(muscular part)

posterior papillary
muscles of right ventricle

right ventricle

apex of hear

myocardium

A

visceral layer of serous pericardium

HEART(VII)

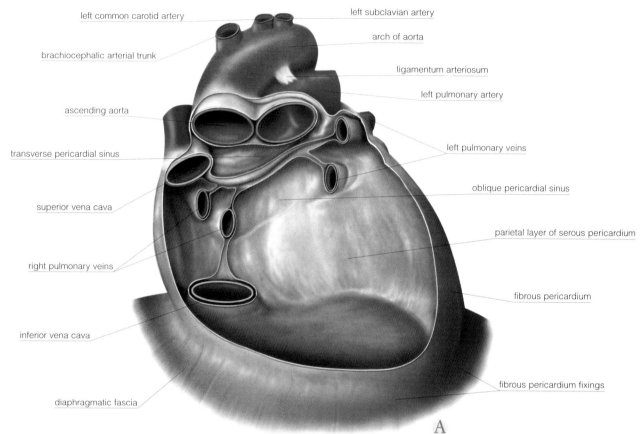

left common carotid artery

left subclavian artery

brachiocephalic arterial trunk

arch of aorta

ligamentum arteriosum

left pulmonary artery

ascending aorta

transverse pericardial sinus

left pulmonary veins

superior vena cava

oblique pericardial sinus

parietal layer of serous pericardium

right pulmonary veins

fibrous pericardium

inferior vena cava

fibrous pericardium fixings

diaphragmatic fascia

A

PERICARDIUM. ANTERIOR VIEW

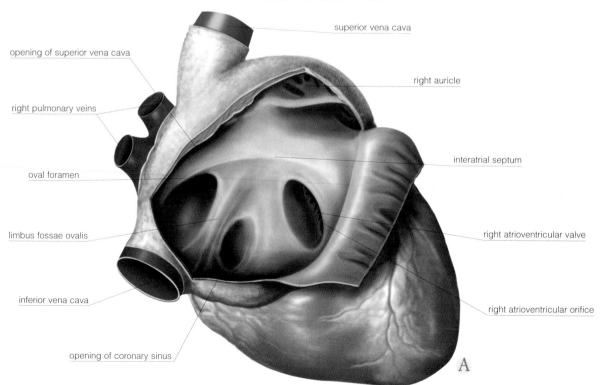

superior vena cava

opening of superior vena cava

right auricle

right pulmonary veins

interatrial septum

oval foramen

limbus fossae ovalis

right atrioventricular valve

inferior vena cava

right atrioventricular orifice

opening of coronary sinus

A

RIGHT ATRIUM of NEWBORN. ANTERIOR VIEW

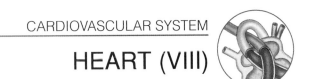

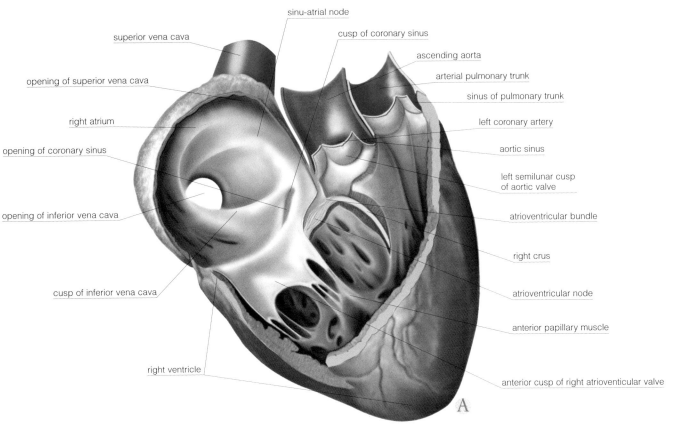

sinu-atrial node

cusp of coronary sinus

superior vena cava

ascending aorta

opening of superior vena cava

arterial pulmonary trunk

sinus of pulmonary trunk

right atrium

left coronary artery

opening of coronary sinus

aortic sinus

left semilunar cusp
of aortic valve

opening of inferior vena cava

atrioventricular bundle

right crus

atrioventricular node

cusp of inferior vena cava

anterior papillary muscle

right ventricle

anterior cusp of right atrioventicular valve

A

RIGHT ATRIUM and VENTRICLE. ANTERIOR VIEW

269

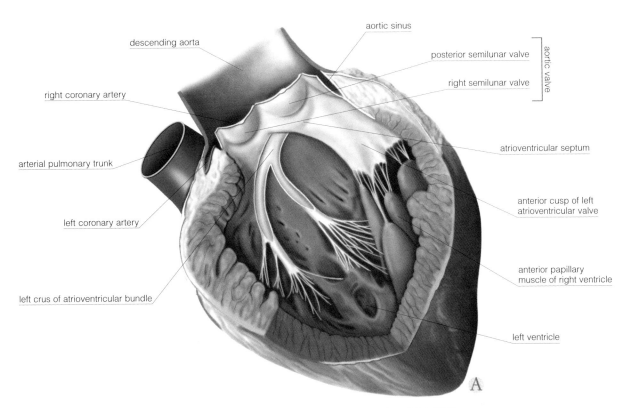

aortic sinus

descending aorta

posterior semilunar valve

aortic valve

right semilunar valve

right coronary artery

atrioventricular septum

arterial pulmonary trunk

anterior cusp of left
atrioventricular valve

left coronary artery

anterior papillary
muscle of right ventricle

left crus of atrioventricular bundle

left ventricle

A

LEFT VENTRICLE. ANTERIOR VIEW

HEART (IX). LEFT CORONARY ARTERY
ANTERIOR VIEW. STERNOCOSTAL LAYER

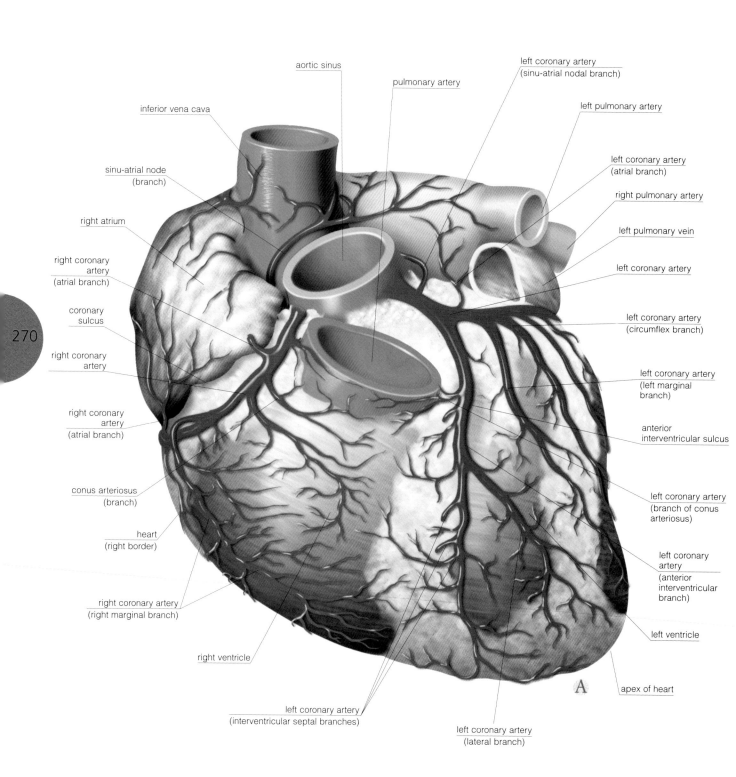

aortic sinus

pulmonary artery

left coronary artery
(sinu-atrial nodal branch)

inferior vena cava

left pulmonary artery

sinu-atrial node
(branch)

left coronary artery
(atrial branch)

right atrium

right pulmonary artery

right coronary
artery
(atrial branch)

left pulmonary vein

left coronary artery

coronary
sulcus

left coronary artery
(circumflex branch)

right coronary
artery

left coronary artery
(left marginal
branch)

right coronary
artery
(atrial branch)

anterior
interventricular sulcus

conus arteriosus
(branch)

left coronary artery
(branch of conus
arteriosus)

heart
(right border)

left coronary
artery
(anterior
interventricular
branch)

right coronary artery
(right marginal branch)

left ventricle

right ventricle

A

apex of heart

left coronary artery
(interventricular septal branches)

left coronary artery
(lateral branch)

270

HEART (X). RIGHT CORONARY ARTERY

POSTERIOR VIEW. DIAPHRAGMATIC LAYER

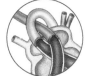

right coronary artery

The right coronary artery originates in the aorta, immediately to the high of the edge of the right semi-lunar valve and the corresponding aortic sinus. Its route heads downwards, towards and rightwards. It involves three segments:
1. Pre-auricular
2. Infra-auricular
3. Inter-ventricular posterior (here the artery is denominated posterior branch) it has a caliber of 3 to 4mm in the healthy adult.

The right coronary artery irrigates:
- The atrium or the right auricle.
- The three right fourths and inferior of the right ventricle included the posterior papillary muscle.
- The right half of the inferior face of the left ventricle.
- The posterior third of the inter-ventricular partition.
- The cardiac conduction nodes (variable).
- The atrioventricular fascicle, or auriculoventricular (variable)

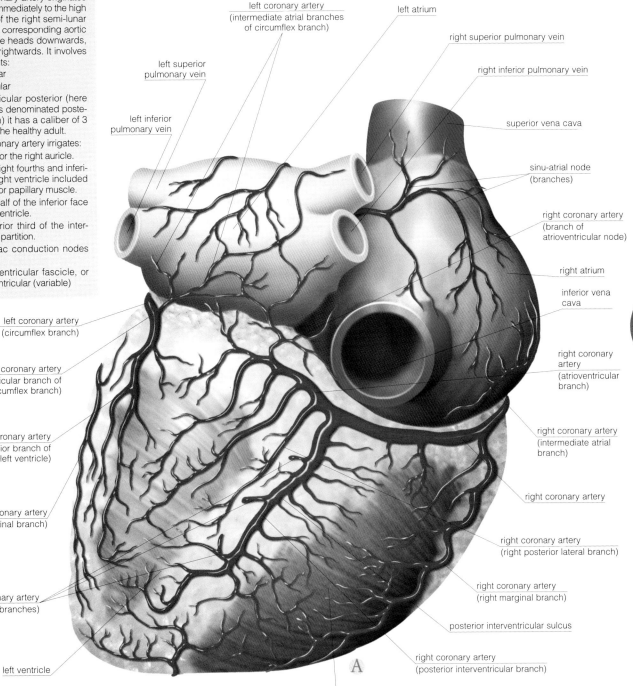

left coronary artery
(intermediate atrial branches
of circumflex branch)

left atrium

right superior pulmonary vein

right inferior pulmonary vein

left superior
pulmonary vein

superior vena cava

left inferior
pulmonary vein

sinu-atrial node
(branches)

right coronary artery
(branch of
atrioventricular node)

right atrium

inferior vena
cava

left coronary artery
(circumflex branch)

right coronary
artery
(atrioventricular
branch)

left coronary artery
(atrioventricular branch of
circumflex branch)

left coronary artery
(posterior branch of
left ventricle)

right coronary artery
(intermediate atrial
branch)

right coronary artery

left coronary artery
(left marginal branch)

right coronary artery
(right posterior lateral branch)

right coronary artery
(right marginal branch)

right coronary artery
nterventricular branches)

posterior interventricular sulcus

left ventricle

right coronary artery
(posterior interventricular branch)

A

right ventricle

HEART (XI)

INTERVAL VIEW

INTERNAL VIEW

heart cavities

The heart has four cavities: two atriums, or two auricles, and two ventricles. These cavities get full and get empty of blood, regulated by valves that opens or closes in an ordered and coordinated way. The heart gets relaxed and constrict rhythmically at all moment. The energy that develops in these contractions makes that the blood that is expelled acquires such pressure that is able to reach all parts of the human body, includes the farthest and even the most hidden corners.

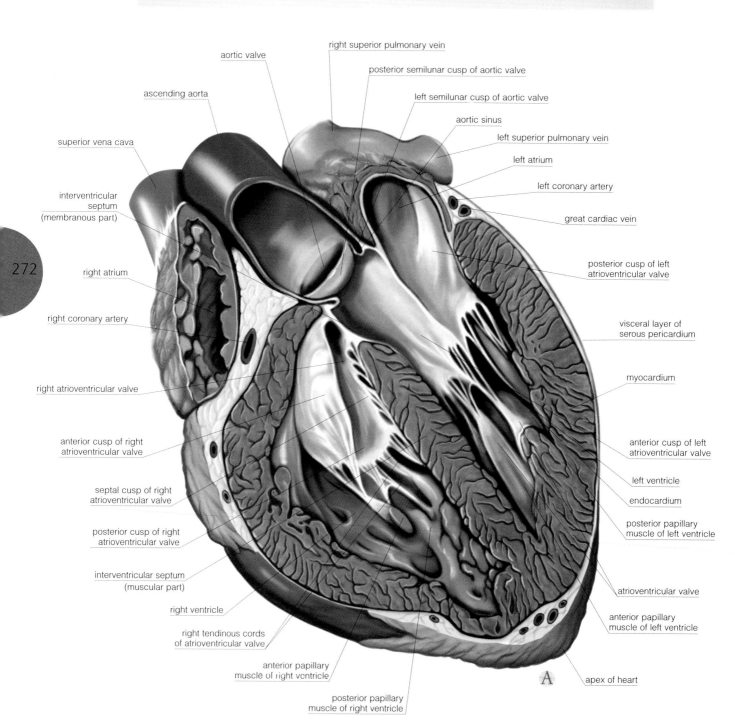

Labels:
aortic valve
right superior pulmonary vein
posterior semilunar cusp of aortic valve
ascending aorta
left semilunar cusp of aortic valve
aortic sinus
superior vena cava
left superior pulmonary vein
left atrium
interventricular septum (membranous part)
left coronary artery
great cardiac vein
right atrium
posterior cusp of left atrioventricular valve
right coronary artery
visceral layer of serous pericardium
right atrioventricular valve
myocardium
anterior cusp of right atrioventricular valve
anterior cusp of left atrioventricular valve
septal cusp of right atrioventricular valve
left ventricle
endocardium
posterior cusp of right atrioventricular valve
posterior papillary muscle of left ventricle
interventricular septum (muscular part)
atrioventricular valve
right ventricle
anterior papillary muscle of left ventricle
right tendinous cords of atrioventricular valve
anterior papillary muscle of right ventricle
apex of heart
posterior papillary muscle of right ventricle

HEART (XII)
INTERNAL VIEW

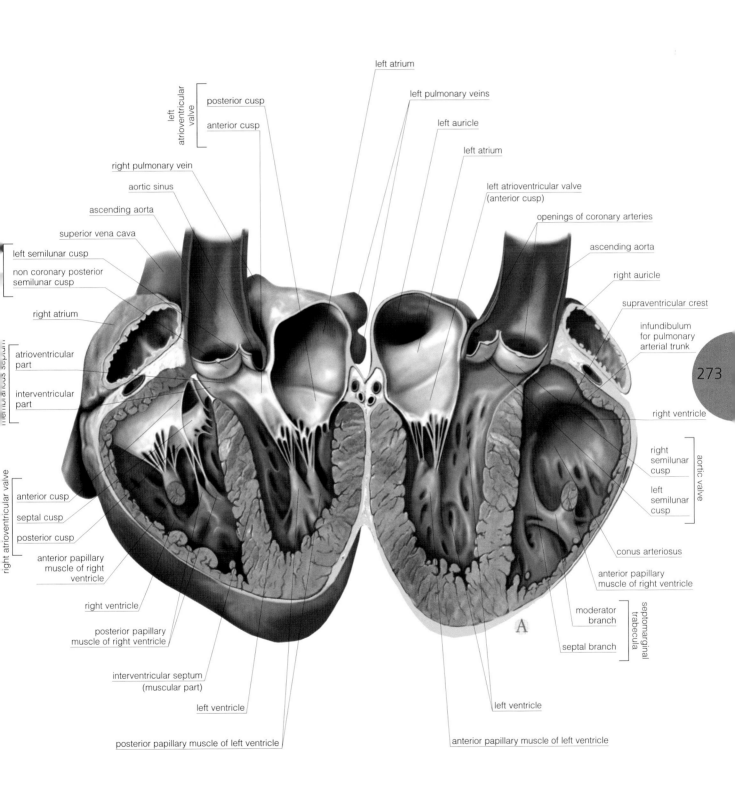

left atrium

left pulmonary veins

left auricle

left atrium

posterior cusp

anterior cusp

left
atrioventricular
valve

right pulmonary vein

aortic sinus

ascending aorta

superior vena cava

left semilunar cusp

non coronary posterior
semilunar cusp

right atrium

atrioventricular
part

interventricular
part

left atrioventricular valve
(anterior cusp)

openings of coronary arteries

ascending aorta

right auricle

supraventricular crest

infundibulum
for pulmonary
arterial trunk

right ventricle

right
semilunar
cusp

left
semilunar
cusp

aortic valve

conus arteriosus

anterior papillary
muscle of right ventricle

moderator
branch

septal branch

septomarginal
trabecula

right atrioventricular valve

anterior cusp

septal cusp

posterior cusp

anterior papillary
muscle of right
ventricle

right ventricle

posterior papillary
muscle of right ventricle

interventricular septum
(muscular part)

left ventricle

posterior papillary muscle of left ventricle

left ventricle

anterior papillary muscle of left ventricle

273

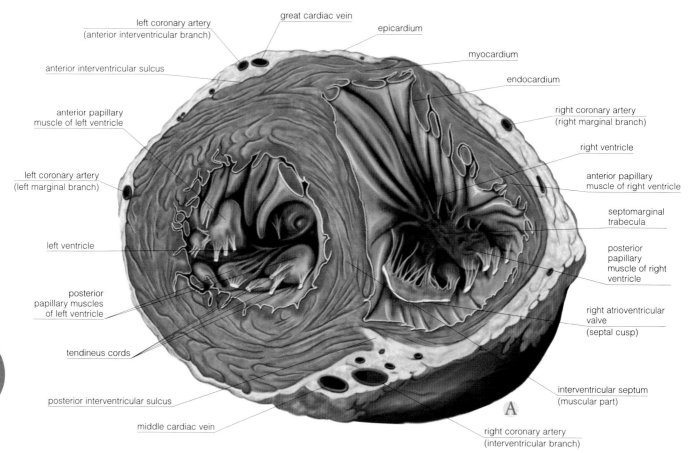

left coronary artery
(anterior interventricular branch)

great cardiac vein

epicardium

myocardium

endocardium

anterior interventricular sulcus

anterior papillary
muscle of left ventricle

right coronary artery
(right marginal branch)

right ventricle

left coronary artery
(left marginal branch)

anterior papillary
muscle of right ventricle

septomarginal
trabecula

left ventricle

posterior
papillary
muscle of right
ventricle

posterior
papillary muscles
of left ventricle

right atrioventricular
valve
(septal cusp)

tendineus cords

interventricular septum
(muscular part)

posterior interventricular sulcus

middle cardiac vein

right coronary artery
(interventricular branch)

RIGHT and LEFT VENTRICLES. TRANSVERSE SECTION

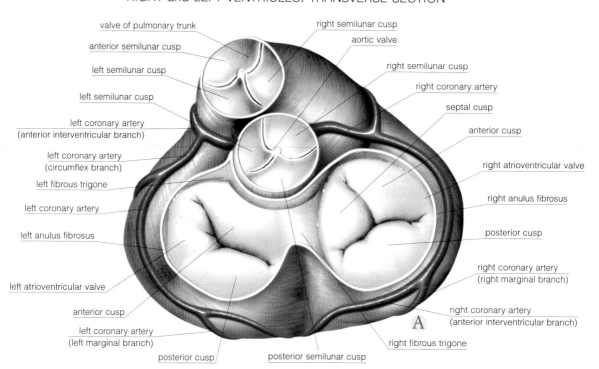

valve of pulmonary trunk

right semilunar cusp

aortic valve

anterior semilunar cusp

left semilunar cusp

right semilunar cusp

right coronary artery

left semilunar cusp

septal cusp

left coronary artery
(anterior interventricular branch)

anterior cusp

left coronary artery
(circumflex branch)

right atrioventricular valve

left fibrous trigone

right anulus fibrosus

left coronary artery

left anulus fibrosus

posterior cusp

right coronary artery
(right marginal branch)

left atrioventricular valve

anterior cusp

right coronary artery
(anterior interventricular branch)

left coronary artery
(left marginal branch)

right fibrous trigone

posterior cusp

posterior semilunar cusp

CARDIAC VALVES. SUPERIOR VIEW

274

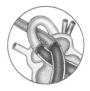

HEART (XIV). VALVES in SYSTOLE and DIASTOLE

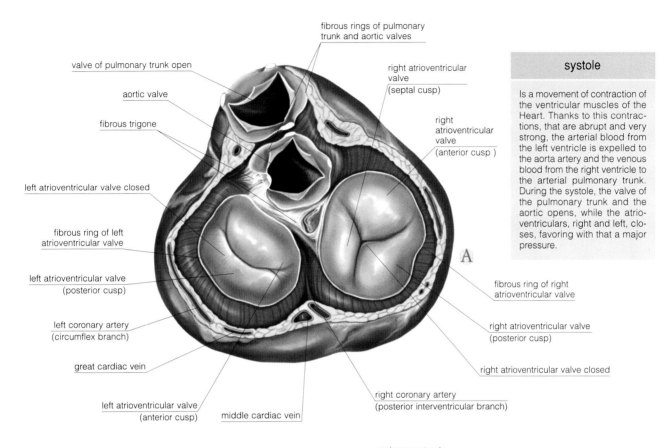

fibrous rings of pulmonary trunk and aortic valves

valve of pulmonary trunk open

aortic valve

fibrous trigone

left atrioventricular valve closed

fibrous ring of left atrioventricular valve

left atrioventricular valve (posterior cusp)

left coronary artery (circumflex branch)

great cardiac vein

left atrioventricular valve (anterior cusp)

middle cardiac vein

right atrioventricular valve (septal cusp)

right atrioventricular valve (anterior cusp)

fibrous ring of right atrioventricular valve

right atrioventricular valve (posterior cusp)

right atrioventricular valve closed

right coronary artery (posterior interventricular branch)

systole

Is a movement of contraction of the ventricular muscles of the Heart. Thanks to this contractions, that are abrupt and very strong, the arterial blood from the left ventricle is expelled to the aorta artery and the venous blood from the right ventricle to the arterial pulmonary trunk. During the systole, the valve of the pulmonary trunk and the aortic opens, while the atrioventriculars, right and left, closes, favoring with that a major pressure.

A

275

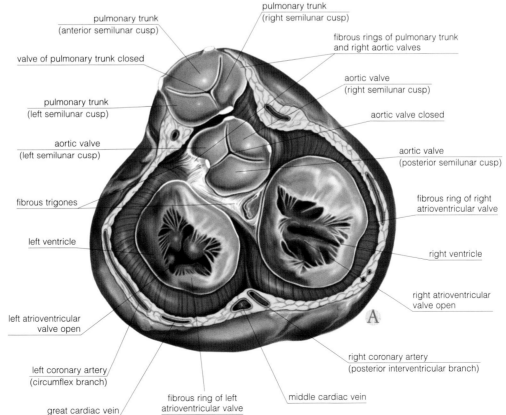

pulmonary trunk (anterior semilunar cusp)

valve of pulmonary trunk closed

pulmonary trunk (left semilunar cusp)

aortic valve (left semilunar cusp)

fibrous trigones

left ventricle

left atrioventricular valve open

left coronary artery (circumflex branch)

great cardiac vein

fibrous ring of left atrioventricular valve

pulmonary trunk (right semilunar cusp)

fibrous rings of pulmonary trunk and right aortic valves

aortic valve (right semilunar cusp)

aortic valve closed

aortic valve (posterior semilunar cusp)

fibrous ring of right atrioventricular valve

right ventricle

right atrioventricular valve open

right coronary artery (posterior interventricular branch)

middle cardiac vein

A

diastole

Is a movement of relaxation of the ventricles, thanks to this allows the pass to the left ventricle of the arterial blood that comes from the left atrium and to the right ventricle the venous blood that comes from the right atrium. Contrary that happens in the systole, in the diastole the atrioventricular valves right and left, remain open, while the ones of the pulmonary trunk and the aortic remain closed, which favors the filling of ventricles. In her could be appreciate two phases: isometric and isotonic.

HEART (XV). SEMILUNAR VALVES

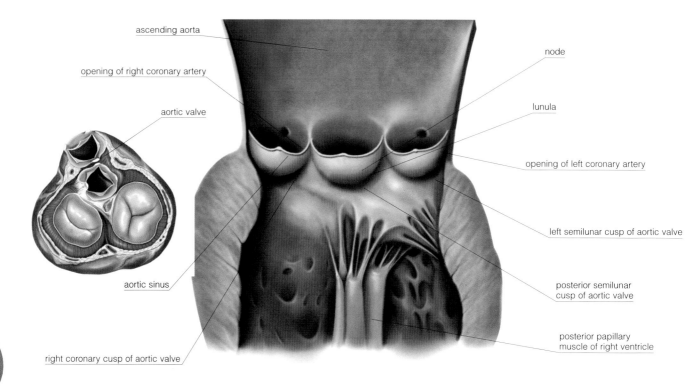

ascending aorta

opening of right coronary artery

aortic valve

node

lunula

opening of left coronary artery

left semilunar cusp of aortic valve

posterior semilunar cusp of aortic valve

posterior papillary muscle of right ventricle

aortic sinus

right coronary cusp of aortic valve

AORTIC VALVE

A

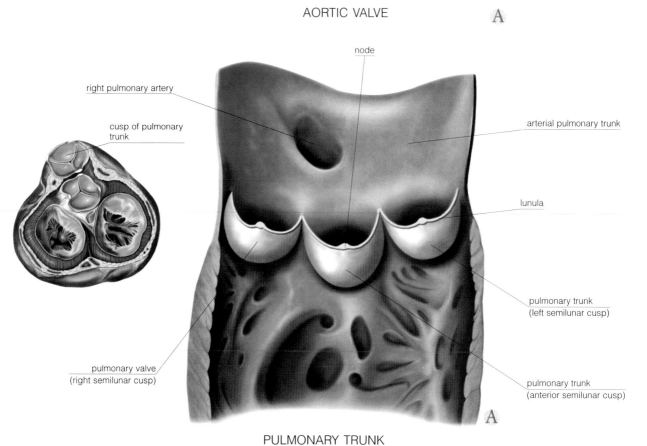

node

right pulmonary artery

cusp of pulmonary trunk

arterial pulmonary trunk

lunula

pulmonary trunk (left semilunar cusp)

pulmonary valve (right semilunar cusp)

pulmonary trunk (anterior semilunar cusp)

A

PULMONARY TRUNK

HEARD (XVI). ATRIOVENTRICULAR VALVES

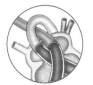

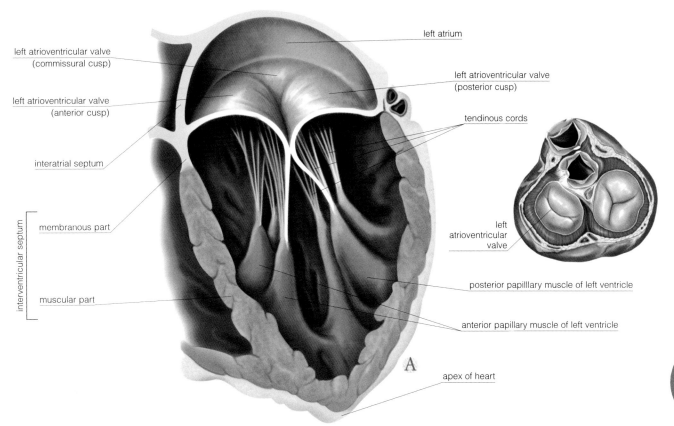

left atrium

left atrioventricular valve
(commissural cusp)

left atrioventricular valve
(posterior cusp)

left atrioventricular valve
(anterior cusp)

tendinous cords

interatrial septum

interventricular septum

membranous part

left
atrioventricular
valve

muscular part

posterior papilllary muscle of left ventricle

anterior papillary muscle of left ventricle

A

apex of heart

277

LEFT ATRIOVENTRICULAR VALVE

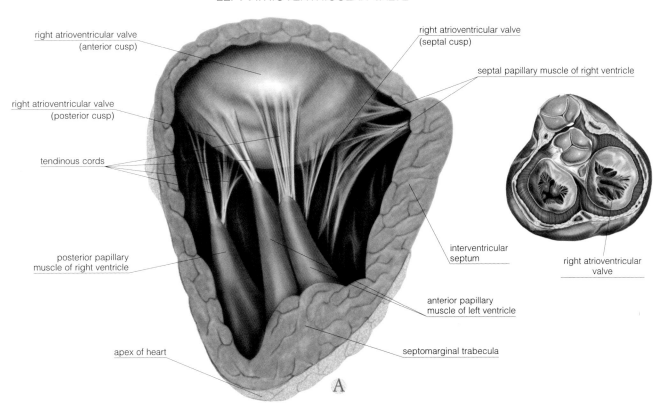

right atrioventricular valve
(anterior cusp)

right atrioventricular valve
(septal cusp)

septal papillary muscle of right ventricle

right atrioventricular valve
(posterior cusp)

tendinous cords

posterior papillary
muscle of right ventricle

interventricular
septum

right atrioventricular
valve

anterior papillary
muscle of left ventricle

apex of heart

septomarginal trabecula

A

RIGHT ATRIOVENTRICULAR VALVE

BLOOD VESSELS

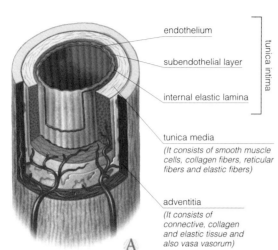

endothelium

subendothelial layer — tunica intima

internal elastic lamina

tunica media
(It consists of smooth muscle cells, collagen fibers, reticular fibers and elastic fibers)

adventitia
(It consists of connective, collagen and elastic tissue and also vasa vasorum)

A

MUSCULAR ARTERY

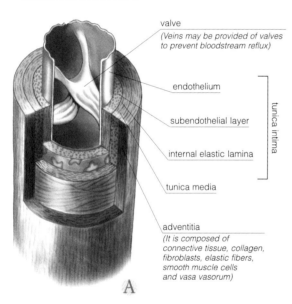

valve
(Veins may be provided of valves to prevent bloodstream reflux)

endothelium

subendothelial layer — tunica intima

internal elastic lamina

tunica media

adventitia
(It is composed of connective tissue, collagen, fibroblasts, elastic fibers, smooth muscle cells and vasa vasorum)

A

GREAT VEIN

A

DIFFERENCES BETWEEN ARTERIES and VEINS

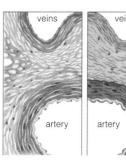

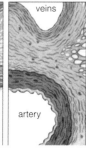

veins

veins

artery

artery

Artery walls are more muscular and their tunica media is thicker than veins and has more elastic tissue while veins adventitious layer is thicker than arteries. The vasa vasorum of adventitious layer are introduced into outer zones of tunica media and provide nutritive substances in their cells.

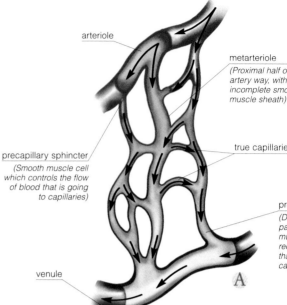

arteriole

metarteriole
(Proximal half of central artery way, with incomplete smooth muscle sheath)

precapillary sphincter
(Smooth muscle cell which controls the flow of blood that is going to capillaries)

true capillaries

preferable path
(Distal half of central path. It lacks smooth muscle cells and receives the blood that comes from capillary bed)

venule

A

BLOOD CAPILLARY NETWORK

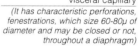

continous capillary
(It lacks fenestrations. Substances which are transported pass through endothelial cell in both directions inside pinocitic vesicles)

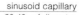

visceral capillary
(It has characteristic perforations, fenestrations, which size 60-80µ of diameter and may be closed or not, throughout a diaphragm)

sinusoid capillary
(Its light is wide -30-40µ of diameter- and is provided of multiple fenestrations and a discontinuous basal lamina, but it lacks of pinocitic vesicles. Endothelial contiguous cells of sinusoids use to overlap incompletely)

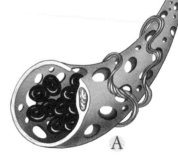

A

BLOOD VESSELS

(They are composed of a simple flat epithelium rolled in a narrow cylinder 8-10µ of diameter)

VASCULAR ANASTOMOSIS (I)

vascular anastomosis

The arteriovenous anastomosis is a complex framework of vases, which function is to guarantee the circulation of blood through all the organism, reaching even the most hidden corners of most difficult access. Consist of two big families of vases or conducts: The arterial net (arteries, arterioles and capillaries) in charge of the transport of the oxygenated blood that comes from the heart, and the venous net (veins, venules and capillaries) that takes care of pick the blood that contains carbon dioxide, substances various and materials of disposal, useless or harmful, to carry it to the heart and to the lungs to be depurated (oxygenated) and becomes suitable to restart the circuit through the arterial net. Thanks to the arteriovenous net all the cells of the organism can keep alive and active, and with this the human body could function correctly.

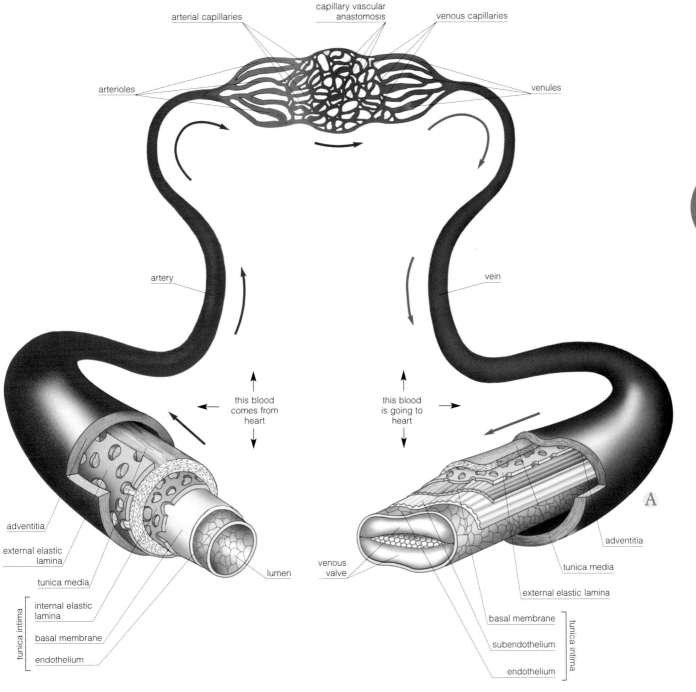

VASCULAR ANASTOMOSIS (II)

ARTERY, VEIN and BLOOD VESSELS.STRUCTURE

artery

The arteries are the sanguineous conducts that transport the blood that has been oxygenated in the lungs (or arterial blood) and that is impulse from the heart to all the corners of the organism with the object of keeping the cells alive and with them the diverse organs and thus guarantee its perfect functioning. For that, form a net (arterial net) in which there are big arteries, that derived in normal arteries, these in arterioles, of smaller caliber and these in arterial capillaries, according to the volume of blood that each of them transport.

vein

The veins are sanguineous conducts that transports to the heart and then to the lungs the blood loaded with refused substances and harmful for the organism, with the end of being purified. This blood is collected by the venules, that meantime have been collected from the capillaries, that have flown into them. Contrary to what happens in the arterial net, the venous net originates in the extremities and its components (capillaries, venues and veins) converge to the lungs and the heart.

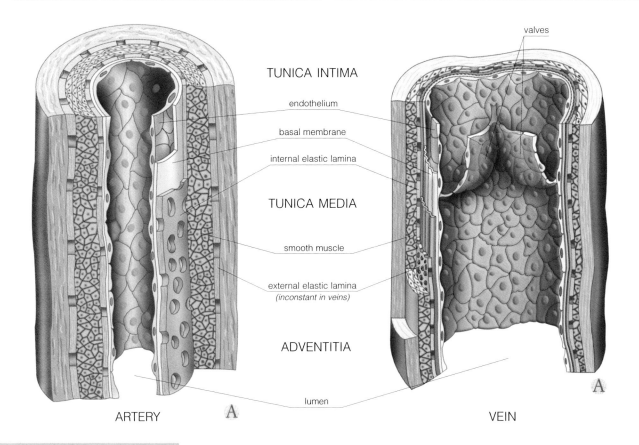

TUNICA INTIMA

endothelium

basal membrane

internal elastic lamina

TUNICA MEDIA

smooth muscle

external elastic lamina
(inconstant in veins)

ADVENTITIA

valves

lumen

ARTERY

VEIN

blood vessel

The sanguineous capillaries are microscopic ramifications in which derived the arteries and veins after have reduced its light up to its minimal expression. The arterial capillaries are continuation of the arterioles. Through them the blood coming from the heart can reach to all the cells of the organism, wherever they are, and provide them the oxygen and other nutritive substances to revitalize them. For their part, they have been expelling the carbon dioxide and other harmful substances. The arterial capillaries transform themselves in venous capillaries, inverting the sense of the way and also the function: pick the dismissed elements and form the venous net and with this, begins the return journey to the heart and the lung. The venous capillaries flow into the venules.

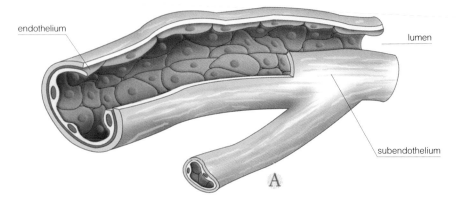

endothelium

lumen

subendothelium

BLOOD VESSEL

280

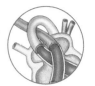

VASCULAR ANASTOMOSIS (III)

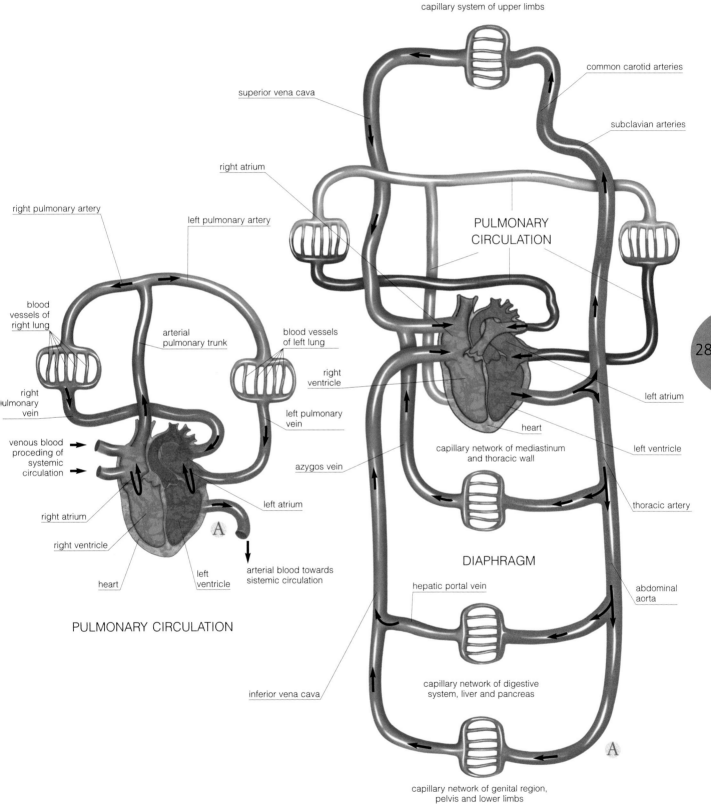

capillary system of upper limbs

common carotid arteries

superior vena cava

subclavian arteries

right atrium

PULMONARY
CIRCULATION

right pulmonary artery

left pulmonary artery

blood
vessels of
right lung

arterial
pulmonary trunk

blood vessels
of left lung

right
ventricle

right
pulmonary
vein

left pulmonary
vein

left atrium

left ventricle

venous blood
proceding of
systemic
circulation

azygos vein

heart

capillary network of mediastinum
and thoracic wall

thoracic artery

right atrium

right ventricle

left atrium

DIAPHRAGM

abdominal
aorta

heart

left
ventricle

hepatic portal vein

A

arterial blood towards
sistemic circulation

PULMONARY CIRCULATION

inferior vena cava

capillary network of digestive
system, liver and pancreas

A

281

capillary network of genital region,
pelvis and lower limbs

SYSTEMIC CIRCULATION

ARTERIAL SYSTEM (I). SYSTEMIC CIRCULATION

MAIN VESSELS

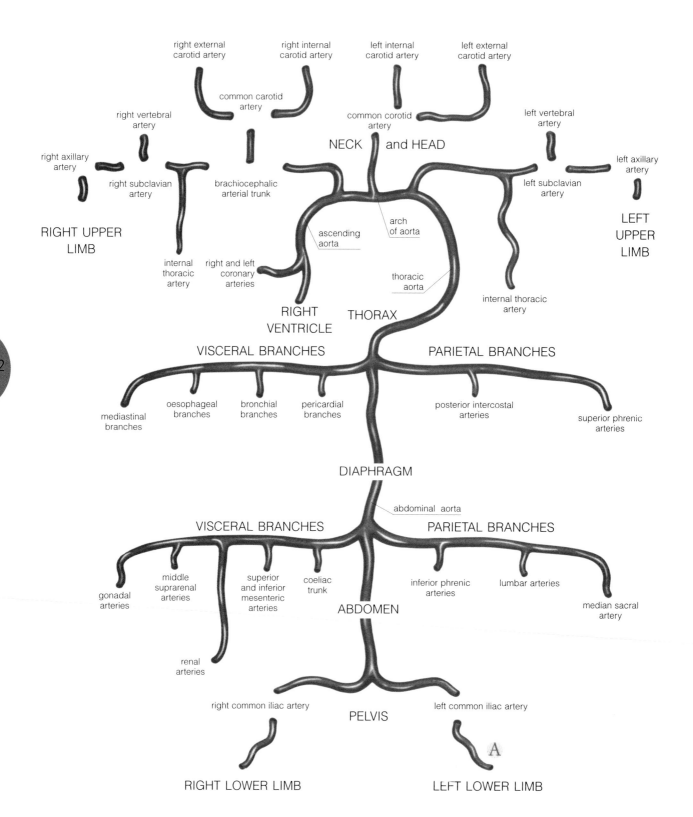

right external
carotid artery

right internal
carotid artery

left internal
carotid artery

left external
carotid artery

common carotid
artery

right vertebral
artery

common corotid
artery

left vertebral
artery

NECK   and HEAD

right axillary
artery

left axillary
artery

right subclavian
artery

brachiocephalic
arterial trunk

left subclavian
artery

RIGHT UPPER
LIMB

arch
of aorta

LEFT
UPPER
LIMB

ascending
aorta

internal
thoracic
artery

right and left
coronary
arteries

thoracic
aorta

internal thoracic
artery

RIGHT
VENTRICLE

THORAX

VISCERAL BRANCHES

PARIETAL BRANCHES

mediastinal
branches

oesophageal
branches

bronchial
branches

pericardial
branches

posterior intercostal
arteries

superior phrenic
arteries

DIAPHRAGM

abdominal aorta

VISCERAL BRANCHES

PARIETAL BRANCHES

gonadal
arteries

middle
suprarenal
arteries

superior
and inferior
mesenteric
arteries

coeliac
trunk

inferior phrenic
arteries

lumbar arteries

median sacral
artery

ABDOMEN

renal
arteries

right common iliac artery

left common iliac artery

PELVIS

A

RIGHT LOWER LIMB

LEFT LOWER LIMB

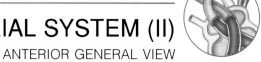

ARTERIAL SYSTEM (II)

ANTERIOR GENERAL VIEW

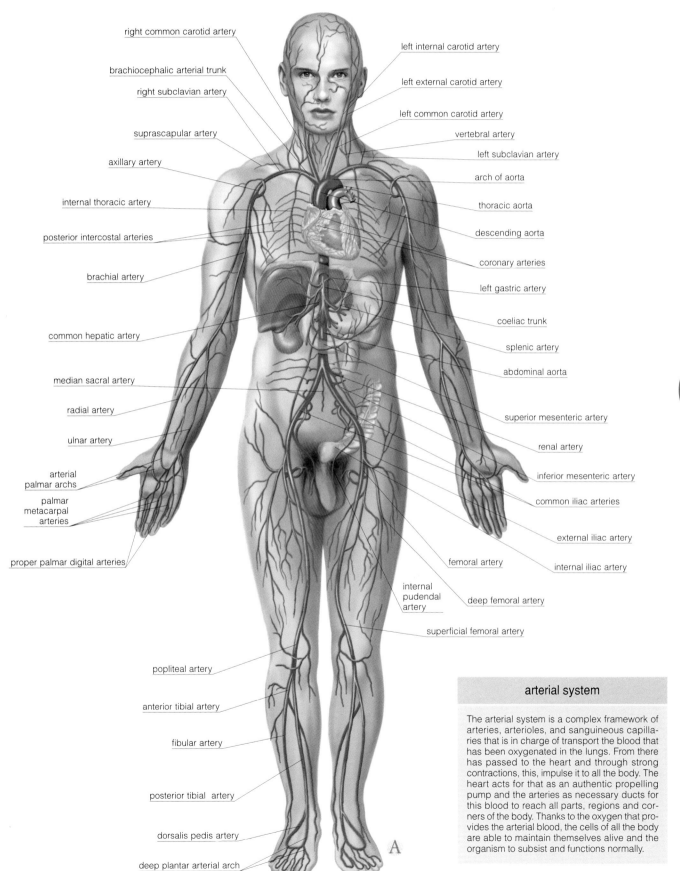

right common carotid artery

brachiocephalic arterial trunk

right subclavian artery

suprascapular artery

axillary artery

internal thoracic artery

posterior intercostal arteries

brachial artery

common hepatic artery

median sacral artery

radial artery

ulnar artery

arterial palmar archs

palmar metacarpal arteries

proper palmar digital arteries

popliteal artery

anterior tibial artery

fibular artery

posterior tibial artery

dorsalis pedis artery

deep plantar arterial arch

left internal carotid artery

left external carotid artery

left common carotid artery

vertebral artery

left subclavian artery

arch of aorta

thoracic aorta

descending aorta

coronary arteries

left gastric artery

coeliac trunk

splenic artery

abdominal aorta

superior mesenteric artery

renal artery

inferior mesenteric artery

common iliac arteries

external iliac artery

internal iliac artery

femoral artery

deep femoral artery

internal pudendal artery

superficial femoral artery

A

283

arterial system

The arterial system is a complex framework of arteries, arterioles, and sanguineous capillaries that is in charge of transport the blood that has been oxygenated in the lungs. From there has passed to the heart and through strong contractions, this, impulse it to all the body. The heart acts for that as an authentic propelling pump and the arteries as necessary ducts for this blood to reach all parts, regions and corners of the body. Thanks to the oxygen that provides the arterial blood, the cells of all the body are able to maintain themselves alive and the organism to subsist and functions normally.

ARTERIAL SYSTEM (III). NECK and HEAD (I)

FRONTAL VIEW

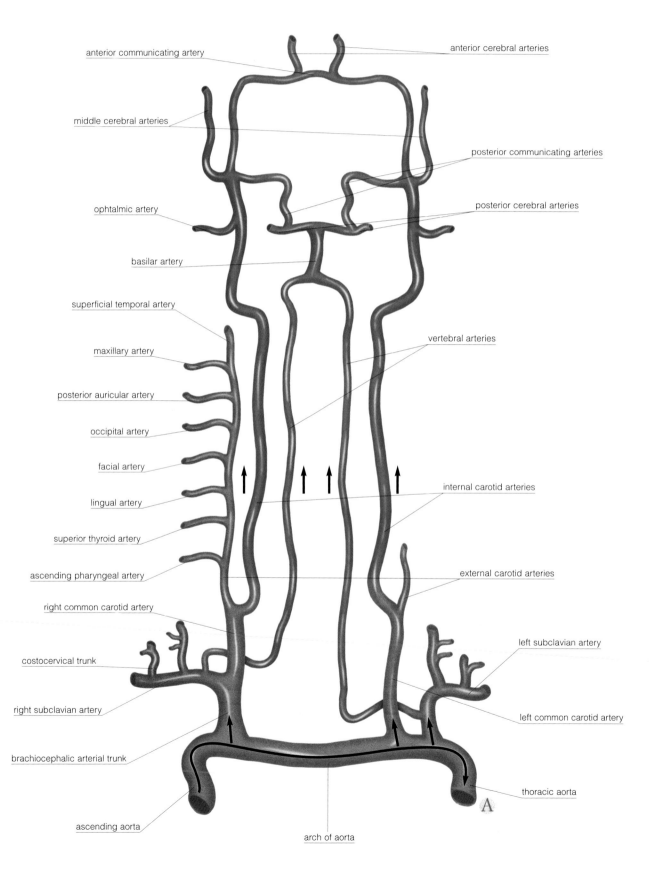

anterior communicating artery

anterior cerebral arteries

middle cerebral arteries

posterior communicating arteries

ophtalmic artery

posterior cerebral arteries

basilar artery

superficial temporal artery

maxillary artery

vertebral arteries

posterior auricular artery

occipital artery

facial artery

internal carotid arteries

lingual artery

superior thyroid artery

ascending pharyngeal artery

external carotid arteries

right common carotid artery

costocervical trunk

left subclavian artery

right subclavian artery

left common carotid artery

brachiocephalic arterial trunk

thoracic aorta

ascending aorta

A

arch of aorta

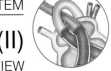

ARTERIAL SYSTEM (IV). NECK and HEAD (II)

FRONTAL VIEW

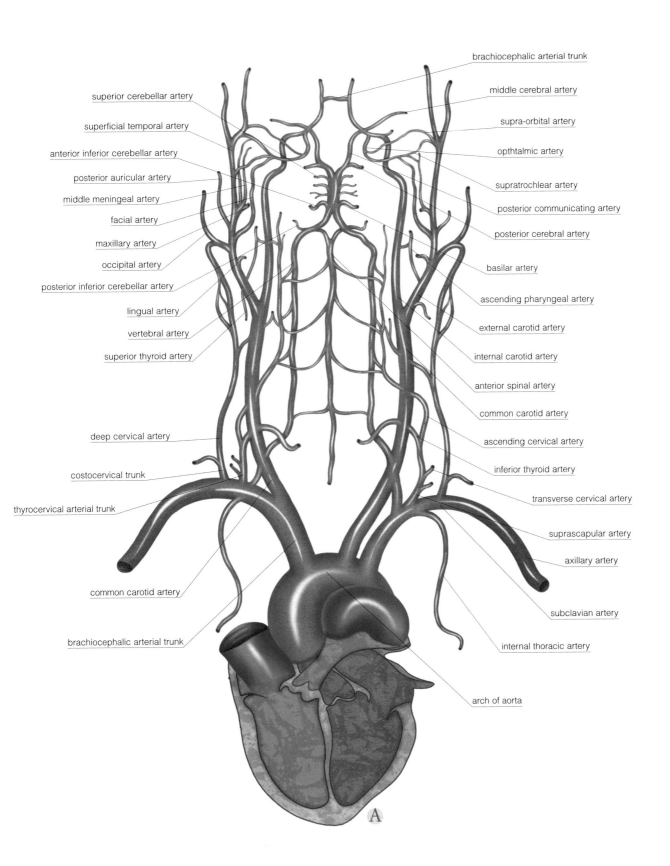

brachiocephalic arterial trunk

middle cerebral artery

supra-orbital artery

opthtalmic artery

supratrochlear artery

posterior communicating artery

posterior cerebral artery

basilar artery

ascending pharyngeal artery

external carotid artery

internal carotid artery

anterior spinal artery

common carotid artery

ascending cervical artery

inferior thyroid artery

transverse cervical artery

suprascapular artery

axillary artery

subclavian artery

internal thoracic artery

arch of aorta

superior cerebellar artery

superficial temporal artery

anterior inferior cerebellar artery

posterior auricular artery

middle meningeal artery

facial artery

maxillary artery

occipital artery

posterior inferior cerebellar artery

lingual artery

vertebral artery

superior thyroid artery

deep cervical artery

costocervical trunk

thyrocervical arterial trunk

common carotid artery

brachiocephalic arterial trunk

285

A

ARTERIAL SYSTEM (V). NECK and HEAD (III)

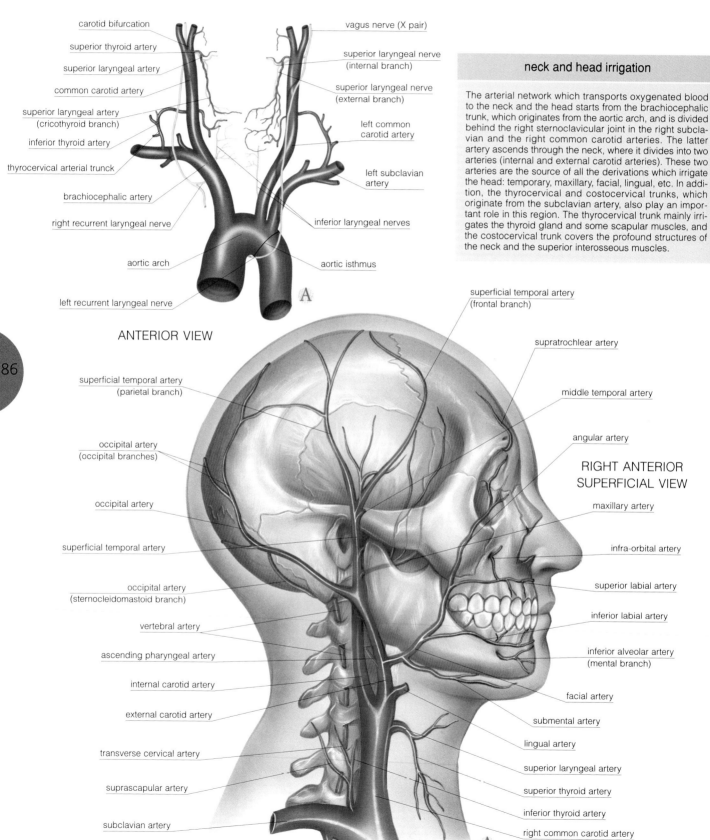

carotid bifurcation

superior thyroid artery

superior laryngeal artery

common carotid artery

superior laryngeal artery
(cricothyroid branch)

inferior thyroid artery

thyrocervical arterial trunk

brachiocephalic artery

right recurrent laryngeal nerve

aortic arch

left recurrent laryngeal nerve

vagus nerve (X pair)

superior laryngeal nerve
(internal branch)

superior laryngeal nerve
(external branch)

left common
carotid artery

left subclavian
artery

inferior laryngeal nerves

aortic isthmus

ANTERIOR VIEW

neck and head irrigation

The arterial network which transports oxygenated blood to the neck and the head starts from the brachiocephalic trunk, which originates from the aortic arch, and is divided behind the right sternoclavicular joint in the right subclavian and the right common carotid arteries. The latter artery ascends through the neck, where it divides into two arteries (internal and external carotid arteries). These two arteries are the source of all the derivations which irrigate the head: temporary, maxillary, facial, lingual, etc. In addition, the thyrocervical and costocervical trunks, which originate from the subclavian artery, also play an important role in this region. The thyrocervical trunk mainly irrigates the thyroid gland and some scapular muscles, and the costocervical trunk covers the profound structures of the neck and the superior interosseous muscles.

superficial temporal artery
(frontal branch)

supratrochlear artery

middle temporal artery

angular artery

**RIGHT ANTERIOR
SUPERFICIAL VIEW**

superficial temporal artery
(parietal branch)

occipital artery
(occipital branches)

occipital artery

superficial temporal artery

occipital artery
(sternocleidomastoid branch)

vertebral artery

ascending pharyngeal artery

internal carotid artery

external carotid artery

transverse cervical artery

suprascapular artery

subclavian artery

maxillary artery

infra-orbital artery

superior labial artery

inferior labial artery

inferior alveolar artery
(mental branch)

facial artery

submental artery

lingual artery

superior laryngeal artery

superior thyroid artery

inferior thyroid artery

right common carotid artery

brachiocephalic arterial trunk

ARTERIAL SYSTEM (VI). NECK and HEAD (IV)

LEFT SUPERFICIAL LATERAL VIEW

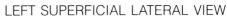

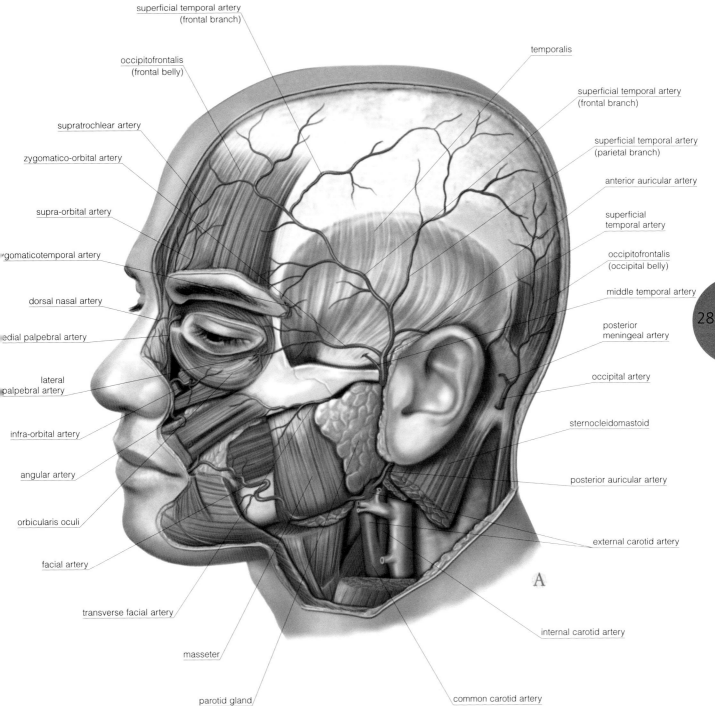

superficial temporal artery
(frontal branch)

occipitofrontalis
(frontal belly)

supratrochlear artery

zygomatico-orbital artery

supra-orbital artery

zygomaticotemporal artery

dorsal nasal artery

medial palpebral artery

lateral
palpebral artery

infra-orbital artery

angular artery

orbicularis oculi

facial artery

transverse facial artery

masseter

parotid gland

temporalis

superficial temporal artery
(frontal branch)

superficial temporal artery
(parietal branch)

anterior auricular artery

superficial
temporal artery

occipitofrontalis
(occipital belly)

middle temporal artery

posterior
meningeal artery

occipital artery

sternocleidomastoid

posterior auricular artery

external carotid artery

internal carotid artery

common carotid artery

A

287

ARTERIAL SYSTEM (VII). NECK and HEAD (V)
LEFT LATERAL DEEP VIEW

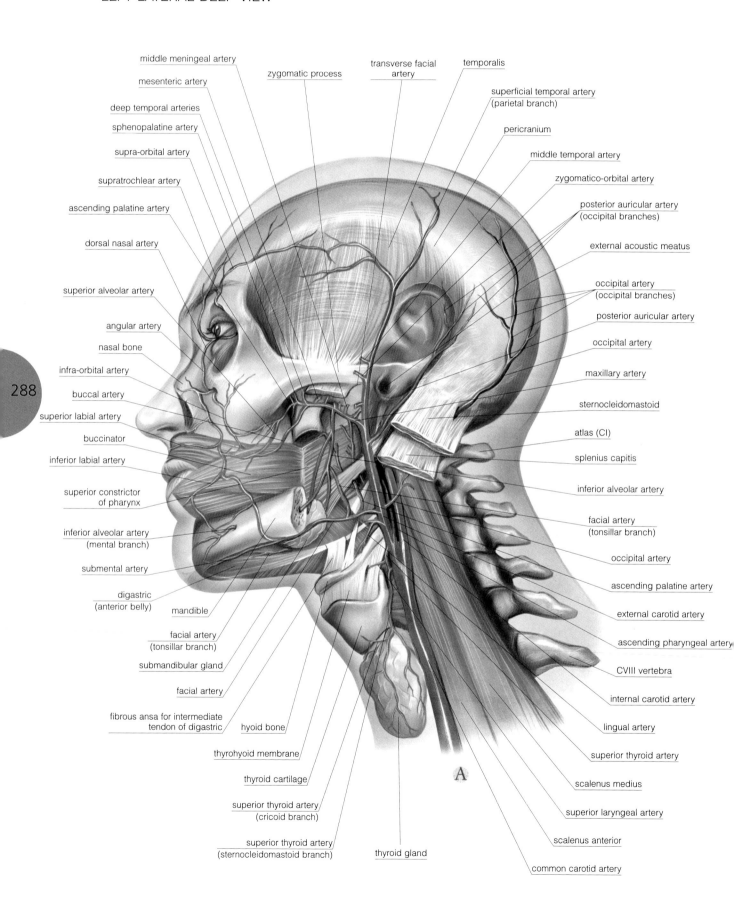

middle meningeal artery

mesenteric artery

deep temporal arteries

sphenopalatine artery

supra-orbital artery

supratrochlear artery

ascending palatine artery

dorsal nasal artery

superior alveolar artery

angular artery

nasal bone

infra-orbital artery

buccal artery

superior labial artery

buccinator

inferior labial artery

superior constrictor of pharynx

inferior alveolar artery (mental branch)

submental artery

digastric (anterior belly)

mandible

facial artery (tonsillar branch)

submandibular gland

facial artery

fibrous ansa for intermediate tendon of digastric

hyoid bone

thyrohyoid membrane

thyroid cartilage

superior thyroid artery (cricoid branch)

superior thyroid artery (sternocleidomastoid branch)

thyroid gland

zygomatic process

transverse facial artery

temporalis

superficial temporal artery (parietal branch)

pericranium

middle temporal artery

zygomatico-orbital artery

posterior auricular artery (occipital branches)

external acoustic meatus

occipital artery (occipital branches)

posterior auricular artery

occipital artery

maxillary artery

sternocleidomastoid

atlas (CI)

splenius capitis

inferior alveolar artery

facial artery (tonsillar branch)

occipital artery

ascending palatine artery

external carotid artery

ascending pharyngeal artery

CVIII vertebra

internal carotid artery

lingual artery

superior thyroid artery

scalenus medius

superior laryngeal artery

scalenus anterior

common carotid artery

288

A

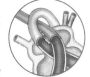

ARTERIAL SYSTEM (VIII). NECK and HEAD (VI)
LEFT DEEP LATERAL VIEW

irrigation of the pharyngeal region

This region is irrigated by the ascendant pharyngeal branch of the external carotid, the ascendant pala-tine, the tonsilar branch of the facial artery, the descendant palatine and pharyngeal branches of the internal maxillary artery. The terminal branches of the external carotid artery irrigate the structures of the face and associated fossas. The superficial temporal artery has a longitudinal course towards the tempo-ral fossa, being easily palpable superficially. The maxillary artery introduces itself in the zygomatic foss and in its short journey emits several branches for the orbital fosses, nasals, oral cavity and meninges.

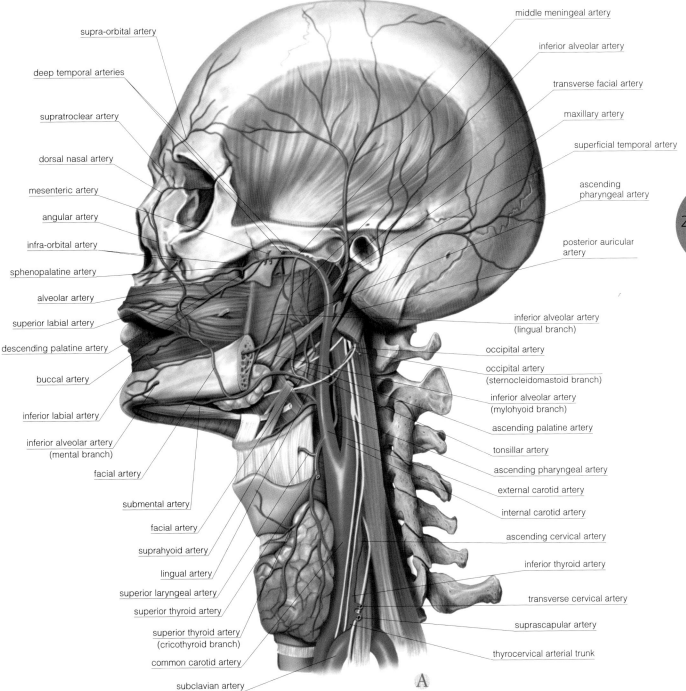

289

- supra-orbital artery
- deep temporal arteries
- supratroclear artery
- dorsal nasal artery
- mesenteric artery
- angular artery
- infra-orbital artery
- sphenopalatine artery
- alveolar artery
- superior labial artery
- descending palatine artery
- buccal artery
- inferior labial artery
- inferior alveolar artery (mental branch)
- facial artery
- submental artery
- facial artery
- suprahyoid artery
- lingual artery
- superior laryngeal artery
- superior thyroid artery
- superior thyroid artery (cricothyroid branch)
- common carotid artery
- subclavian artery

- middle meningeal artery
- inferior alveolar artery
- transverse facial artery
- maxillary artery
- superficial temporal artery
- ascending pharyngeal artery
- posterior auricular artery
- inferior alveolar artery (lingual branch)
- occipital artery
- occipital artery (sternocleidomastoid branch)
- inferior alveolar artery (mylohyoid branch)
- ascending palatine artery
- tonsillar artery
- ascending pharyngeal artery
- external carotid artery
- internal carotid artery
- ascending cervical artery
- inferior thyroid artery
- transverse cervical artery
- suprascapular artery
- thyrocervical arterial trunk

A

ARTERIAL SYSTEM (IX). BRAIN (I)
INFERIOR VIEW

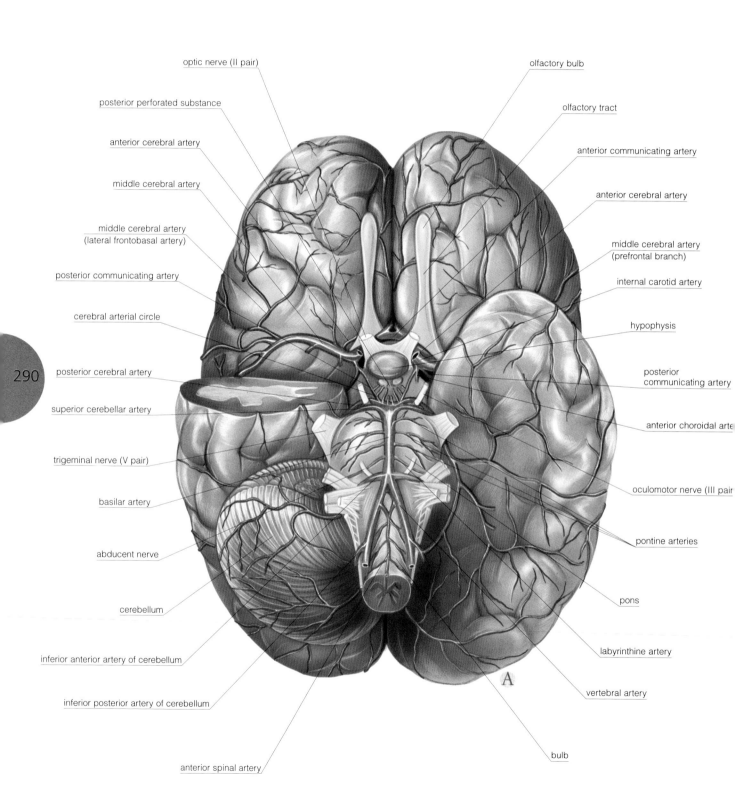

optic nerve (II pair)

posterior perforated substance

anterior cerebral artery

middle cerebral artery

middle cerebral artery
(lateral frontobasal artery)

posterior communicating artery

cerebral arterial circle

290

posterior cerebral artery

superior cerebellar artery

trigeminal nerve (V pair)

basilar artery

abducent nerve

cerebellum

inferior anterior artery of cerebellum

inferior posterior artery of cerebellum

anterior spinal artery

olfactory bulb

olfactory tract

anterior communicating artery

anterior cerebral artery

middle cerebral artery
(prefrontal branch)

internal carotid artery

hypophysis

posterior
communicating artery

anterior choroidal arte

oculomotor nerve (III pair

pontine arteries

pons

labyrinthine artery

vertebral artery

bulb

A

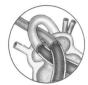

ARTERIAL SYSTEM (X). BRAIN (II)

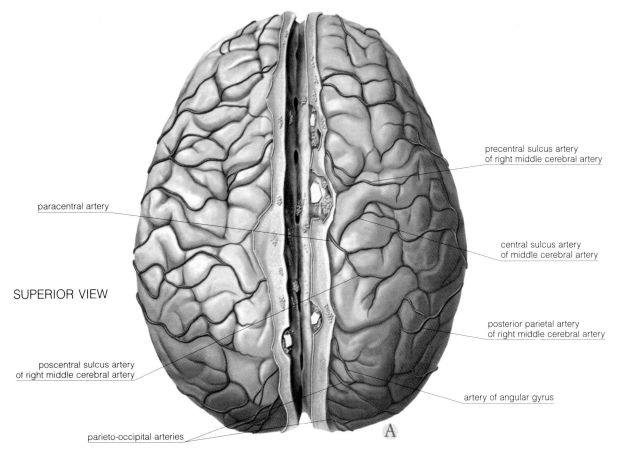

precentral sulcus artery
of right middle cerebral artery

paracentral artery

central sulcus artery
of middle cerebral artery

SUPERIOR VIEW

posterior parietal artery
of right middle cerebral artery

poscentral sulcus artery
of right middle cerebral artery

artery of angular gyrus

parieto-occipital arteries

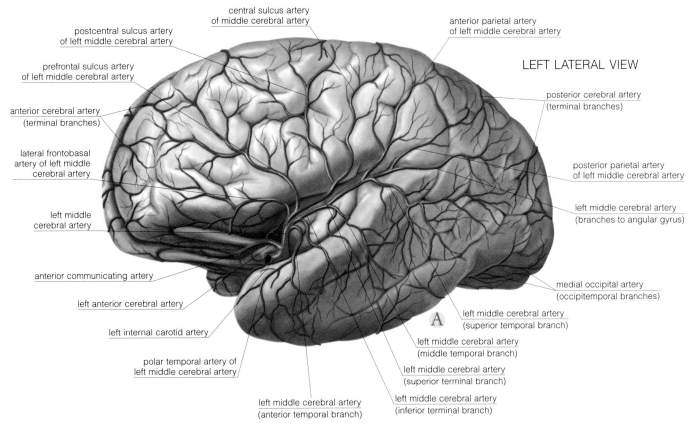

central sulcus artery
of middle cerebral artery

postcentral sulcus artery
of left middle cerebral artery

anterior parietal artery
of left middle cerebral artery

prefrontal sulcus artery
of left middle cerebral artery

LEFT LATERAL VIEW

posterior cerebral artery
(terminal branches)

anterior cerebral artery
(terminal branches)

lateral frontobasal
artery of left middle
cerebral artery

posterior parietal artery
of left middle cerebral artery

left middle
cerebral artery

left middle cerebral artery
(branches to angular gyrus)

anterior communicating artery

medial occipital artery
(occipitemporal branches)

left anterior cerebral artery

left middle cerebral artery
(superior temporal branch)

left internal carotid artery

left middle cerebral artery
(middle temporal branch)

polar temporal artery of
left middle cerebral artery

left middle cerebral artery
(superior terminal branch)

left middle cerebral artery
(anterior temporal branch)

left middle cerebral artery
(inferior terminal branch)

ARTERIAL SYSTEM (XI). BRAIN (III)

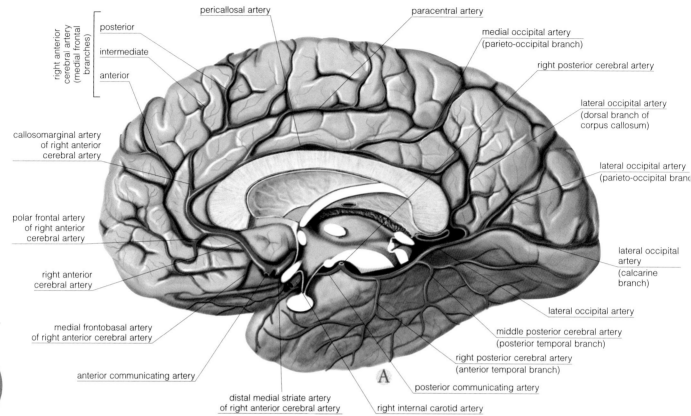

right anterior cerebral artery (medial frontal branches)
- posterior
- intermediate
- anterior

pericallosal artery

paracentral artery

medial occipital artery (parieto-occipital branch)

right posterior cerebral artery

lateral occipital artery (dorsal branch of corpus callosum)

lateral occipital artery (parieto-occipital branch)

callosomarginal artery of right anterior cerebral artery

lateral occipital artery (calcarine branch)

polar frontal artery of right anterior cerebral artery

right anterior cerebral artery

lateral occipital artery

middle posterior cerebral artery (posterior temporal branch)

right posterior cerebral artery (anterior temporal branch)

medial frontobasal artery of right anterior cerebral artery

posterior communicating artery

anterior communicating artery

distal medial striate artery of right anterior cerebral artery

right internal carotid artery

MEDIAL VIEW

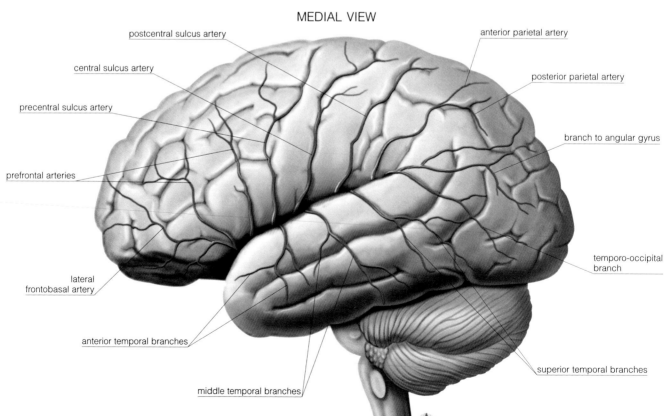

postcentral sulcus artery

anterior parietal artery

central sulcus artery

posterior parietal artery

precentral sulcus artery

branch to angular gyrus

prefrontal arteries

temporo-occipital branch

lateral frontobasal artery

anterior temporal branches

superior temporal branches

middle temporal branches

RIGHT MIDDLE CEREBRAL ARTERY

ARTERIAL SYSTEM (XII). BRAIN (IV)
SAGITTAL and MEDIAL SECTIONS

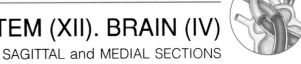

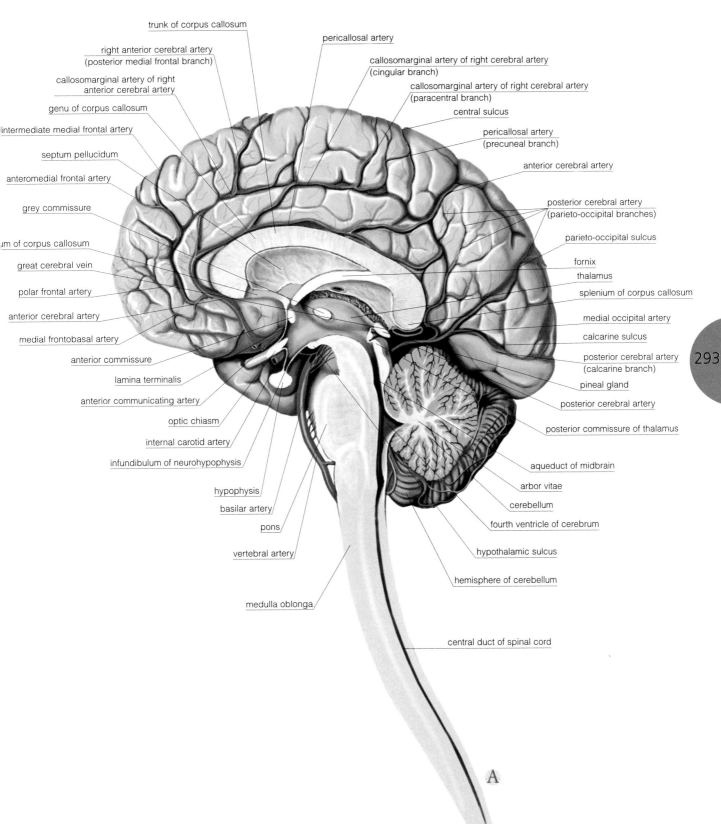

trunk of corpus callosum

pericallosal artery

right anterior cerebral artery
(posterior medial frontal branch)

callosomarginal artery of right cerebral artery
(cingular branch)

callosomarginal artery of right
anterior cerebral artery

callosomarginal artery of right cerebral artery
(paracentral branch)

genu of corpus callosum

central sulcus

intermediate medial frontal artery

pericallosal artery
(precuneal branch)

septum pellucidum

anteromedial frontal artery

anterior cerebral artery

grey commissure

posterior cerebral artery
(parieto-occipital branches)

um of corpus callosum

parieto-occipital sulcus

great cerebral vein

fornix

thalamus

polar frontal artery

splenium of corpus callosum

anterior cerebral artery

medial occipital artery

medial frontobasal artery

calcarine sulcus

anterior commissure

posterior cerebral artery
(calcarine branch)

lamina terminalis

pineal gland

anterior communicating artery

posterior cerebral artery

optic chiasm

posterior commissure of thalamus

internal carotid artery

aqueduct of midbrain

infundibulum of neurohypophysis

arbor vitae

hypophysis

cerebellum

basilar artery

fourth ventricle of cerebrum

pons

hypothalamic sulcus

vertebral artery

hemisphere of cerebellum

medulla oblonga

central duct of spinal cord

293

A

294

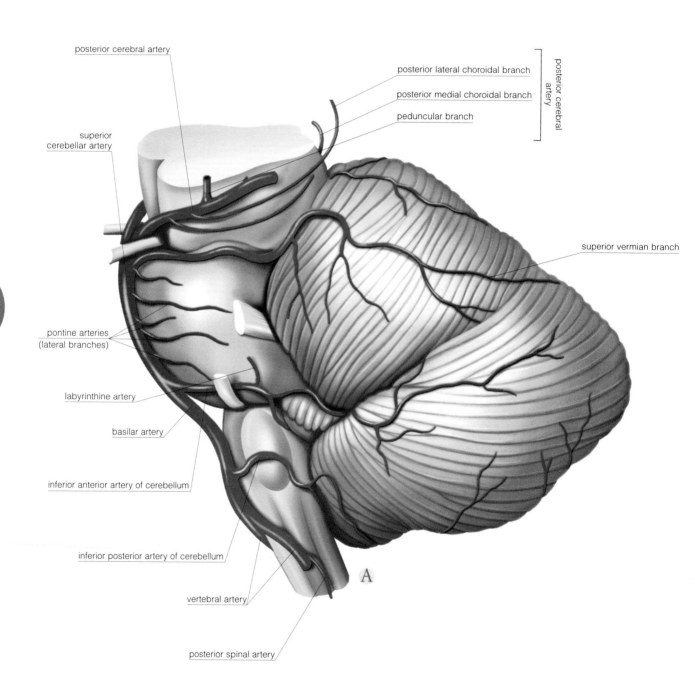

posterior cerebral artery

posterior lateral choroidal branch

posterior medial choroidal branch

peduncular branch

posterior cerebral artery

superior cerebellar artery

superior vermian branch

pontine arteries (lateral branches)

labyrinthine artery

basilar artery

inferior anterior artery of cerebellum

inferior posterior artery of cerebellum

vertebral artery

posterior spinal artery

A

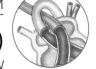

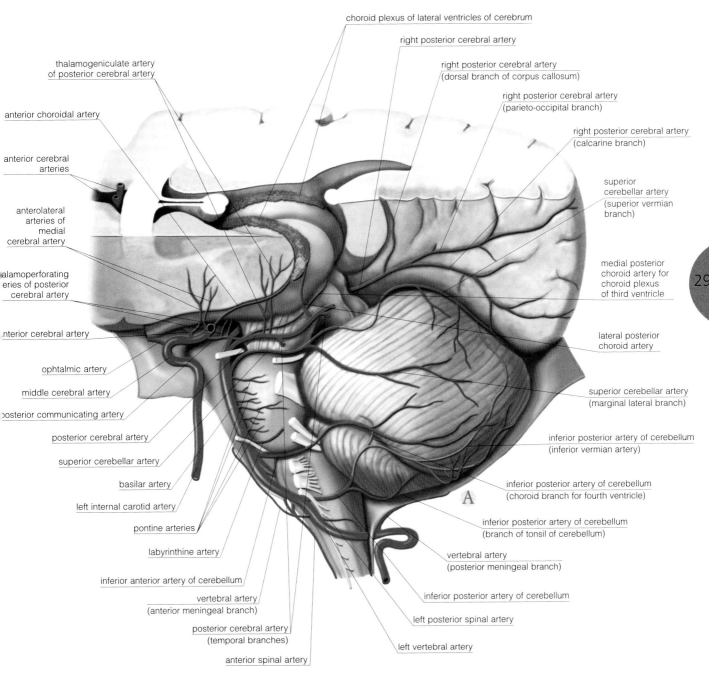

choroid plexus of lateral ventricles of cerebrum

right posterior cerebral artery

right posterior cerebral artery
(dorsal branch of corpus callosum)

right posterior cerebral artery
(parieto-occipital branch)

right posterior cerebral artery
(calcarine branch)

superior
cerebellar artery
(superior vermian
branch)

medial posterior
choroid artery for
choroid plexus
of third ventricle

lateral posterior
choroid artery

superior cerebellar artery
(marginal lateral branch)

inferior posterior artery of cerebellum
(inferior vermian artery)

inferior posterior artery of cerebellum
(choroid branch for fourth ventricle)

inferior posterior artery of cerebellum
(branch of tonsil of cerebellum)

vertebral artery
(posterior meningeal branch)

inferior posterior artery of cerebellum

left posterior spinal artery

left vertebral artery

thalamogeniculate artery
of posterior cerebral artery

anterior choroidal artery

anterior cerebral
arteries

anterolateral
arteries of
medial
cerebral artery

alamoperforating
eries of posterior
cerebral artery

nterior cerebral artery

ophtalmic artery

middle cerebral artery

osterior communicating artery

posterior cerebral artery

superior cerebellar artery

basilar artery

left internal carotid artery

pontine arteries

labyrinthine artery

inferior anterior artery of cerebellum

vertebral artery
(anterior meningeal branch)

posterior cerebral artery
(temporal branches)

anterior spinal artery

A

295

ARTERIAL SYSTEM (XV). BRAIN (VII). BASE

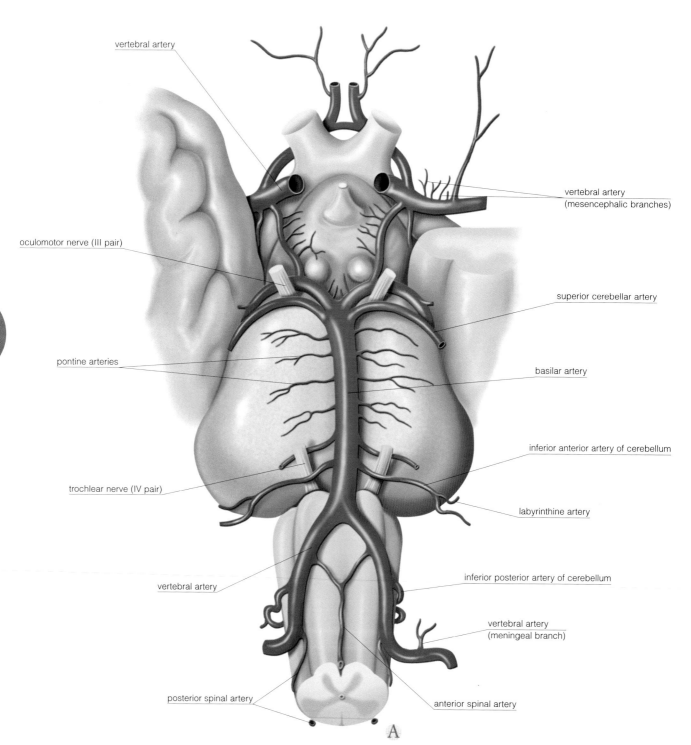

vertebral artery

vertebral artery
(mesencephalic branches)

oculomotor nerve (III pair)

superior cerebellar artery

pontine arteries

basilar artery

inferior anterior artery of cerebellum

trochlear nerve (IV pair)

labyrinthine artery

inferior posterior artery of cerebellum

vertebral artery

vertebral artery
(meningeal branch)

posterior spinal artery

anterior spinal artery

A

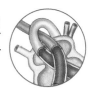

ARTERIAL SYSTEM (XVI). VERTEBRAL ARTERY

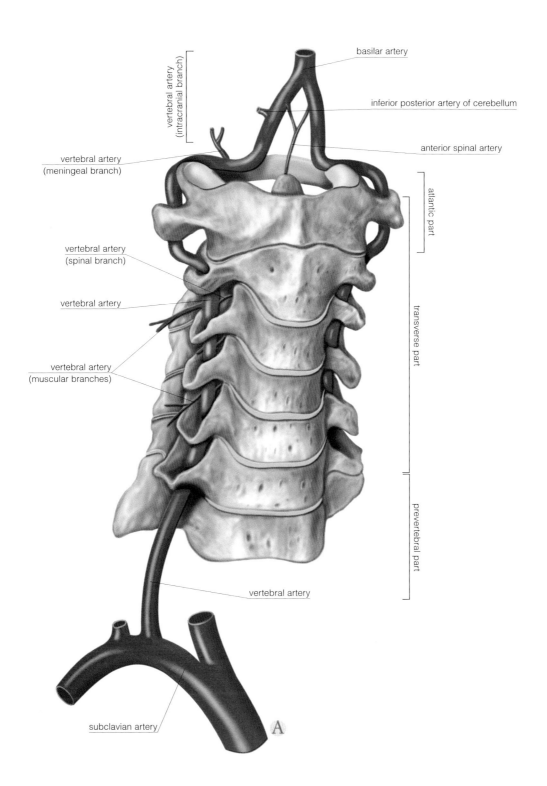

vertebral artery
(intracranial branch)

basilar artery

inferior posterior artery of cerebellum

vertebral artery
(meningeal branch)

anterior spinal artery

atlantic part

vertebral artery
(spinal branch)

vertebral artery

transverse part

vertebral artery
(muscular branches)

prevertebral part

vertebral artery

subclavian artery

A

297

ARTERIAL SYSTEM (XVII). TONGUE

INFERIOR ANTERIOR VIEW

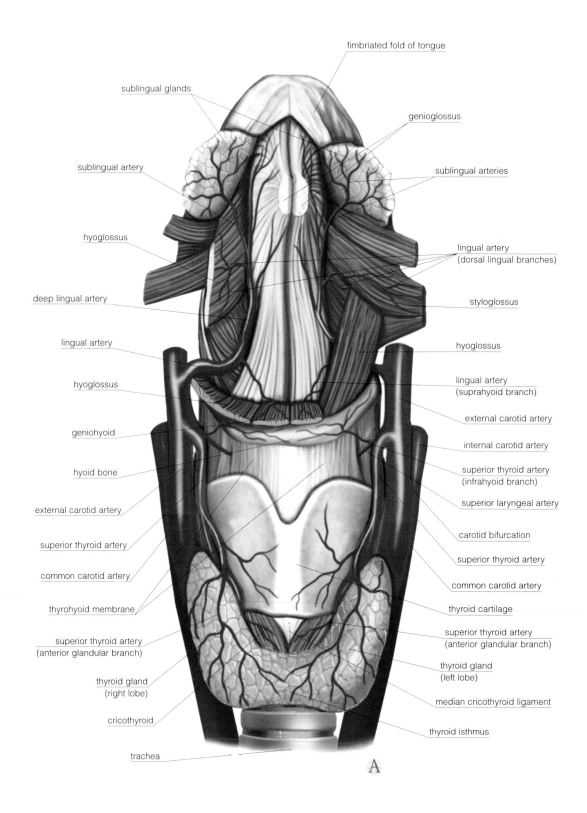

fimbriated fold of tongue

sublingual glands

genioglossus

sublingual artery

sublingual arteries

hyoglossus

lingual artery
(dorsal lingual branches)

deep lingual artery

styloglossus

lingual artery

hyoglossus

hyoglossus

lingual artery
(suprahyoid branch)

geniohyoid

external carotid artery

internal carotid artery

hyoid bone

superior thyroid artery
(infrahyoid branch)

external carotid artery

superior laryngeal artery

superior thyroid artery

carotid bifurcation

common carotid artery

superior thyroid artery

thyrohyoid membrane

common carotid artery

thyroid cartilage

superior thyroid artery
(anterior glandular branch)

superior thyroid artery
(anterior glandular branch)

thyroid gland
(right lobe)

thyroid gland
(left lobe)

median cricothyroid ligament

cricothyroid

thyroid isthmus

trachea

A

298

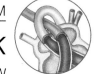

ARTERIAL SYSTEM (XVIII). NECK
EXTERNAL CAROTID and SUBCLAVIAN ARTERIES. POSTERIOR VIEW

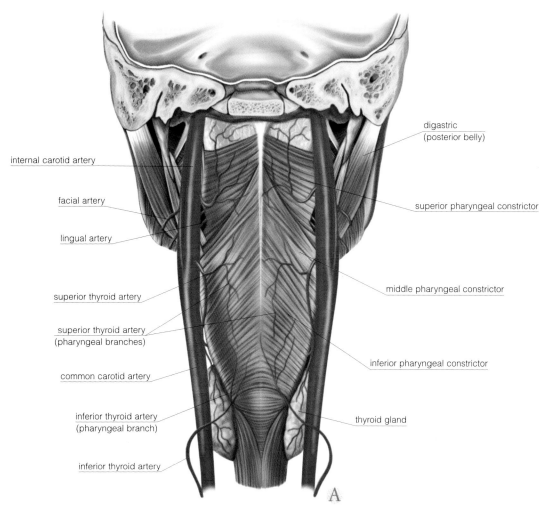

internal carotid artery

facial artery

lingual artery

superior thyroid artery

superior thyroid artery
(pharyngeal branches)

common carotid artery

inferior thyroid artery
(pharyngeal branch)

inferior thyroid artery

digastric
(posterior belly)

superior pharyngeal constrictor

middle pharyngeal constrictor

inferior pharyngeal constrictor

thyroid gland

A

299

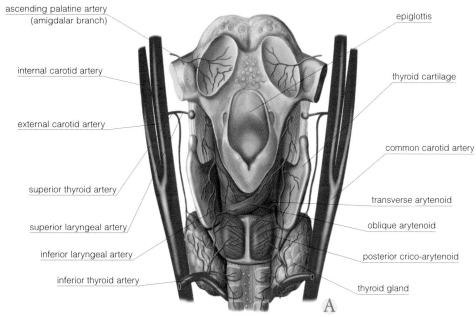

ascending palatine artery
(amigdalar branch)

internal carotid artery

external carotid artery

superior thyroid artery

superior laryngeal artery

inferior laryngeal artery

inferior thyroid artery

epiglottis

thyroid cartilage

common carotid artery

transverse arytenoid

oblique arytenoid

posterior crico-arytenoid

thyroid gland

A

ARTERIAL SYSTEM (XIX). THORACIC WALL

ANTERIOR VIEW

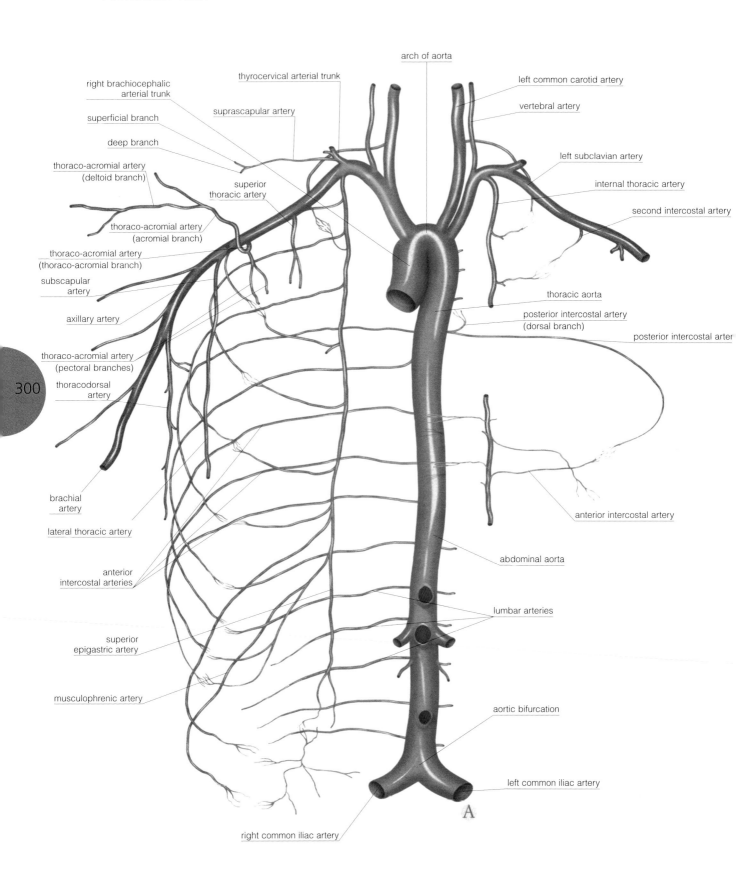

arch of aorta

thyrocervical arterial trunk

left common carotid artery

right brachiocephalic arterial trunk

vertebral artery

superficial branch

suprascapular artery

deep branch

left subclavian artery

thoraco-acromial artery (deltoid branch)

superior thoracic artery

internal thoracic artery

thoraco-acromial artery (acromial branch)

second intercostal artery

thoraco-acromial artery (thoraco-acromial branch)

subscapular artery

thoracic aorta

axillary artery

posterior intercostal artery (dorsal branch)

posterior intercostal arter

thoraco-acromial artery (pectoral branches)

thoracodorsal artery

brachial artery

lateral thoracic artery

anterior intercostal arteries

anterior intercostal artery

superior epigastric artery

abdominal aorta

lumbar arteries

musculophrenic artery

aortic bifurcation

left common iliac artery

A

right common iliac artery

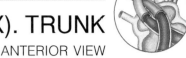

ARTERIAL SYSTEM (XX). TRUNK
ANTERIOR VIEW

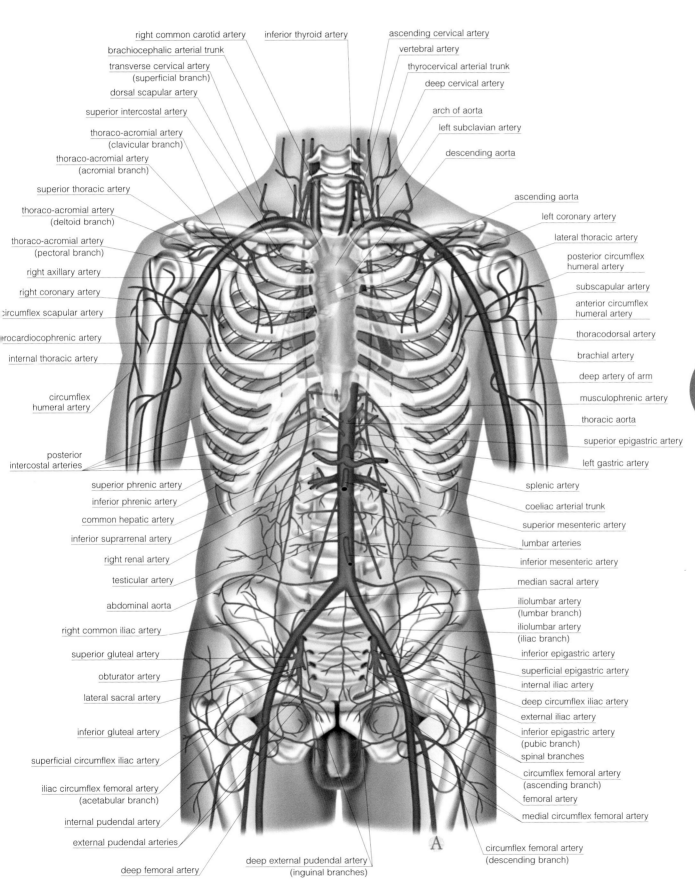

right common carotid artery

brachiocephalic arterial trunk

transverse cervical artery
(superficial branch)

dorsal scapular artery

superior intercostal artery

thoraco-acromial artery
(clavicular branch)

thoraco-acromial artery
(acromial branch)

superior thoracic artery

thoraco-acromial artery
(deltoid branch)

thoraco-acromial artery
(pectoral branch)

right axillary artery

right coronary artery

circumflex scapular artery

pericardiocophrenic artery

internal thoracic artery

circumflex
humeral artery

posterior
intercostal arteries

superior phrenic artery

inferior phrenic artery

common hepatic artery

inferior suprarrenal artery

right renal artery

testicular artery

abdominal aorta

right common iliac artery

superior gluteal artery

obturator artery

lateral sacral artery

inferior gluteal artery

superficial circumflex iliac artery

iliac circumflex femoral artery
(acetabular branch)

internal pudendal artery

external pudendal arteries

deep femoral artery

inferior thyroid artery

deep external pudendal artery
(inguinal branches)

A

ascending cervical artery

vertebral artery

thyrocervical arterial trunk

deep cervical artery

arch of aorta

left subclavian artery

descending aorta

ascending aorta

left coronary artery

lateral thoracic artery

posterior circumflex
humeral artery

subscapular artery

anterior circumflex
humeral artery

thoracodorsal artery

brachial artery

deep artery of arm

musculophrenic artery

thoracic aorta

superior epigastric artery

left gastric artery

splenic artery

coeliac arterial trunk

superior mesenteric artery

lumbar arteries

inferior mesenteric artery

median sacral artery

iliolumbar artery
(lumbar branch)

iliolumbar artery
(iliac branch)

inferior epigastric artery

superficial epigastric artery

internal iliac artery

deep circumflex iliac artery

external iliac artery

inferior epigastric artery
(pubic branch)

spinal branches

circumflex femoral artery
(ascending branch)

femoral artery

medial circumflex femoral artery

circumflex femoral artery
(descending branch)

301

ARTERIAL SYSTEM (XXI). PULMONARY ARTERIES

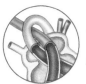

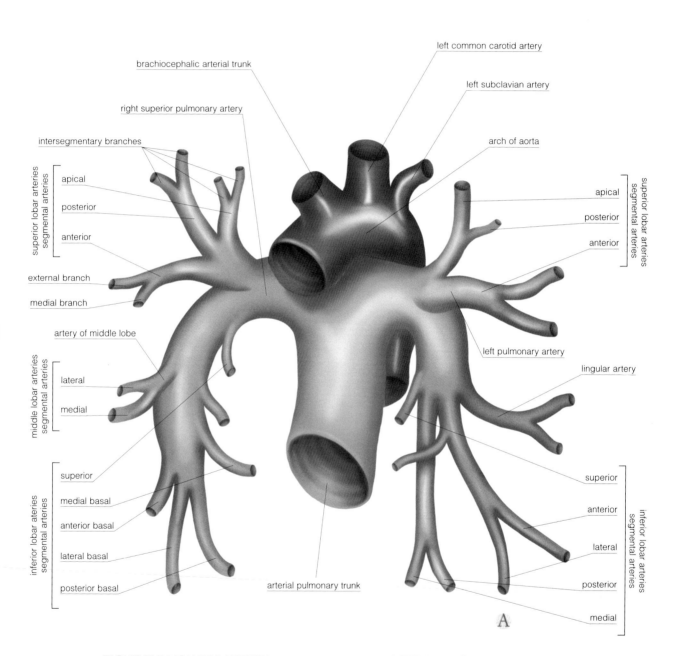

brachiocephalic arterial trunk

left common carotid artery

right superior pulmonary artery

left subclavian artery

intersegmentary branches

arch of aorta

superior lobar arteries segmental arteries

apical

posterior

anterior

external branch

medial branch

superior lobar arteries segmental arteries

apical

posterior

anterior

artery of middle lobe

left pulmonary artery

middle lobar arteries segmental arteries

lateral

medial

lingular artery

inferior lobar arteries segmental arteries

superior

medial basal

anterior basal

lateral basal

posterior basal

inferior lobar arteries segmental arteries

superior

anterior

lateral

posterior

medial

arterial pulmonary trunk

A

RIGHT PULMONARY ARTERY

LEFT PULMONARY ARTERY

302

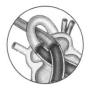

ARTERIAL SYSTEM (XXII). COELIAC TRUNK

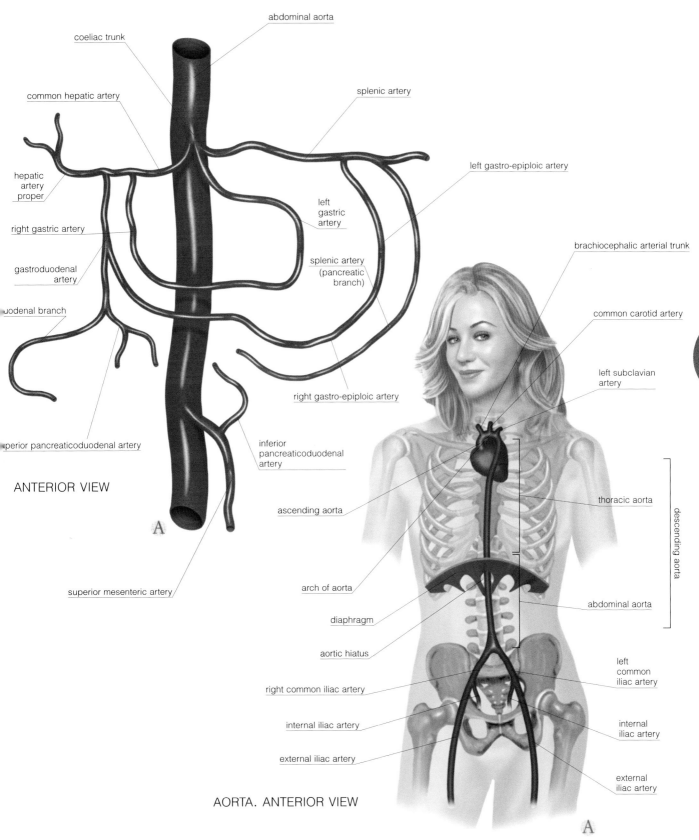

abdominal aorta

coeliac trunk

splenic artery

common hepatic artery

left gastro-epiploic artery

hepatic
artery
proper

left
gastric
artery

right gastric artery

brachiocephalic arterial trunk

gastroduodenal
artery

splenic artery
(pancreatic
branch)

common carotid artery

uodenal branch

left subclavian
artery

303

perior pancreaticoduodenal artery

right gastro-epiploic artery

ANTERIOR VIEW

inferior
pancreaticoduodenal
artery

thoracic aorta

A

descending aorta

ascending aorta

superior mesenteric artery

arch of aorta

abdominal aorta

diaphragm

aortic hiatus

left
common
iliac artery

right common iliac artery

internal iliac artery

internal
iliac artery

external iliac artery

external
iliac artery

AORTA. ANTERIOR VIEW

A

ARTERIAL SYSTEM (XXIII). OESOPHAGUS

ANTERIOR VIEW

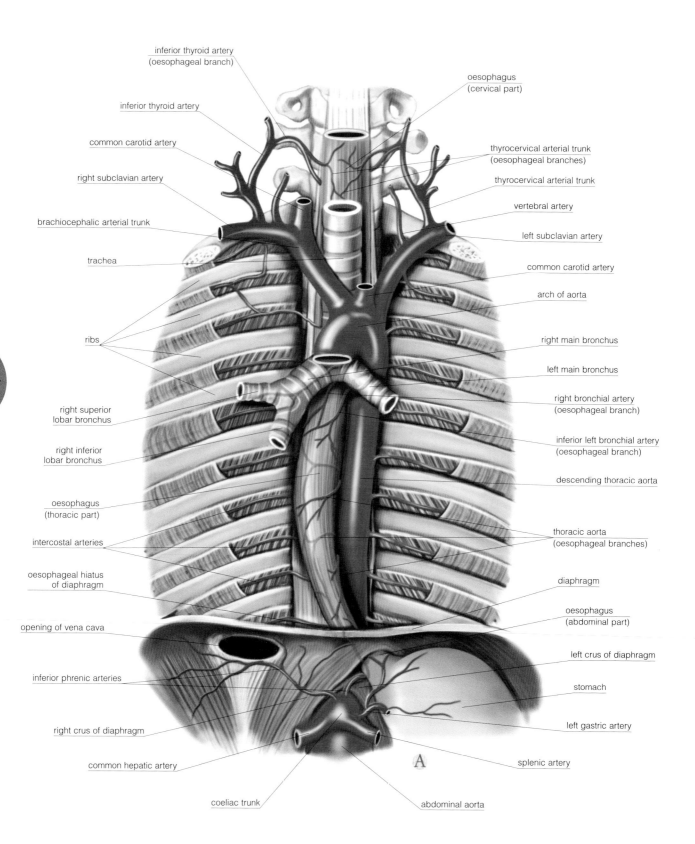

inferior thyroid artery
(oesophageal branch)

inferior thyroid artery

common carotid artery

right subclavian artery

brachiocephalic arterial trunk

trachea

ribs

right superior
lobar bronchus

right inferior
lobar bronchus

oesophagus
(thoracic part)

intercostal arteries

oesophageal hiatus
of diaphragm

opening of vena cava

inferior phrenic arteries

right crus of diaphragm

common hepatic artery

coeliac trunk

oesophagus
(cervical part)

thyrocervical arterial trunk
(oesophageal branches)

thyrocervical arterial trunk

vertebral artery

left subclavian artery

common carotid artery

arch of aorta

right main bronchus

left main bronchus

right bronchial artery
(oesophageal branch)

inferior left bronchial artery
(oesophageal branch)

descending thoracic aorta

thoracic aorta
(oesophageal branches)

diaphragm

oesophagus
(abdominal part)

left crus of diaphragm

stomach

left gastric artery

splenic artery

abdominal aorta

A

304

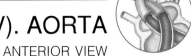

ARTERIAL SYSTEM (XXIV). AORTA
ANTERIOR VIEW

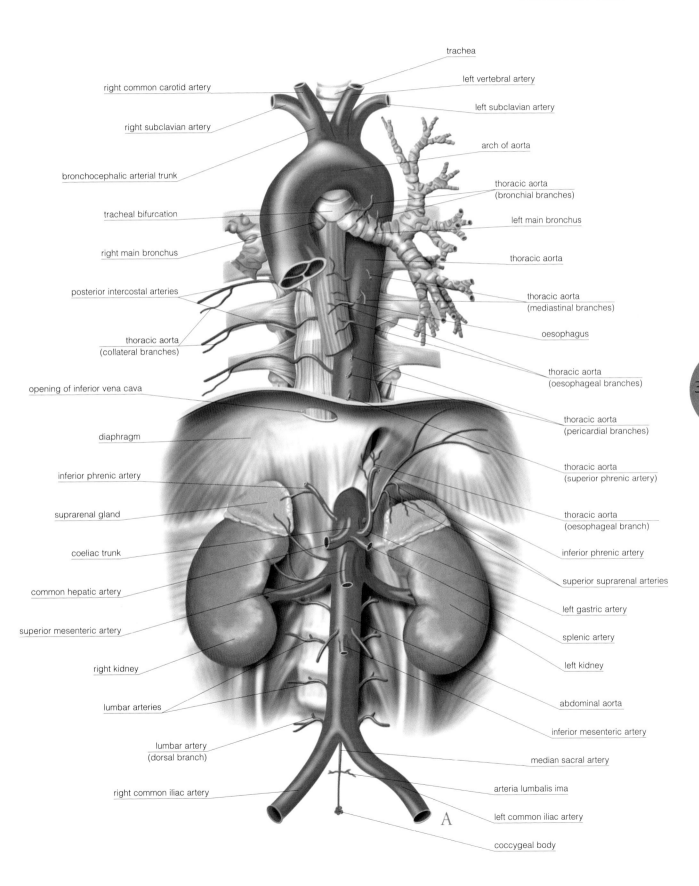

trachea

right common carotid artery

left vertebral artery

right subclavian artery

left subclavian artery

arch of aorta

bronchocephalic arterial trunk

thoracic aorta
(bronchial branches)

tracheal bifurcation

left main bronchus

right main bronchus

thoracic aorta

posterior intercostal arteries

thoracic aorta
(mediastinal branches)

thoracic aorta
(collateral branches)

oesophagus

opening of inferior vena cava

thoracic aorta
(oesophageal branches)

diaphragm

thoracic aorta
(pericardial branches)

inferior phrenic artery

thoracic aorta
(superior phrenic artery)

suprarenal gland

thoracic aorta
(oesophageal branch)

coeliac trunk

inferior phrenic artery

common hepatic artery

superior suprarenal arteries

superior mesenteric artery

left gastric artery

right kidney

splenic artery

lumbar arteries

left kidney

lumbar artery
(dorsal branch)

abdominal aorta

right common iliac artery

inferior mesenteric artery

median sacral artery

arteria lumbalis ima

left common iliac artery

coccygeal body

A

305

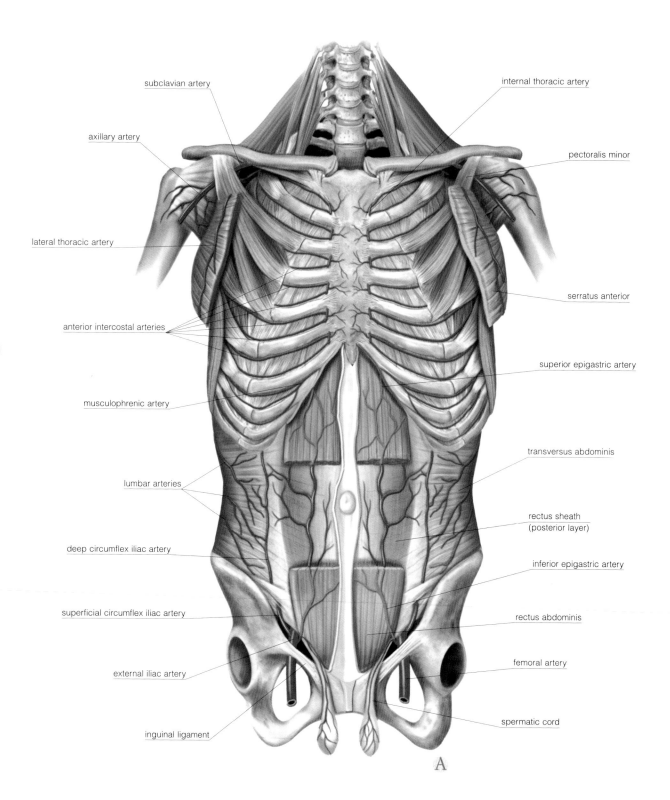

subclavian artery

internal thoracic artery

axillary artery

pectoralis minor

lateral thoracic artery

serratus anterior

anterior intercostal arteries

superior epigastric artery

musculophrenic artery

transversus abdominis

lumbar arteries

rectus sheath
(posterior layer)

deep circumflex iliac artery

inferior epigastric artery

superficial circumflex iliac artery

rectus abdominis

external iliac artery

femoral artery

spermatic cord

inguinal ligament

A

ARTERIAL SYSTEM (XXVI). ABDOMINAL WALL
POSTERIOR VIEW

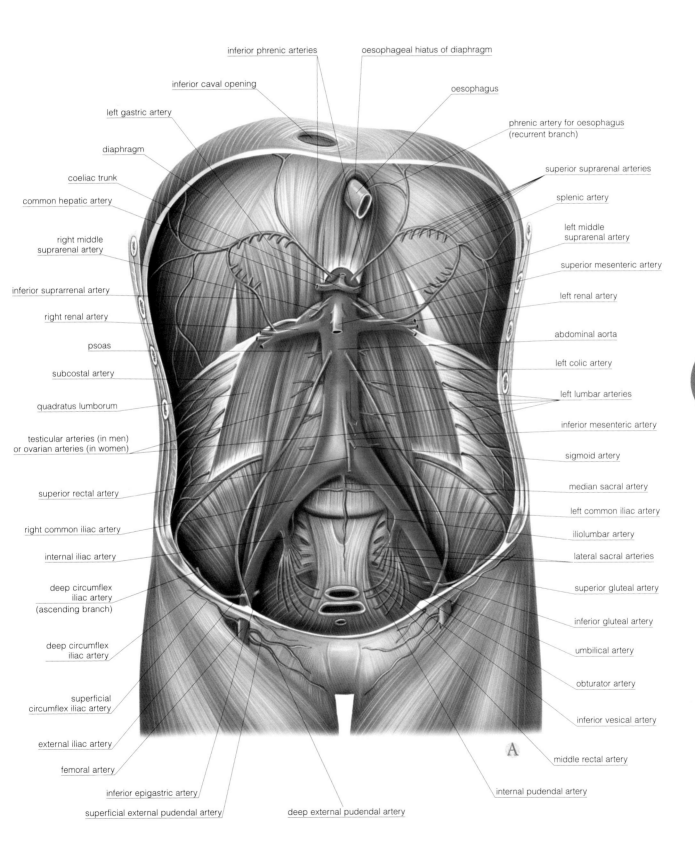

inferior phrenic arteries

oesophageal hiatus of diaphragm

inferior caval opening

oesophagus

left gastric artery

phrenic artery for oesophagus
(recurrent branch)

diaphragm

superior suprarenal arteries

coeliac trunk

splenic artery

common hepatic artery

left middle
suprarenal artery

right middle
suprarenal artery

superior mesenteric artery

inferior suprarrenal artery

left renal artery

right renal artery

abdominal aorta

psoas

left colic artery

subcostal artery

left lumbar arteries

quadratus lumborum

inferior mesenteric artery

testicular arteries (in men)
or ovarian arteries (in women)

sigmoid artery

superior rectal artery

median sacral artery

left common iliac artery

right common iliac artery

iliolumbar artery

internal iliac artery

lateral sacral arteries

deep circumflex
iliac artery
(ascending branch)

superior gluteal artery

inferior gluteal artery

deep circumflex
iliac artery

umbilical artery

superficial
circumflex iliac artery

obturator artery

inferior vesical artery

external iliac artery

femoral artery

A

middle rectal artery

inferior epigastric artery

internal pudendal artery

superficial external pudendal artery

deep external pudendal artery

307

ARTERIAL SYSTEM (XXVII). ABDOMEN

ANTERIOR VIEW

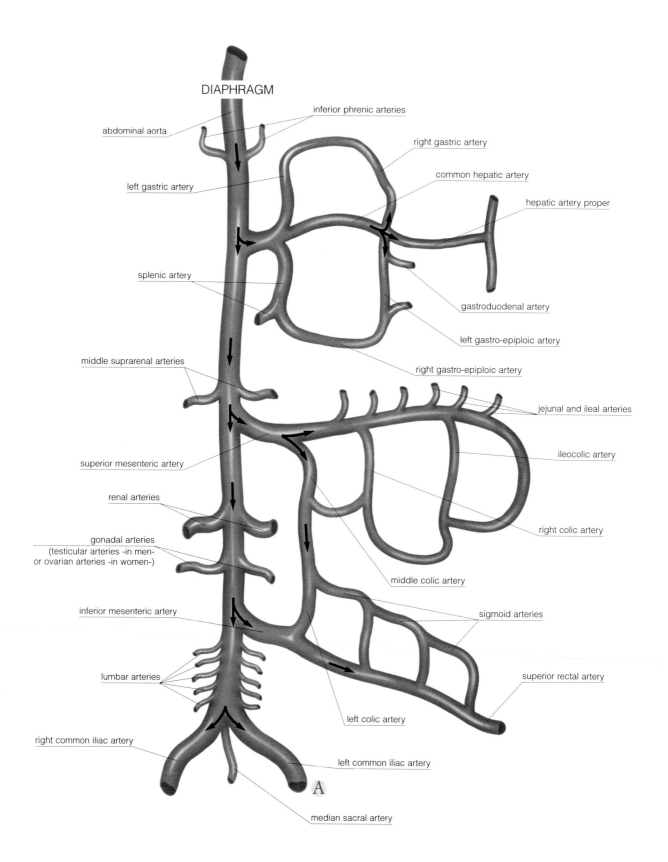

DIAPHRAGM

inferior phrenic arteries

abdominal aorta

right gastric artery

left gastric artery

common hepatic artery

hepatic artery proper

splenic artery

gastroduodenal artery

left gastro-epiploic artery

middle suprarenal arteries

right gastro-epiploic artery

jejunal and ileal arteries

ileocolic artery

superior mesenteric artery

renal arteries

right colic artery

gonadal arteries
(testicular arteries -in men-
or ovarian arteries -in women-)

middle colic artery

inferior mesenteric artery

sigmoid arteries

lumbar arteries

superior rectal artery

left colic artery

right common iliac artery

left common iliac artery

A

median sacral artery

308

ARTERIAL SYSTEM (XXVIII). STOMACH
ANTERIOR VIEW

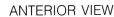

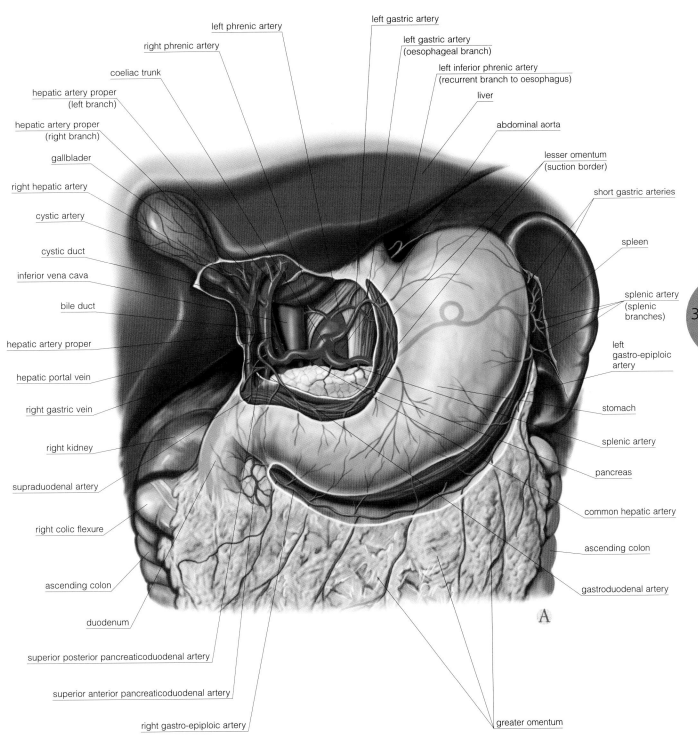

left phrenic artery

left gastric artery

right phrenic artery

left gastric artery
(oesophageal branch)

coeliac trunk

left inferior phrenic artery
(recurrent branch to oesophagus)

hepatic artery proper
(left branch)

liver

hepatic artery proper
(right branch)

abdominal aorta

gallblader

lesser omentum
(suction border)

right hepatic artery

short gastric arteries

cystic artery

spleen

cystic duct

inferior vena cava

splenic artery
(splenic
branches)

bile duct

309

hepatic artery proper

left
gastro-epiploic
artery

hepatic portal vein

right gastric vein

stomach

right kidney

splenic artery

supraduodenal artery

pancreas

right colic flexure

common hepatic artery

ascending colon

ascending colon

gastroduodenal artery

duodenum

superior posterior pancreaticoduodenal artery

A

superior anterior pancreaticoduodenal artery

right gastro-epiploic artery

greater omentum

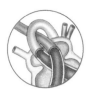

ARTERIAL SYSTEM (XXIX)
LARGE and SMALL INTESTINES (I)
ANTERIOR VIEW

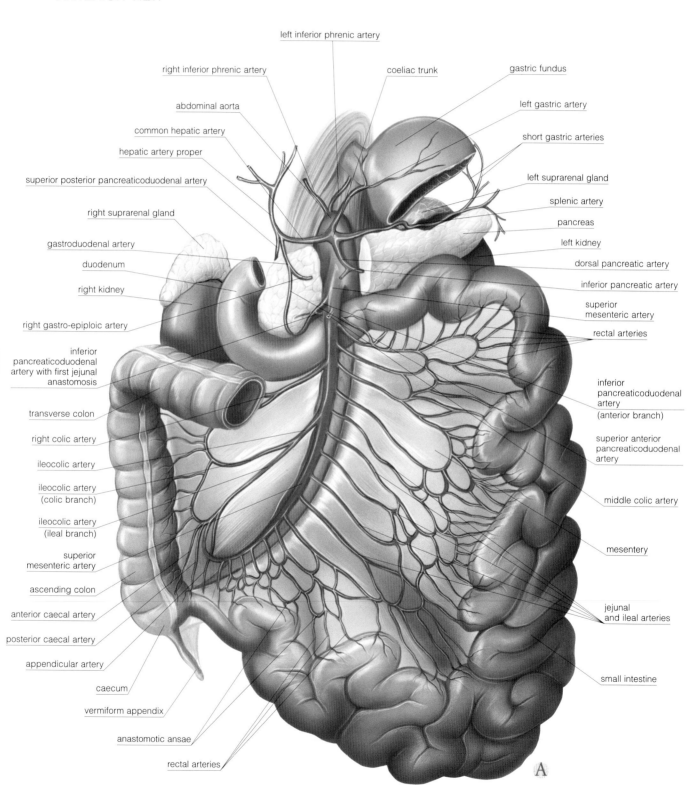

left inferior phrenic artery

right inferior phrenic artery

coeliac trunk

gastric fundus

abdominal aorta

left gastric artery

common hepatic artery

short gastric arteries

hepatic artery proper

superior posterior pancreaticoduodenal artery

left suprarenal gland

right suprarenal gland

splenic artery

pancreas

gastroduodenal artery

left kidney

duodenum

dorsal pancreatic artery

right kidney

inferior pancreatic artery

right gastro-epiploic artery

superior mesenteric artery

rectal arteries

inferior pancreaticoduodenal artery with first jejunal anastomosis

inferior pancreaticoduodenal artery (anterior branch)

transverse colon

superior anterior pancreaticoduodenal artery

right colic artery

ileocolic artery

ileocolic artery (colic branch)

middle colic artery

ileocolic artery (ileal branch)

superior mesenteric artery

mesentery

ascending colon

anterior caecal artery

jejunal and ileal arteries

posterior caecal artery

appendicular artery

caecum

small intestine

vermiform appendix

anastomotic ansae

rectal arteries

310

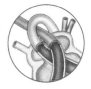

ARTERIAL SYSTEM (XXX)
LARGE and SMALL INTESTINES (II)
ANTERIOR VIEW

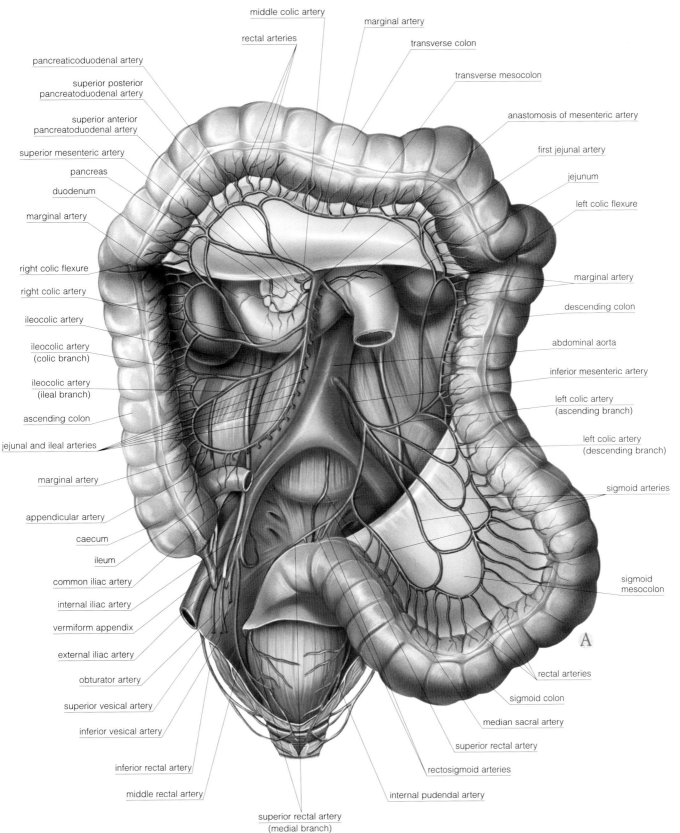

middle colic artery

rectal arteries

marginal artery

transverse colon

transverse mesocolon

pancreaticoduodenal artery

superior posterior pancreatoduodenal artery

anastomosis of mesenteric artery

first jejunal artery

superior anterior pancreatoduodenal artery

jejunum

superior mesenteric artery

pancreas

left colic flexure

duodenum

marginal artery

right colic flexure

marginal artery

right colic artery

descending colon

ileocolic artery

ileocolic artery (colic branch)

abdominal aorta

inferior mesenteric artery

ileocolic artery (ileal branch)

left colic artery (ascending branch)

ascending colon

jejunal and ileal arteries

left colic artery (descending branch)

marginal artery

sigmoid arteries

appendicular artery

caecum

ileum

sigmoid mesocolon

common iliac artery

internal iliac artery

vermiform appendix

external iliac artery

obturator artery

A

superior vesical artery

rectal arteries

inferior vesical artery

sigmoid colon

median sacral artery

inferior rectal artery

superior rectal artery

middle rectal artery

rectosigmoid arteries

internal pudendal artery

superior rectal artery (medial branch)

311

ARTERIAL SYSTEM (XXXI)
GASTRO-INTESTINAL TRACT
ANTERIOR VIEW

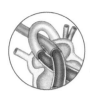

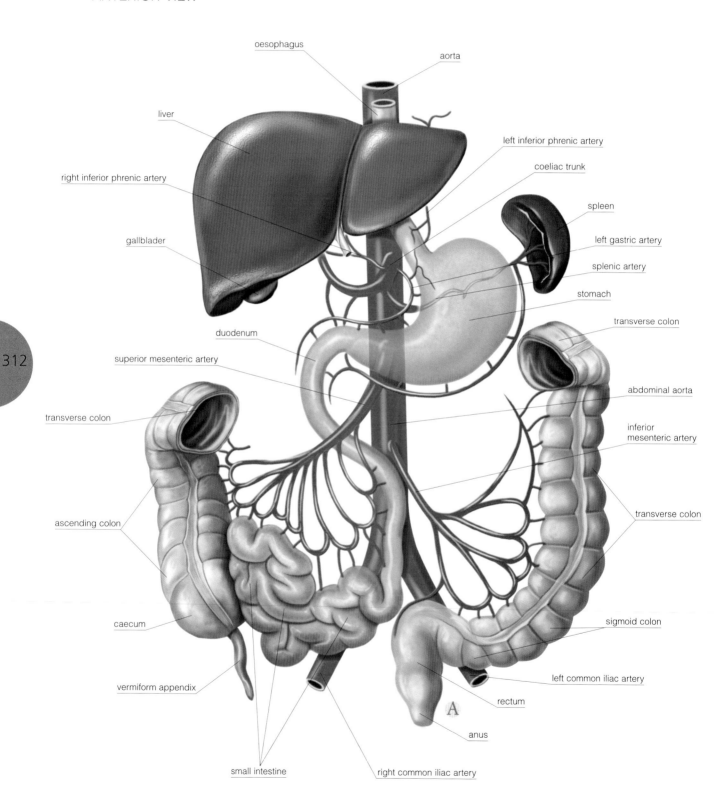

312

oesophagus

aorta

liver

left inferior phrenic artery

coeliac trunk

right inferior phrenic artery

spleen

left gastric artery

gallblader

splenic artery

stomach

transverse colon

duodenum

superior mesenteric artery

abdominal aorta

transverse colon

inferior
mesenteric artery

ascending colon

transverse colon

caecum

sigmoid colon

vermiform appendix

left common iliac artery

rectum

anus

small intestine

right common iliac artery

A

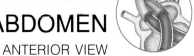

ARTERIAL SYSTEM (XXXII). TRUNK and ABDOMEN
ANTERIOR VIEW

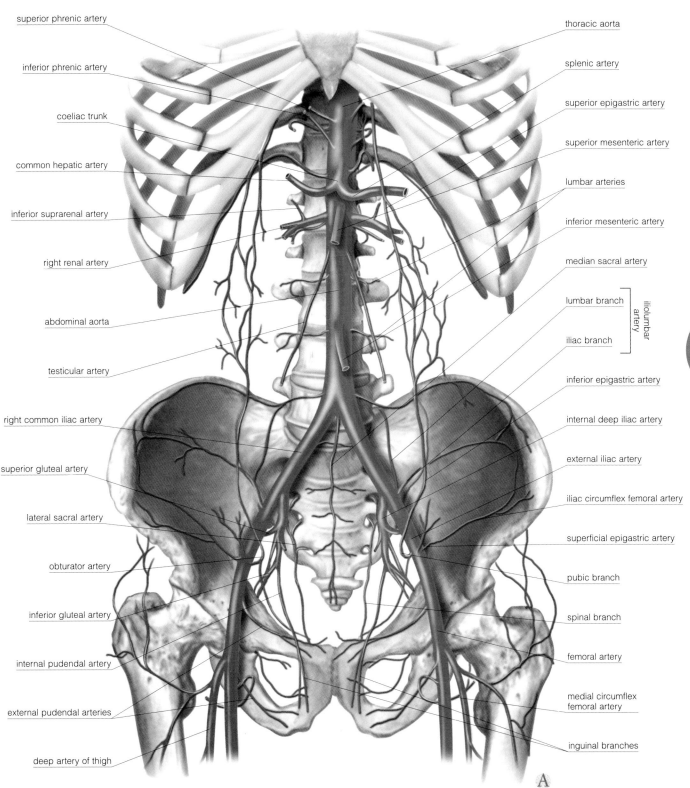

superior phrenic artery

inferior phrenic artery

coeliac trunk

common hepatic artery

inferior suprarenal artery

right renal artery

abdominal aorta

testicular artery

right common iliac artery

superior gluteal artery

lateral sacral artery

obturator artery

inferior gluteal artery

internal pudendal artery

external pudendal arteries

deep artery of thigh

thoracic aorta

splenic artery

superior epigastric artery

superior mesenteric artery

lumbar arteries

inferior mesenteric artery

median sacral artery

lumbar branch

iliac branch

iliolumbar artery

inferior epigastric artery

internal deep iliac artery

external iliac artery

iliac circumflex femoral artery

superficial epigastric artery

pubic branch

spinal branch

femoral artery

medial circumflex femoral artery

inguinal branches

313

A

ARTERIAL SYSTEM (XXXIII). ABDOMEN

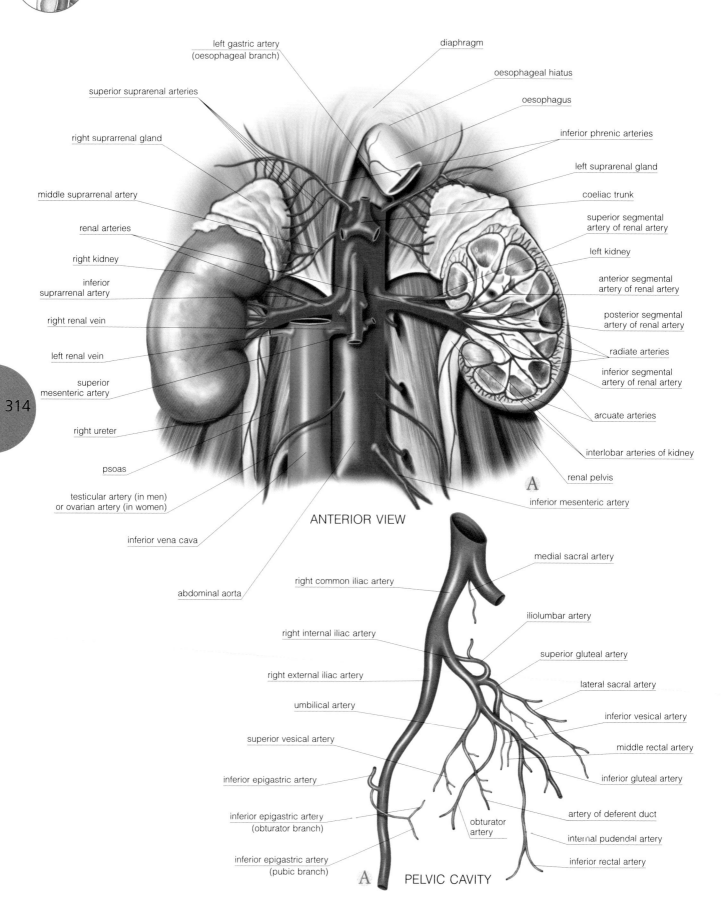

left gastric artery (oesophageal branch)

superior suprarenal arteries

right suprarrenal gland

middle suprarrenal artery

renal arteries

right kidney

inferior suprarrenal artery

right renal vein

left renal vein

superior mesenteric artery

right ureter

psoas

testicular artery (in men) or ovarian artery (in women)

inferior vena cava

abdominal aorta

diaphragm

oesophageal hiatus

oesophagus

inferior phrenic arteries

left suprarenal gland

coeliac trunk

superior segmental artery of renal artery

left kidney

anterior segmental artery of renal artery

posterior segmental artery of renal artery

radiate arteries

inferior segmental artery of renal artery

arcuate arteries

interlobar arteries of kidney

renal pelvis

inferior mesenteric artery

A

ANTERIOR VIEW

right common iliac artery

right internal iliac artery

right external iliac artery

umbilical artery

superior vesical artery

inferior epigastric artery

inferior epigastric artery (obturator branch)

inferior epigastric artery (pubic branch)

medial sacral artery

iliolumbar artery

superior gluteal artery

lateral sacral artery

inferior vesical artery

middle rectal artery

inferior gluteal artery

artery of deferent duct

internal pudendal artery

inferior rectal artery

obturator artery

A   PELVIC CAVITY

314

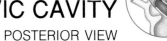

ARTERIAL SYSTEM (XXXIV). PELVIC CAVITY

POSTERIOR VIEW

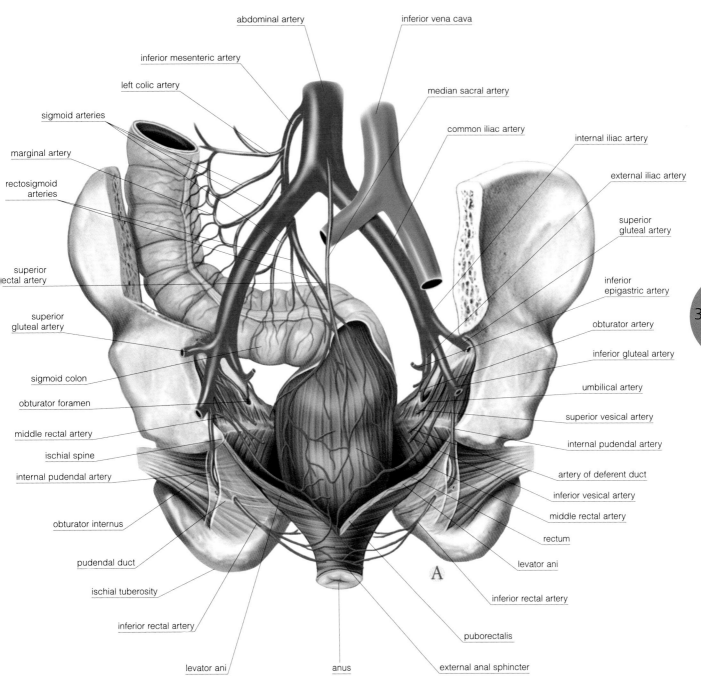

abdominal artery

inferior vena cava

inferior mesenteric artery

median sacral artery

left colic artery

common iliac artery

sigmoid arteries

internal iliac artery

marginal artery

external iliac artery

rectosigmoid arteries

superior gluteal artery

superior rectal artery

inferior epigastric artery

superior gluteal artery

obturator artery

sigmoid colon

inferior gluteal artery

obturator foramen

umbilical artery

middle rectal artery

superior vesical artery

ischial spine

internal pudendal artery

internal pudendal artery

artery of deferent duct

inferior vesical artery

obturator internus

middle rectal artery

rectum

pudendal duct

levator ani

ischial tuberosity

inferior rectal artery

inferior rectal artery

puborectalis

levator ani

anus

external anal sphincter

A

315

ARTERIAL SYSTEM (XXXV). THORAX and UPPER LIMB

RIGHT UPPER LIMB. ANTERIOR VIEW

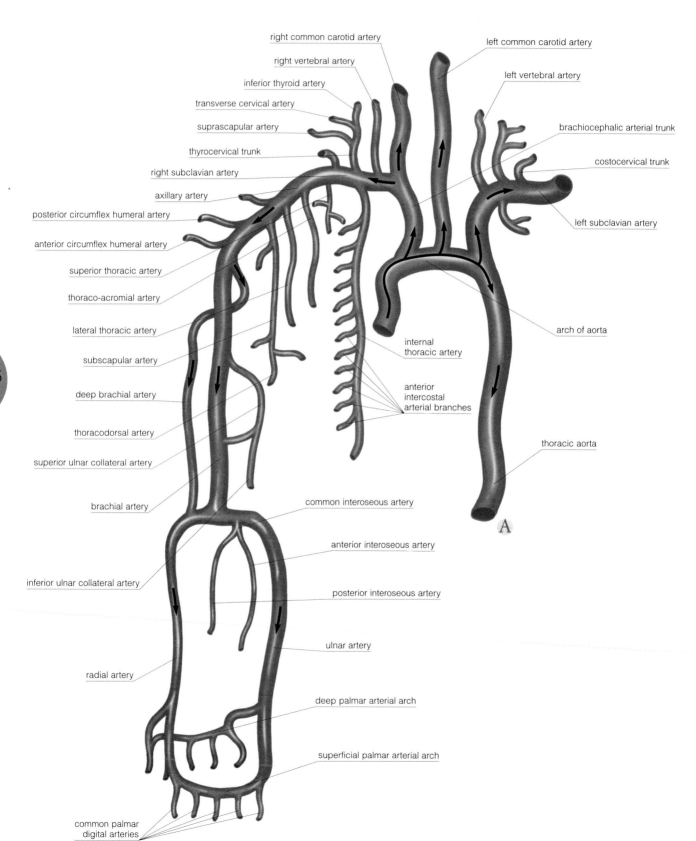

right common carotid artery

right vertebral artery

inferior thyroid artery

transverse cervical artery

suprascapular artery

thyrocervical trunk

right subclavian artery

axillary artery

posterior circumflex humeral artery

anterior circumflex humeral artery

superior thoracic artery

thoraco-acromial artery

lateral thoracic artery

subscapular artery

deep brachial artery

thoracodorsal artery

superior ulnar collateral artery

brachial artery

inferior ulnar collateral artery

radial artery

common palmar
digital arteries

left common carotid artery

left vertebral artery

brachiocephalic arterial trunk

costocervical trunk

left subclavian artery

arch of aorta

internal
thoracic artery

anterior
intercostal
arterial branches

thoracic aorta

A

common interoseous artery

anterior interoseous artery

posterior interoseous artery

ulnar artery

deep palmar arterial arch

superficial palmar arterial arch

316

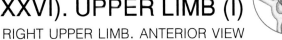

ARTERIAL SYSTEM (XXXVI). UPPER LIMB (I)

RIGHT UPPER LIMB. ANTERIOR VIEW

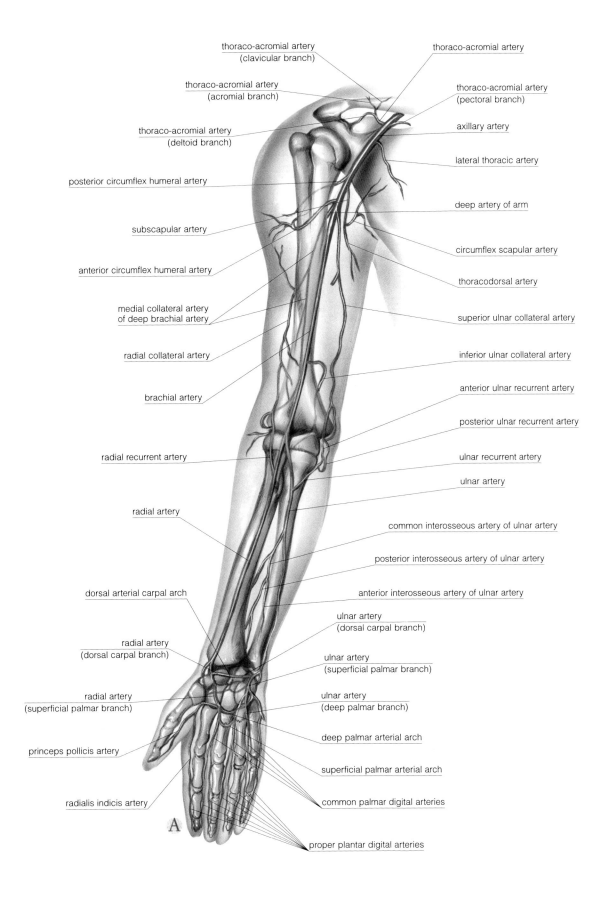

thoraco-acromial artery
(clavicular branch)

thoraco-acromial artery

thoraco-acromial artery
(acromial branch)

thoraco-acromial artery
(pectoral branch)

thoraco-acromial artery
(deltoid branch)

axillary artery

lateral thoracic artery

posterior circumflex humeral artery

deep artery of arm

subscapular artery

circumflex scapular artery

anterior circumflex humeral artery

thoracodorsal artery

medial collateral artery
of deep brachial artery

superior ulnar collateral artery

radial collateral artery

inferior ulnar collateral artery

anterior ulnar recurrent artery

brachial artery

posterior ulnar recurrent artery

radial recurrent artery

ulnar recurrent artery

ulnar artery

radial artery

common interosseous artery of ulnar artery

posterior interosseous artery of ulnar artery

dorsal arterial carpal arch

anterior interosseous artery of ulnar artery

ulnar artery
(dorsal carpal branch)

radial artery
(dorsal carpal branch)

ulnar artery
(superficial palmar branch)

radial artery
(superficial palmar branch)

ulnar artery
(deep palmar branch)

deep palmar arterial arch

princeps pollicis artery

superficial palmar arterial arch

common palmar digital arteries

radialis indicis artery

A

proper plantar digital arteries

ARTERIAL SYSTEM (XXXIX). UPPER LIMB (IV). ARM (I)

RIGHT UPPER LIMB. ANTERIOR VIEW

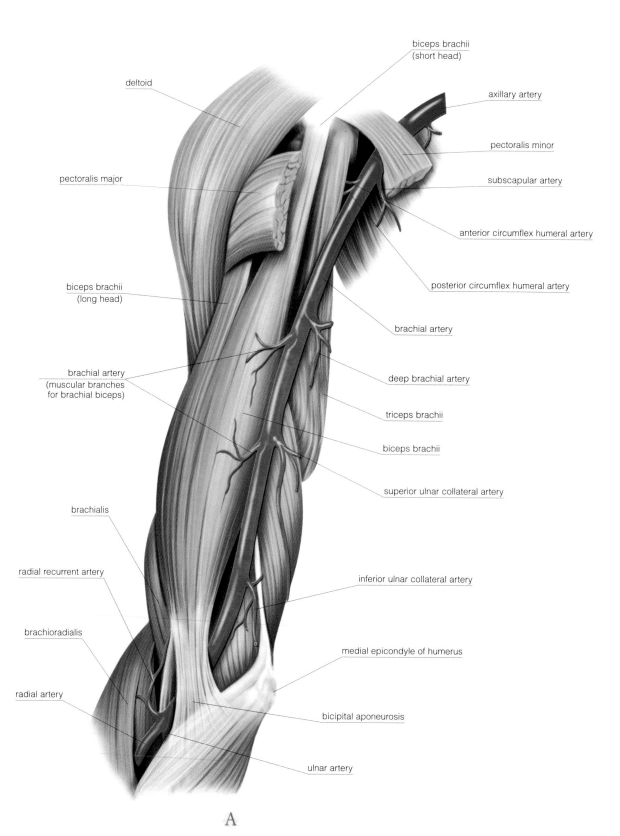

biceps brachii (short head)

axillary artery

deltoid

pectoralis minor

subscapular artery

pectoralis major

anterior circumflex humeral artery

posterior circumflex humeral artery

biceps brachii (long head)

brachial artery

brachial artery (muscular branches for brachial biceps)

deep brachial artery

triceps brachii

biceps brachii

superior ulnar collateral artery

brachialis

radial recurrent artery

inferior ulnar collateral artery

brachioradialis

medial epicondyle of humerus

radial artery

bicipital aponeurosis

ulnar artery

A

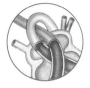

ARTERIAL SYSTEM (XL). UPPER LIMB (V). ARM (II)

RIGHT UPPER LIMB. ANTERIOR VIEW

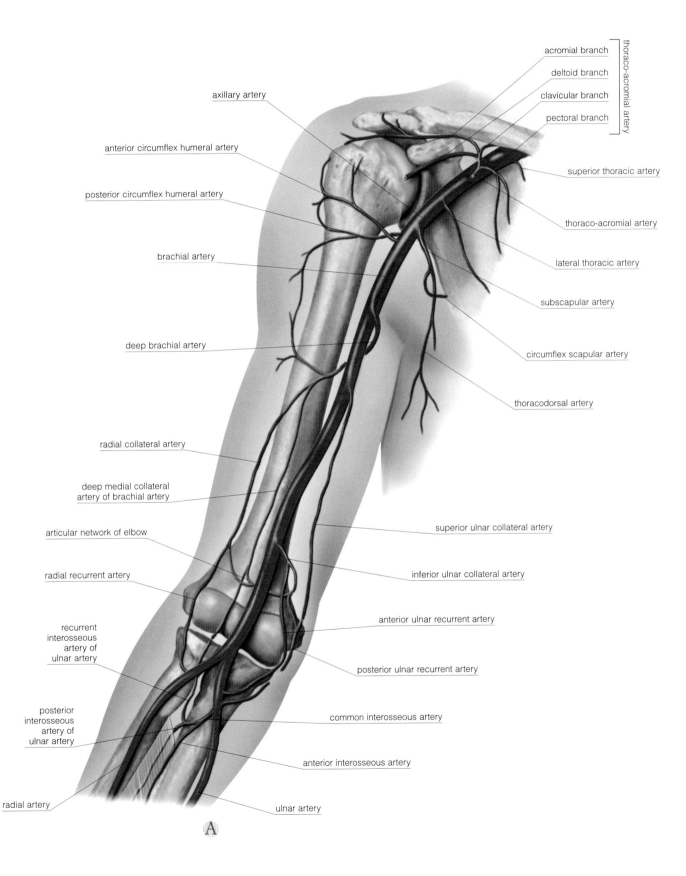

acromial branch
deltoid branch
clavicular branch
pectoral branch
thoraco-acromial artery

axillary artery

anterior circumflex humeral artery

posterior circumflex humeral artery

brachial artery

deep brachial artery

superior thoracic artery

thoraco-acromial artery

lateral thoracic artery

subscapular artery

circumflex scapular artery

thoracodorsal artery

radial collateral artery

deep medial collateral
artery of brachial artery

articular network of elbow

radial recurrent artery

recurrent
interosseous
artery of
ulnar artery

posterior
interosseous
artery of
ulnar artery

radial artery

superior ulnar collateral artery

inferior ulnar collateral artery

anterior ulnar recurrent artery

posterior ulnar recurrent artery

common interosseous artery

anterior interosseous artery

ulnar artery

321

A

ARTERIAL SYSTEM (XLI). UPPER LIMB (VI). FOREARM

RIGHT UPPER LIMB. ANTERIOR VIEW

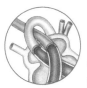

322

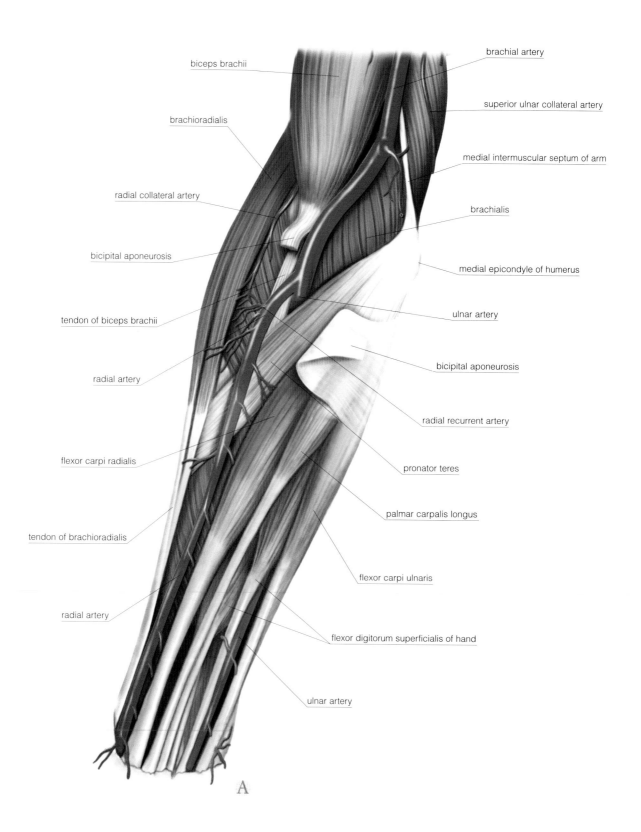

biceps brachii

brachial artery

brachioradialis

superior ulnar collateral artery

radial collateral artery

medial intermuscular septum of arm

bicipital aponeurosis

brachialis

tendon of biceps brachii

medial epicondyle of humerus

radial artery

ulnar artery

flexor carpi radialis

bicipital aponeurosis

tendon of brachioradialis

radial recurrent artery

radial artery

pronator teres

palmar carpalis longus

flexor carpi ulnaris

flexor digitorum superficialis of hand

ulnar artery

A

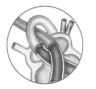

ARTERIAL SYSTEM (XLII). UPPER LIMB (VII). HAND (I)

RIGHT UPPER LIMB. SUPERFICIAL PALMAR VIEW

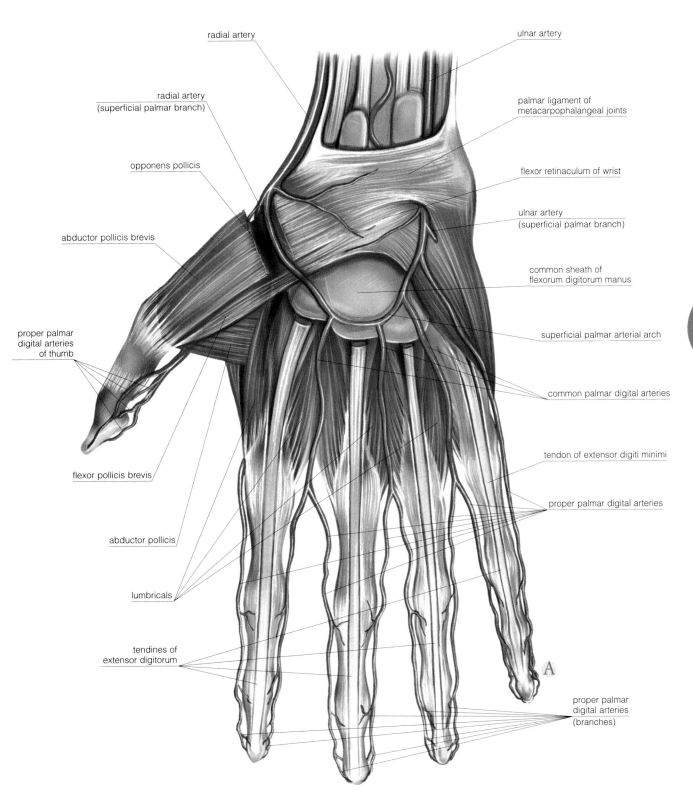

radial artery

ulnar artery

radial artery
(superficial palmar branch)

palmar ligament of
metacarpophalangeal joints

opponens pollicis

flexor retinaculum of wrist

abductor pollicis brevis

ulnar artery
(superficial palmar branch)

common sheath of
flexorum digitorum manus

proper palmar
digital arteries
of thumb

superficial palmar arterial arch

common palmar digital arteries

flexor pollicis brevis

tendon of extensor digiti minimi

proper palmar digital arteries

abductor pollicis

lumbricals

tendines of
extensor digitorum

A

proper palmar
digital arteries
(branches)

323

ARTERIAL SYSTEM (XLIII). UPPER LIMB (VIII). HAND (II)
RIGHT UPPER LIMB. DEEP PALMAR VIEW

324

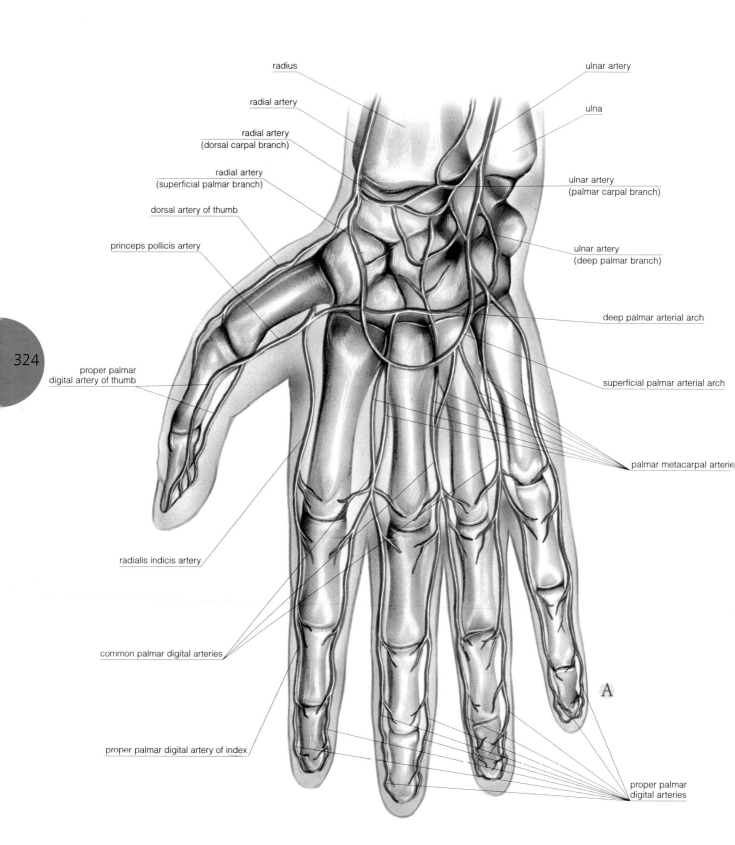

radius

radial artery

radial artery
(dorsal carpal branch)

radial artery
(superficial palmar branch)

dorsal artery of thumb

princeps pollicis artery

proper palmar
digital artery of thumb

radialis indicis artery

common palmar digital arteries

proper palmar digital artery of index

ulnar artery

ulna

ulnar artery
(palmar carpal branch)

ulnar artery
(deep palmar branch)

deep palmar arterial arch

superficial palmar arterial arch

palmar metacarpal arterie

A

proper palmar
digital arteries

ARTERIAL SYSTEM (XLIV). UPPER LIMB (IX). HAND (III)

RIGHT UPPER LIMB. DORSAL VIEW

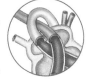

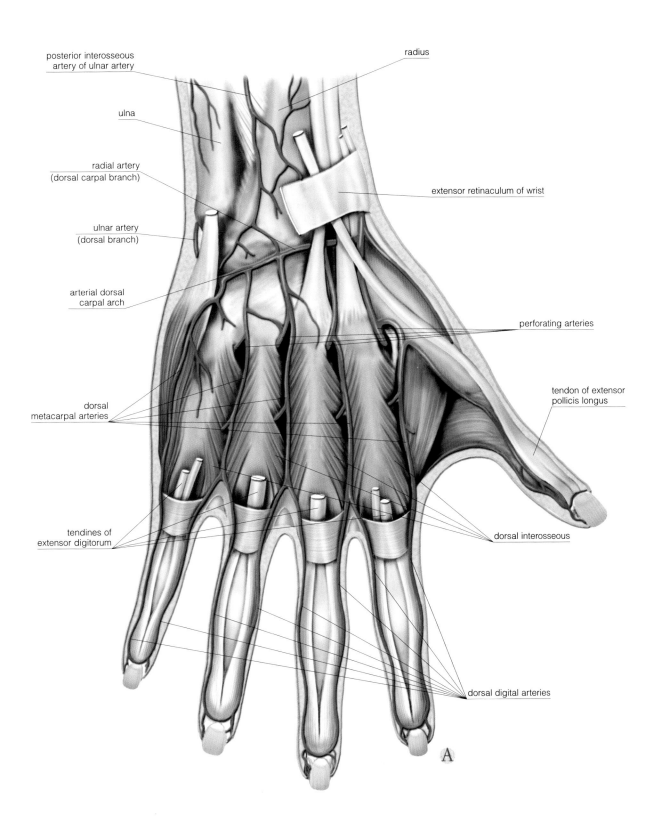

posterior interosseous
artery of ulnar artery

radius

ulna

radial artery
(dorsal carpal branch)

extensor retinaculum of wrist

ulnar artery
(dorsal branch)

arterial dorsal
carpal arch

perforating arteries

tendon of extensor
pollicis longus

dorsal
metacarpal arteries

tendines of
extensor digitorum

dorsal interosseous

dorsal digital arteries

A

325

ARTERIAL SYSTEM (XLV)
PELVIC REGION and LOWER LIMB
RIGHT LOWER LIMB. ANTERIOR VIEW

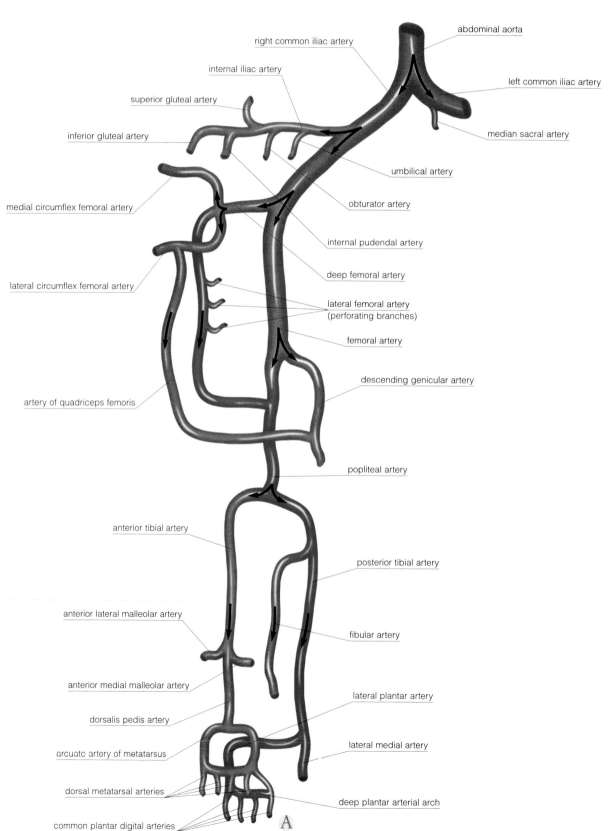

right common iliac artery

abdominal aorta

internal iliac artery

left common iliac artery

superior gluteal artery

inferior gluteal artery

median sacral artery

umbilical artery

medial circumflex femoral artery

obturator artery

internal pudendal artery

lateral circumflex femoral artery

deep femoral artery

lateral femoral artery
(perforating branches)

femoral artery

descending genicular artery

artery of quadriceps femoris

popliteal artery

anterior tibial artery

posterior tibial artery

anterior lateral malleolar artery

fibular artery

anterior medial malleolar artery

lateral plantar artery

dorsalis pedis artery

lateral medial artery

arcuate artery of metatarsus

dorsal metatarsal arteries

deep plantar arterial arch

common plantar digital arteries

A

ARTERIAL SYSTEM (XLVI). LOWER LIMB (I)

RIGHT LOWER LIMB. ANTERIOR VIEW

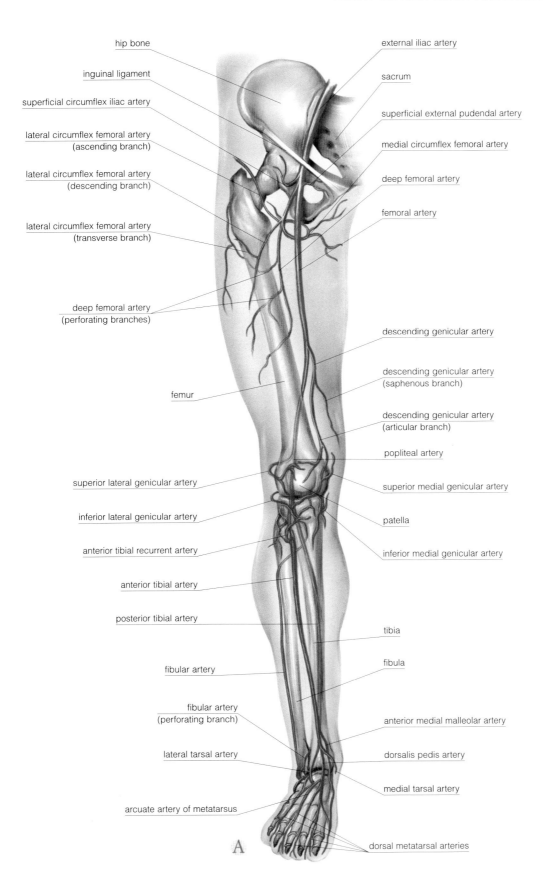

hip bone

inguinal ligament

superficial circumflex iliac artery

lateral circumflex femoral artery
(ascending branch)

lateral circumflex femoral artery
(descending branch)

lateral circumflex femoral artery
(transverse branch)

deep femoral artery
(perforating branches)

femur

superior lateral genicular artery

inferior lateral genicular artery

anterior tibial recurrent artery

anterior tibial artery

posterior tibial artery

fibular artery

fibular artery
(perforating branch)

lateral tarsal artery

arcuate artery of metatarsus

external iliac artery

sacrum

superficial external pudendal artery

medial circumflex femoral artery

deep femoral artery

femoral artery

descending genicular artery

descending genicular artery
(saphenous branch)

descending genicular artery
(articular branch)

popliteal artery

superior medial genicular artery

patella

inferior medial genicular artery

tibia

fibula

anterior medial malleolar artery

dorsalis pedis artery

medial tarsal artery

dorsal metatarsal arteries

A

327

ARTERIAL SYSTEM (XLVII). LOWER LIMB (II)

RIGHT LOWER LIMB

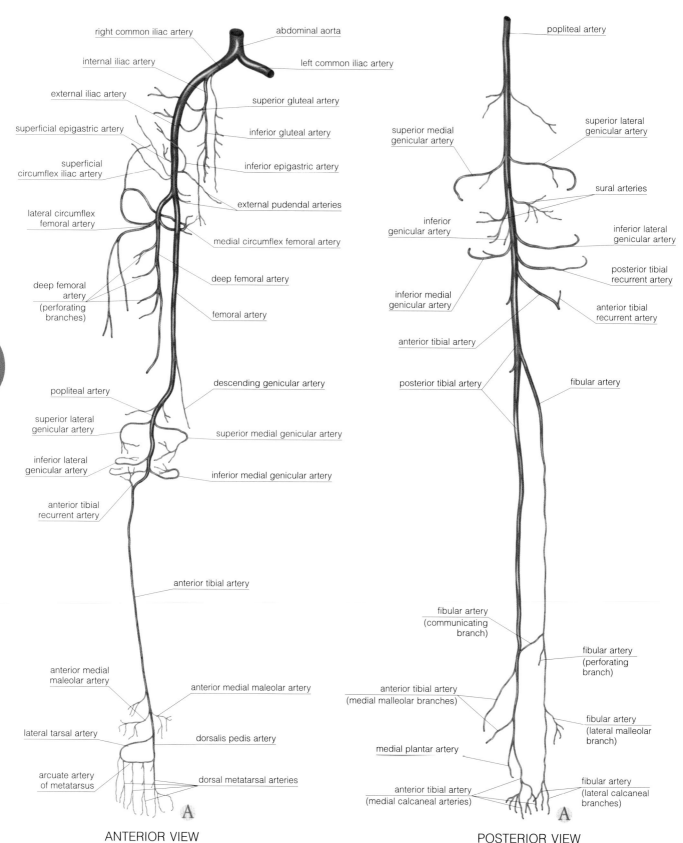

right common iliac artery

abdominal aorta

internal iliac artery

left common iliac artery

external iliac artery

superior gluteal artery

superficial epigastric artery

inferior gluteal artery

superficial circumflex iliac artery

inferior epigastric artery

lateral circumflex femoral artery

external pudendal arteries

medial circumflex femoral artery

deep femoral artery (perforating branches)

deep femoral artery

femoral artery

popliteal artery

descending genicular artery

superior lateral genicular artery

superior medial genicular artery

inferior lateral genicular artery

inferior medial genicular artery

anterior tibial recurrent artery

anterior tibial artery

anterior medial maleolar artery

anterior medial maleolar artery

lateral tarsal artery

dorsalis pedis artery

arcuate artery of metatarsus

dorsal metatarsal arteries

ANTERIOR VIEW

popliteal artery

superior medial genicular artery

superior lateral genicular artery

sural arteries

inferior genicular artery

inferior lateral genicular artery

posterior tibial recurrent artery

inferior medial genicular artery

anterior tibial recurrent artery

anterior tibial artery

posterior tibial artery

fibular artery

fibular artery (communicating branch)

fibular artery (perforating branch)

anterior tibial artery (medial malleolar branches)

fibular artery (lateral malleolar branch)

medial plantar artery

anterior tibial artery (medial calcaneal arteries)

fibular artery (lateral calcaneal branches)

POSTERIOR VIEW

328

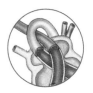

ARTERIAL SYSTEM (XLVIII). LOWER LIMB (III)
GLUTEAL REGION and THIGH

RIGHT LOWER LIMB. POSTERIOR VIEW

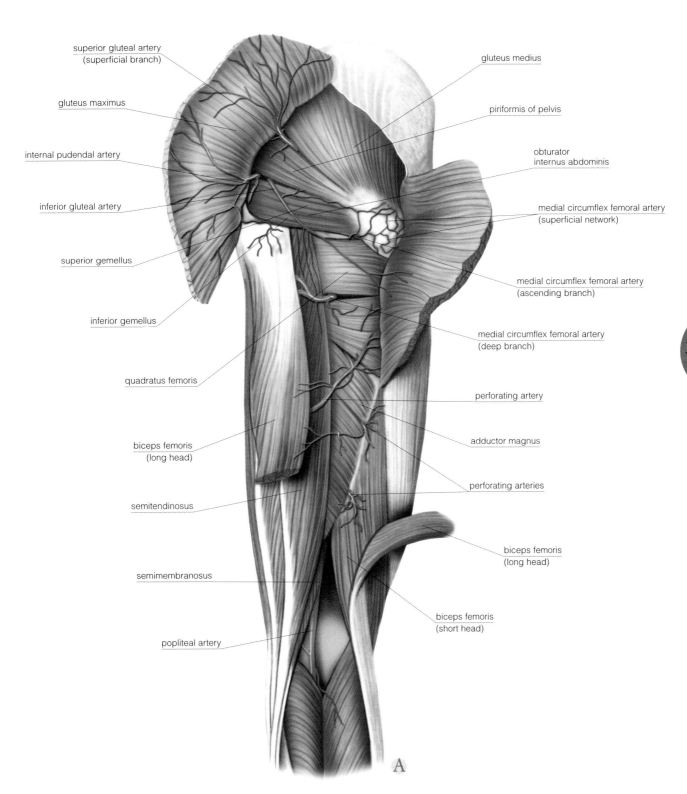

superior gluteal artery
(superficial branch)

gluteus maximus

internal pudendal artery

inferior gluteal artery

superior gemellus

inferior gemellus

quadratus femoris

biceps femoris
(long head)

semitendinosus

semimembranosus

popliteal artery

gluteus medius

piriformis of pelvis

obturator
internus abdominis

medial circumflex femoral artery
(superficial network)

medial circumflex femoral artery
(ascending branch)

medial circumflex femoral artery
(deep branch)

perforating artery

adductor magnus

perforating arteries

biceps femoris
(long head)

biceps femoris
(short head)

A

329

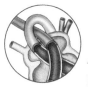

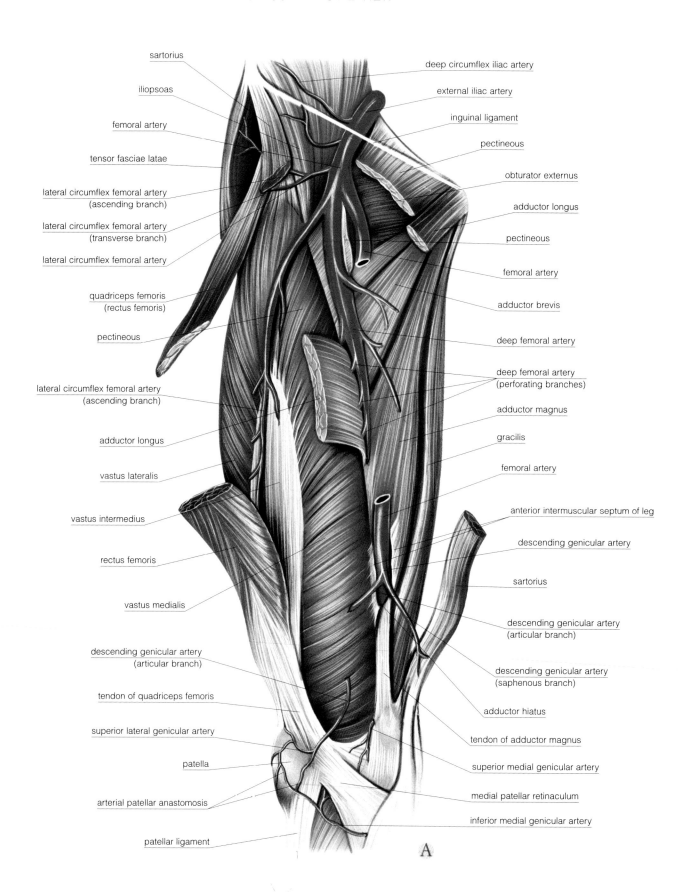

sartorius

iliopsoas

femoral artery

tensor fasciae latae

lateral circumflex femoral artery
(ascending branch)

lateral circumflex femoral artery
(transverse branch)

lateral circumflex femoral artery

quadriceps femoris
(rectus femoris)

pectineous

lateral circumflex femoral artery
(ascending branch)

adductor longus

vastus lateralis

vastus intermedius

rectus femoris

vastus medialis

descending genicular artery
(articular branch)

tendon of quadriceps femoris

superior lateral genicular artery

patella

arterial patellar anastomosis

patellar ligament

deep circumflex iliac artery

external iliac artery

inguinal ligament

pectineous

obturator externus

adductor longus

pectineous

femoral artery

adductor brevis

deep femoral artery

deep femoral artery
(perforating branches)

adductor magnus

gracilis

femoral artery

anterior intermuscular septum of leg

descending genicular artery

sartorius

descending genicular artery
(articular branch)

descending genicular artery
(saphenous branch)

adductor hiatus

tendon of adductor magnus

superior medial genicular artery

medial patellar retinaculum

inferior medial genicular artery

A

330

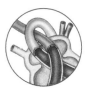

ARTERIAL SYSTEM (L). LOWER LIMB (V). THIGH (II)

RIGHT LOWER LIMB. ANTERIOR DEEP VIEW

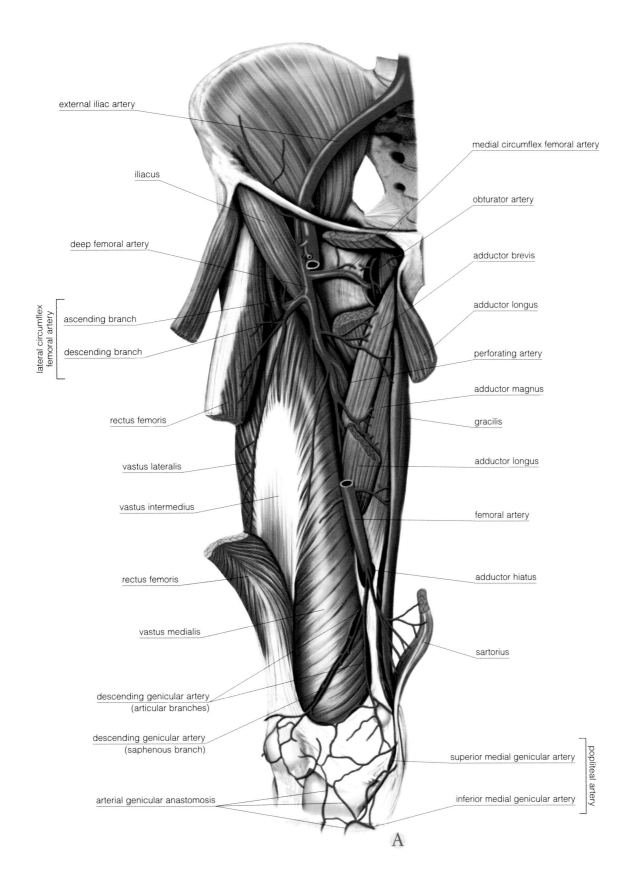

external iliac artery

iliacus

deep femoral artery

lateral circumflex femoral artery
- ascending branch
- descending branch

rectus femoris

vastus lateralis

vastus intermedius

rectus femoris

vastus medialis

descending genicular artery
(articular branches)

descending genicular artery
(saphenous branch)

arterial genicular anastomosis

medial circumflex femoral artery

obturator artery

adductor brevis

adductor longus

perforating artery

adductor magnus

gracilis

adductor longus

femoral artery

adductor hiatus

sartorius

superior medial genicular artery

inferior medial genicular artery

popliteal artery

A

331

ARTERIAL SYSTEM (LI). LOWER LIMB (VI). HIP

RIGHT LOWER LIMB. ANTERIOR VIEW

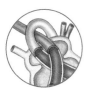

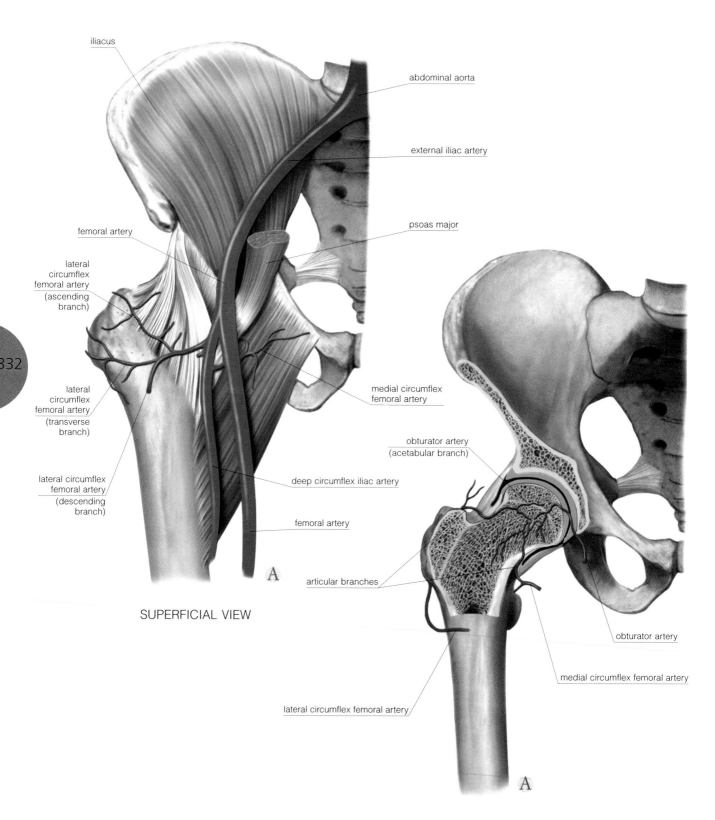

iliacus

abdominal aorta

external iliac artery

femoral artery

psoas major

lateral circumflex femoral artery (ascending branch)

lateral circumflex femoral artery (transverse branch)

medial circumflex femoral artery

lateral circumflex femoral artery (descending branch)

deep circumflex iliac artery

obturator artery (acetabular branch)

femoral artery

articular branches

obturator artery

medial circumflex femoral artery

lateral circumflex femoral artery

SUPERFICIAL VIEW

A

A

DEEP VIEW

332

ARTERIAL SYSTEM (LII). LOWER LIMB (VII)

RIGHT LOWER LIMB. ANTERIOR VIEW

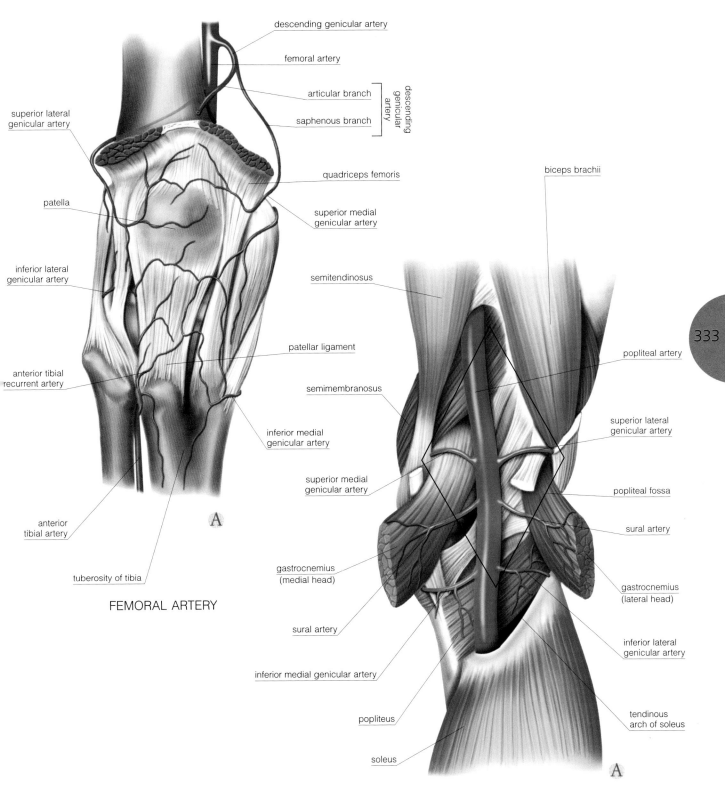

descending genicular artery

femoral artery

articular branch

saphenous branch

descending genicular artery

superior lateral genicular artery

patella

inferior lateral genicular artery

anterior tibial recurrent artery

anterior tibial artery

tuberosity of tibia

quadriceps femoris

superior medial genicular artery

biceps brachii

semitendinosus

patellar ligament

semimembranosus

superior medial genicular artery

inferior medial genicular artery

gastrocnemius (medial head)

sural artery

inferior medial genicular artery

popliteus

soleus

popliteal artery

superior lateral genicular artery

popliteal fossa

sural artery

gastrocnemius (lateral head)

inferior lateral genicular artery

tendinous arch of soleus

FEMORAL ARTERY

POPLITEAL ARTERY

333

ARTERIAL SYSTEM (LIII). LOWER LIMB (VIII). LEG (I)

RIGHT LOWER LIMB. ANTERIOR VIEW

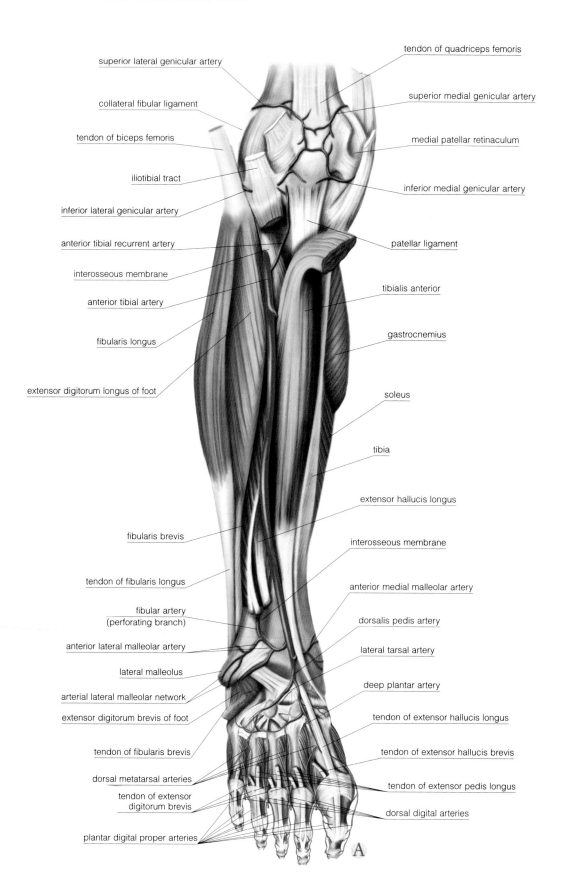

superior lateral genicular artery

collateral fibular ligament

tendon of biceps femoris

iliotibial tract

inferior lateral genicular artery

anterior tibial recurrent artery

interosseous membrane

anterior tibial artery

fibularis longus

extensor digitorum longus of foot

334

fibularis brevis

tendon of fibularis longus

fibular artery
(perforating branch)

anterior lateral malleolar artery

lateral malleolus

arterial lateral malleolar network

extensor digitorum brevis of foot

tendon of fibularis brevis

dorsal metatarsal arteries

tendon of extensor
digitorum brevis

plantar digital proper arteries

tendon of quadriceps femoris

superior medial genicular artery

medial patellar retinaculum

inferior medial genicular artery

patellar ligament

tibialis anterior

gastrocnemius

soleus

tibia

extensor hallucis longus

interosseous membrane

anterior medial malleolar artery

dorsalis pedis artery

lateral tarsal artery

deep plantar artery

tendon of extensor hallucis longus

tendon of extensor hallucis brevis

tendon of extensor pedis longus

dorsal digital arteries

A

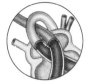

ARTERIAL SYSTEM (LIV). LOWER LIMB (IX). LEG (II)

RIGHT LOWER LIMB. POSTERIOR VIEW

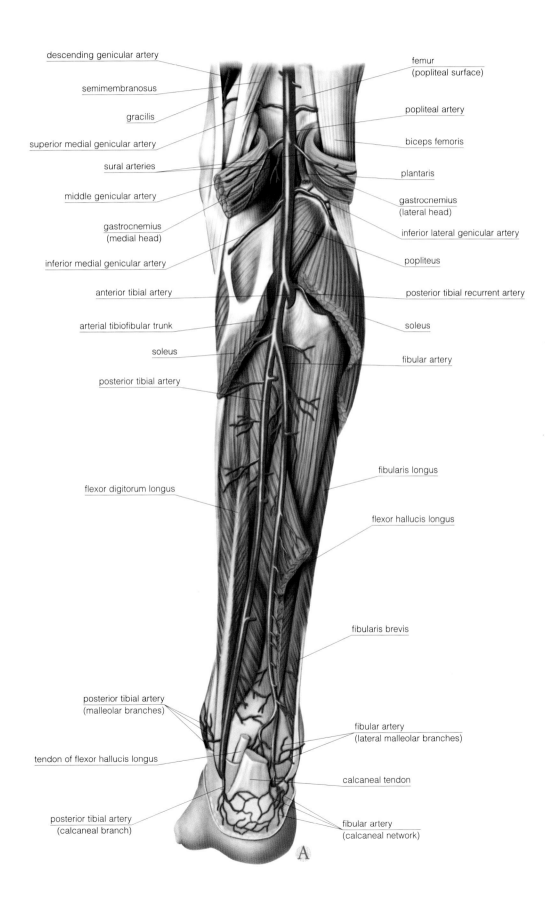

descending genicular artery

semimembranosus

gracilis

superior medial genicular artery

sural arteries

middle genicular artery

gastrocnemius
(medial head)

inferior medial genicular artery

anterior tibial artery

arterial tibiofibular trunk

soleus

posterior tibial artery

flexor digitorum longus

posterior tibial artery
(malleolar branches)

tendon of flexor hallucis longus

posterior tibial artery
(calcaneal branch)

femur
(popliteal surface)

popliteal artery

biceps femoris

plantaris

gastrocnemius
(lateral head)

inferior lateral genicular artery

popliteus

posterior tibial recurrent artery

soleus

fibular artery

fibularis longus

flexor hallucis longus

fibularis brevis

fibular artery
(lateral malleolar branches)

calcaneal tendon

fibular artery
(calcaneal network)

A

335

336

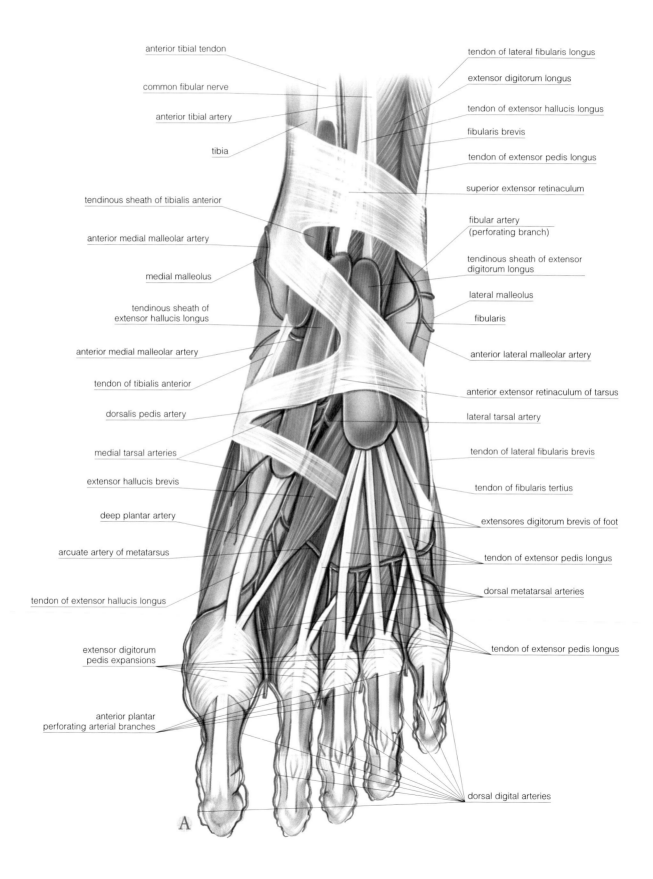

anterior tibial tendon

common fibular nerve

anterior tibial artery

tibia

tendinous sheath of tibialis anterior

anterior medial malleolar artery

medial malleolus

tendinous sheath of
extensor hallucis longus

anterior medial malleolar artery

tendon of tibialis anterior

dorsalis pedis artery

medial tarsal arteries

extensor hallucis brevis

deep plantar artery

arcuate artery of metatarsus

tendon of extensor hallucis longus

extensor digitorum
pedis expansions

anterior plantar
perforating arterial branches

tendon of lateral fibularis longus

extensor digitorum longus

tendon of extensor hallucis longus

fibularis brevis

tendon of extensor pedis longus

superior extensor retinaculum

fibular artery
(perforating branch)

tendinous sheath of extensor
digitorum longus

lateral malleolus

fibularis

anterior lateral malleolar artery

anterior extensor retinaculum of tarsus

lateral tarsal artery

tendon of lateral fibularis brevis

tendon of fibularis tertius

extensores digitorum brevis of foot

tendon of extensor pedis longus

dorsal metatarsal arteries

tendon of extensor pedis longus

dorsal digital arteries

A

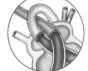

ARTERIAL SYSTEM (LVI). LOWER LIMB (XI). FOOT (II)

LEFT LOWER LIMB. DORSAL DEEP VIEW

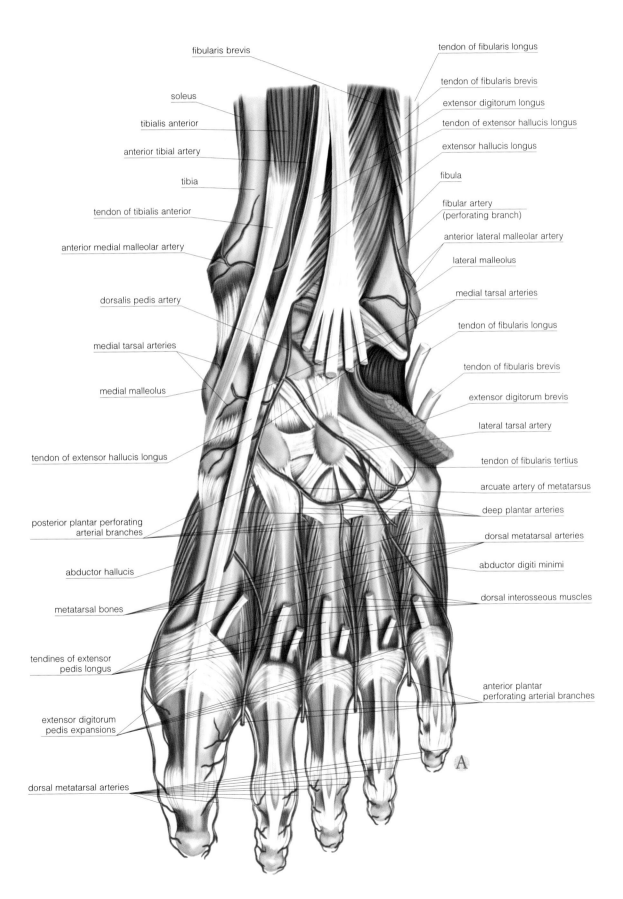

fibularis brevis

soleus

tibialis anterior

anterior tibial artery

tibia

tendon of tibialis anterior

anterior medial malleolar artery

dorsalis pedis artery

medial tarsal arteries

medial malleolus

tendon of extensor hallucis longus

posterior plantar perforating
arterial branches

abductor hallucis

metatarsal bones

tendines of extensor
pedis longus

extensor digitorum
pedis expansions

dorsal metatarsal arteries

tendon of fibularis longus

tendon of fibularis brevis

extensor digitorum longus

tendon of extensor hallucis longus

extensor hallucis longus

fibula

fibular artery
(perforating branch)

anterior lateral malleolar artery

lateral malleolus

medial tarsal arteries

tendon of fibularis longus

tendon of fibularis brevis

extensor digitorum brevis

lateral tarsal artery

tendon of fibularis tertius

arcuate artery of metatarsus

deep plantar arteries

dorsal metatarsal arteries

abductor digiti minimi

dorsal interosseous muscles

anterior plantar
perforating arterial branches

A

ARTERIAL SYSTEM (LVII). LOWER LIMB (XII). FOOT (III)
LEFT LOWER LIMB. DORSAL VIEW

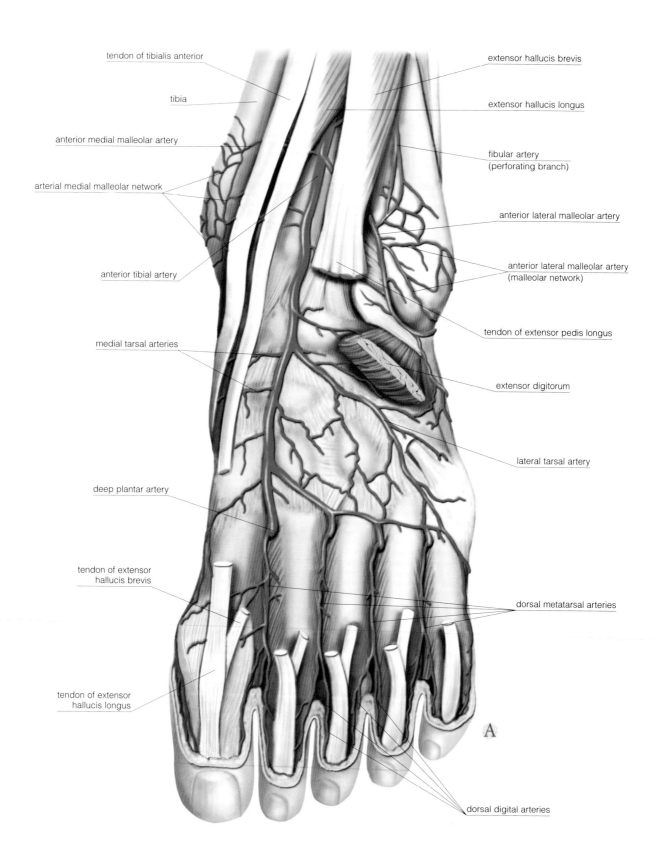

tendon of tibialis anterior

tibia

anterior medial malleolar artery

arterial medial malleolar network

anterior tibial artery

medial tarsal arteries

deep plantar artery

tendon of extensor
hallucis brevis

tendon of extensor
hallucis longus

extensor hallucis brevis

extensor hallucis longus

fibular artery
(perforating branch)

anterior lateral malleolar artery

anterior lateral malleolar artery
(malleolar network)

tendon of extensor pedis longus

extensor digitorum

lateral tarsal artery

dorsal metatarsal arteries

dorsal digital arteries

A

338

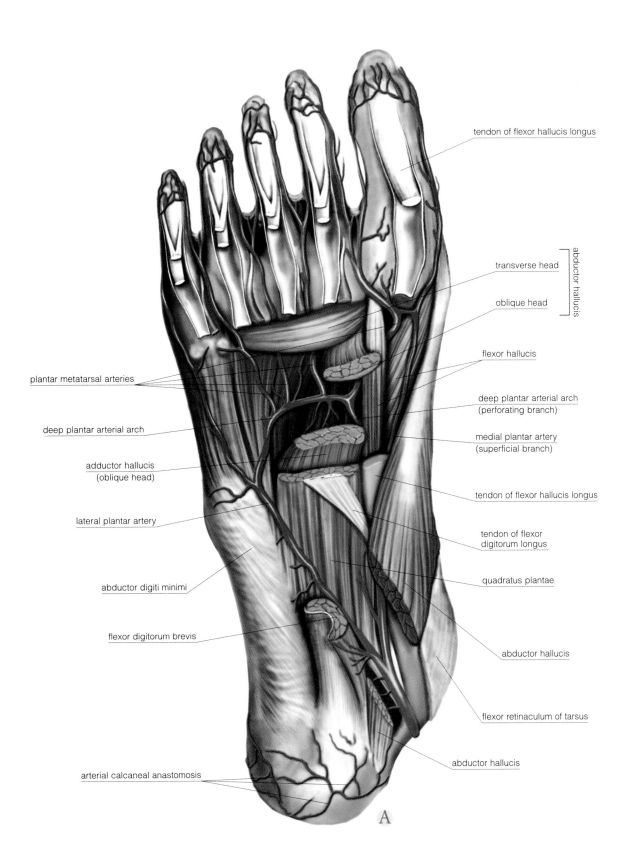

tendon of flexor hallucis longus

transverse head
oblique head
abductor hallucis

flexor hallucis

deep plantar arterial arch
(perforating branch)

medial plantar artery
(superficial branch)

tendon of flexor hallucis longus

tendon of flexor
digitorum longus

quadratus plantae

abductor hallucis

flexor retinaculum of tarsus

abductor hallucis

plantar metatarsal arteries

deep plantar arterial arch

adductor hallucis
(oblique head)

lateral plantar artery

abductor digiti minimi

flexor digitorum brevis

arterial calcaneal anastomosis

A

VASCULAR ANASTOMOSIS (I). PELVIC CAVITY (I)

MALE SEX. LEFT LATERAL VIEW

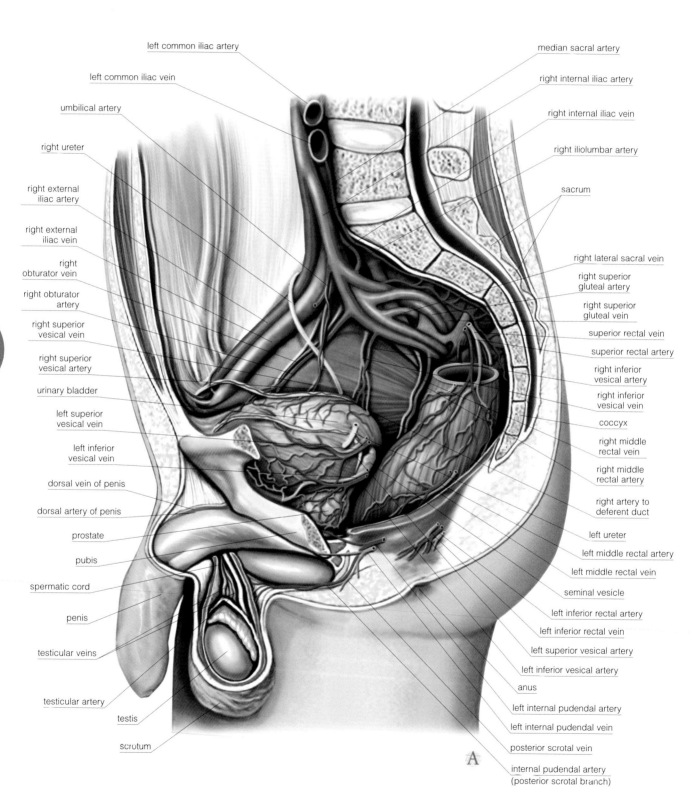

left common iliac artery

left common iliac vein

umbilical artery

right ureter

right external iliac artery

right external iliac vein

right obturator vein

right obturator artery

right superior vesical vein

right superior vesical artery

urinary bladder

left superior vesical vein

left inferior vesical vein

dorsal vein of penis

dorsal artery of penis

prostate

pubis

spermatic cord

penis

testicular veins

testicular artery

testis

scrotum

median sacral artery

right internal iliac artery

right internal iliac vein

right iliolumbar artery

sacrum

right lateral sacral vein

right superior gluteal artery

right superior gluteal vein

superior rectal vein

superior rectal artery

right inferior vesical artery

right inferior vesical vein

coccyx

right middle rectal vein

right middle rectal artery

right artery to deferent duct

left ureter

left middle rectal artery

left middle rectal vein

seminal vesicle

left inferior rectal artery

left inferior rectal vein

left superior vesical artery

left inferior vesical artery

anus

left internal pudendal artery

left internal pudendal vein

posterior scrotal vein

internal pudendal artery (posterior scrotal branch)

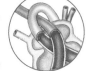

VASCULAR ANASTOMOSIS (II). PELVIC CAVITY (II)

FEMALE SEX. LEFT LATERAL VIEW

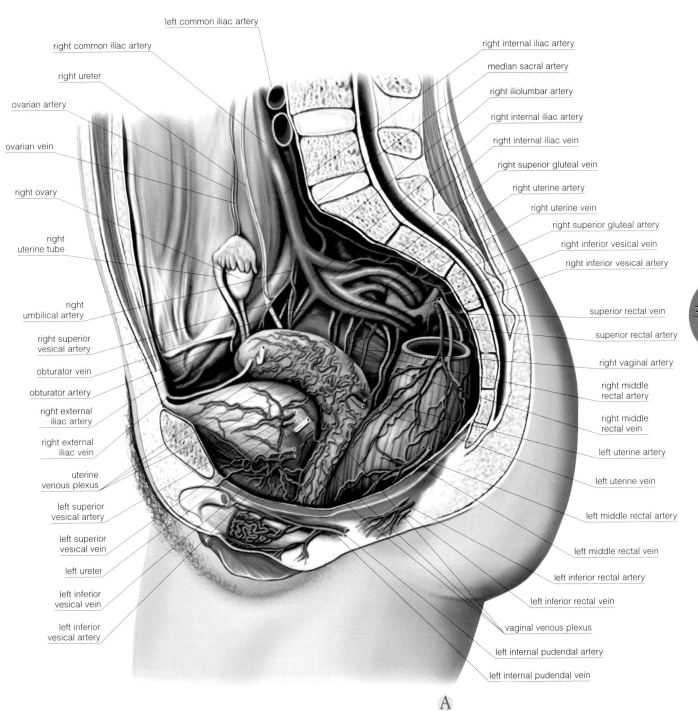

left common iliac artery

right common iliac artery

right ureter

ovarian artery

ovarian vein

right ovary

right uterine tube

right umbilical artery

right superior vesical artery

obturator vein

obturator artery

right external iliac artery

right external iliac vein

uterine venous plexus

left superior vesical artery

left superior vesical vein

left ureter

left inferior vesical vein

left inferior vesical artery

right internal iliac artery

median sacral artery

right iliolumbar artery

right internal iliac artery

right internal iliac vein

right superior gluteal vein

right uterine artery

right uterine vein

right superior gluteal artery

right inferior vesical vein

right inferior vesical artery

superior rectal vein

superior rectal artery

right vaginal artery

right middle rectal artery

right middle rectal vein

left uterine artery

left uterine vein

left middle rectal artery

left middle rectal vein

left inferior rectal artery

left inferior rectal vein

vaginal venous plexus

left internal pudendal artery

left internal pudendal vein

341

A

VENOUS SYSTEM (I)

ANTERIOR GENERAL VIEW

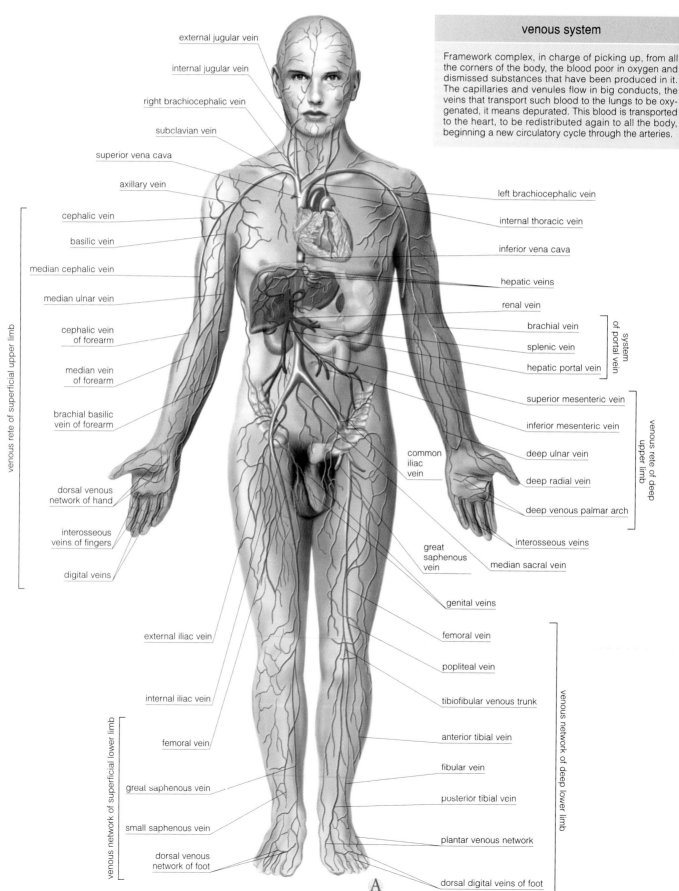

venous system

Framework complex, in charge of picking up, from all the corners of the body, the blood poor in oxygen and dismissed substances that have been produced in it. The capillaries and venules flow in big conducts, the veins that transport such blood to the lungs to be oxygenated, it means depurated. This blood is transported to the heart, to be redistributed again to all the body, beginning a new circulatory cycle through the arteries.

external jugular vein

internal jugular vein

right brachiocephalic vein

subclavian vein

superior vena cava

axillary vein

cephalic vein

basilic vein

median cephalic vein

median ulnar vein

cephalic vein of forearm

median vein of forearm

brachial basilic vein of forearm

dorsal venous network of hand

interosseous veins of fingers

digital veins

venous rete of superficial upper limb

left brachiocephalic vein

internal thoracic vein

inferior vena cava

hepatic veins

renal vein

brachial vein

splenic vein

hepatic portal vein

system of portal vein

superior mesenteric vein

inferior mesenteric vein

deep ulnar vein

deep radial vein

deep venous palmar arch

interosseous veins

median sacral vein

venous rete of deep upper limb

common iliac vein

great saphenous vein

genital veins

femoral vein

popliteal vein

tibiofibular venous trunk

anterior tibial vein

fibular vein

posterior tibial vein

plantar venous network

venous network of deep lower limb

external iliac vein

internal iliac vein

femoral vein

great saphenous vein

small saphenous vein

dorsal venous network of foot

venous network of superficial lower limb

dorsal digital veins of foot

342

A

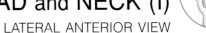

VENOUS SYSTEM (II). HEAD and NECK (I)

LATERAL ANTERIOR VIEW

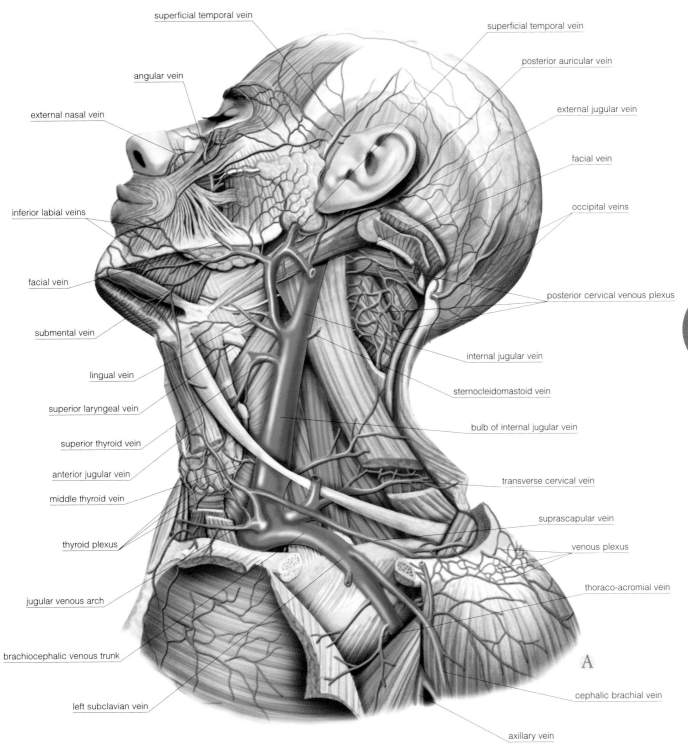

superficial temporal vein

angular vein

external nasal vein

inferior labial veins

facial vein

submental vein

lingual vein

superior laryngeal vein

superior thyroid vein

anterior jugular vein

middle thyroid vein

thyroid plexus

jugular venous arch

brachiocephalic venous trunk

left subclavian vein

superficial temporal vein

posterior auricular vein

external jugular vein

facial vein

occipital veins

posterior cervical venous plexus

internal jugular vein

sternocleidomastoid vein

bulb of internal jugular vein

transverse cervical vein

suprascapular vein

venous plexus

thoraco-acromial vein

cephalic brachial vein

axillary vein

343

A

VENOUS SYSTEM (III). HEAD and NECK (II)

ANTERIOR VIEW

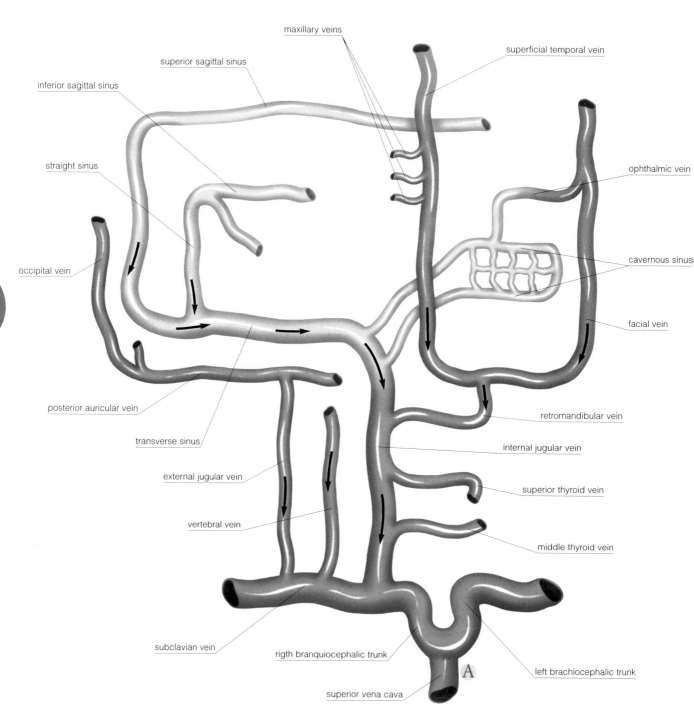

maxillary veins

superficial temporal vein

superior sagittal sinus

inferior sagittal sinus

ophthalmic vein

straight sinus

cavernous sinus

occipital vein

facial vein

posterior auricular vein

retromandibular vein

transverse sinus

internal jugular vein

external jugular vein

superior thyroid vein

vertebral vein

middle thyroid vein

subclavian vein

rigth branquiocephalic trunk

left brachiocephalic trunk

superior vena cava

A

344

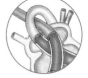

VENOUS SYSTEM (IV). HEAD and NECK (III)

LEFT LATERAL VIEW

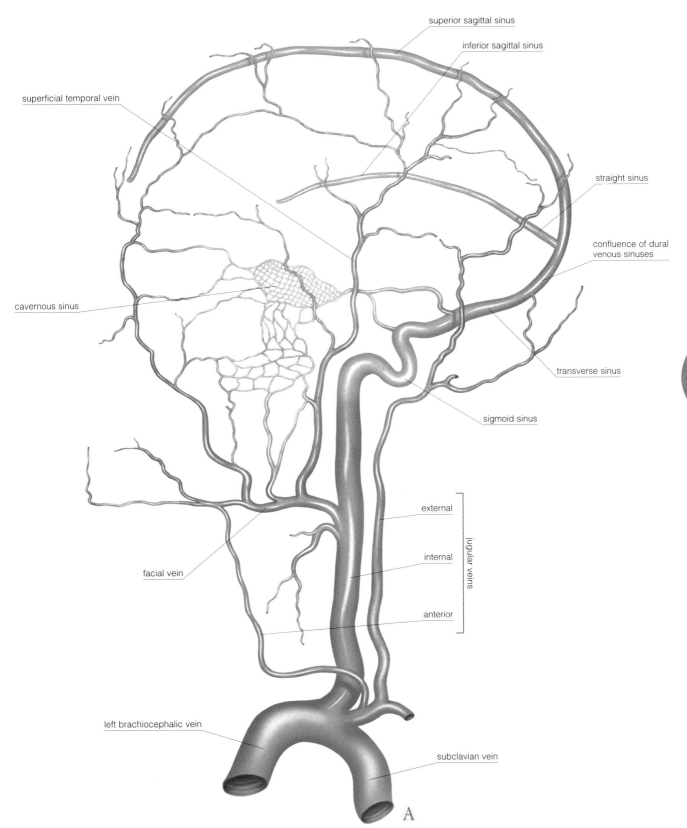

superior sagittal sinus

inferior sagittal sinus

superficial temporal vein

straight sinus

confluence of dural venous sinuses

cavernous sinus

transverse sinus

sigmoid sinus

external

internal

anterior

jugular veins

facial vein

left brachiocephalic vein

subclavian vein

A

345

VENOUS SYSTEM (V). HEAD and NECK (IV)

LEFT LATERAL VIEW

346

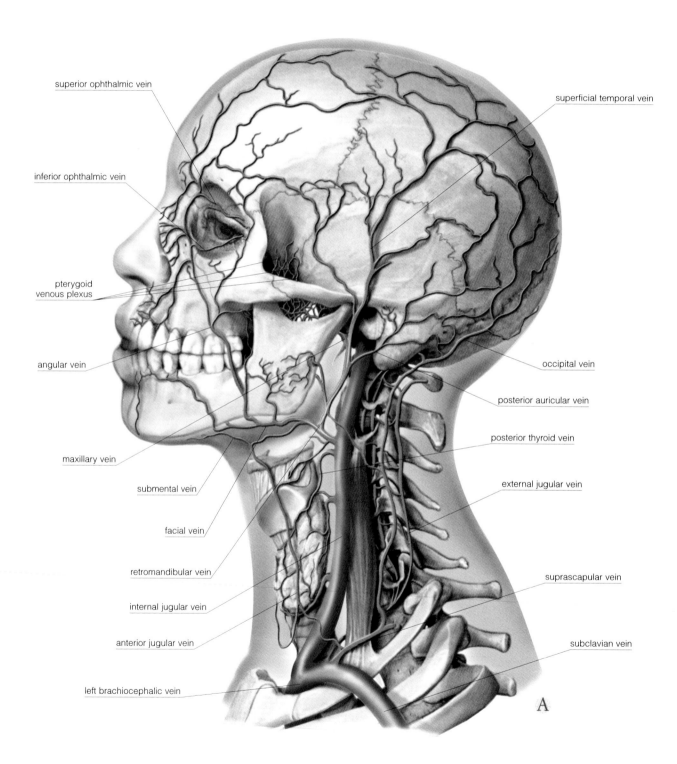

superior ophthalmic vein

superficial temporal vein

inferior ophthalmic vein

pterygoid
venous plexus

angular vein

occipital vein

posterior auricular vein

posterior thyroid vein

maxillary vein

external jugular vein

submental vein

facial vein

retromandibular vein

suprascapular vein

internal jugular vein

anterior jugular vein

subclavian vein

left brachiocephalic vein

A

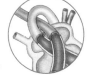

VENOUS SYSTEM (VI). HEAD and NECK (V)

LEFT LATERAL VIEW

drainage of the pharyngeal region

The veins of the pharynx form a exterior plexus and one over the constrictor muscles and the fascia pharyngobasilar, being this fascia inmediatelly under the mucous membrane. These plexus flow in the pterygoid plexus and the internal jugular vein. The facial vein, before flows in the internal jugular vein, generally it anastomoses itself with the ophthalmic veins, picks the blood from the face and receives the flows of the retromandibular vein, which tributaries are the superficial temporal veins and the pterigoid plexus. Often there is an anastomosis between the retromandibular vein and the external jugular.

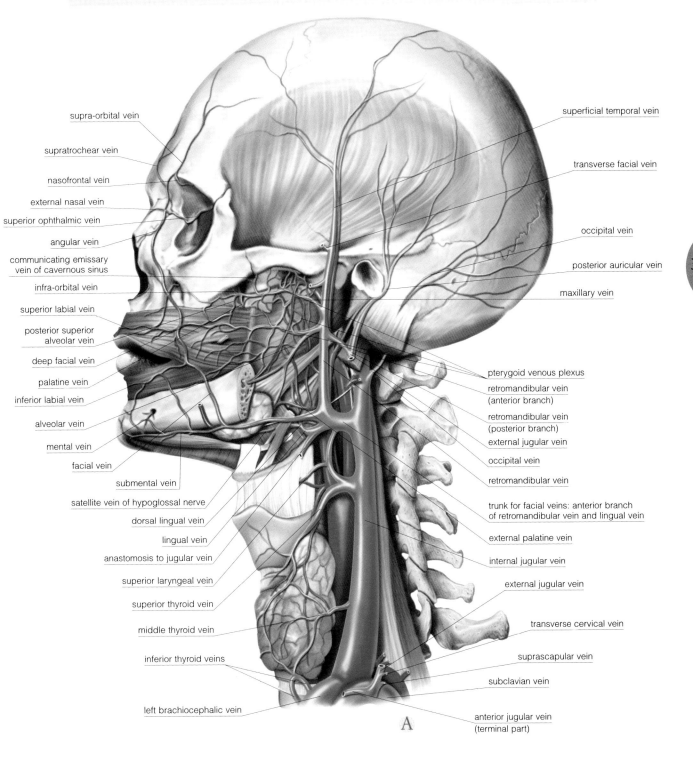

supra-orbital vein

supratrochear vein

nasofrontal vein

external nasal vein

superior ophthalmic vein

angular vein

communicating emissary
vein of cavernous sinus

infra-orbital vein

superior labial vein

posterior superior
alveolar vein

deep facial vein

palatine vein

inferior labial vein

alveolar vein

mental vein

facial vein

submental vein

satellite vein of hypoglossal nerve

dorsal lingual vein

lingual vein

anastomosis to jugular vein

superior laryngeal vein

superior thyroid vein

middle thyroid vein

inferior thyroid veins

left brachiocephalic vein

superficial temporal vein

transverse facial vein

occipital vein

posterior auricular vein

maxillary vein

pterygoid venous plexus

retromandibular vein
(anterior branch)

retromandibular vein
(posterior branch)

external jugular vein

occipital vein

retromandibular vein

trunk for facial veins: anterior branch
of retromandibular vein and lingual vein

external palatine vein

internal jugular vein

external jugular vein

transverse cervical vein

suprascapular vein

subclavian vein

anterior jugular vein
(terminal part)

347

A

VENOUS SYSTEM (VII). HEAD and NECK (VI)

RIGHT LATERAL SUPERFICIAL VIEW

drainage of head and neck

Are three the pair of veins that picks the major part of the blood of the head and the neck: the external jugular veins -that flow in the subclavian veins-, the internal jugular veins -that are the biggest veins of the head and the neck- and the vertebral veins- that drain the cervical veins, the spinal medulla and some small muscles of the neck and pour out in the brachiocephalic trunk-. Even though most of the veian and arteries of this zone are denominated in the same way (facial, occipital, temporal superficial, etc.). Their communications and their routes are substantially different.

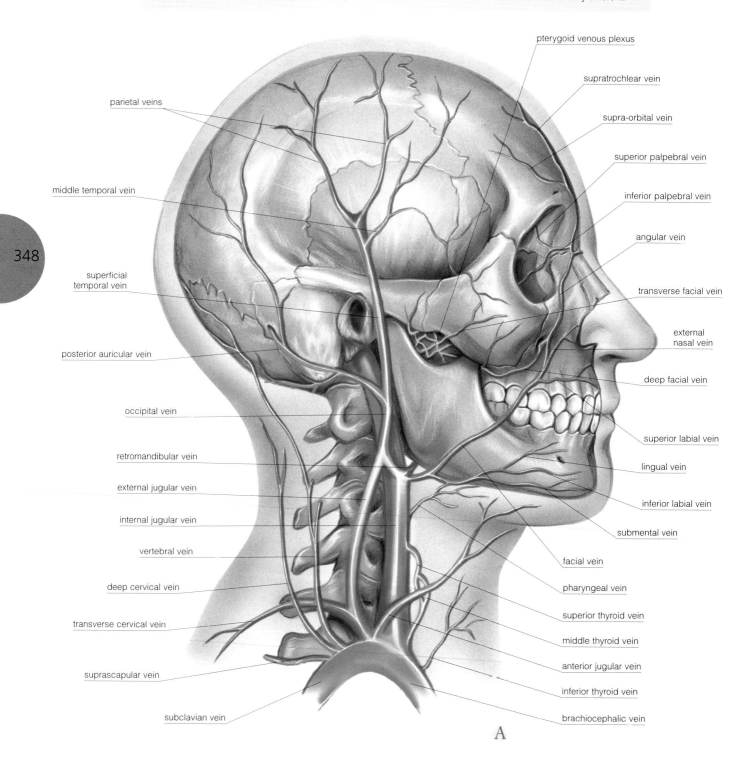

pterygoid venous plexus

supratrochlear vein

supra-orbital vein

superior palpebral vein

inferior palpebral vein

angular vein

transverse facial vein

external nasal vein

deep facial vein

superior labial vein

lingual vein

inferior labial vein

submental vein

facial vein

pharyngeal vein

superior thyroid vein

middle thyroid vein

anterior jugular vein

inferior thyroid vein

brachiocephalic vein

parietal veins

middle temporal vein

superficial temporal vein

posterior auricular vein

occipital vein

retromandibular vein

external jugular vein

internal jugular vein

vertebral vein

deep cervical vein

transverse cervical vein

suprascapular vein

subclavian vein

348

A

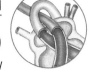

VENOUS SYSTEM (VIII). HEAD and NECK (VII)
LEFT LATERAL DEEP VIEW

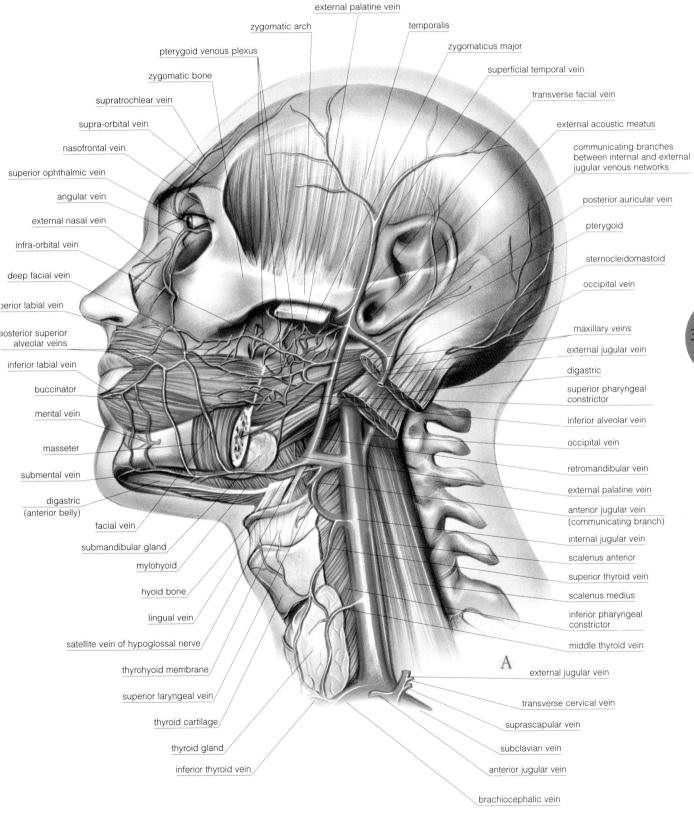

external palatine vein

zygomatic arch

temporalis

pterygoid venous plexus

zygomaticus major

zygomatic bone

superficial temporal vein

supratrochlear vein

transverse facial vein

supra-orbital vein

external acoustic meatus

nasofrontal vein

communicating branches between internal and external jugular venous networks

superior ophthalmic vein

angular vein

posterior auricular vein

external nasal vein

pterygoid

infra-orbital vein

sternocleidomastoid

deep facial vein

occipital vein

perior labial vein

maxillary veins

posterior superior alveolar veins

external jugular vein

digastric

inferior labial vein

superior pharyngeal constrictor

buccinator

inferior alveolar vein

mental vein

occipital vein

masseter

retromandibular vein

submental vein

external palatine vein

digastric (anterior belly)

anterior jugular vein (communicating branch)

facial vein

internal jugular vein

submandibular gland

scalenus anterior

mylohyoid

superior thyroid vein

hyoid bone

scalenus medius

lingual vein

inferior pharyngeal constrictor

satellite vein of hypoglossal nerve

middle thyroid vein

thyrohyoid membrane

A

external jugular vein

superior laryngeal vein

transverse cervical vein

thyroid cartilage

suprascapular vein

thyroid gland

subclavian vein

inferior thyroid vein

anterior jugular vein

brachiocephalic vein

349

VENOUS SYSTEM (IX). HEAD and NECK (VIII)

LEFT LATERAL SUPERFICIAL VIEW

350

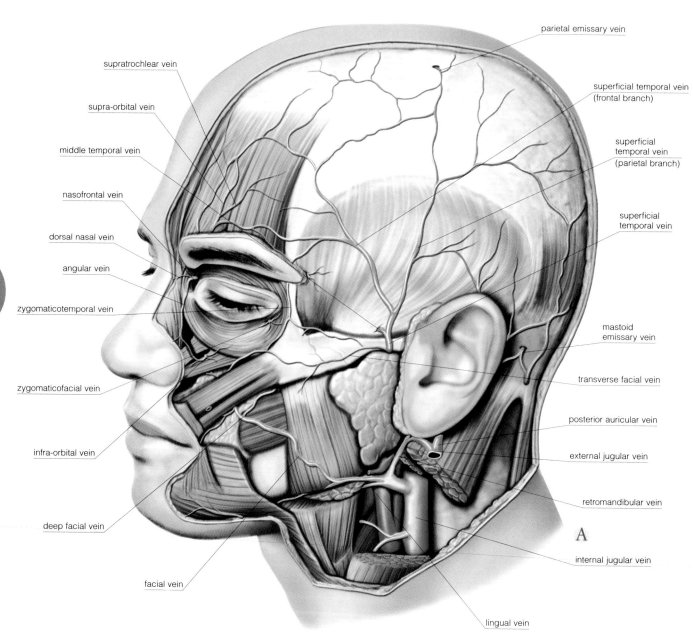

parietal emissary vein

supratrochlear vein

superficial temporal vein
(frontal branch)

supra-orbital vein

superficial
temporal vein
(parietal branch)

middle temporal vein

nasofrontal vein

superficial
temporal vein

dorsal nasal vein

angular vein

zygomaticotemporal vein

mastoid
emissary vein

zygomaticofacial vein

transverse facial vein

posterior auricular vein

external jugular vein

infra-orbital vein

retromandibular vein

deep facial vein

A

internal jugular vein

facial vein

lingual vein

VENOUS SYSTEM (X). HEAD and NECK (IX)

LEFT LATERAL VIEW

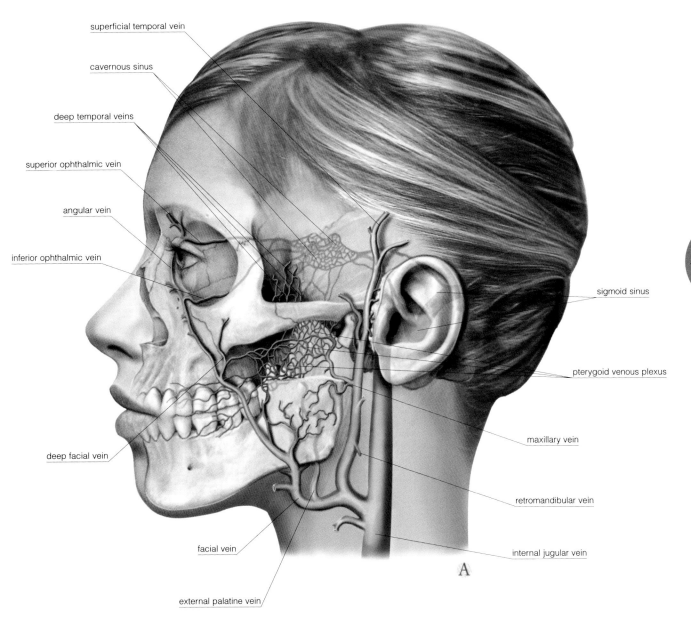

superficial temporal vein

cavernous sinus

deep temporal veins

superior ophthalmic vein

angular vein

inferior ophthalmic vein

sigmoid sinus

pterygoid venous plexus

maxillary vein

deep facial vein

retromandibular vein

facial vein

internal jugular vein

A

external palatine vein

351

VENOUS SYSTEM (XI). BRAIN

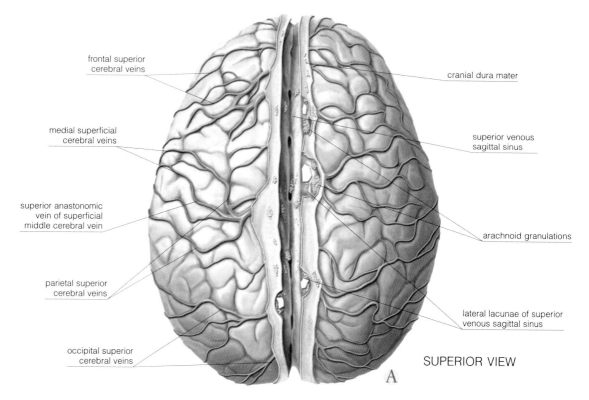

frontal superior cerebral veins

cranial dura mater

medial superficial cerebral veins

superior venous sagittal sinus

superior anastonomic vein of superficial middle cerebral vein

arachnoid granulations

parietal superior cerebral veins

lateral lacunae of superior venous sagittal sinus

occipital superior cerebral veins

SUPERIOR VIEW

A

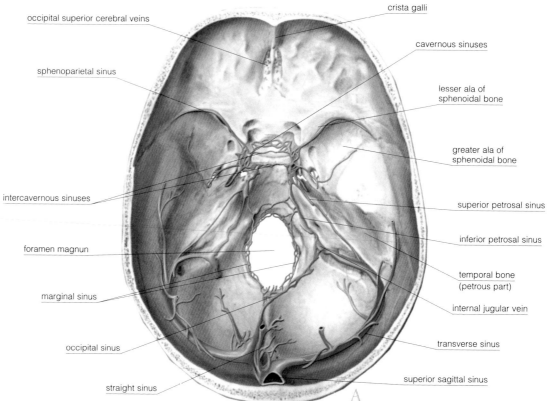

occipital superior cerebral veins

crista galli

sphenoparietal sinus

cavernous sinuses

lesser ala of sphenoidal bone

greater ala of sphenoidal bone

intercavernous sinuses

superior petrosal sinus

inferior petrosal sinus

foramen magnun

temporal bone (petrous part)

marginal sinus

internal jugular vein

occipital sinus

transverse sinus

superior sagittal sinus

straight sinus

A

CRANIAL BASE. DURAL VENOUS SINUSES
SUPERIOR VIEW

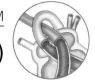

VENOUS SYSTEM (XII)

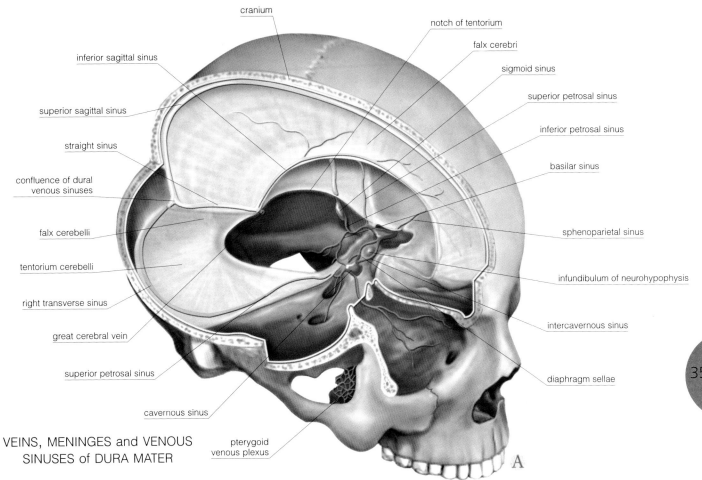

cranium

notch of tentorium

falx cerebri

inferior sagittal sinus

sigmoid sinus

superior petrosal sinus

superior sagittal sinus

inferior petrosal sinus

straight sinus

basilar sinus

confluence of dural
venous sinuses

sphenoparietal sinus

falx cerebelli

tentorium cerebelli

infundibulum of neurohypophysis

right transverse sinus

intercavernous sinus

great cerebral vein

diaphragm sellae

superior petrosal sinus

353

cavernous sinus

**VEINS, MENINGES and VENOUS
SINUSES of DURA MATER**

pterygoid
venous plexus

A

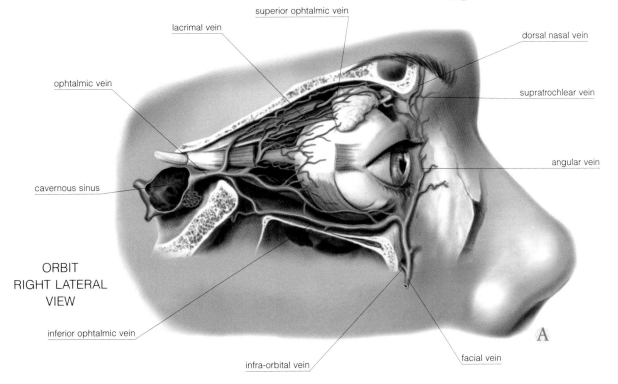

superior ophtalmic vein

lacrimal vein

dorsal nasal vein

ophtalmic vein

supratrochlear vein

angular vein

cavernous sinus

**ORBIT
RIGHT LATERAL
VIEW**

A

inferior ophtalmic vein

infra-orbital vein

facial vein

VENOUS SYSTEM (XIII). UPPER LIMB and THORAX

RIGHT UPPER LIMB. ANTERIOR VIEW

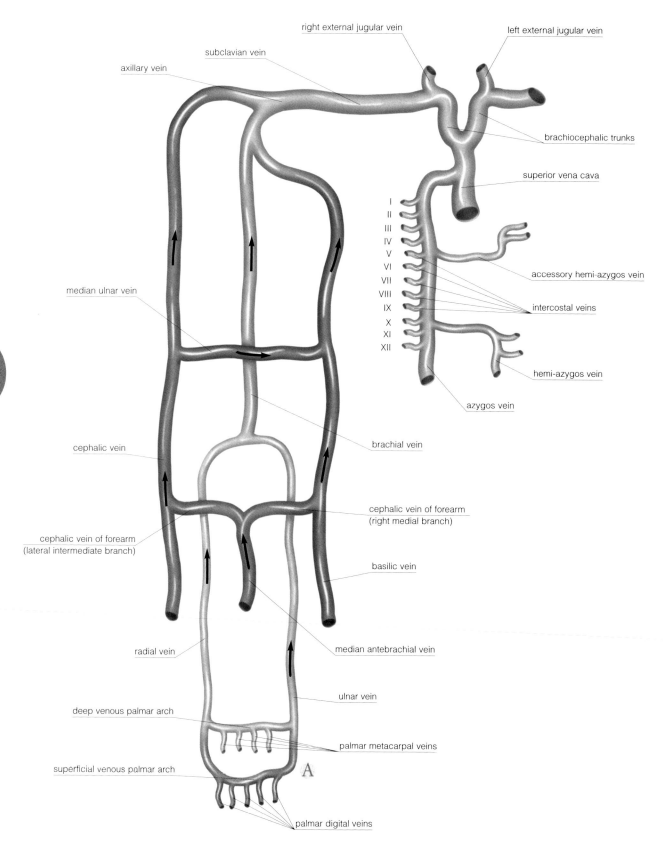

right external jugular vein

left external jugular vein

subclavian vein

axillary vein

brachiocephalic trunks

superior vena cava

I
II
III
IV
V
VI
VII
VIII
IX
X
XI
XII

accessory hemi-azygos vein

intercostal veins

median ulnar vein

hemi-azygos vein

azygos vein

cephalic vein

brachial vein

cephalic vein of forearm
(right medial branch)

cephalic vein of forearm
(lateral intermediate branch)

basilic vein

radial vein

median antebrachial vein

ulnar vein

deep venous palmar arch

palmar metacarpal veins

superficial venous palmar arch

A

palmar digital veins

354

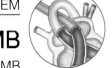

VENOUS SYSTEM (XIV). LOWER LIMB

RIGHT LOWER LIMB

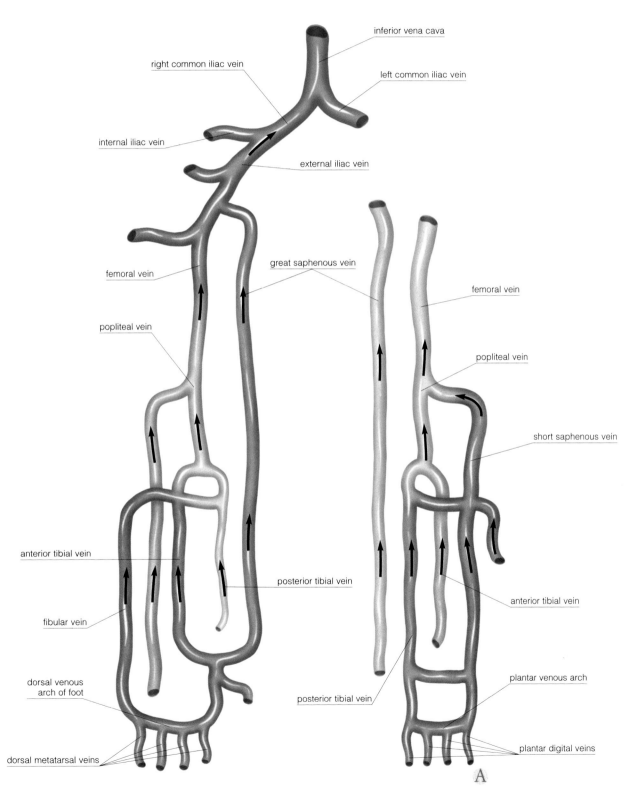

inferior vena cava

right common iliac vein

left common iliac vein

internal iliac vein

external iliac vein

great saphenous vein

femoral vein

femoral vein

popliteal vein

popliteal vein

short saphenous vein

anterior tibial vein

posterior tibial vein

anterior tibial vein

fibular vein

dorsal venous
arch of foot

plantar venous arch

posterior tibial vein

dorsal metatarsal veins

plantar digital veins

A

ANTERIOR VIEW

POSTERIOR VIEW

VENOUS SYSTEM (XV). UPPER LIMB (I)

RIGHT UPPER LIMB. DORSAL VIEW

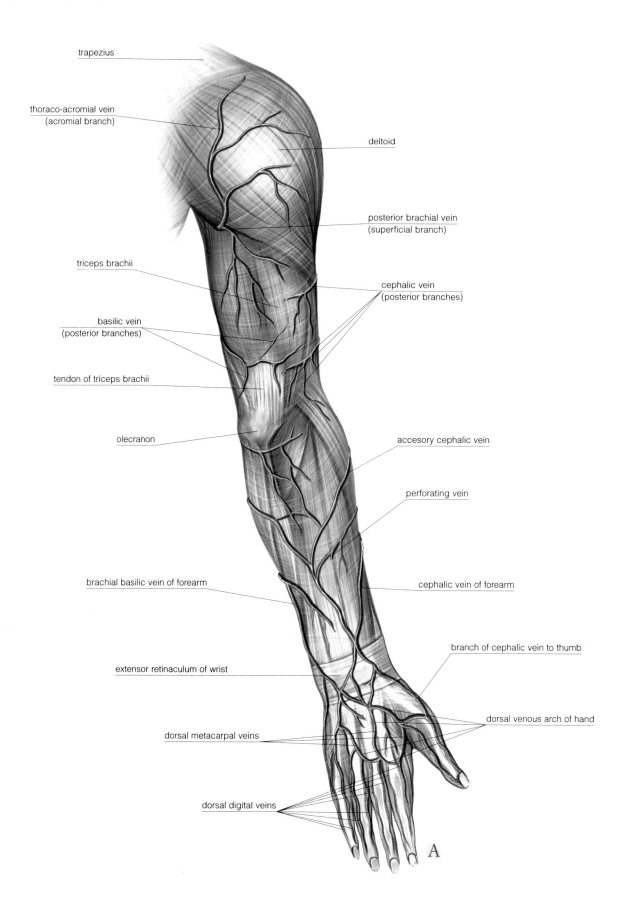

trapezius

thoraco-acromial vein
(acromial branch)

deltoid

posterior brachial vein
(superficial branch)

triceps brachii

cephalic vein
(posterior branches)

basilic vein
(posterior branches)

tendon of tríceps brachii

olecranon

accesory cephalic vein

perforating vein

brachial basilic vein of forearm

cephalic vein of forearm

branch of cephalic vein to thumb

extensor retinaculum of wrist

dorsal venous arch of hand

dorsal metacarpal veins

dorsal digital veins

A

356

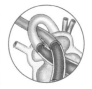

VENOUS SYSTEM (XVI). UPPER LIMB (II)

RIGHT UPPER LIMB. PALMAR VIEW

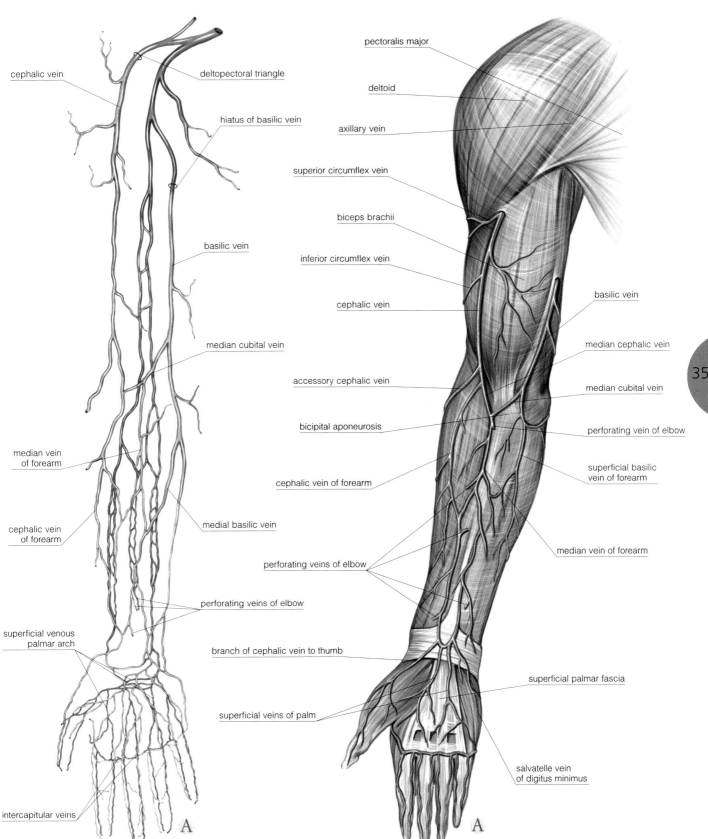

cephalic vein

deltopectoral triangle

hiatus of basilic vein

basilic vein

median cubital vein

median vein
of forearm

cephalic vein
of forearm

medial basilic vein

perforating veins of elbow

perforating veins of elbow

superficial venous
palmar arch

branch of cephalic vein to thumb

superficial veins of palm

intercapitular veins

A

pectoralis major

deltoid

axillary vein

superior circumflex vein

biceps brachii

inferior circumflex vein

cephalic vein

accessory cephalic vein

bicipital aponeurosis

cephalic vein of forearm

basilic vein

median cephalic vein

median cubital vein

perforating vein of elbow

superficial basilic
vein of forearm

median vein of forearm

superficial palmar fascia

salvatelle vein
of digitus minimus

A

357

VENOUS SYSTEM (XVII). UPPER LIMB (III). HAND (I)

RIGHT UPPER LIMB. PALMAR VIEW

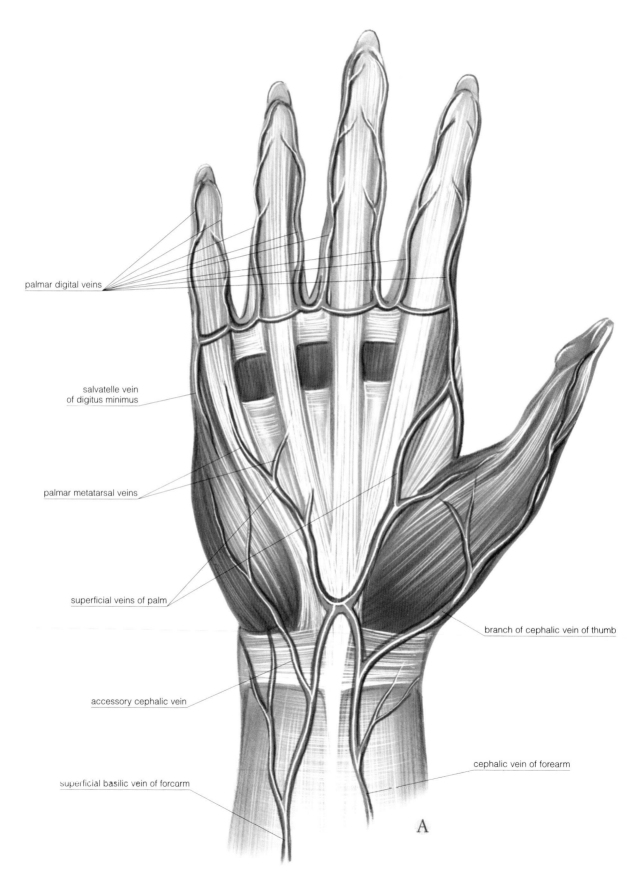

palmar digital veins

salvatelle vein
of digitus minimus

palmar metatarsal veins

superficial veins of palm

branch of cephalic vein of thumb

accessory cephalic vein

cephalic vein of forearm

superficial basilic vein of forearm

A

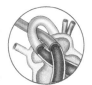

VENOUS SYSTEM (XVIII). UPPER LIMB (IV). HAND (II)

RIGHT UPPER LIMB. DORSAL VIEW

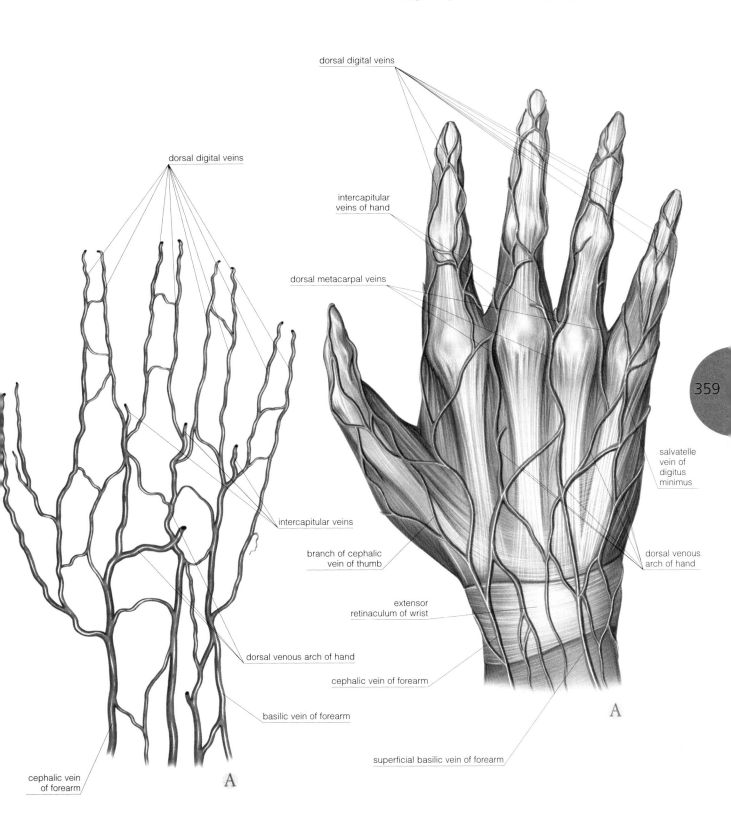

dorsal digital veins

dorsal digital veins

intercapitular
veins of hand

dorsal metacarpal veins

intercapitular veins

branch of cephalic
vein of thumb

extensor
retinaculum of wrist

dorsal venous arch of hand

cephalic vein of forearm

basilic vein of forearm

salvatelle
vein of
digitus
minimus

dorsal venous
arch of hand

superficial basilic vein of forearm

cephalic vein
of forearm

359

A

A

VENOUS SYSTEM (XIX). UPPER LIMB (V)

RIGHT UPPER LIMB. ANTERIOR VIEW

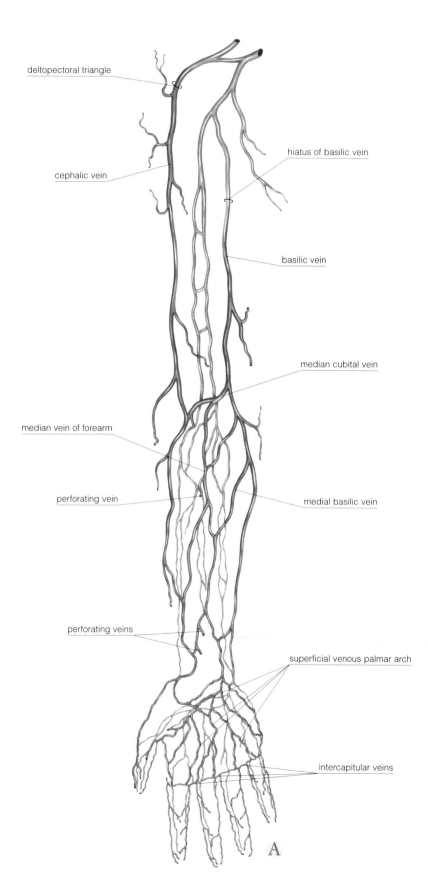

deltopectoral triangle

cephalic vein

hiatus of basilic vein

basilic vein

median cubital vein

median vein of forearm

perforating vein

medial basilic vein

perforating veins

superficial venous palmar arch

intercapitular veins

A

360

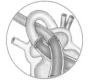

VENOUS SYSTEM (XX). LOWER LIMB (I)

RIGHT LOWER LIMB. ANTERIOR DEEP VIEW

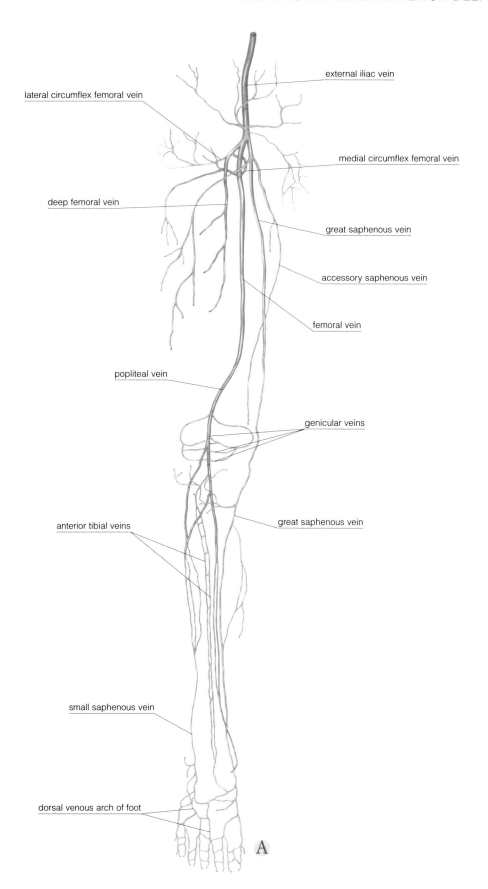

external iliac vein

lateral circumflex femoral vein

medial circumflex femoral vein

deep femoral vein

great saphenous vein

accessory saphenous vein

femoral vein

popliteal vein

genicular veins

great saphenous vein

anterior tibial veins

small saphenous vein

dorsal venous arch of foot

A

361

VENOUS SYSTEM (XXI). LOWER LIMB (II)

RIGHT LOWER LIMB. ANTERIOR SUPERFICIAL VIEW

362

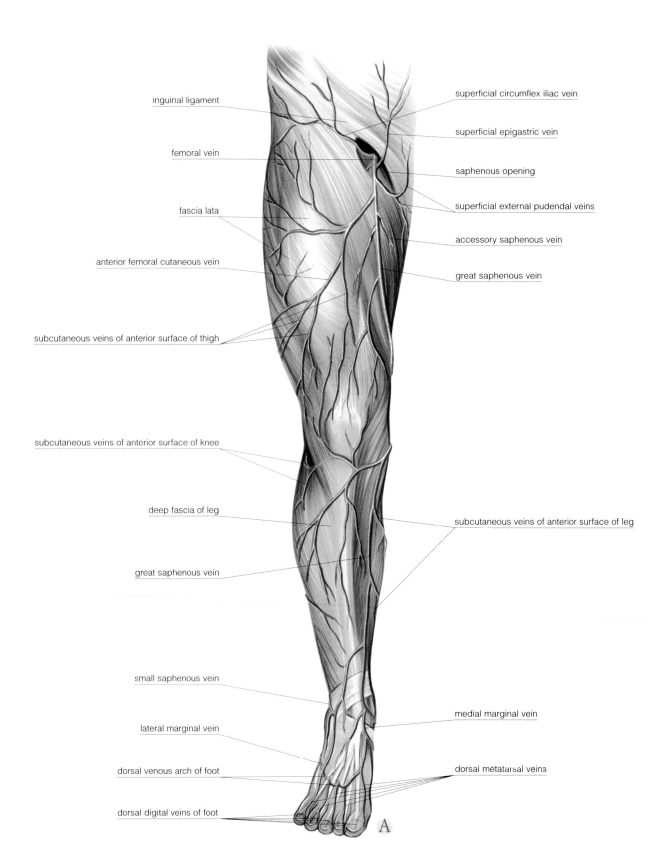

inguinal ligament

femoral vein

fascia lata

anterior femoral cutaneous vein

subcutaneous veins of anterior surface of thigh

subcutaneous veins of anterior surface of knee

deep fascia of leg

great saphenous vein

small saphenous vein

lateral marginal vein

dorsal venous arch of foot

dorsal digital veins of foot

superficial circumflex iliac vein

superficial epigastric vein

saphenous opening

superficial external pudendal veins

accessory saphenous vein

great saphenous vein

subcutaneous veins of anterior surface of leg

medial marginal vein

dorsal metatarsal veins

A

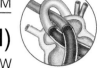

VENOUS SYSTEM (XXII). LOWER LIMB (III)

RIGHT LOWER LIMB. POSTERIOR SUPERFICIAL VIEW

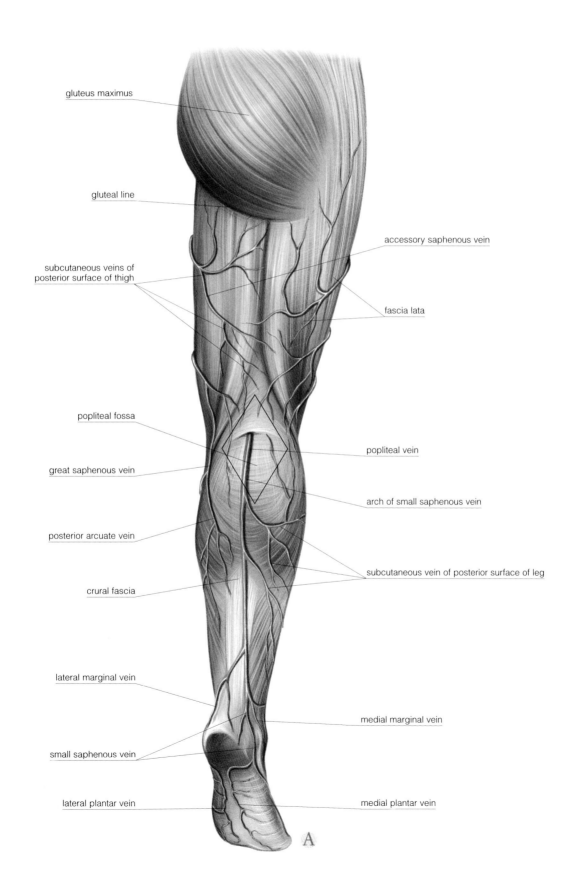

gluteus maximus

gluteal line

accessory saphenous vein

subcutaneous veins of
posterior surface of thigh

fascia lata

popliteal fossa

popliteal vein

great saphenous vein

arch of small saphenous vein

posterior arcuate vein

subcutaneous vein of posterior surface of leg

crural fascia

lateral marginal vein

medial marginal vein

small saphenous vein

lateral plantar vein

medial plantar vein

A

363

VENOUS SYSTEM (XXIII). MALE PELVIS
ANTERIOR VIEW

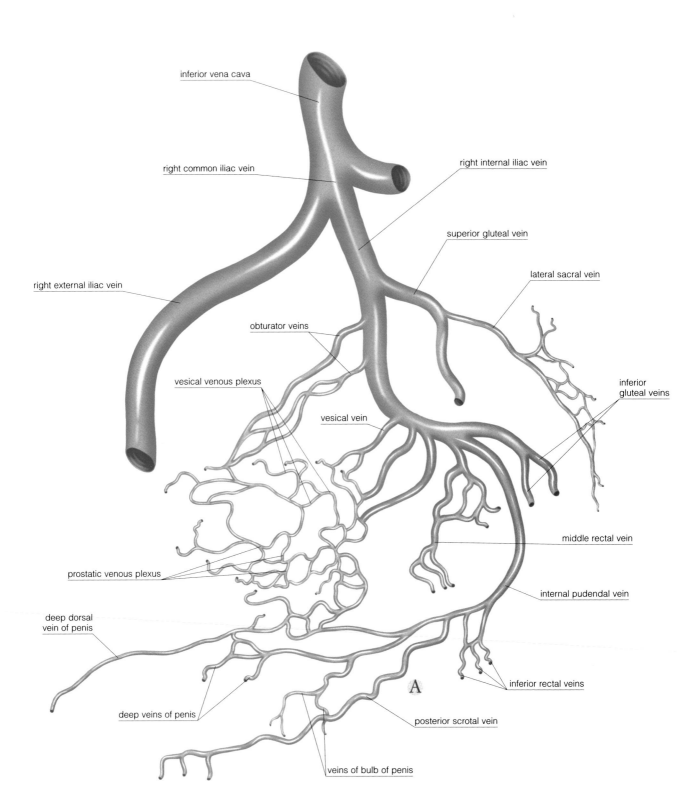

inferior vena cava

right common iliac vein

right internal iliac vein

superior gluteal vein

lateral sacral vein

right external iliac vein

obturator veins

vesical venous plexus

inferior gluteal veins

vesical vein

middle rectal vein

prostatic venous plexus

internal pudendal vein

deep dorsal vein of penis

inferior rectal veins

deep veins of penis

A

posterior scrotal vein

veins of bulb of penis

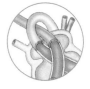

VENOUS SYSTEM (XXIV). PELVIS
POSTERIOR VIEW

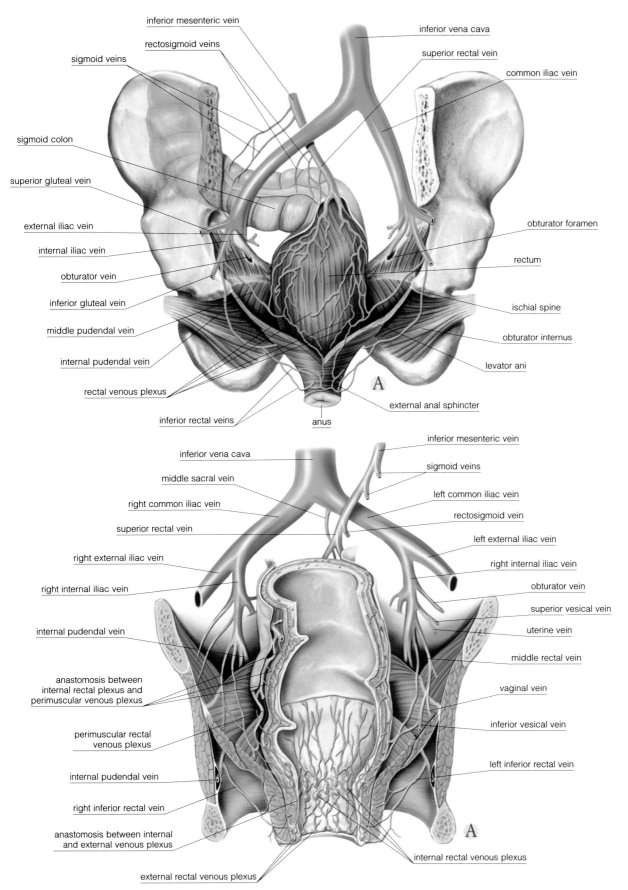

inferior mesenteric vein

rectosigmoid veins

sigmoid veins

sigmoid colon

superior gluteal vein

external iliac vein

internal iliac vein

obturator vein

inferior gluteal vein

middle pudendal vein

internal pudendal vein

rectal venous plexus

inferior rectal veins

anus

inferior vena cava

superior rectal vein

common iliac vein

obturator foramen

rectum

ischial spine

obturator internus

levator ani

external anal sphincter

A

inferior mesenteric vein

inferior vena cava

sigmoid veins

middle sacral vein

left common iliac vein

right common iliac vein

rectosigmoid vein

superior rectal vein

left external iliac vein

right external iliac vein

right internal iliac vein

right internal iliac vein

obturator vein

internal pudendal vein

superior vesical vein

uterine vein

anastomosis between
internal rectal plexus and
perimuscular venous plexus

middle rectal vein

vaginal vein

perimuscular rectal
venous plexus

inferior vesical vein

internal pudendal vein

left inferior rectal vein

right inferior rectal vein

anastomosis between internal
and external venous plexus

internal rectal venous plexus

external rectal venous plexus

A

VENOUS SYSTEM (XXV). VERTEBRAL VENOUS PLEXUS
POSTERIOR VIEW

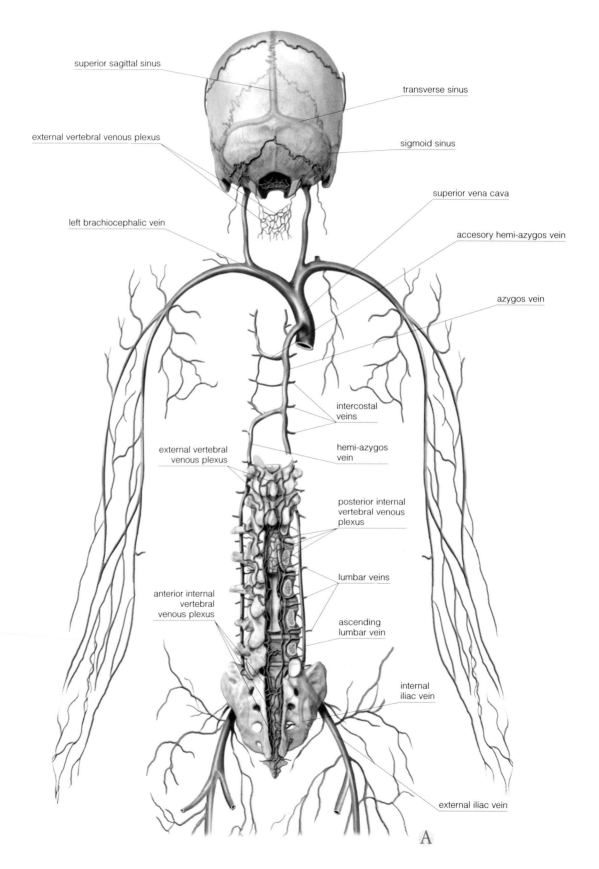

superior sagittal sinus

transverse sinus

external vertebral venous plexus

sigmoid sinus

superior vena cava

left brachiocephalic vein

accesory hemi-azygos vein

azygos vein

intercostal veins

external vertebral venous plexus

hemi-azygos vein

posterior internal vertebral venous plexus

lumbar veins

anterior internal vertebral venous plexus

ascending lumbar vein

internal iliac vein

external iliac vein

A

366

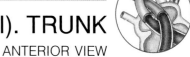

VENOUS SYSTEM (XXVI). TRUNK
ANTERIOR VIEW

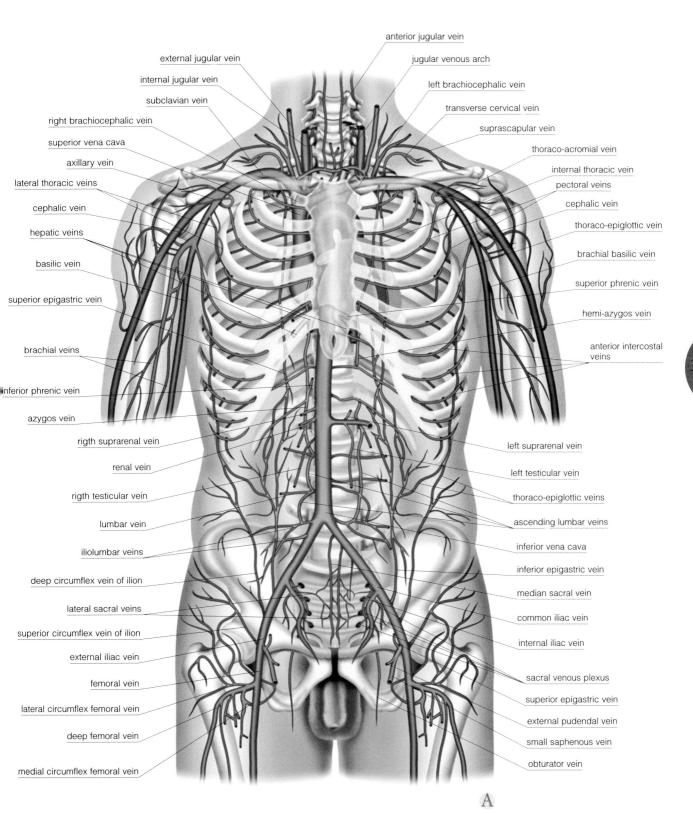

anterior jugular vein

external jugular vein

jugular venous arch

internal jugular vein

left brachiocephalic vein

subclavian vein

transverse cervical vein

right brachiocephalic vein

suprascapular vein

superior vena cava

thoraco-acromial vein

axillary vein

internal thoracic vein

lateral thoracic veins

pectoral veins

cephalic vein

cephalic vein

hepatic veins

thoraco-epiglottic vein

basilic vein

brachial basilic vein

superior epigastric vein

superior phrenic vein

hemi-azygos vein

brachial veins

anterior intercostal veins

inferior phrenic vein

367

azygos vein

rigth suprarenal vein

left suprarenal vein

renal vein

left testicular vein

rigth testicular vein

thoraco-epiglottic veins

lumbar vein

ascending lumbar veins

iliolumbar veins

inferior vena cava

deep circumflex vein of ilion

inferior epigastric vein

median sacral vein

lateral sacral veins

common iliac vein

superior circumflex vein of ilion

internal iliac vein

external iliac vein

sacral venous plexus

femoral vein

superior epigastric vein

lateral circumflex femoral vein

external pudendal vein

deep femoral vein

small saphenous vein

medial circumflex femoral vein

obturator vein

A

VENOUS SYSTEM (XXVII). VENA CAVA and FLOWINGS

FEMALE SEX. ANTERIOR VIEW

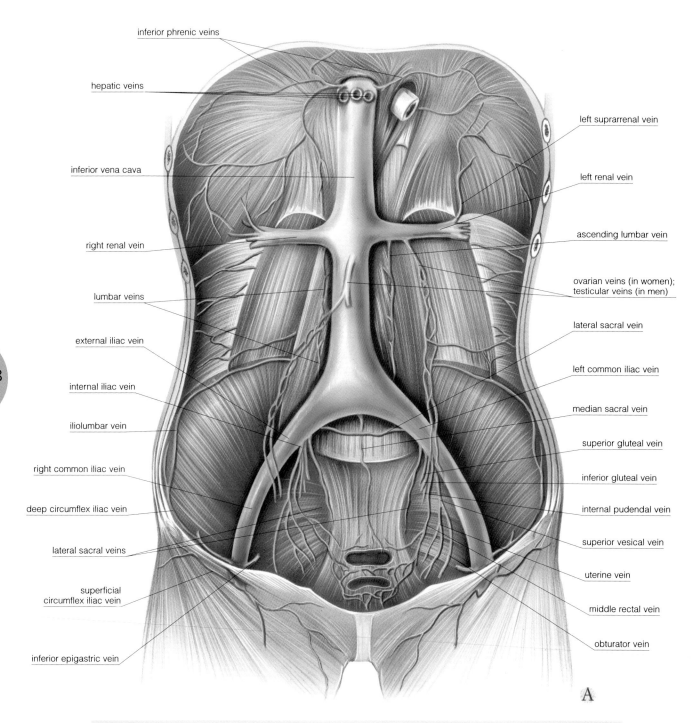

inferior phrenic veins

hepatic veins

inferior vena cava

right renal vein

lumbar veins

external iliac vein

internal iliac vein

iliolumbar vein

right common iliac vein

deep circumflex iliac vein

lateral sacral veins

superficial
circumflex iliac vein

inferior epigastric vein

left suprarrenal vein

left renal vein

ascending lumbar vein

ovarian veins (in women);
testicular veins (in men)

lateral sacral vein

left common iliac vein

median sacral vein

superior gluteal vein

inferior gluteal vein

internal pudendal vein

superior vesical vein

uterine vein

middle rectal vein

obturator vein

A

vena cava

Venous duct of major caliber, where at the end goes to flow all the venous blood, that will be poured out in the right atrium. The venous net is formed for a series of ducts that begins being tiny (capillaries) and then flow in other ducts of major caliber (venules) which, at the same time, pour out in others bigger (veins). Also the veins, in the way of their journey, goes growing progressively of caliber to increase their capacity and with that be able to receive a caudal of blood every time major, until flow in big ducts in which a great quantity of blood pass by. Among these last conducts, the cava veins are the most important. Thus the vena cava superior picks all the venous blood from the superior half of the body and the vena cava inferior does the same with the inferior half. Both flow in the right atrium of the heart, from where will pass to the lungs to be oxygenated and then come back to be expelled for all the body.

VENOUS SYSTEM (XXVIII)
THORAX and ABDOMEN (I). ANTERIOR WALL
MALE SEX. ANTERIOR VIEW

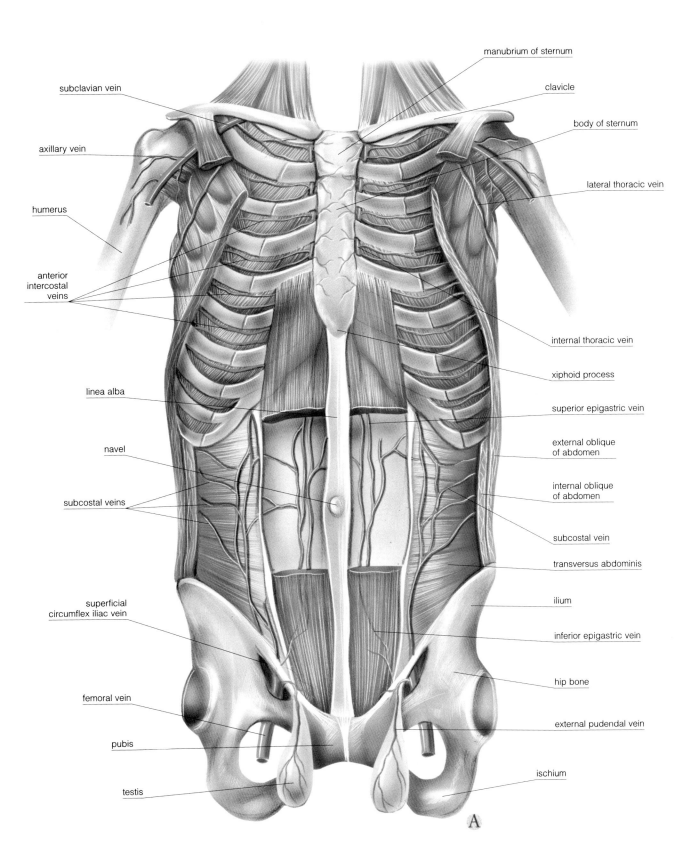

manubrium of sternum

subclavian vein

clavicle

axillary vein

body of sternum

humerus

lateral thoracic vein

anterior
intercostal
veins

internal thoracic vein

369

xiphoid process

linea alba

superior epigastric vein

external oblique
of abdomen

navel

internal oblique
of abdomen

subcostal veins

subcostal vein

transversus abdominis

superficial
circumflex iliac vein

ilium

inferior epigastric vein

femoral vein

hip bone

pubis

external pudendal vein

testis

ischium

A

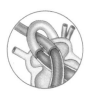

VENOUS SYSTEM (XXIX)
THORAX and ABDOMEN (II). COSTAL NETWORK (I)
ANTERIOR VIEW

370

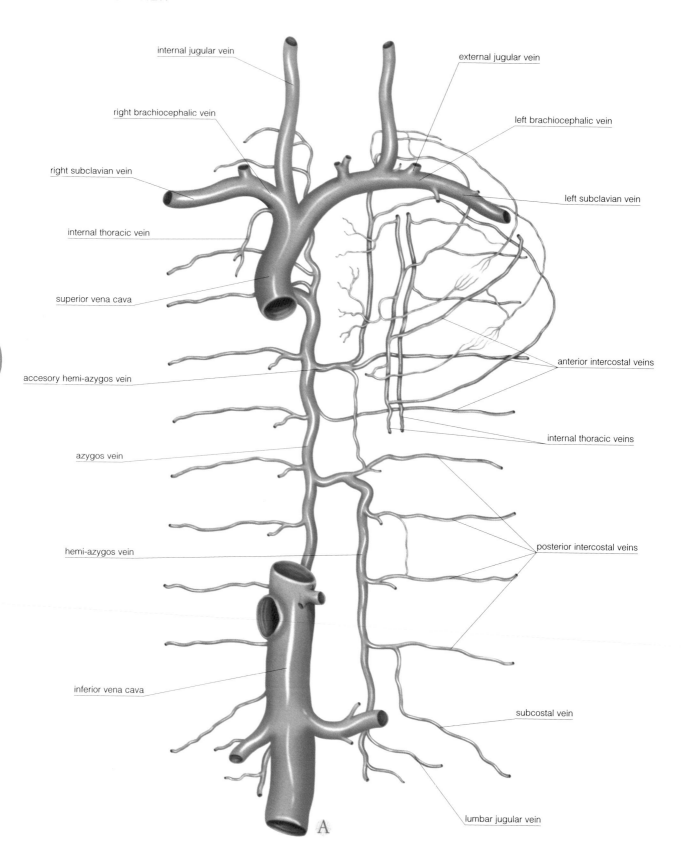

internal jugular vein

external jugular vein

right brachiocephalic vein

left brachiocephalic vein

right subclavian vein

left subclavian vein

internal thoracic vein

superior vena cava

anterior intercostal veins

accesory hemi-azygos vein

internal thoracic veins

azygos vein

hemi-azygos vein

posterior intercostal veins

inferior vena cava

subcostal vein

lumbar jugular vein

A

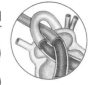

VENOUS SYSTEM (XXX)
THORAX and ABDOMEN (III). COSTAL NETWORK (II)
ANTERIOR VIEW

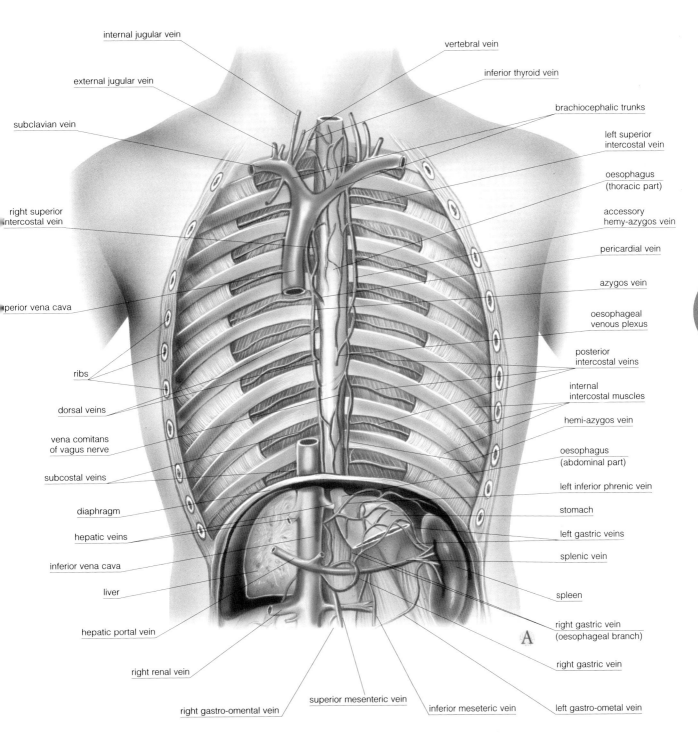

internal jugular vein

vertebral vein

inferior thyroid vein

external jugular vein

brachiocephalic trunks

subclavian vein

left superior
intercostal vein

right superior
intercostal vein

oesophagus
(thoracic part)

accessory
hemy-azygos vein

pericardial vein

azygos vein

perior vena cava

oesophageal
venous plexus

ribs

posterior
intercostal veins

dorsal veins

internal
intercostal muscles

vena comitans
of vagus nerve

hemi-azygos vein

subcostal veins

oesophagus
(abdominal part)

diaphragm

left inferior phrenic vein

hepatic veins

stomach

inferior vena cava

left gastric veins

liver

splenic vein

hepatic portal vein

spleen

right gastric vein
(oesophageal branch)

right renal vein

A

right gastric vein

right gastro-omental vein

superior mesenteric vein

inferior meseteric vein

left gastro-ometal vein

VENOUS SYSTEM (XXXI). AZYGOS VEIN NETWORK

ANTERIOR VIEW

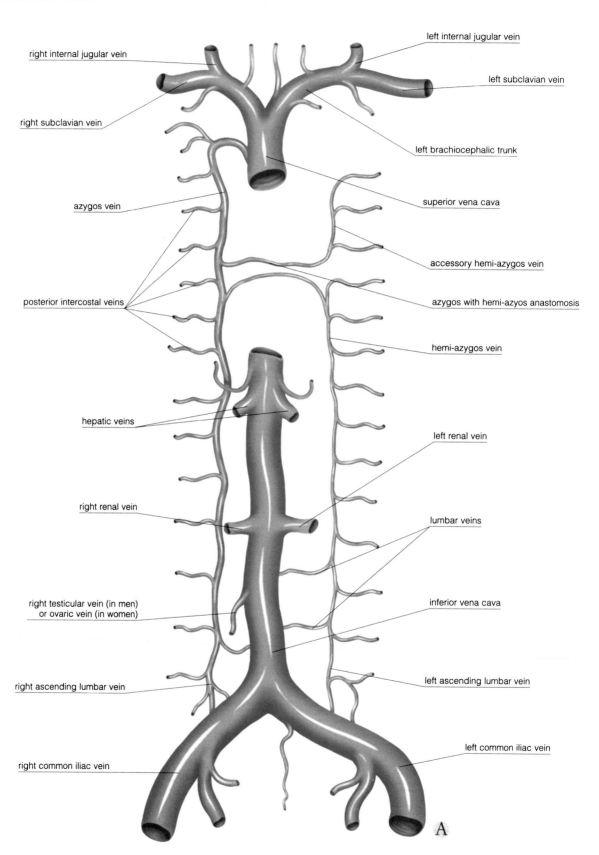

right internal jugular vein

left internal jugular vein

right subclavian vein

left subclavian vein

left brachiocephalic trunk

azygos vein

superior vena cava

accessory hemi-azygos vein

posterior intercostal veins

azygos with hemi-azyos anastomosis

hemi-azygos vein

hepatic veins

left renal vein

right renal vein

lumbar veins

right testicular vein (in men)
or ovaric vein (in women)

inferior vena cava

right ascending lumbar vein

left ascending lumbar vein

left common iliac vein

right common iliac vein

A

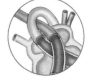

VENOUS SYSTEM (XXXII). THORAX

ANTERIOR VIEW

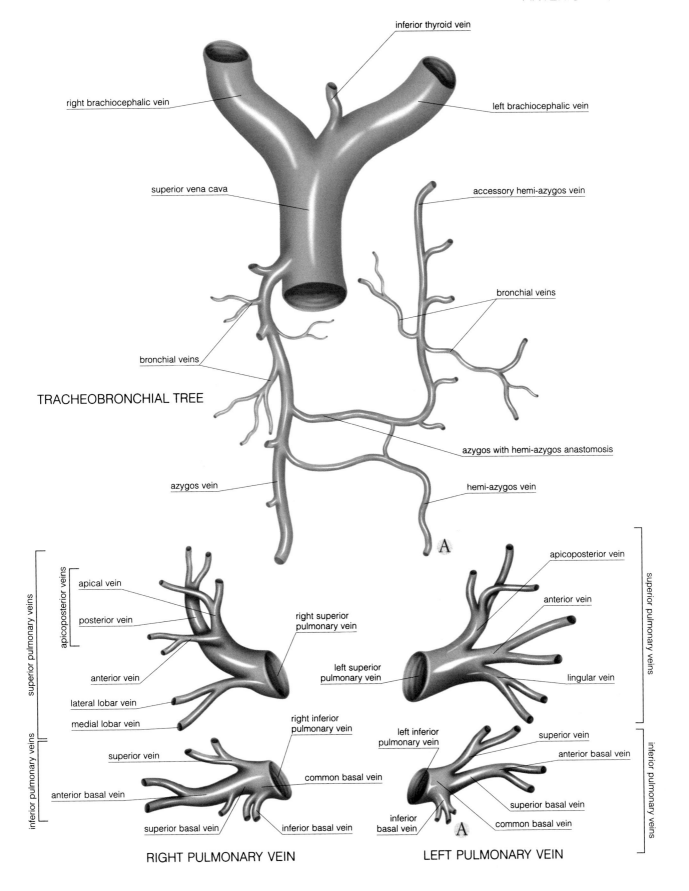

inferior thyroid vein

right brachiocephalic vein

left brachiocephalic vein

superior vena cava

accessory hemi-azygos vein

bronchial veins

TRACHEOBRONCHIAL TREE

bronchial veins

azygos with hemi-azygos anastomosis

azygos vein

hemi-azygos vein

superior pulmonary veins

apicoposterior veins

apical vein

posterior vein

right superior pulmonary vein

apicoposterior vein

anterior vein

anterior vein

left superior pulmonary vein

lateral lobar vein

medial lobar vein

lingular vein

inferior pulmonary veins

superior pulmonary veins

right inferior pulmonary vein

left inferior pulmonary vein

superior vein

superior vein

anterior basal vein

common basal vein

anterior basal vein

superior basal vein

inferior basal vein

inferior basal vein

superior basal vein

common basal vein

inferior pulmonary veins

RIGHT PULMONARY VEIN

LEFT PULMONARY VEIN

373

VENOUS SYSTEM (XXXIII). OESOPHAGUS
ANTERIOR VIEW

374

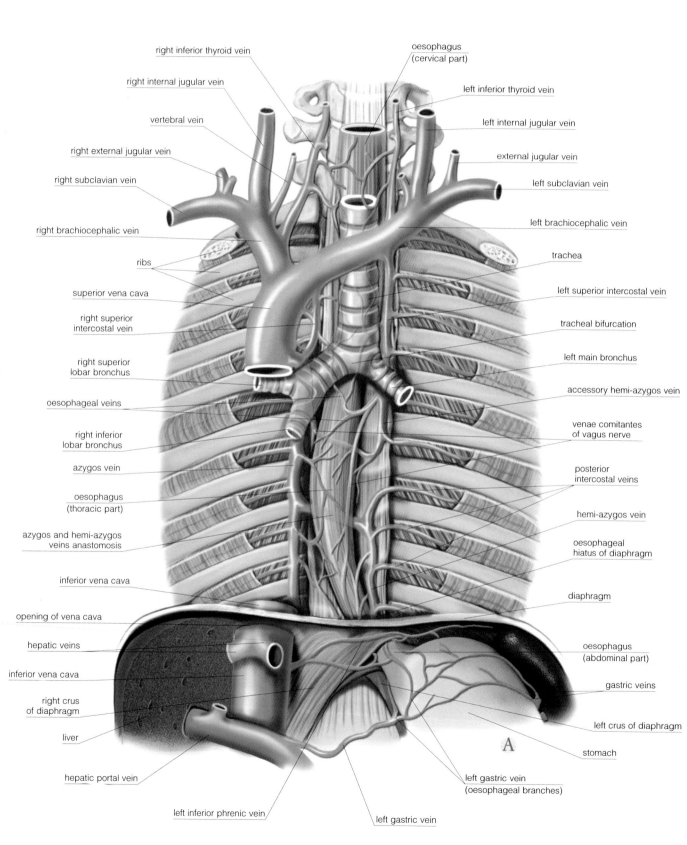

right inferior thyroid vein

right internal jugular vein

vertebral vein

right external jugular vein

right subclavian vein

right brachiocephalic vein

ribs

superior vena cava

right superior intercostal vein

right superior lobar bronchus

oesophageal veins

right inferior lobar bronchus

azygos vein

oesophagus (thoracic part)

azygos and hemi-azygos veins anastomosis

inferior vena cava

opening of vena cava

hepatic veins

inferior vena cava

right crus of diaphragm

liver

hepatic portal vein

left inferior phrenic vein

left gastric vein

oesophagus (cervical part)

left inferior thyroid vein

left internal jugular vein

external jugular vein

left subclavian vein

left brachiocephalic vein

trachea

left superior intercostal vein

tracheal bifurcation

left main bronchus

accessory hemi-azygos vein

venae comitantes of vagus nerve

posterior intercostal veins

hemi-azygos vein

oesophageal hiatus of diaphragm

diaphragm

oesophagus (abdominal part)

gastric veins

left crus of diaphragm

stomach

left gastric vein (oesophageal branches)

A

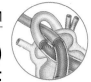

VENOUS SYSTEM (XXXIV)
TRACHEOBRONCHIAL TREE
ANTERIOR VIEW

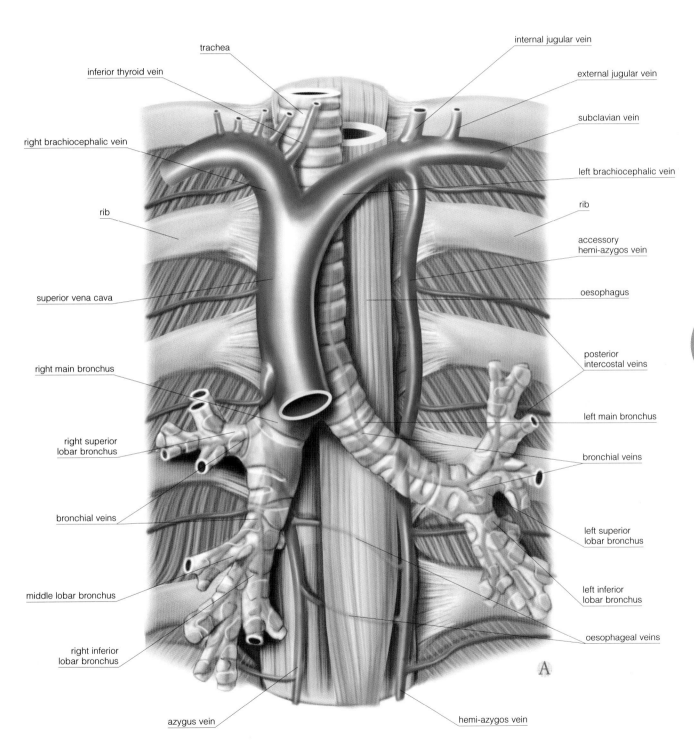

trachea

internal jugular vein

inferior thyroid vein

external jugular vein

subclavian vein

right brachiocephalic vein

left brachiocephalic vein

rib

rib

accessory
hemi-azygos vein

superior vena cava

oesophagus

posterior
intercostal veins

right main bronchus

left main bronchus

right superior
lobar bronchus

bronchial veins

bronchial veins

left superior
lobar bronchus

middle lobar bronchus

left inferior
lobar bronchus

right inferior
lobar bronchus

oesophageal veins

azygus vein

hemi-azygos vein

375

VENOUS SYSTEM (XXXV). INTERCOSTAL VEINS and VERTEBRAL VENOUS PLEXUS

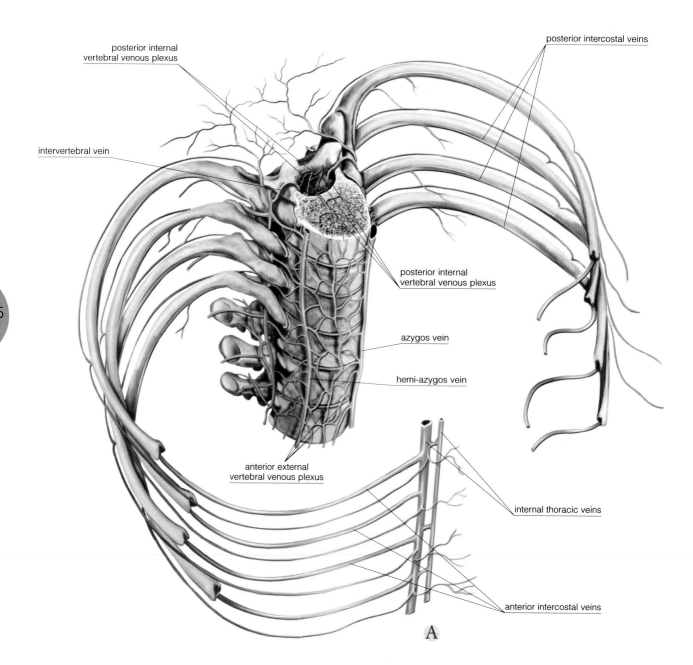

posterior intercostal veins

posterior internal vertebral venous plexus

intervertebral vein

posterior internal vertebral venous plexus

azygos vein

hemi-azygos vein

anterior external vertebral venous plexus

internal thoracic veins

anterior intercostal veins

A

ANTERIOR SUPERIOR VIEW

VENOUS SYSTEM (XXXVI). ABDOMEN
ANTERIOR VIEW

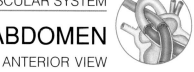

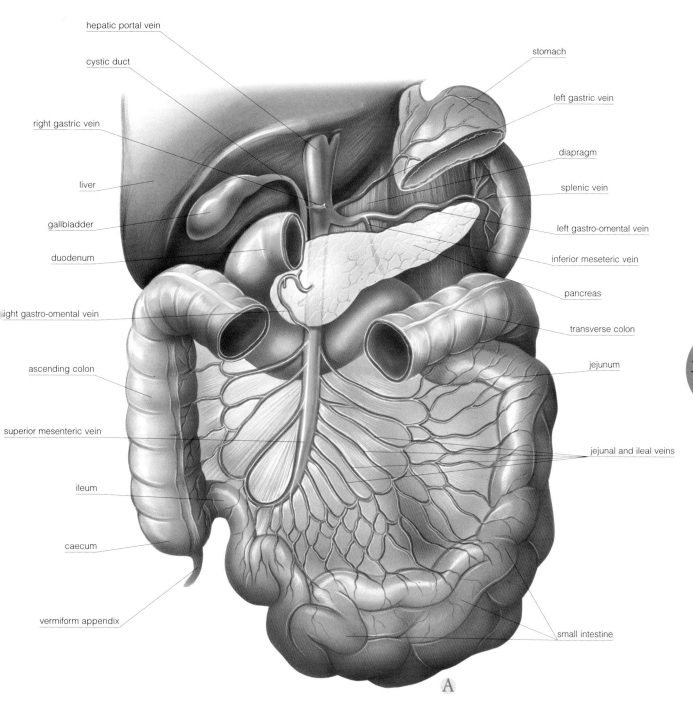

hepatic portal vein

cystic duct

right gastric vein

liver

gallbladder

duodenum

ight gastro-omental vein

ascending colon

superior mesenteric vein

ileum

caecum

vermiform appendix

stomach

left gastric vein

diapragm

splenic vein

left gastro-omental vein

inferior meseteric vein

pancreas

transverse colon

jejunum

jejunal and ileal veins

small intestine

A

drainage of the digestive system

The blood that drains the digestive apparatus is picked up by the portal vein that transports it to the liver to purify it and then bring it back to the circuit of the systemic circulation through the hepatic veins. In the drainage of the digestive apparatus have a fundamental role the mesenteric veins superior and inferior and also the splenic vein. Thus the mesenteric superior drains the small intestine, a part of the large and the stomach. The mesenteric inferior drains the distal zones of the large intestine and the rectum; before joins with the mesenteric superior, it joins with the splenic. This one collects the blood from the spleen and one part of the stomach and the pancreas; after that joins with the mesenteric superior to form the portal hepatic vein that flow in the liver, giving origin to the denominated portal system.

VENOUS SYSTEM (XXXVII)
PORTAL VEIN NETWORK (I). DISTRIBUTION
ANTERIOR VIEW

378

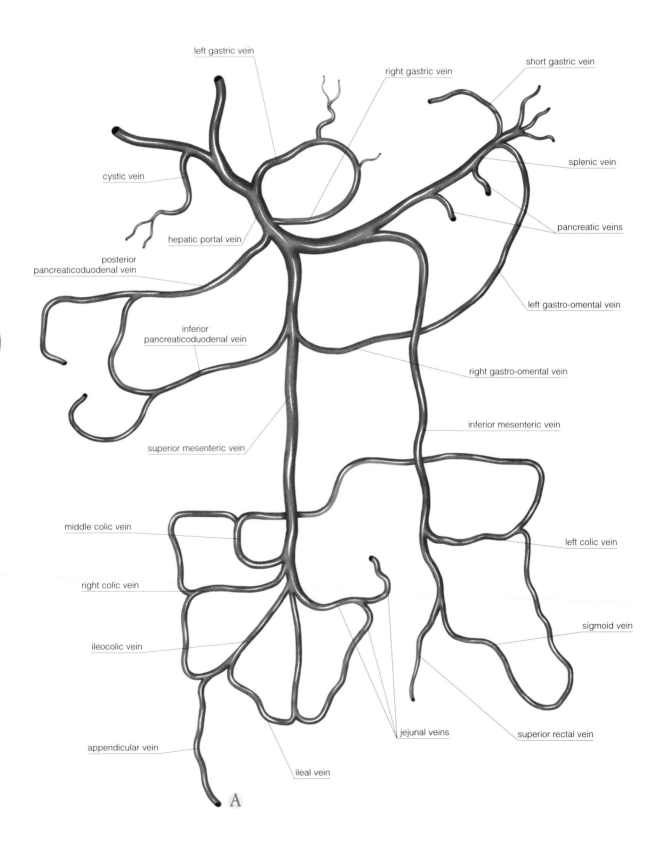

left gastric vein

right gastric vein

short gastric vein

cystic vein

splenic vein

hepatic portal vein

pancreatic veins

posterior pancreaticoduodenal vein

left gastro-omental vein

inferior pancreaticoduodenal vein

right gastro-omental vein

inferior mesenteric vein

superior mesenteric vein

middle colic vein

left colic vein

right colic vein

sigmoid vein

ileocolic vein

jejunal veins

superior rectal vein

appendicular vein

ileal vein

A

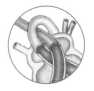

VENOUS SYSTEM (XXXVIII). PORTAL VEIN NETWORK (II) COLLATERAL VESSELS

ANTERIOR VIEW

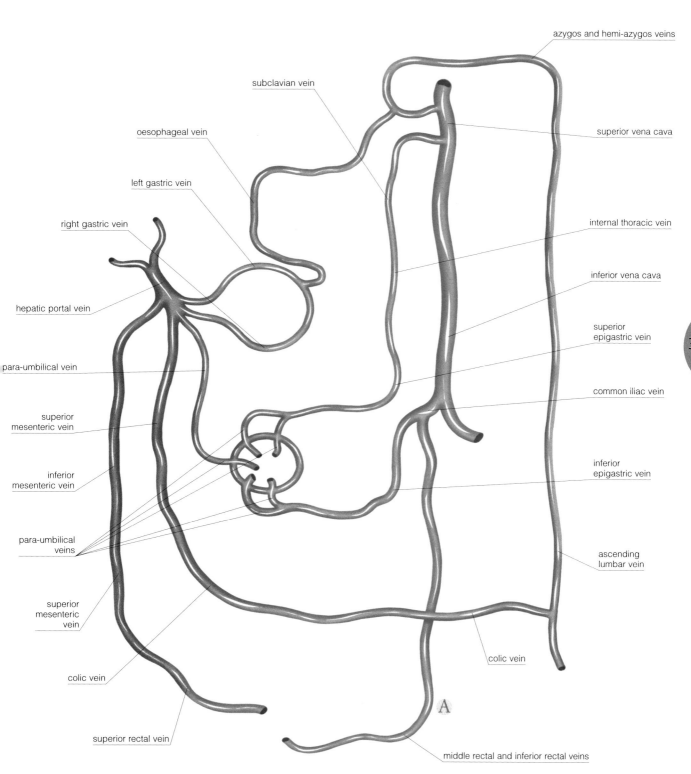

azygos and hemi-azygos veins

subclavian vein

oesophageal vein

left gastric vein

right gastric vein

hepatic portal vein

para-umbilical vein

superior mesenteric vein

inferior mesenteric vein

para-umbilical veins

superior mesenteric vein

colic vein

superior rectal vein

superior vena cava

internal thoracic vein

inferior vena cava

superior epigastric vein

common iliac vein

inferior epigastric vein

ascending lumbar vein

colic vein

middle rectal and inferior rectal veins

A

379

VENOUS SYSTEM (XXXIX). ABDOMEN

ANTERIOR VIEW

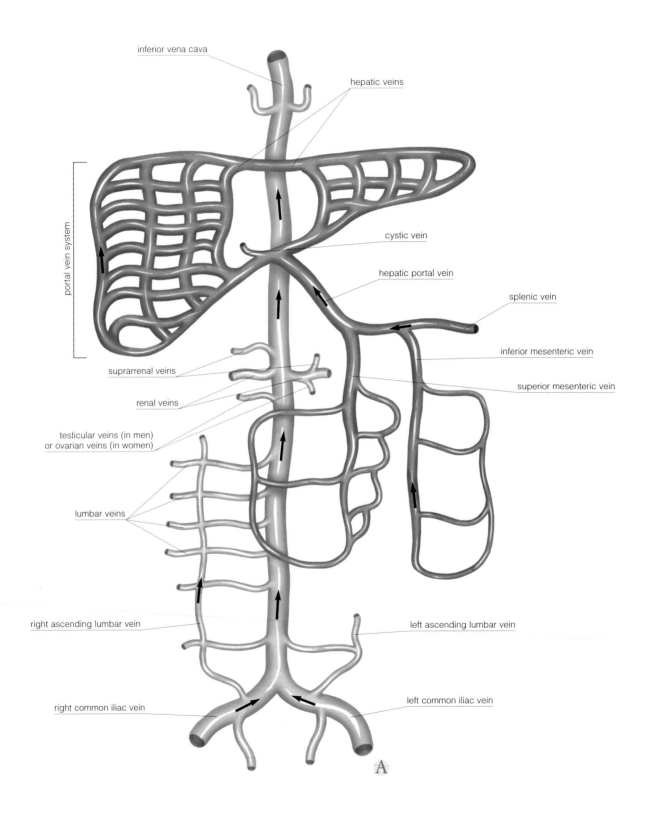

inferior vena cava

hepatic veins

portal vein system

cystic vein

hepatic portal vein

splenic vein

inferior mesenteric vein

superior mesenteric vein

suprarrenal veins

renal veins

testicular veins (in men)
or ovarian veins (in women)

lumbar veins

right ascending lumbar vein

left ascending lumbar vein

right common iliac vein

left common iliac vein

380

A

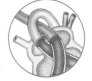

VENOUS SYSTEM (XL). PORTAL VEIN and FLOWINGS
ANTERIOR VIEW

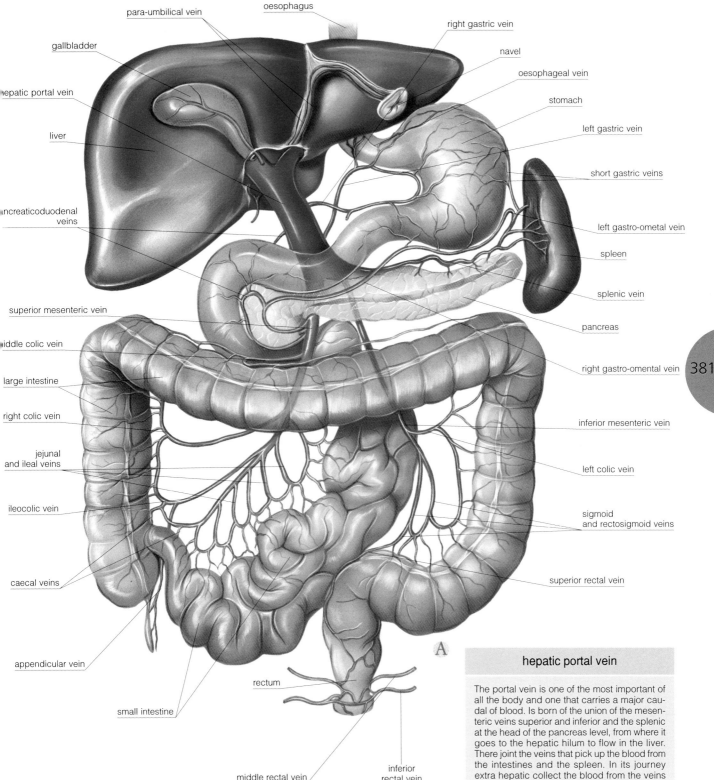

para-umbilical vein

oesophagus

right gastric vein

navel

oesophageal vein

gallbladder

stomach

hepatic portal vein

left gastric vein

liver

short gastric veins

pancreaticoduodenal veins

left gastro-ometal vein

spleen

splenic vein

superior mesenteric vein

pancreas

middle colic vein

large intestine

right gastro-omental vein

right colic vein

inferior mesenteric vein

jejunal and ileal veins

left colic vein

ileocolic vein

sigmoid and rectosigmoid veins

caecal veins

superior rectal vein

appendicular vein

A

rectum

small intestine

middle rectal vein

inferior rectal vein

381

hepatic portal vein

The portal vein is one of the most important of all the body and one that carries a major cau-dal of blood. Is born of the union of the mesen-teric veins superior and inferior and the splenic at the head of the pancreas level, from where it goes to the hepatic hilum to flow in the liver. There joint the veins that pick up the blood from the intestines and the spleen. In its journey extra hepatic collect the blood from the veins of the stomach, from the gallbladder, the umbi-lical region and from the pancreas. It penetra-tes in the liver, where it ramifies forming a thick and complex net, and afterwards, comes back to the systemic circulation.

VENOUS SYSTEM (XLI). HEPATIC VESSELS and DUCTS

hepatic portal circulation

In general, is denominated portal circulation to the sanguineous system that origins from a vein to other passing through a net of capillaries that mediates between them. That´s what happens precisely with the portal vein that forms an own circuit. Thus, after collecting the blood that have been poured out by the gastrointestinal, mesenteric, superior and inferior and splenic veins, it introduces in the liver, where derives in multiple capillaries (sinusoid of the liver). In this hepatic journey process and depurate the substances that carries the blood and that have entered in the organism through the digestive tube. These capillaries then will be joining to form the hepatic vein, that goes out from the liver to flow in the inferior vena cava.

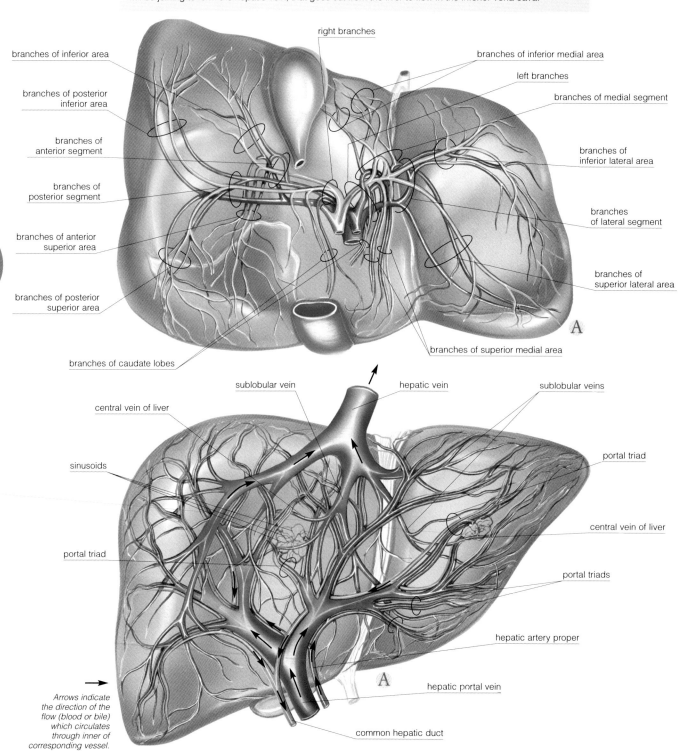

right branches

branches of inferior area

branches of inferior medial area

branches of posterior inferior area

left branches

branches of medial segment

branches of anterior segment

branches of inferior lateral area

branches of posterior segment

branches of lateral segment

branches of anterior superior area

branches of superior lateral area

branches of posterior superior area

branches of superior medial area

A

branches of caudate lobes

sublobular vein

hepatic vein

sublobular veins

central vein of liver

portal triad

sinusoids

central vein of liver

portal triad

portal triads

hepatic artery proper

A

hepatic portal vein

Arrows indicate the direction of the flow (blood or bile) which circulates through inner of corresponding vessel.

common hepatic duct

382

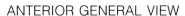

LYMPHOID SYSTEM (I)

ANTERIOR GENERAL VIEW

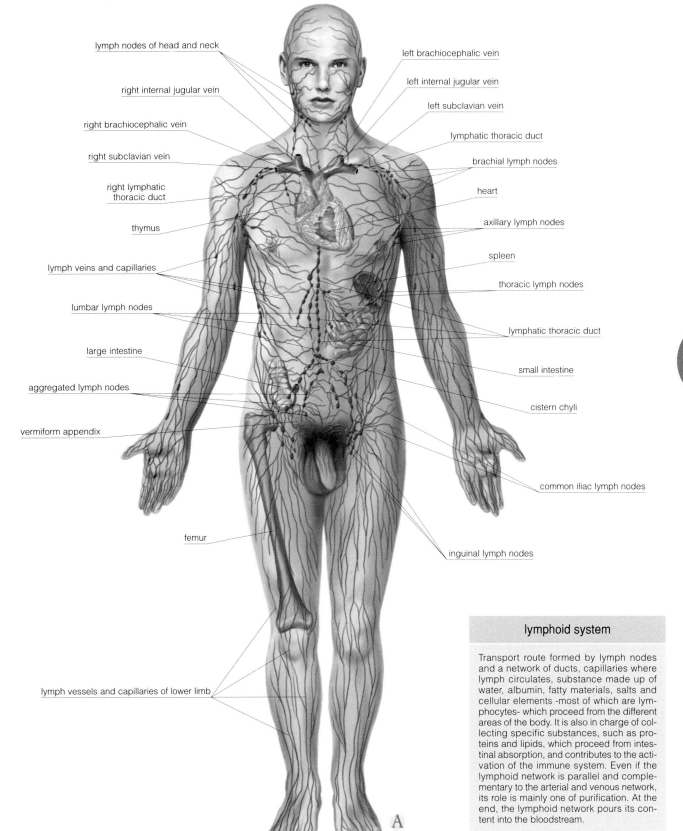

lymph nodes of head and neck

right internal jugular vein

right brachiocephalic vein

right subclavian vein

right lymphatic thoracic duct

thymus

lymph veins and capillaries

lumbar lymph nodes

large intestine

aggregated lymph nodes

vermiform appendix

femur

lymph vessels and capillaries of lower limb

left brachiocephalic vein

left internal jugular vein

left subclavian vein

lymphatic thoracic duct

brachial lymph nodes

heart

axillary lymph nodes

spleen

thoracic lymph nodes

lymphatic thoracic duct

small intestine

cistern chyli

common iliac lymph nodes

inguinal lymph nodes

383

A

lymphoid system

Transport route formed by lymph nodes and a network of ducts, capillaries where lymph circulates, substance made up of water, albumin, fatty materials, salts and cellular elements -most of which are lymphocytes- which proceed from the different areas of the body. It is also in charge of collecting specific substances, such as proteins and lipids, which proceed from intestinal absorption, and contributes to the activation of the immune system. Even if the lymphoid network is parallel and complementary to the arterial and venous network, its role is mainly one of purification. At the end, the lymphoid network pours its content into the bloodstream.

LYMPHOID SYSTEM (II). LYMPH NODE and CAPILLARY

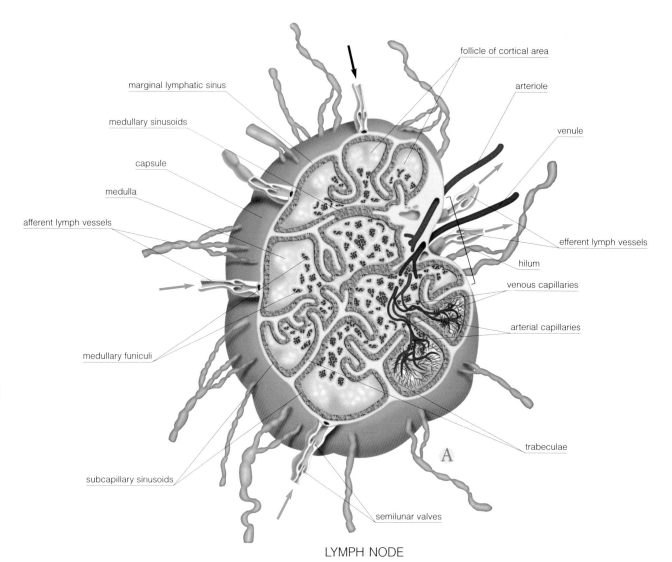

marginal lymphatic sinus

medullary sinusoids

capsule

medulla

afferent lymph vessels

medullary funiculi

subcapillary sinusoids

follicle of cortical area

arteriole

venule

efferent lymph vessels

hilum

venous capillaries

arterial capillaries

trabeculae

semilunar valves

LYMPH NODE

lymph node

The lymphatic ganglia are nodules spread in groups for all over the body, both in the superficial plane as in the deep, between the lymphatic net. There are about 600 in all the body, its shape is like a bean and its size vary substantially (from 1 to 25mm long) according to the importance of its activity. Near the mammary glands, armpits and the crotches is concentrated big agglomerations of ganglia. To them goes the lymph. Its function is acts like a filter. Thus, as such lymph gets into by an extreme of the ganglion, given by the afferent vessels, the strange substances that carries got caught by the reticular fibers of the sinusoids. The macrophages eliminate some substances by phagocitosis while the lymphocytes are in charge of destroying other substances through immunologic mechanisms. The lymph, once filtered comes out of the ganglion through the efferent vessels to return to the lymphatic net.

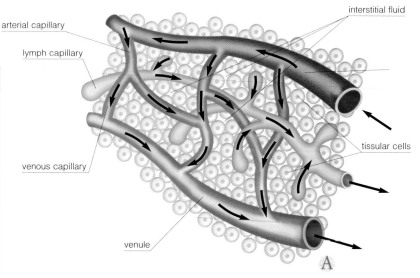

arterial capillary

lymph capillary

venous capillary

venule

interstitial fluid

tissular cells

LYMPHATIC CAPILLARY

LYMPHOID SYSTEM (III). LYMPHATIC CIRCULATION

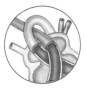

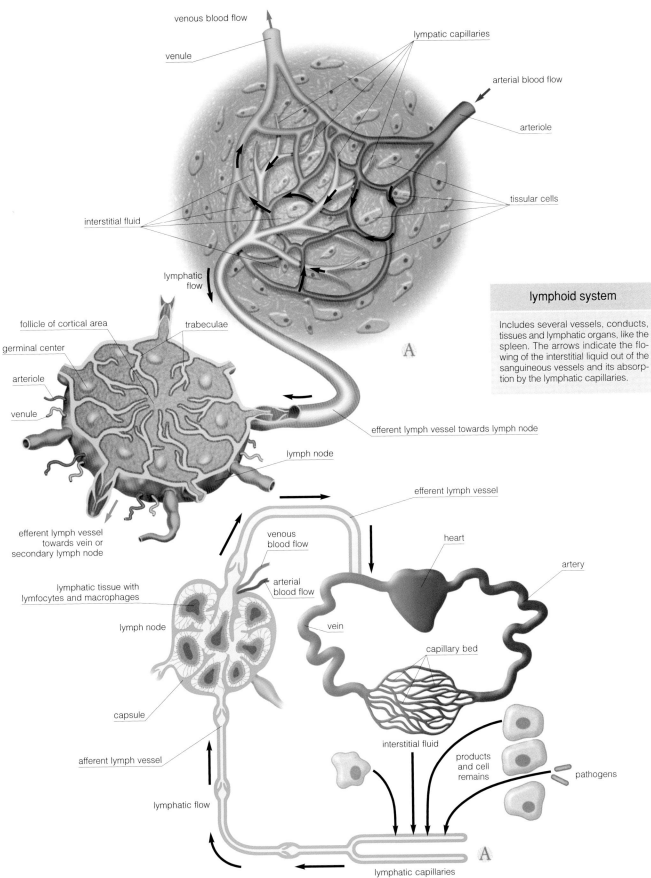

venous blood flow

venule

lympatic capillaries

arterial blood flow

arteriole

tissular cells

interstitial fluid

lymphatic flow

lymphoid system

Includes several vessels, conducts, tissues and lymphatic organs, like the spleen. The arrows indicate the flowing of the interstitial liquid out of the sanguineous vessels and its absorption by the lymphatic capillaries.

385

follicle of cortical area

trabeculae

germinal center

arteriole

venule

efferent lymph vessel towards lymph node

lymph node

efferent lymph vessel towards vein or secondary lymph node

efferent lymph vessel

heart

artery

lymphatic tissue with lymfocytes and macrophages

venous blood flow

arterial blood flow

vein

lymph node

capsule

capillary bed

interstitial fluid

afferent lymph vessel

products and cell remains

pathogens

lymphatic flow

lymphatic capillaries

LYMPHOID SYSTEM (IV). LYMPHATIC DRAINAGE (I)

RIGHT LATERAL GENERAL VIEW

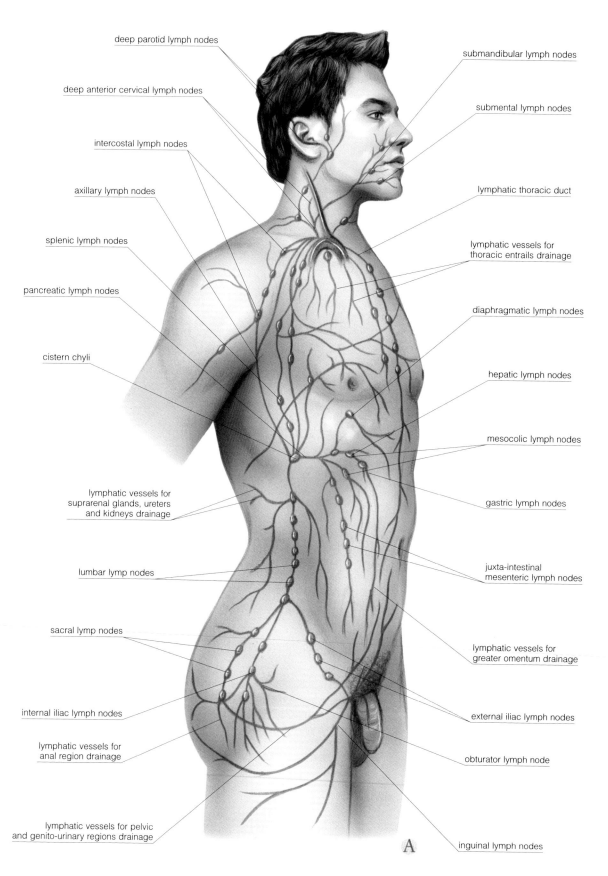

deep parotid lymph nodes

deep anterior cervical lymph nodes

intercostal lymph nodes

axillary lymph nodes

splenic lymph nodes

pancreatic lymph nodes

cistern chyli

lymphatic vessels for
suprarenal glands, ureters
and kidneys drainage

lumbar lymp nodes

sacral lymp nodes

internal iliac lymph nodes

lymphatic vessels for
anal region drainage

lymphatic vessels for pelvic
and genito-urinary regions drainage

submandibular lymph nodes

submental lymph nodes

lymphatic thoracic duct

lymphatic vessels for
thoracic entrails drainage

diaphragmatic lymph nodes

hepatic lymph nodes

mesocolic lymph nodes

gastric lymph nodes

juxta-intestinal
mesenteric lymph nodes

lymphatic vessels for
greater omentum drainage

external iliac lymph nodes

obturator lymph node

inguinal lymph nodes

A

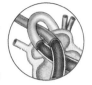

LYMPHOID SYSTEM (V). LYMPHATIC DRAINAGE (II)

FRONTAL GENERAL VIEW

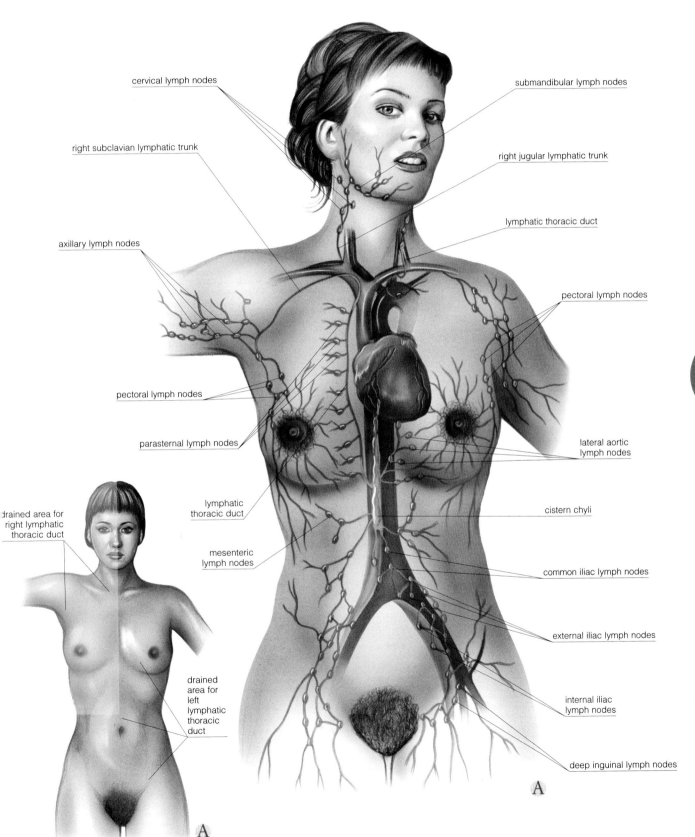

cervical lymph nodes

submandibular lymph nodes

right subclavian lymphatic trunk

right jugular lymphatic trunk

lymphatic thoracic duct

axillary lymph nodes

pectoral lymph nodes

pectoral lymph nodes

parasternal lymph nodes

lateral aortic
lymph nodes

drained area for
right lymphatic
thoracic duct

lymphatic
thoracic duct

cistern chyli

mesenteric
lymph nodes

common iliac lymph nodes

external iliac lymph nodes

drained
area for
left
lymphatic
thoracic
duct

internal iliac
lymph nodes

deep inguinal lymph nodes

A

A

387

LYMPHOID SYSTEM (VI)

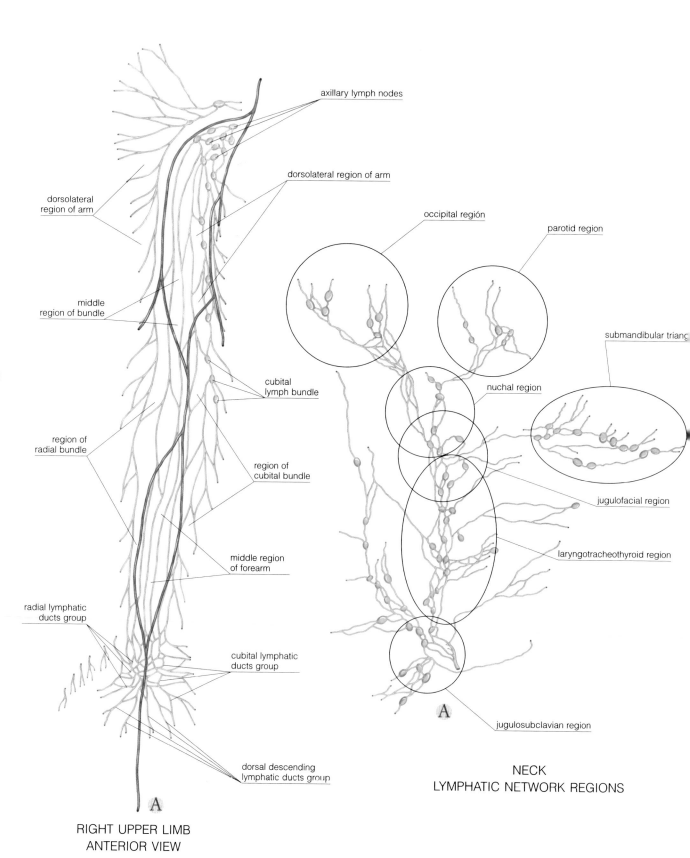

axillary lymph nodes

dorsolateral region of arm

dorsolateral
region of arm

occipital región

parotid region

middle
region of bundle

submandibular triang

cubital
lymph bundle

nuchal region

region of
radial bundle

region of
cubital bundle

jugulofacial region

laryngotracheothyroid region

middle region
of forearm

radial lymphatic
ducts group

cubital lymphatic
ducts group

dorsal descending
lymphatic ducts group

jugulosubclavian region

A

A

RIGHT UPPER LIMB
ANTERIOR VIEW

NECK
LYMPHATIC NETWORK REGIONS

388

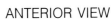

LYMPHOID SYSTEM (VII). NECK, AXILLA and ARM

ANTERIOR VIEW

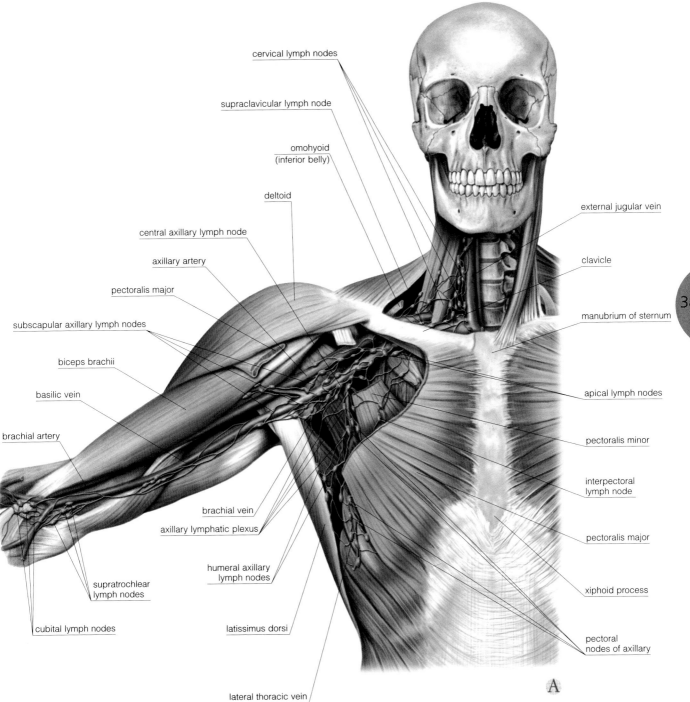

cervical lymph nodes

supraclavicular lymph node

omohyoid
(inferior belly)

deltoid

central axillary lymph node

axillary artery

pectoralis major

subscapular axillary lymph nodes

biceps brachii

basilic vein

brachial artery

brachial vein

axillary lymphatic plexus

humeral axillary
lymph nodes

supratrochlear
lymph nodes

cubital lymph nodes

latissimus dorsi

lateral thoracic vein

external jugular vein

clavicle

manubrium of sternum

apical lymph nodes

pectoralis minor

interpectoral
lymph node

pectoralis major

xiphoid process

pectoral
nodes of axillary

A

LYMPHOID SYSTEM (VIII)
MEDIASTINUM and THORACIC CAVITY
ANTERIOR VIEW

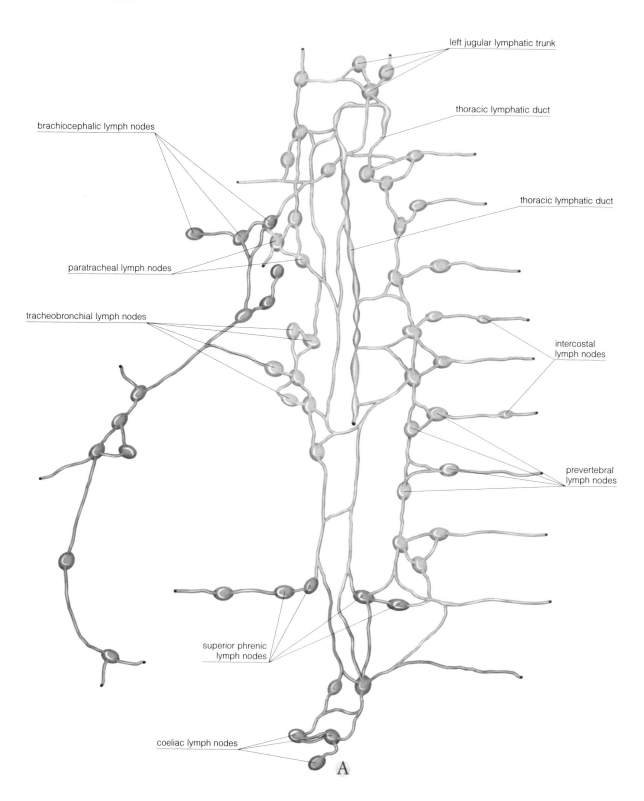

left jugular lymphatic trunk

thoracic lymphatic duct

brachiocephalic lymph nodes

thoracic lymphatic duct

paratracheal lymph nodes

tracheobronchial lymph nodes

intercostal lymph nodes

prevertebral lymph nodes

superior phrenic lymph nodes

coeliac lymph nodes

A

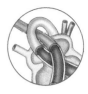

LYMPHOID SYSTEM (IX)
TRACHEA and BRONCHIAL TREE
ANTERIOR VIEW

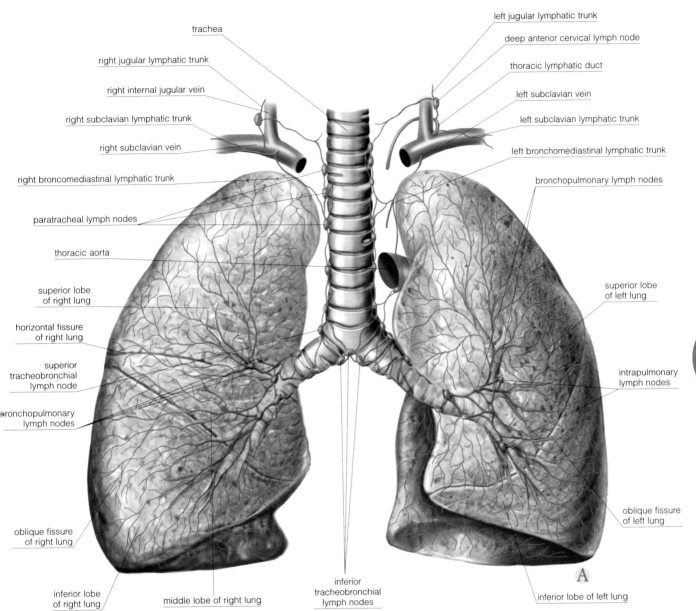

trachea

right jugular lymphatic trunk

right internal jugular vein

right subclavian lymphatic trunk

right subclavian vein

right broncomediastinal lymphatic trunk

paratracheal lymph nodes

thoracic aorta

superior lobe of right lung

horizontal fissure of right lung

superior tracheobronchial lymph node

bronchopulmonary lymph nodes

oblique fissure of right lung

inferior lobe of right lung

middle lobe of right lung

inferior tracheobronchial lymph nodes

left jugular lymphatic trunk

deep anterior cervical lymph node

thoracic lymphatic duct

left subclavian vein

left subclavian lymphatic trunk

left bronchomediastinal lymphatic trunk

bronchopulmonary lymph nodes

superior lobe of left lung

intrapulmonary lymph nodes

oblique fissure of left lung

inferior lobe of left lung

A

391

lymphatic drainage of the lungs

The lymphatic drainage of the lungs is carried out by the deep lymphatic vessels or peri-bronchial and by the superficial lymphatic vessels or segmental. The deep lymphatic vessels run following the conjunctive peri-bronchial tissues and posses ganglionary stations. From inside to outside are found the bronco-pulmonary ganglia that are located in the places of division of the lobar and segmental bronchus and then the trachea-bronchial ganglion inferior and superior that are located to the level of the main bronchus and the tracheal bifurcation. The superficial lymphatic vessels are originated in the lymphatic capillaries of the conjunctive tissue sub-pleural and in the partitions of conjunctive tissue inter-lobular and inter-segmental and join around the pulmonary alveolus to continue to the lymphatic trachea-bronchial ganglia. The efferent vessels of the trachea-bronchial ganglia (ganglia that receive the lymphatic pulmonary drainage from the deep and superficial lymphatic vessels) extend along the trachea to join to similar vessels coming from the parasternal and branchio-cephalic ganglia and form the right and left bronchomediastinal trunks. These trunks flow in the deep veins of the base of the neck or in the lymphatic right trunk, or in the thoracic conduct.

LYMPHOID SYSTEM (X). SMALL INTESTINE
ANTERIOR VIEW

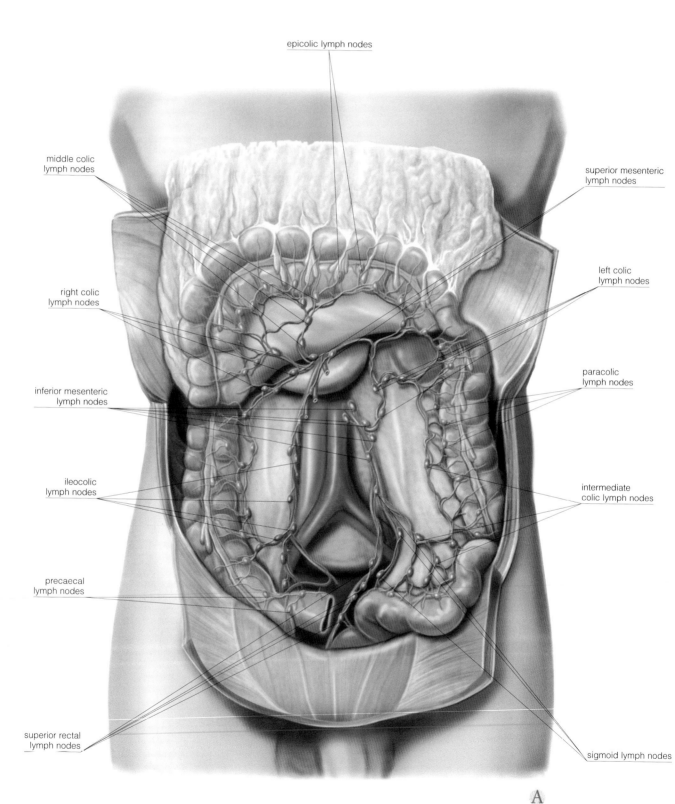

epicolic lymph nodes

middle colic
lymph nodes

superior mesenteric
lymph nodes

right colic
lymph nodes

left colic
lymph nodes

inferior mesenteric
lymph nodes

paracolic
lymph nodes

ileocolic
lymph nodes

intermediate
colic lymph nodes

precaecal
lymph nodes

superior rectal
lymph nodes

sigmoid lymph nodes

A

392

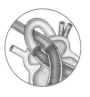

LYMPHOID SYSTEM (XI). POSTERIOR WALL
of ABDOMEN
ANTERIOR VIEW

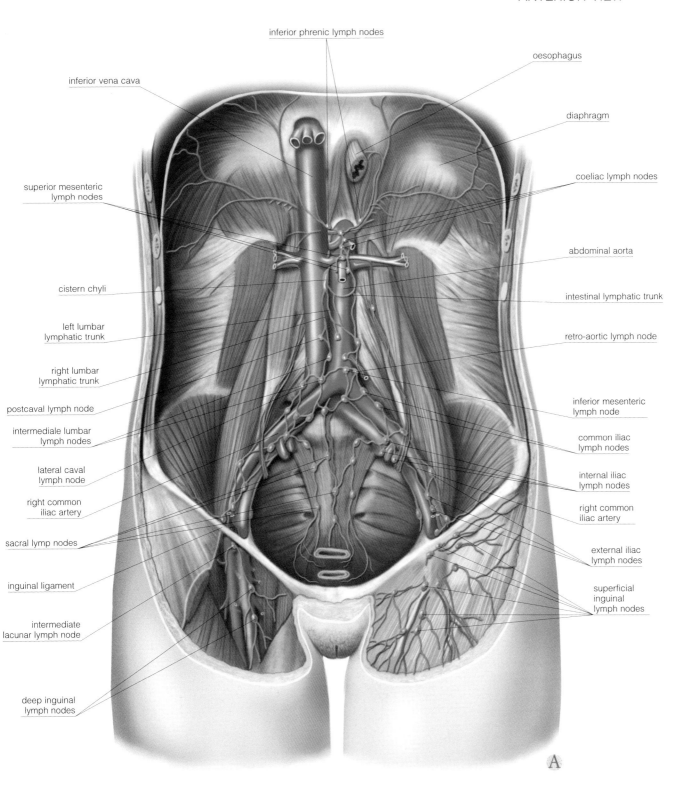

inferior phrenic lymph nodes

oesophagus

inferior vena cava

diaphragm

coeliac lymph nodes

superior mesenteric
lymph nodes

abdominal aorta

cistern chyli

intestinal lymphatic trunk

left lumbar
lymphatic trunk

retro-aortic lymph node

393

right lumbar
lymphatic trunk

inferior mesenteric
lymph node

postcaval lymph node

common iliac
lymph nodes

intermediale lumbar
lymph nodes

internal iliac
lymph nodes

lateral caval
lymph node

right common
iliac artery

right common
iliac artery

sacral lymp nodes

external iliac
lymph nodes

inguinal ligament

superficial
inguinal
lymph nodes

intermediate
lacunar lymph node

deep inguinal
lymph nodes

A

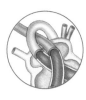

LYMPHOID SYSTEM (XII)
ABDOMINOGENITAL REGION (I)

MALE SEX. ANTERIOR VIEW

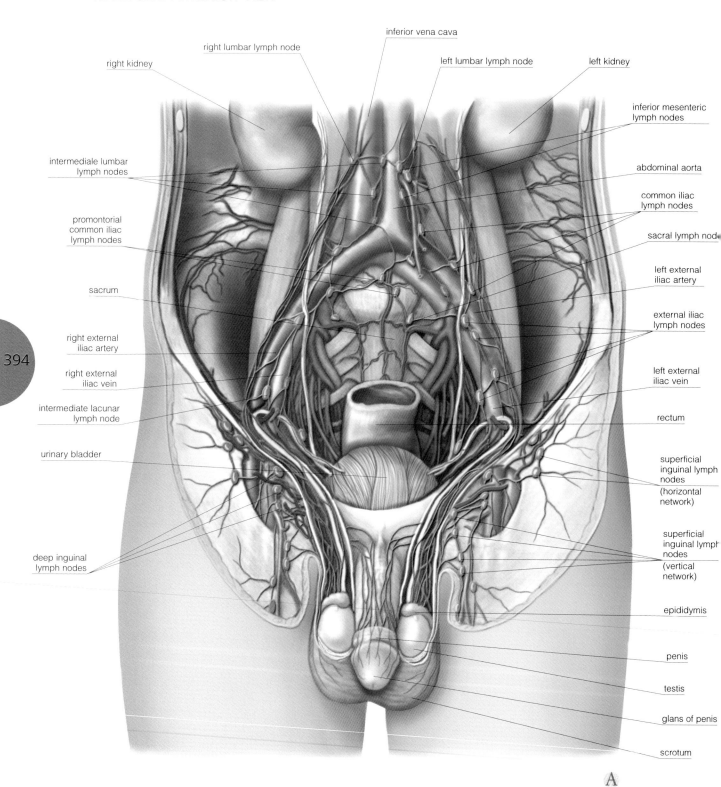

inferior vena cava

right lumbar lymph node

left lumbar lymph node

right kidney

left kidney

inferior mesenteric lymph nodes

intermediale lumbar lymph nodes

abdominal aorta

common iliac lymph nodes

promontorial common iliac lymph nodes

sacral lymph node

left external iliac artery

sacrum

external iliac lymph nodes

right external iliac artery

left external iliac vein

right external iliac vein

rectum

intermediate lacunar lymph node

urinary bladder

superficial inguinal lymph nodes (horizontal network)

superficial inguinal lymph nodes (vertical network)

deep inguinal lymph nodes

epididymis

penis

testis

glans of penis

scrotum

394

A

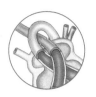

LYMPHOID SYSTEM (XIII)
ABDOMINOGENITAL REGION (II)
FEMALE SEX. ANTERIOR VIEW

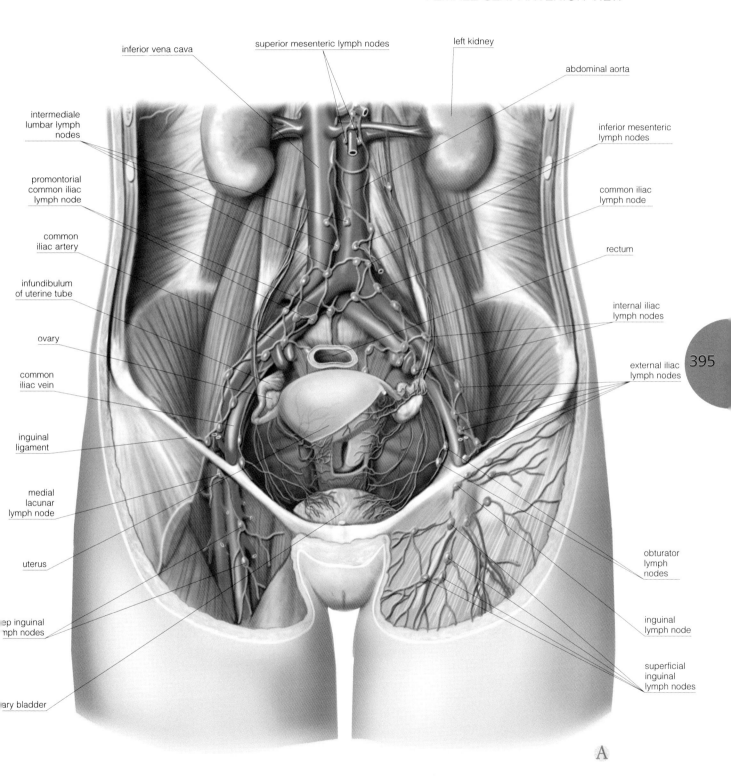

inferior vena cava

superior mesenteric lymph nodes

left kidney

abdominal aorta

intermediale lumbar lymph nodes

inferior mesenteric lymph nodes

promontorial common iliac lymph node

common iliac lymph node

common iliac artery

rectum

infundibulum of uterine tube

internal iliac lymph nodes

ovary

external iliac lymph nodes

common iliac vein

395

inguinal ligament

medial lacunar lymph node

obturator lymph nodes

uterus

inguinal lymph node

ep inguinal mph nodes

superficial inguinal lymph nodes

ary bladder

A

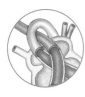

LYMPHOID SYSTEM (XIV). SPLEEN, PANCREAS and DUODENUM

ANTERIOR VIEW

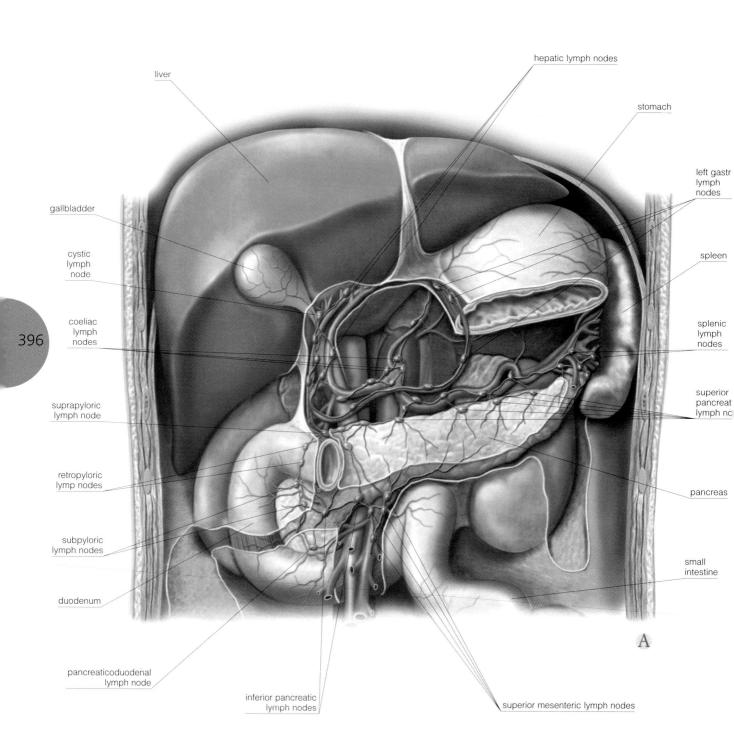

hepatic lymph nodes

liver

stomach

left gastr
lymph
nodes

gallbladder

cystic
lymph
node

spleen

396

coeliac
lymph
nodes

splenic
lymph
nodes

superior
pancreat
lymph nc

suprapyloric
lymph node

retropyloric
lymp nodes

pancreas

subpyloric
lymph nodes

small
intestine

duodenum

A

pancreaticoduodenal
lymph node

inferior pancreatic
lymph nodes

superior mesenteric lymph nodes

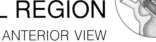

LYMPHOID SYSTEM (XV). INGUINAL REGION

ANTERIOR VIEW

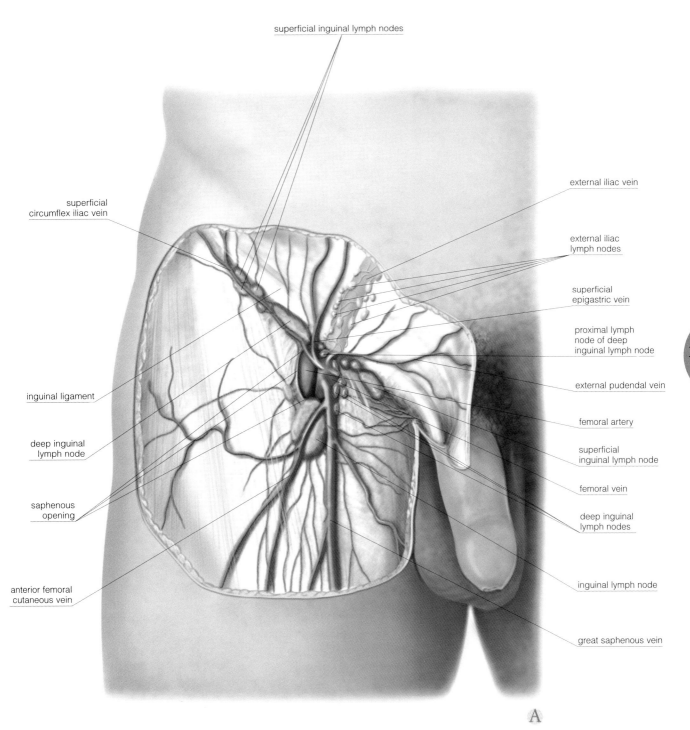

superficial inguinal lymph nodes

external iliac vein

external iliac lymph nodes

superficial epigastric vein

proximal lymph node of deep inguinal lymph node

external pudendal vein

femoral artery

superficial inguinal lymph node

femoral vein

deep inguinal lymph nodes

inguinal lymph node

great saphenous vein

superficial circumflex iliac vein

inguinal ligament

deep inguinal lymph node

saphenous opening

anterior femoral cutaneous vein

397

A

LYMPHOID SYSTEM (XVI). GENERAL PATHS

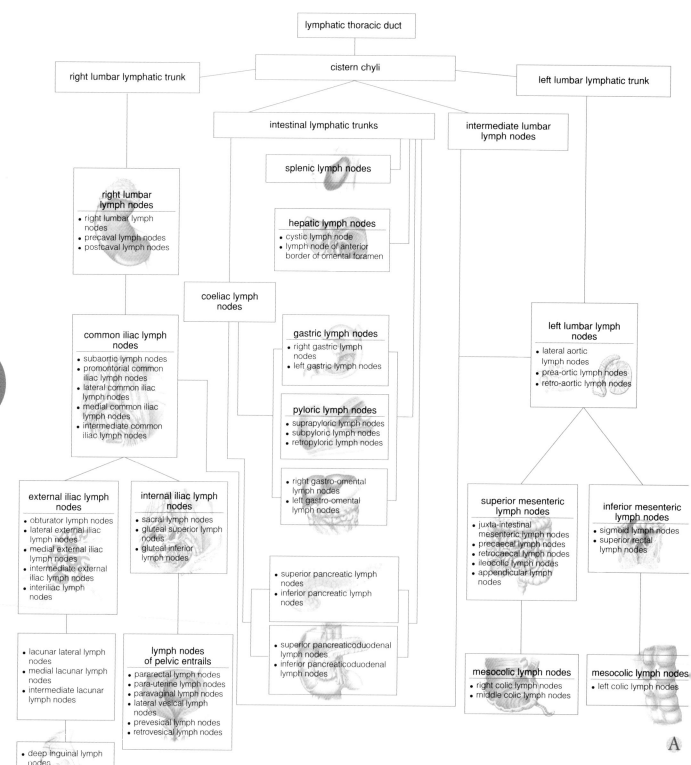

lymphatic thoracic duct

cistern chyli

right lumbar lymphatic trunk

left lumbar lymphatic trunk

intestinal lymphatic trunks

intermediate lumbar lymph nodes

splenic lymph nodes

right lumbar lymph nodes
- right lumbar lymph nodes
- precaval lymph nodes
- postcaval lymph nodes

hepatic lymph nodes
- cystic lymph node
- lymph node of anterior border of omental foramen

coeliac lymph nodes

common iliac lymph nodes
- subaortic lymph nodes
- promontorial common iliac lymph nodes
- lateral common iliac lymph nodes
- medial common iliac lymph nodes
- intermediate common iliac lymph nodes

gastric lymph nodes
- right gastric lymph nodes
- left gastric lymph nodes

left lumbar lymph nodes
- lateral aortic lymph nodes
- prea-ortic lymph nodes
- retro-aortic lymph nodes

pyloric lymph nodes
- suprapyloric lymph nodes
- subpyloric lymph nodes
- retropyloric lymph nodes

- right gastro-omental lymph nodes
- left gastro-omental lymph nodes

external iliac lymph nodes
- obturator lymph nodes
- lateral external iliac lymph nodes
- medial external iliac lymph nodes
- intermediate external iliac lymph nodes
- interiliac lymph nodes

internal iliac lymph nodes
- sacral lymph nodes
- gluteal superior lymph nodes
- gluteal inferior lymph nodes

superior mesenteric lymph nodes
- juxta-intestinal mesenteric lymph nodes
- precaecal lymph nodes
- retrocaecal lymph nodes
- ileocolic lymph nodes
- appendicular lymph nodes

inferior mesenteric lymph nodes
- sigmoid lymph nodes
- superior rectal lymph nodes

- superior pancreatic lymph nodes
- inferior pancreatic lymph nodes

- lacunar lateral lymph nodes
- medial lacunar lymph nodes
- intermediate lacunar lymph nodes

lymph nodes of pelvic entrails
- pararectal lymph nodes
- para-uterine lymph nodes
- paravaginal lymph nodes
- lateral vesical lymph nodes
- prevesical lymph nodes
- retrovesical lymph nodes

- superior pancreaticoduodenal lymph nodes
- inferior pancreaticoduodenal lymph nodes

mesocolic lymph nodes
- right colic lymph nodes
- middle colic lymph nodes

mesocolic lymph nodes
- left colic lymph nodes

- deep inguinal lymph nodes

- superficial inguinal lymph nodes

A

DIGESTIVE SYSTEM

Includes the group of organs which intervene in digestion and convert ingested food into molecules, which are small enough to be absorbed and to enter the human body. This is achieved through five essential processes: ingestion, fragmentation, digestion, absorption and elimination of waste products. Therefore, the role of the digestive system is essentially nutritional.

Basically, the digestive system is composed of a long tract, approximately 12m long. The following parts can be differentiated: mouth (where food is ingested and where the first digestion- or oral fragmentation-takes place), pharynx (muscular membranous duct which collaborates with deglution), oesophagus (its role is to transport and to lubricate, therefore, it segregates mucous in its distal third), stomach (where fragmentation ends and gastric digestion takes place, aided by an abundant secretion of gastric juices, which are rich in hydrochloric acid and ferments; the final result is a liquid substance called chime), small intestine (which performs chemical digestion with its diverse elements, multiple secretions and movements, the small intestine disintegrates food into the basic substances it is made up of, with the purpose of absorbing it, the surface of the small intestine walls is large, and thus has a great capacity to absorb), and large intestine (lacking in enzyme secreting glands. Its purpose is to utilize some substances which are still useful, mostly water, as well as collect the resulting residue, using it to form fecal matter). The tract ends up in the anus.

The fecal matter, that is to say, the residue which results from the digestive process, is expelled.

For digestion to work correctly, the digestive tract is assisted by a series of attachments, especially teeth (which grind food mixed with saliva, and with the help of tongue movements, make up the alimentary bolus), salivary glands (which segregate saliva, which includes mucous, enzymes such as lysozyme and amylase, antibodies and organic ions), the liver (a very large viscera which segregates bile and is very important for the digestion and absorption of fat), the gallbladder (where bile is secreted by the liver before it enters the duodenum), and the pancreas (gland which is both endocrine and exocrine, which segregates pancreatic juice, rich in enzymes, which ends up in the duodenum).

These organs and structures ensure that the ingested food is broken down into its basic components. They also ensure that nutritional substances are obtained from the ingested food, and are absorbed by the body. These substances are necessary for the correct maintenance and functioning of the body.

A

DIGESTIVE SYSTEM

ANTERIOR GENERAL VIEW

digestive system

The human body needs a group of substances for its survival (essentially carbohydrates, fats and proteins). These substances, when correctly transformed, can be assimilated and converted into elements which can be used for cell maintenance. This function is carried out through the digestive system, which is a long tract, approximately 12 meters long, which starts in the oral cleft and ends in the anus.

400

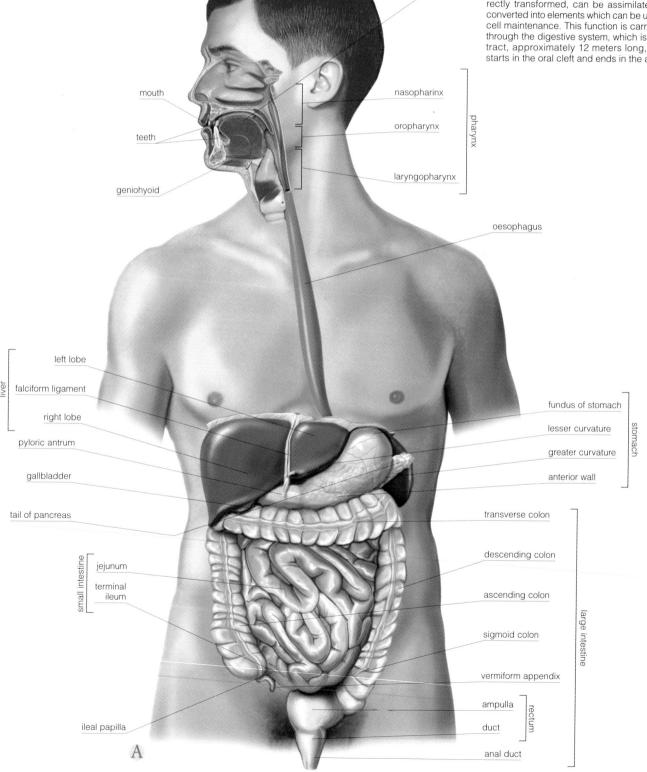

tongue

mouth

teeth

geniohyoid

nasopharinx

oropharynx

laryngopharynx

pharynx

oesophagus

liver

left lobe

falciform ligament

right lobe

pyloric antrum

gallbladder

tail of pancreas

small intestine

jejunum

terminal ileum

ileal papilla

A

fundus of stomach

lesser curvature

greater curvature

anterior wall

stomach

transverse colon

descending colon

ascending colon

sigmoid colon

vermiform appendix

large intestine

ampulla

duct

rectum

anal duct

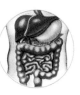

PHASES of the DIGESTIVE PROCESS

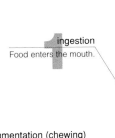

ingestion
Food enters the mouth.

fragmentation (chewing)
Process where food is ground down by the mouth and is insalivated until a mass is formed (alimentary bolus). This phase lasts approximately 1 minute.

fragmentation (salivation)
Process where food which enters the mouth is mixed with the saliva secreted by the salivary glands (mainly the parotid, submandibular and sublingual glands), which helps break down food enzymatically. It lasts approximately 60 seconds.

deglutition and propulsion
Once food is ground down and insalivated, a mass is formed (alimentary bolus) which is swallowed (pushed towards the oesophagus) through the pharynx, which pushes food through muscle contractions. It lasts approximately 2-3 seconds.

gastric digestion
When the alimentary bolus reaches the stomach, fragmentation is finalized and food which is ground down undergoes the action of the juices secreted by the stomach. These juices degrade food until they break it down into very small pieces. Some, not all, of these pieces will be suitable to be absorbed the digestive tract mucous. This process lasts approximately 2-4 hours.

digestion (bile action)
The liver, as it metabolizes, produces bile, which a substance that is poured into the duodenum in order to emulsify certain fats in food and convert them into very small particles which are suitable to be processed by pancreatic enzymes and absorbed in the small intestine. Moreover, bile helps in the transportation and absorption of the resulting products of fat digestion through the mucous of the small intestine.

digestion (action of pancreatic the exocrine secretion)
The pancreas is a gland which secretes a liquid -pancreatic juice- which is very important, since it subjects certain substances in food to a specific chemical action. These substances can be absorbed due to this action.

digestion

Complex, mechanical and enzymatic process, which main function is to make sure the ingested food undergoes a set of transformations, breaking down food into its most fundamental components. Food is then absorbed by the intestinal mucous and is incorporated into the cell mass of the organism. Some of these substances are used as an energy substrate and some others are used in cell formation and maintenance. The human body needs energy to survive and to function. This energy is taken from the ingested food. However, the organism does not absorb food in its natural state. Food undergoes digestion, which is a process with several phases, breaking down food into its basic substances. Food absorbs the beneficial substances and discards unnecessary ones.

nutrient absorption
In the small intestine, food which comes from the stomach and has been broken down is mixed with the bile, the pancreatic juice and the substances secreted by the intestine itself. Thanks to this action, all the substances in food are broken down into the basic elements they are made up of. The organism absorbs the elements it needs. These elements enter the digestive mucous cells and pass to the blood and the lymph. These phases lasts approximately 1 to 4 hours.

401

elimination of residual products (formation of feces)
A liquid is formed with the substances that the organism does not use. Subsequently, a mass -or fecal matter- in the large intestine. The large intestine absorbs water and some substances which are still useful from the fecal matter. Residue is deposited in the rectum. This phase can last from 10 hours to several days.

elimination of residual products (defecation)
When the non-digested substances which result from the entire process turn into the feces, the feces remain in the rectum and are subsequently expelled through the anus. This finalizes the digestion process.

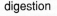
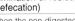

A

ORAL CAVITY and PHARYNX (I)

LEFT SAGITTAL and MEDIAL VIEW

402

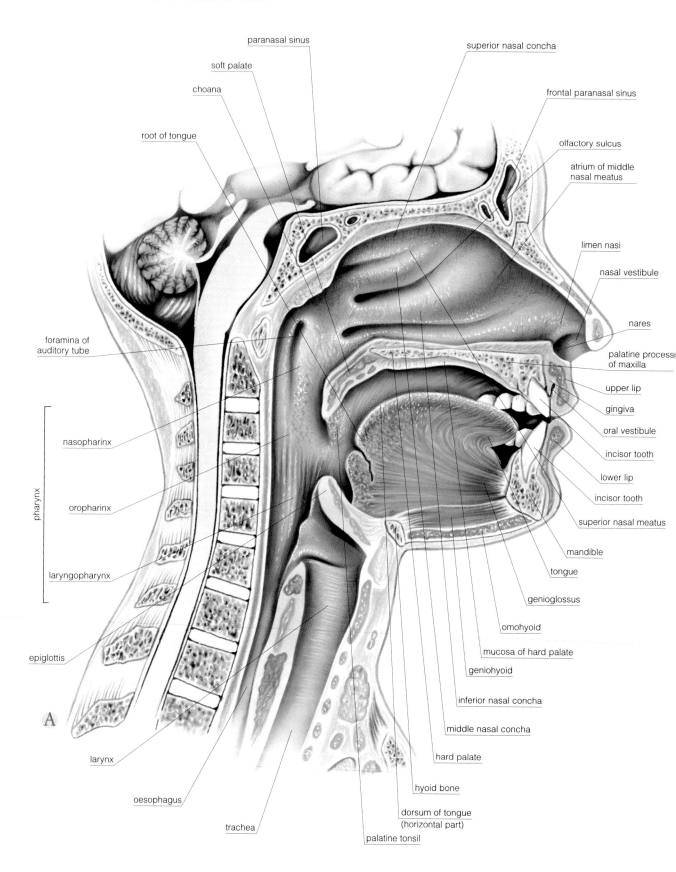

paranasal sinus

soft palate

choana

root of tongue

superior nasal concha

frontal paranasal sinus

olfactory sulcus

atrium of middle
nasal meatus

limen nasi

nasal vestibule

nares

palatine process
of maxilla

upper lip

gingiva

oral vestibule

incisor tooth

lower lip

incisor tooth

superior nasal meatus

mandible

tongue

genioglossus

omohyoid

mucosa of hard palate

geniohyoid

inferior nasal concha

middle nasal concha

hard palate

hyoid bone

dorsum of tongue
(horizontal part)

palatine tonsil

foramina of
auditory tube

pharynx

nasopharinx

oropharinx

laryngopharynx

epiglottis

A

larynx

oesophagus

trachea

ORAL CAVITY and PHARYNX (II)
RIGHT SAGITTAL and MIDDLE VIEW

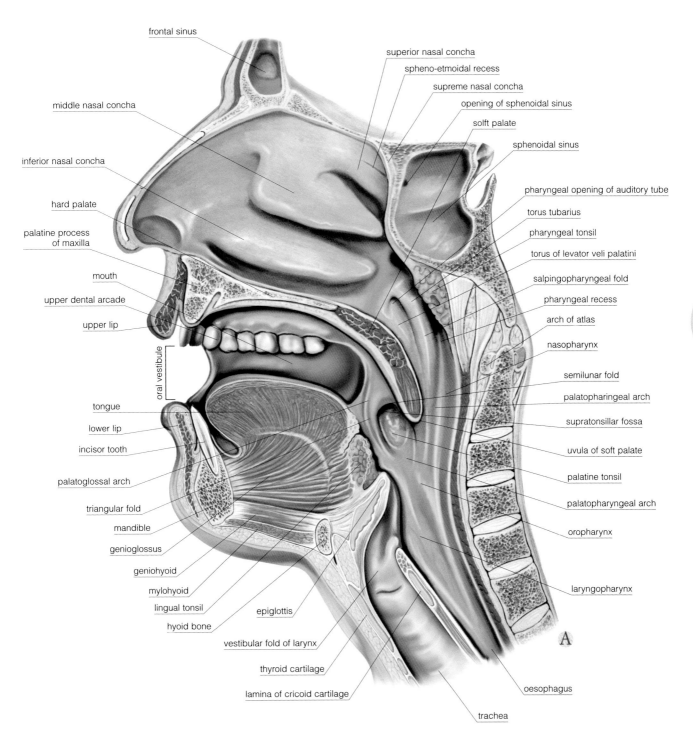

frontal sinus

superior nasal concha

spheno-etmoidal recess

supreme nasal concha

opening of sphenoidal sinus

middle nasal concha

solft palate

sphenoidal sinus

inferior nasal concha

pharyngeal opening of auditory tube

torus tubarius

hard palate

pharyngeal tonsil

palatine process
of maxilla

torus of levator veli palatini

salpingopharyngeal fold

mouth

pharyngeal recess

upper dental arcade

arch of atlas

upper lip

nasopharynx

oral vestibule

semilunar fold

palatopharingeal arch

tongue

supratonsillar fossa

lower lip

uvula of soft palate

incisor tooth

palatine tonsil

palatoglossal arch

palatopharyngeal arch

triangular fold

oropharynx

mandible

genioglossus

geniohyoid

mylohyoid

laryngopharynx

lingual tonsil

epiglottis

hyoid bone

vestibular fold of larynx

thyroid cartilage

oesophagus

lamina of cricoid cartilage

trachea

A

403

404

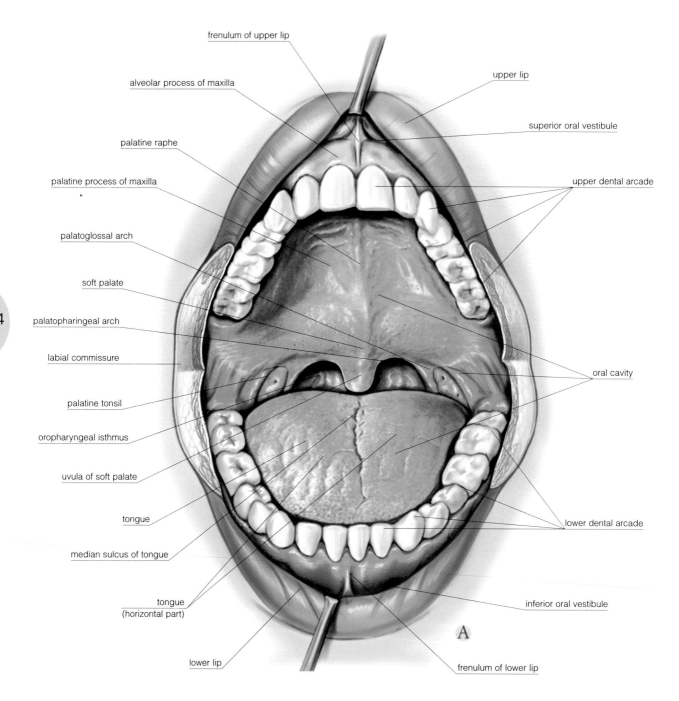

frenulum of upper lip

alveolar process of maxilla

palatine raphe

palatine process of maxilla

palatoglossal arch

soft palate

palatopharingeal arch

labial commissure

palatine tonsil

oropharyngeal isthmus

uvula of soft palate

tongue

median sulcus of tongue

tongue
(horizontal part)

lower lip

upper lip

superior oral vestibule

upper dental arcade

oral cavity

lower dental arcade

inferior oral vestibule

frenulum of lower lip

A

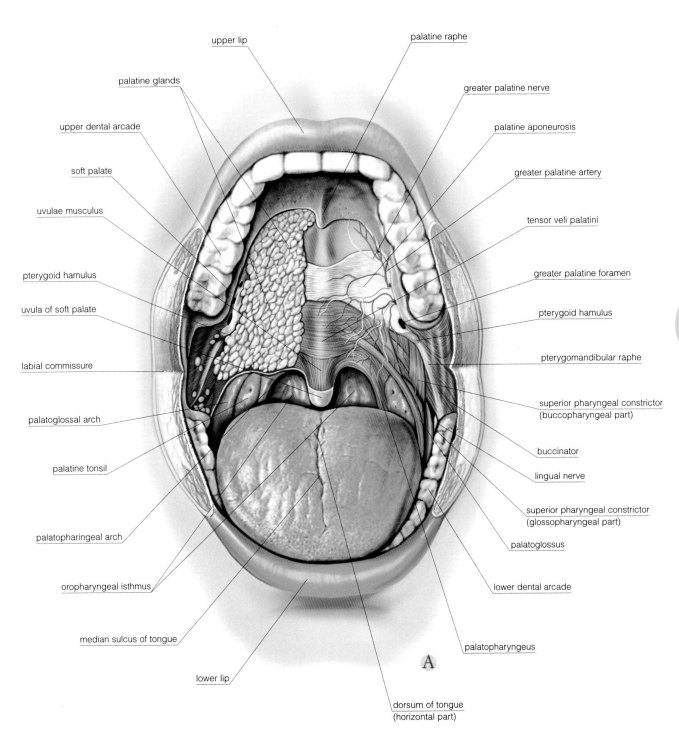

upper lip

palatine raphe

palatine glands

greater palatine nerve

upper dental arcade

palatine aponeurosis

soft palate

greater palatine artery

uvulae musculus

tensor veli palatini

pterygoid hamulus

greater palatine foramen

uvula of soft palate

pterygoid hamulus

labial commissure

pterygomandibular raphe

superior pharyngeal constrictor
(buccopharyngeal part)

palatoglossal arch

buccinator

palatine tonsil

lingual nerve

superior pharyngeal constrictor
(glossopharyngeal part)

palatopharingeal arch

palatoglossus

oropharyngeal isthmus

lower dental arcade

median sulcus of tongue

palatopharyngeus

lower lip

A

dorsum of tongue
(horizontal part)

406

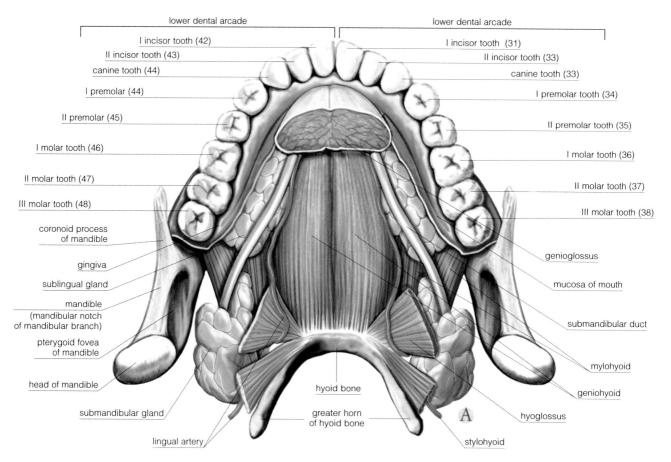

lower dental arcade

I incisor tooth (42)
II incisor tooth (43)
canine tooth (44)
I premolar (44)
II premolar (45)
I molar tooth (46)
II molar tooth (47)
III molar tooth (48)
coronoid process of mandible
gingiva
sublingual gland
mandible (mandibular notch of mandibular branch)
pterygoid fovea of mandible
head of mandible
submandibular gland
lingual artery

lower dental arcade

I incisor tooth (31)
II incisor tooth (33)
canine tooth (33)
I premolar tooth (34)
II premolar tooth (35)
I molar tooth (36)
II molar tooth (37)
III molar tooth (38)
genioglossus
mucosa of mouth
submandibular duct
mylohyoid
geniohyoid
hyoglossus

hyoid bone
greater horn of hyoid bone
stylohyoid

A

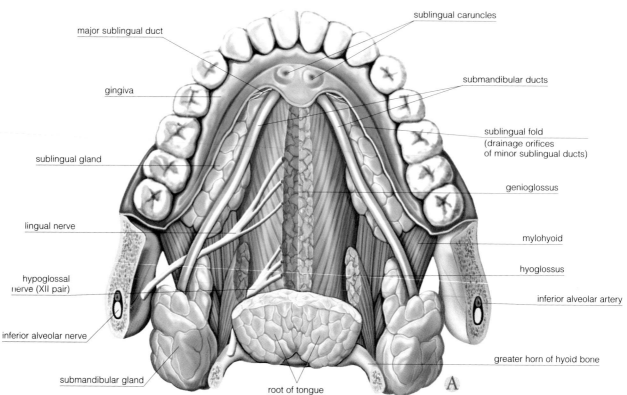

major sublingual duct
gingiva
sublingual gland
lingual nerve
hypoglossal nerve (XII pair)
inferior alveolar nerve
submandibular gland

sublingual caruncles
submandibular ducts
sublingual fold (drainage orifices of minor sublingual ducts)
genioglossus
mylohyoid
hyoglossus
inferior alveolar artery
greater horn of hyoid bone

root of tongue

A

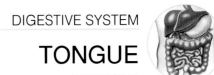

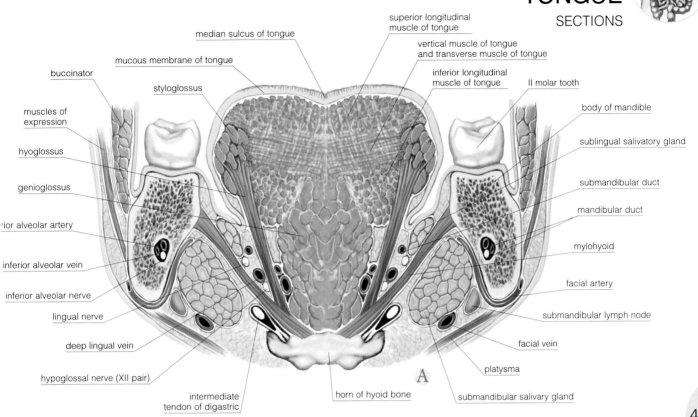

buccinator

muscles of expression

hyoglossus

genioglossus

inferior alveolar artery

inferior alveolar vein

inferior alveolar nerve

lingual nerve

deep lingual vein

hypoglossal nerve (XII pair)

intermediate tendon of digastric

median sulcus of tongue

mucous membrane of tongue

styloglossus

superior longitudinal muscle of tongue

vertical muscle of tongue and transverse muscle of tongue

inferior longitudinal muscle of tongue

II molar tooth

body of mandible

sublingual salivatory gland

submandibular duct

mandibular duct

mylohyoid

facial artery

submandibular lymph node

facial vein

platysma

submandibular salivary gland

horn of hyoid bone

LEVEL of SECOND MOLAR TOOTH. ANTERIOR VIEW

407

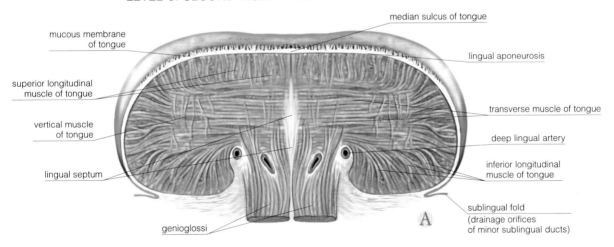

mucous membrane of tongue

superior longitudinal muscle of tongue

vertical muscle of tongue

lingual septum

genioglossi

median sulcus of tongue

lingual aponeurosis

transverse muscle of tongue

deep lingual artery

inferior longitudinal muscle of tongue

sublingual fold (drainage orifices of minor sublingual ducts)

LEVEL of MEDIUM SEGMENT of TONGUE. ANTERIOR VIEW

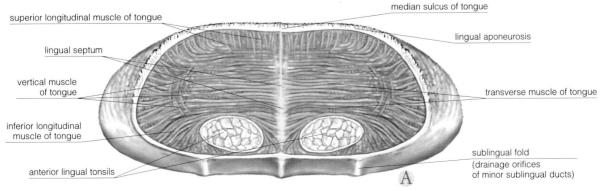

superior longitudinal muscle of tongue

lingual septum

vertical muscle of tongue

inferior longitudinal muscle of tongue

anterior lingual tonsils

median sulcus of tongue

lingual aponeurosis

transverse muscle of tongue

sublingual fold (drainage orifices of minor sublingual ducts)

APEX of TONGUE LEVEL. ANTERIOR VIEW

TONGUE and ORAL FLOOR

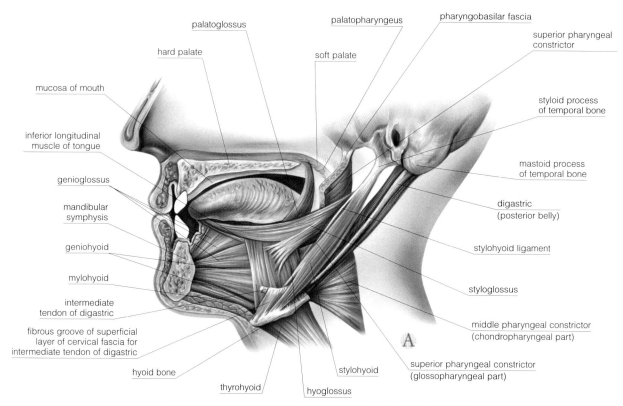

palatoglossus

palatopharyngeus

pharyngobasilar fascia

superior pharyngeal constrictor

hard palate

soft palate

mucosa of mouth

styloid process of temporal bone

inferior longitudinal muscle of tongue

mastoid process of temporal bone

genioglossus

digastric (posterior belly)

mandibular symphysis

stylohyoid ligament

geniohyoid

styloglossus

mylohyoid

intermediate tendon of digastric

middle pharyngeal constrictor (chondropharyngeal part)

fibrous groove of superficial layer of cervical fascia for intermediate tendon of digastric

superior pharyngeal constrictor (glossopharyngeal part)

hyoid bone

stylohyoid

thyrohyoid

hyoglossus

A

EXTRINSIC MUSCLES of TONGUE and ORAL FLOOR
RIGHT LATERAL VIEW

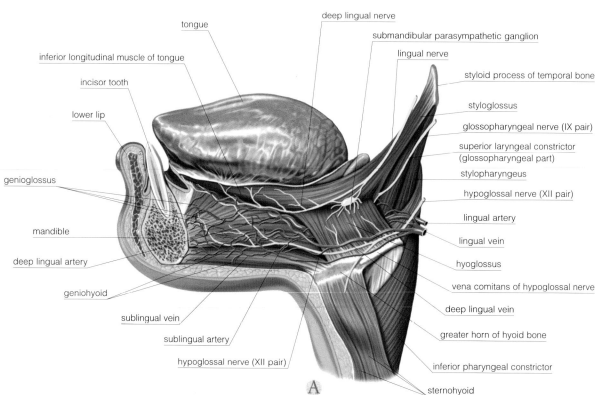

tongue

deep lingual nerve

submandibular parasympathetic ganglion

inferior longitudinal muscle of tongue

lingual nerve

incisor tooth

styloid process of temporal bone

lower lip

styloglossus

glossopharyngeal nerve (IX pair)

superior laryngeal constrictor (glossopharyngeal part)

genioglossus

stylopharyngeus

hypoglossal nerve (XII pair)

lingual artery

mandible

lingual vein

deep lingual artery

hyoglossus

geniohyoid

vena comitans of hypoglossal nerve

deep lingual vein

sublingual vein

greater horn of hyoid bone

sublingual artery

inferior pharyngeal constrictor

hypoglossal nerve (XII pair)

A

sternohyoid

VESSELS and NERVES of TONGUE and ORAL FLOOR
RIGHT LATERAL VIEW

408

TONGUE, ORAL FLOOR and NECK

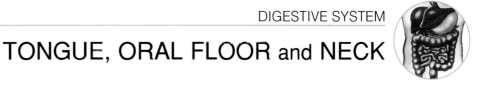

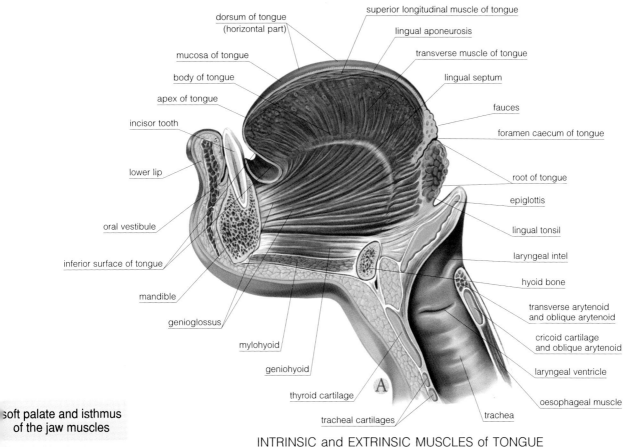

dorsum of tongue
(horizontal part)

mucosa of tongue

body of tongue

apex of tongue

incisor tooth

lower lip

oral vestibule

inferior surface of tongue

mandible

genioglossus

mylohyoid

geniohyoid

thyroid cartilage

tracheal cartilages

superior longitudinal muscle of tongue

lingual aponeurosis

transverse muscle of tongue

lingual septum

fauces

foramen caecum of tongue

root of tongue

epiglottis

lingual tonsil

laryngeal intel

hyoid bone

transverse arytenoid
and oblique arytenoid

cricoid cartilage
and oblique arytenoid

laryngeal ventricle

oesophageal muscle

trachea

INTRINSIC and EXTRINSIC MUSCLES of TONGUE
RIGHT LATERAL VIEW

soft palate and isthmus
of the jaw muscles

- Levator of the soft palate
- Tensor of the soft palate
- Uvulae
- Palatoglossus
- Palatopharingeus

409

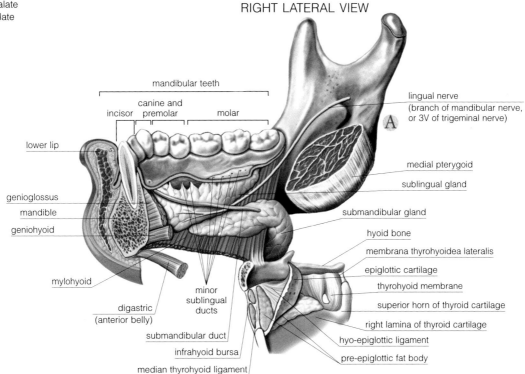

mandibular teeth

canine and
premolar

incisor   molar

lower lip

genioglossus

mandible

geniohyoid

mylohyoid

digastric
(anterior belly)

minor
sublingual
ducts

submandibular duct

infrahyoid bursa

median thyrohyoid ligament

lingual nerve
(branch of mandibular nerve,
or 3V of trigeminal nerve)

medial pterygoid

sublingual gland

submandibular gland

hyoid bone

membrana thyrohyoidea lateralis

epiglottic cartilage

thyrohyoid membrane

superior horn of thyroid cartilage

right lamina of thyroid cartilage

hyo-epiglottic ligament

pre-epiglottic fat body

SUBLINGUAL and SUBMANDIBULAR GLAND
WITH ORAL FLOOR RELATIONS. RIGHT LATERAL VIEW

ORAL REGION and TOPOGRAPHY of GLANDS (I)
LEFT ANTERIOR LATERAL VIEW

410

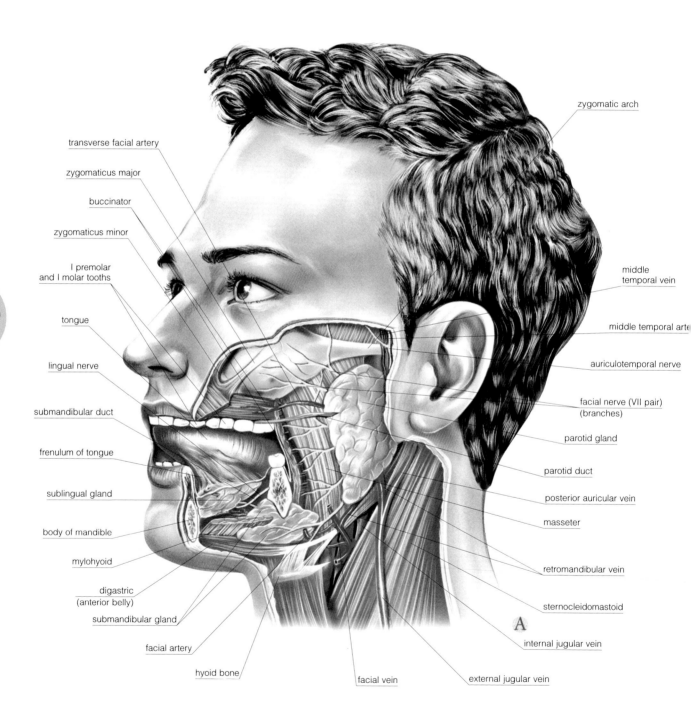

zygomatic arch

transverse facial artery

zygomaticus major

buccinator

zygomaticus minor

I premolar
and I molar tooths

tongue

lingual nerve

submandibular duct

frenulum of tongue

sublingual gland

body of mandible

mylohyoid

digastric
(anterior belly)

submandibular gland

facial artery

hyoid bone

facial vein

middle
temporal vein

middle temporal arte

auriculotemporal nerve

facial nerve (VII pair)
(branches)

parotid gland

parotid duct

posterior auricular vein

masseter

retromandibular vein

sternocleidomastoid

internal jugular vein

external jugular vein

A

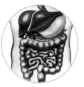

ORAL REGION and TOPOGRAPHY of GLANDS (II)

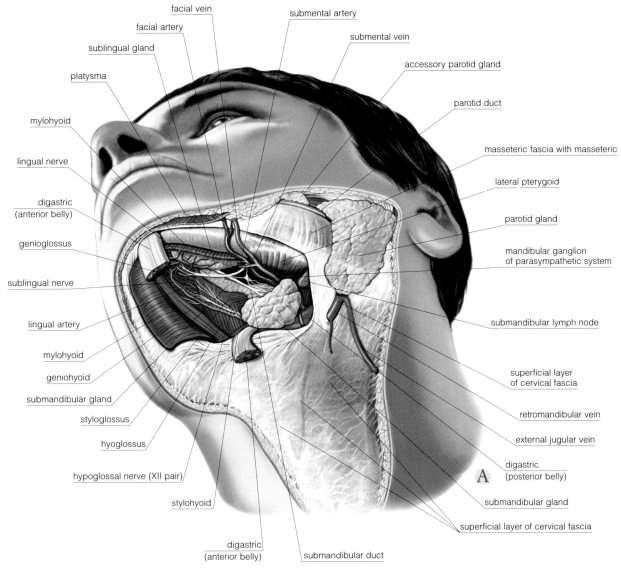

facial vein

facial artery

sublingual gland

platysma

mylohyoid

lingual nerve

digastric
(anterior belly)

genioglossus

sublingual nerve

lingual artery

mylohyoid

geniohyoid

submandibular gland

styloglossus

hyoglossus

hypoglossal nerve (XII pair)

stylohyoid

digastric
(anterior belly)

submental artery

submental vein

accessory parotid gland

parotid duct

masseteric fascia with masseteric

lateral pterygoid

parotid gland

mandibular ganglion
of parasympathetic system

submandibular lymph node

superficial layer
of cervical fascia

retromandibular vein

external jugular vein

digastric
(posterior belly)

submandibular gland

superficial layer of cervical fascia

submandibular duct

A

MAJOR SALIVARY GLANDS FROM ORAL FLOOR. CAUDOCRANIAL VIEW

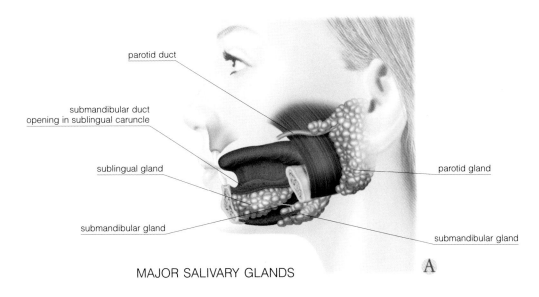

parotid duct

submandibular duct
opening in sublingual caruncle

sublingual gland

submandibular gland

parotid gland

submandibular gland

MAJOR SALIVARY GLANDS

A

TEETH (I). CHILD

dentition

Refers to the set of teeth that a person uses to chew food he ingests, as an initial digestion process. Throughout his life, human beings have two types of teeth. The first is temporary (first dentition, child teeth) and lasts until the age of 5-7. The second dentition is the definite, permanent or secondary set of teeth.

APPROXIMATE TIME of ERUPTION (in months)

CORRELATIVE ORDER of ERUPTION

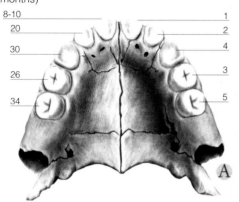

8-10	1
20	2
30	4
26	3
34	5

MAXILLA and PALATINE BONE CAUDOCRANIAL VIEW

maxilla

left	55	54	53	52	51	61	62	63	64	65	right
	85	84	83	82	81	71	72	73	74	75	

mandible

DENTAL FORMULE of IDF (International Dental Federation)

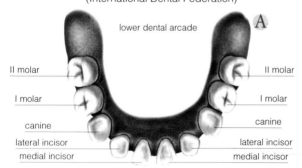

lower dental arcade

II molar		II molar
I molar		I molar
canine		canine
lateral incisor		lateral incisor
medial incisor		medial incisor

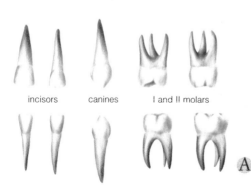

incisors   canines   I and II molars

DECIDOUS TEETH

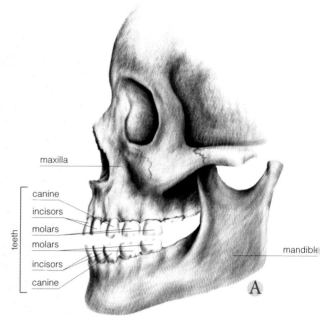

maxilla

teeth
- canine
- incisors
- molars
- molars
- incisors
- canine

mandible

CHILD of 5 YEARS OLD APPROXIMATE

first dentition

First set of teeth in the first years of life of a person. Their duration is limited. A baby is born without teeth. After 6 months of age, teeth start to appear. The first dentition ends between the ages of 30 and 34 months. The first dentition includes 20 teeth which are distributed among the superior and inferior dental arches. At the ages of 5-7, these teeth start to fall off and are replaced by a different set of teeth, which are permanent, and will make up the definite or second dentition.

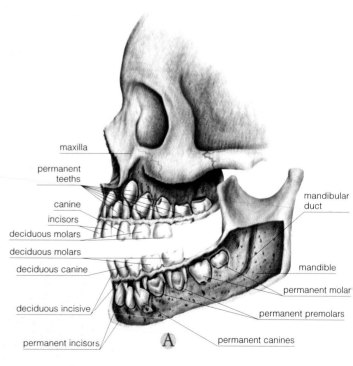

maxilla

permanent teeths

canine

incisors

deciduous molars

deciduous molars

deciduous canine

deciduous incisive

permanent incisors

mandibular duct

mandible

permanent molar

permanent premolars

permanent canines

CHILD of 5 YEARS OLD APPROXIMATE

412

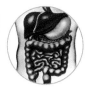

TEETH (II). ADULT

PPROXIMATE TIME ERUPTION (in years)

CORRELATIVE ORDER of ERUPTION

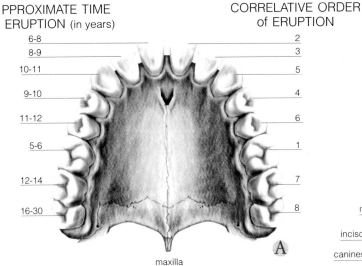

6-8	2
8-9	3
10-11	5
9-10	4
11-12	6
5-6	1
12-14	7
16-30	8

maxilla

Ⓐ

18	17	16	15	14	13	12	11	21	22	23	24	25	26	27	28
48	47	46	45	44	43	42	41	31	32	33	34	35	36	37	38

left   mandible   right

second dentition

Set of teeth which start to come out when the first set of teeth fall off. This process occurs approximately at the ages of 5-7. This is the final dentition, which can be completed during adult life. At times, the third molars, or wisdom teeth, do not come out. It has 32 pieces which are symmetrically laid out and are incrusted in the alveolus, forming a dental arch with 16 teeth (4 incisors, 2 canines, 4 premolars and 6 molars) in the axillary, and other pieces in the mandible.

DENTAL FORMULE of IDF
(International Dental Federation)

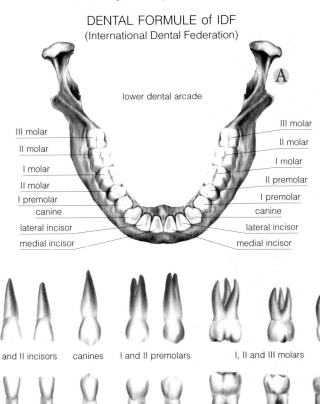

lower dental arcade

Ⓐ

III molar	III molar
II molar	II molar
I molar	I molar
II molar	II premolar
I premolar	I premolar
canine	canine
lateral incisor	lateral incisor
medial incisor	medial incisor

and II incisors   canines   I and II premolars   I, II and III molars   Ⓐ

LEFT PERMANENT TEETH

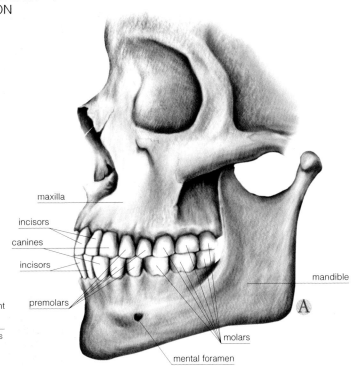

maxilla

incisors

canines

incisors

premolars

mandible

molars

mental foramen

Ⓐ

MAN of 20 YEARS OLD

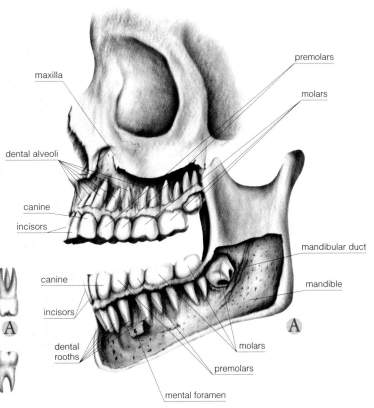

premolars

molars

maxilla

dental alveoli

canine

incisors

canine

incisors

dental rooths

mandibular duct

mandible

molars

premolars

mental foramen

Ⓐ

MAN of 20 YEARS OLD

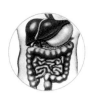

TEETH (III). STRUCTURE of an INCISOR

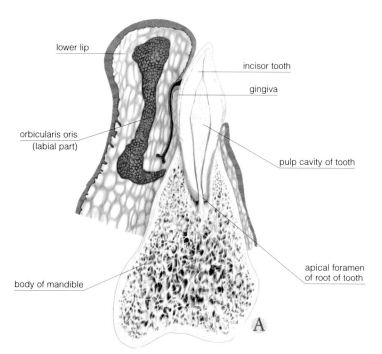

lower lip

incisor tooth

gingiva

orbicularis oris
(labial part)

pulp cavity of tooth

body of mandible

apical foramen
of root of tooth

A

INCISOR and ATTACHED STRUCTURES

teeth

Teeth are structures which are inserted in the dental alveolus (or cavities) which are present in the inferior edge of the maxillary bones, or in the alveolus process, and the superior edge of the mandible, or the mandibular body alveolus. In the final dentition, the person has 32 teeth which are distributed in two arches, superior and inferior. Each arch has 16 teeth. There are four types of teeth. Each one of these types has a specific morphology, according to their function: incisors (four in each arcade, with a cutting function), canines (two in each arcade, with a tearing function), premolars (four in each arcade, with a grinding function), and molars (six in each arcade, with a grinding function).

414

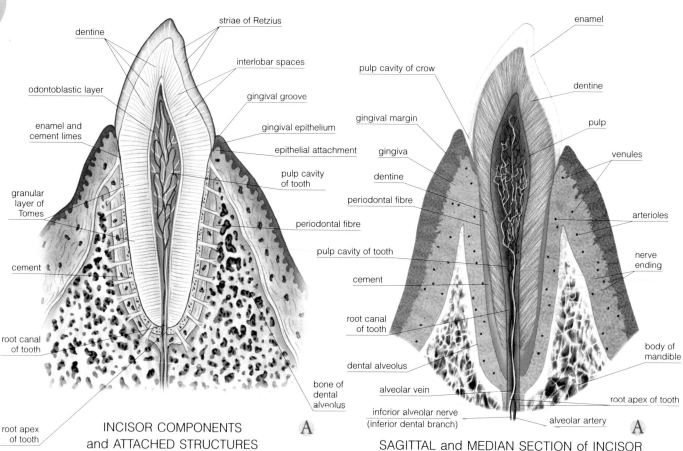

dentine

striae of Retzius

interlobar spaces

odontoblastic layer

gingival groove

gingival epithelium

enamel and
cement limes

epithelial attachment

pulp cavity
of tooth

granular
layer of
Tomes

periodontal fibre

cement

root canal
of tooth

root apex
of tooth

bone of
dental
alveolus

INCISOR COMPONENTS
and ATTACHED STRUCTURES

A

enamel

pulp cavity of crow

dentine

gingival margin

pulp

gingiva

venules

dentine

periodontal fibre

arterioles

pulp cavity of tooth

nerve
ending

cement

root canal
of tooth

body of
mandible

dental alveolus

root apex of tooth

alveolar vein

inferior alveolar nerve
(inferior dental branch)

alveolar artery

A

SAGITTAL and MEDIAN SECTION of INCISOR

TEETH (IV). STRUCTURE of a MOLAR

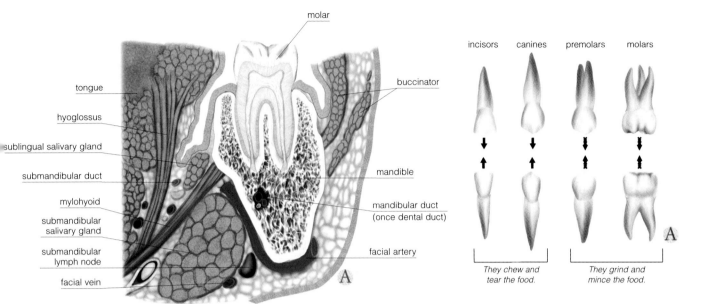

MOLAR and ATTACHED STRUCTURES

molar

tongue

hyoglossus

sublingual salivary gland

submandibular duct

mylohyoid

submandibular salivary gland

submandibular lymph node

facial vein

buccinator

mandible

mandibular duct (once dental duct)

facial artery

incisors   canines   premolars   molars

They chew and tear the food.

They grind and mince the food.

TEETH FUNCTIONS

415

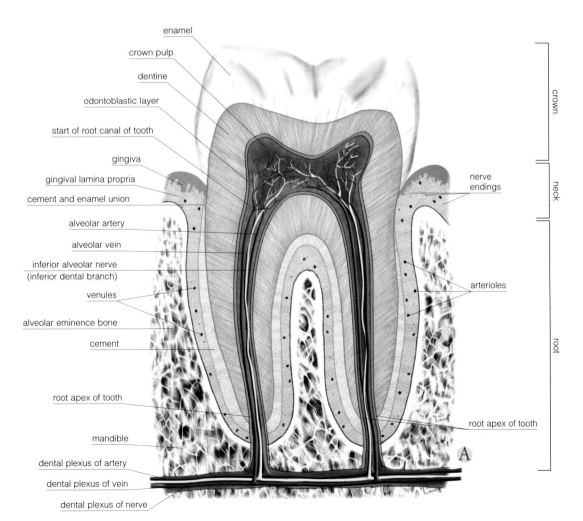

enamel

crown pulp

dentine

odontoblastic layer

start of root canal of tooth

gingiva

gingival lamina propria

cement and enamel union

alveolar artery

alveolar vein

inferior alveolar nerve (inferior dental branch)

venules

alveolar eminence bone

cement

root apex of tooth

mandible

dental plexus of artery

dental plexus of vein

dental plexus of nerve

nerve endings

arterioles

root apex of tooth

crown

neck

root

CORONAL SECTION ACROSS ANTERIOR ROOTS

TONGUE, LARYNX and THYROID

ANTERIOR VIEW of LARYNX, INFERIOR of ORAL and LINGUAL FLOOR

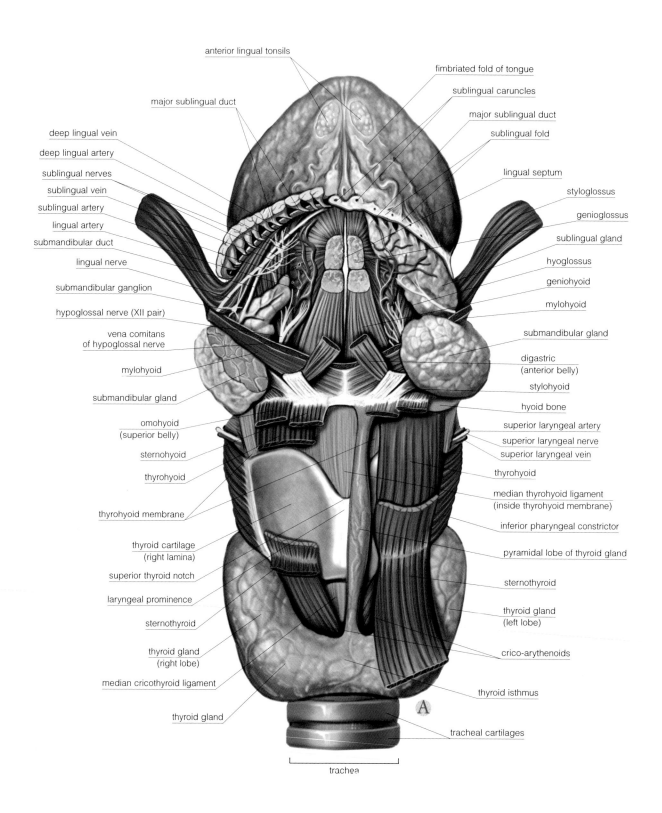

anterior lingual tonsils

fimbriated fold of tongue

major sublingual duct

sublingual caruncles

major sublingual duct

deep lingual vein

sublingual fold

deep lingual artery

sublingual nerves

lingual septum

sublingual vein

styloglossus

sublingual artery

genioglossus

lingual artery

sublingual gland

submandibular duct

hyoglossus

lingual nerve

geniohyoid

submandibular ganglion

mylohyoid

hypoglossal nerve (XII pair)

submandibular gland

vena comitans
of hypoglossal nerve

digastric
(anterior belly)

mylohyoid

stylohyoid

submandibular gland

hyoid bone

omohyoid
(superior belly)

superior laryngeal artery

sternohyoid

superior laryngeal nerve

superior laryngeal vein

thyrohyoid

thyrohyoid

thyrohyoid membrane

median thyrohyoid ligament
(inside thyrohyoid membrane)

inferior pharyngeal constrictor

thyroid cartilage
(right lamina)

pyramidal lobe of thyroid gland

superior thyroid notch

sternothyroid

laryngeal prominence

thyroid gland
(left lobe)

sternothyroid

thyroid gland
(right lobe)

crico-arythenoids

median cricothyroid ligament

thyroid isthmus

thyroid gland

A

tracheal cartilages

trachea

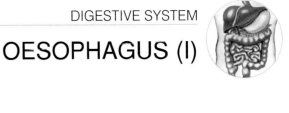
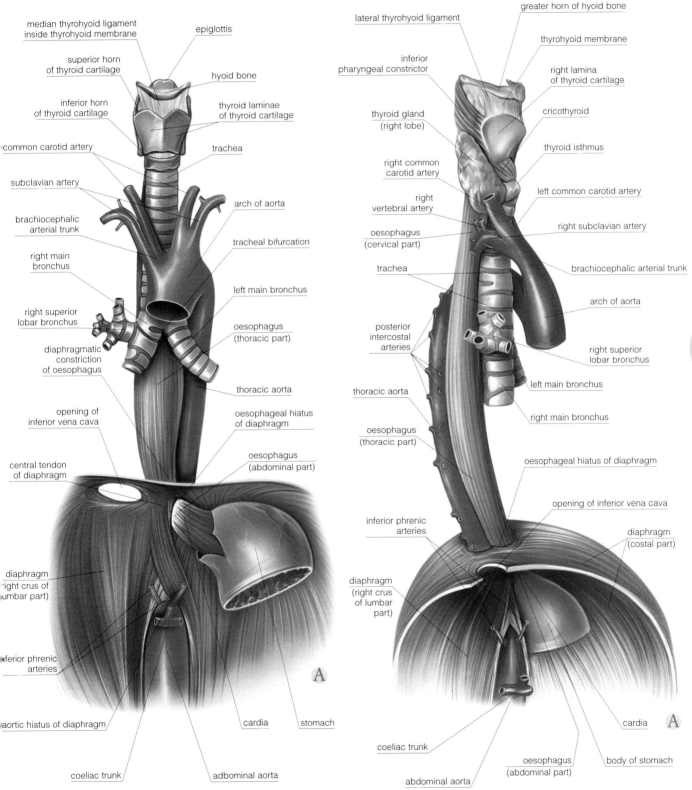

median thyrohyoid ligament inside thyrohyoid membrane

epiglottis

superior horn of thyroid cartilage

hyoid bone

inferior horn of thyroid cartilage

thyroid laminae of thyroid cartilage

common carotid artery

trachea

subclavian artery

arch of aorta

brachiocephalic arterial trunk

tracheal bifurcation

right main bronchus

left main bronchus

right superior lobar bronchus

oesophagus (thoracic part)

diaphragmatic constriction of oesophagus

thoracic aorta

opening of inferior vena cava

oesophageal hiatus of diaphragm

central tendon of diaphragm

oesophagus (abdominal part)

diaphragm (right crus of lumbar part)

inferior phrenic arteries

aortic hiatus of diaphragm

cardia

stomach

coeliac trunk

adbominal aorta

ANTERIOR VIEW

lateral thyrohyoid ligament

greater horn of hyoid bone

thyrohyoid membrane

inferior pharyngeal constrictor

right lamina of thyroid cartilage

thyroid gland (right lobe)

cricothyroid

thyroid isthmus

right common carotid artery

left common carotid artery

right vertebral artery

right subclavian artery

oesophagus (cervical part)

brachiocephalic arterial trunk

trachea

arch of aorta

posterior intercostal arteries

right superior lobar bronchus

thoracic aorta

left main bronchus

oesophagus (thoracic part)

right main bronchus

oesophageal hiatus of diaphragm

opening of inferior vena cava

inferior phrenic arteries

diaphragm (costal part)

diaphragm (right crus of lumbar part)

cardia

coeliac trunk

oesophagus (abdominal part)

body of stomach

abdominal aorta

LATERAL VIEW

OESOPHAGUS and MAIN RELATIONS

OESOPHAGUS (II)

oesophagus

Tubular muscular duct which is part of the digestive tract and extends from the pharynx to the stomach. The oesophagus placing is vertical, and very slightly inclined to the left, and slightly sinuous. The esophagus first curves to the left, then to the right, and again to the left. It travels along a part of the neck and the thoracic cavity, behind the trachea and the heart, and it crosses the diaphragm, in order to start a small route through the abdominal cavity. It is about 25cm long and it has a transverse diameter of approximately 2-3cm. When it contracts, its walls push down food from the pharynx towards the stomach, passing through the inferior edge of the oesophagus, called the cardia. It presents three narrowing parts, a cricoid, an aortic, a bronchial and a diaphragmatic narrowing.

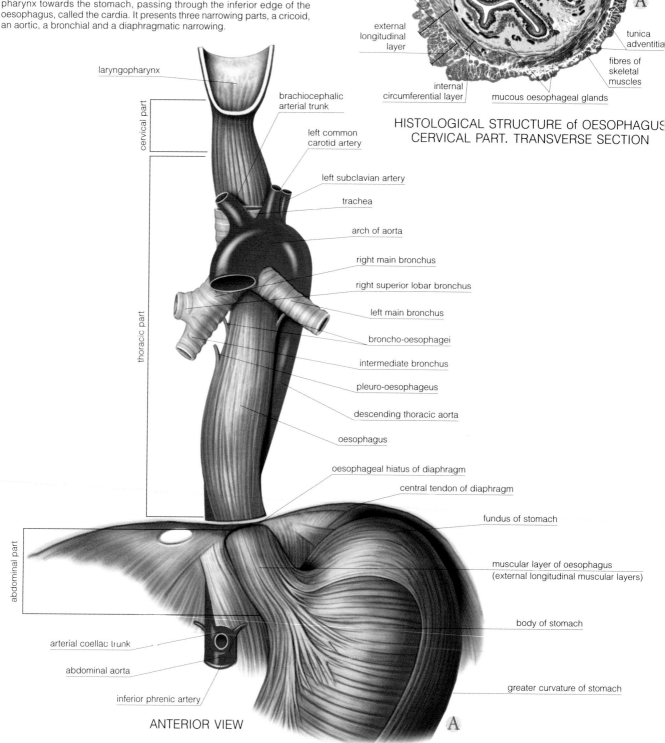

HISTOLOGICAL STRUCTURE of OESOPHAGUS
CERVICAL PART. TRANSVERSE SECTION

squamous epithelium

submucosa

muscular l
of mucosa

lumen

lamin
propr

muscular layer

tunica
adventitia

external
longitudinal
layer

fibres of
skeletal
muscles

internal
circumferential layer

mucous oesophageal glands

laryngopharynx

brachiocephalic
arterial trunk

cervical part

left common
carotid artery

left subclavian artery

trachea

arch of aorta

right main bronchus

right superior lobar bronchus

left main bronchus

broncho-oesophagei

intermediate bronchus

pleuro-oesophageus

descending thoracic aorta

oesophagus

thoracic part

oesophageal hiatus of diaphragm

central tendon of diaphragm

fundus of stomach

muscular layer of oesophagus
(external longitudinal muscular layers)

body of stomach

abdominal part

arterial coeliac trunk

abdominal aorta

greater curvature of stomach

inferior phrenic artery

ANTERIOR VIEW

OESOPHAGUS (III). MEDIASTINAL TRACK
POSTERIOR VIEW

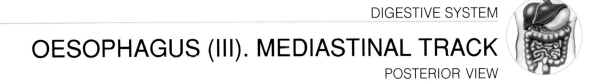

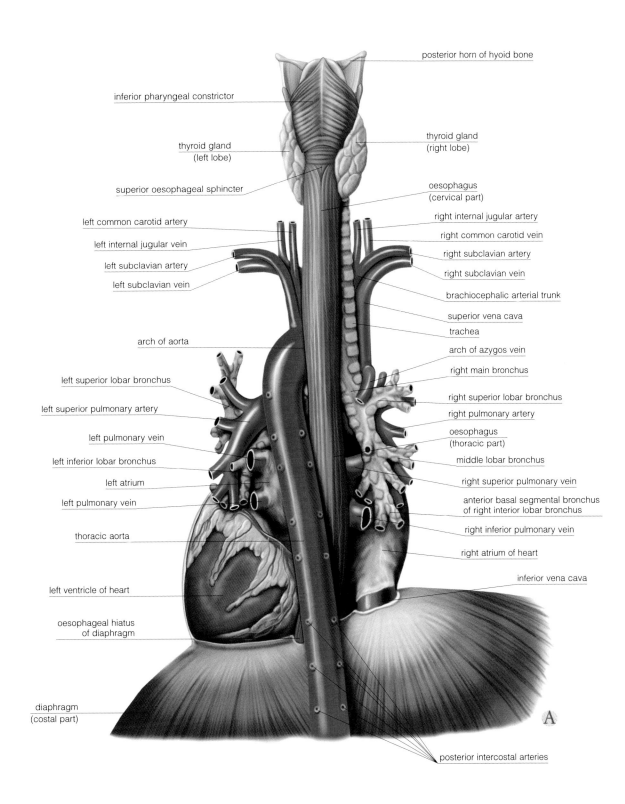

posterior horn of hyoid bone

inferior pharyngeal constrictor

thyroid gland
(right lobe)

thyroid gland
(left lobe)

oesophagus
(cervical part)

superior oesophageal sphincter

right internal jugular artery

left common carotid artery

right common carotid vein

left internal jugular vein

right subclavian artery

left subclavian artery

right subclavian vein

left subclavian vein

brachiocephalic arterial trunk

superior vena cava

trachea

arch of aorta

arch of azygos vein

right main bronchus

left superior lobar bronchus

right superior lobar bronchus

left superior pulmonary artery

right pulmonary artery

oesophagus
(thoracic part)

left pulmonary vein

middle lobar bronchus

left inferior lobar bronchus

left atrium

right superior pulmonary vein

left pulmonary vein

anterior basal segmental bronchus
of right interior lobar bronchus

thoracic aorta

right inferior pulmonary vein

right atrium of heart

left ventricle of heart

inferior vena cava

oesophageal hiatus
of diaphragm

diaphragm
(costal part)

A

posterior intercostal arteries

ABDOMEN and PELVIS (I)

MALE SEX. LEFT SAGITTAL SECTION. LATERAL VIEW

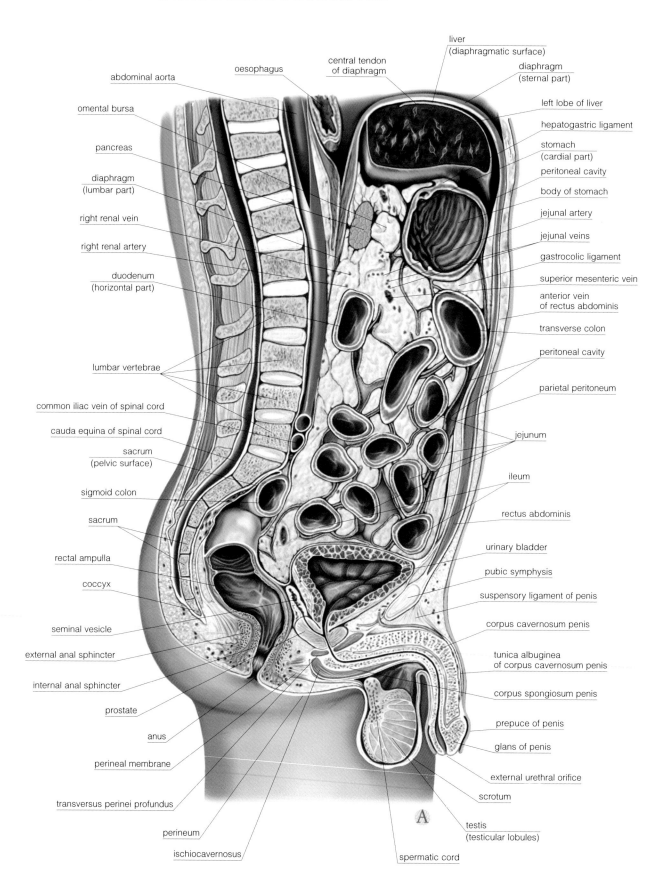

abdominal aorta

omental bursa

pancreas

diaphragm
(lumbar part)

right renal vein

right renal artery

duodenum
(horizontal part)

lumbar vertebrae

common iliac vein of spinal cord

cauda equina of spinal cord

sacrum
(pelvic surface)

sigmoid colon

sacrum

rectal ampulla

coccyx

seminal vesicle

external anal sphincter

internal anal sphincter

prostate

anus

perineal membrane

transversus perinei profundus

perineum

ischiocavernosus

oesophagus

central tendon
of diaphragm

liver
(diaphragmatic surface)

diaphragm
(sternal part)

left lobe of liver

hepatogastric ligament

stomach
(cardial part)

peritoneal cavity

body of stomach

jejunal artery

jejunal veins

gastrocolic ligament

superior mesenteric vein

anterior vein
of rectus abdominis

transverse colon

peritoneal cavity

parietal peritoneum

jejunum

ileum

rectus abdominis

urinary bladder

pubic symphysis

suspensory ligament of penis

corpus cavernosum penis

tunica albuginea
of corpus cavernosum penis

corpus spongiosum penis

prepuce of penis

glans of penis

external urethral orifice

scrotum

testis
(testicular lobules)

spermatic cord

A

420

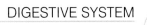

ABDOMEN and PELVIS (II)
FEMALE SEX. RIGHT SAGITTAL SECTION. LATERAL VIEW

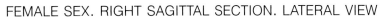

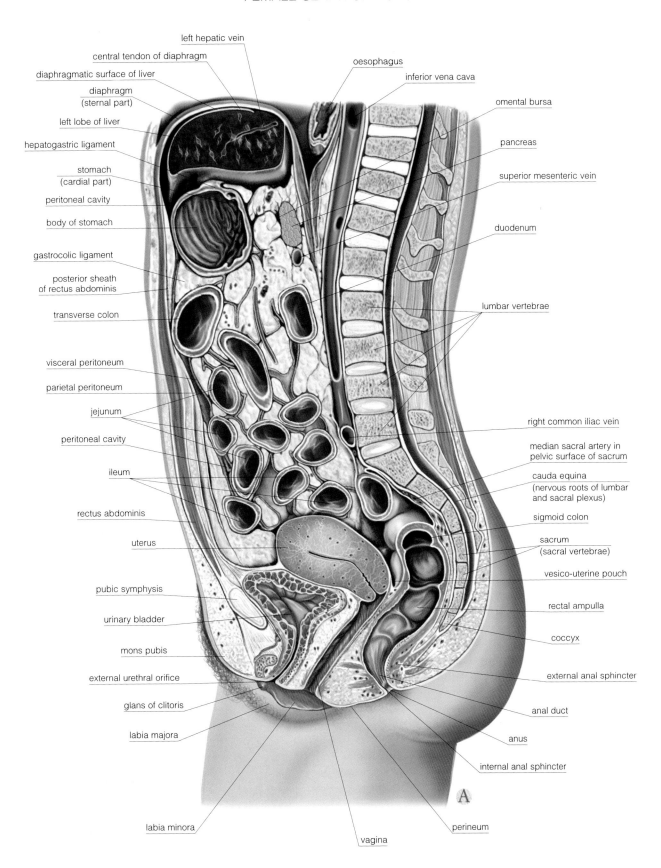

left hepatic vein

central tendon of diaphragm

diaphragmatic surface of liver

diaphragm
(sternal part)

left lobe of liver

hepatogastric ligament

stomach
(cardial part)

peritoneal cavity

body of stomach

gastrocolic ligament

posterior sheath
of rectus abdominis

transverse colon

visceral peritoneum

parietal peritoneum

jejunum

peritoneal cavity

ileum

rectus abdominis

uterus

pubic symphysis

urinary bladder

mons pubis

external urethral orifice

glans of clitoris

labia majora

labia minora

vagina

oesophagus

inferior vena cava

omental bursa

pancreas

superior mesenteric vein

duodenum

lumbar vertebrae

right common iliac vein

median sacral artery in
pelvic surface of sacrum

cauda equina
(nervous roots of lumbar
and sacral plexus)

sigmoid colon

sacrum
(sacral vertebrae)

vesico-uterine pouch

rectal ampulla

coccyx

external anal sphincter

anal duct

anus

internal anal sphincter

perineum

421

A

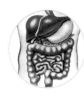

ABDOMINAL and PELVIC ENTRAILS
of DIGESTIVE TRACT and THEIR ATTACHES
ANTERIOR VIEW

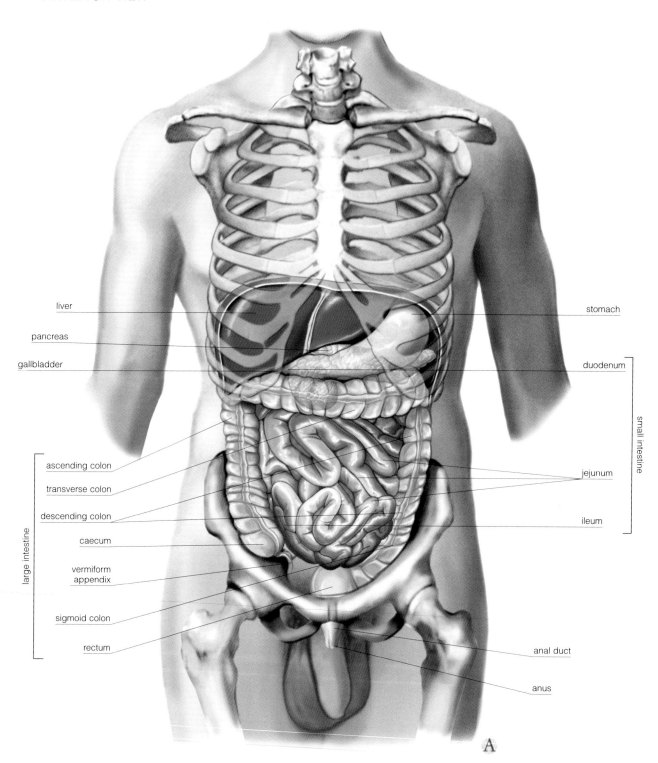

liver

pancreas

gallbladder

ascending colon

transverse colon

descending colon

caecum

vermiform
appendix

sigmoid colon

rectum

large intestine

stomach

duodenum

jejunum

ileum

small intestine

anal duct

anus

A

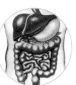

GREATER OMENTUM
ANTERIOR VIEW and RELATIONS

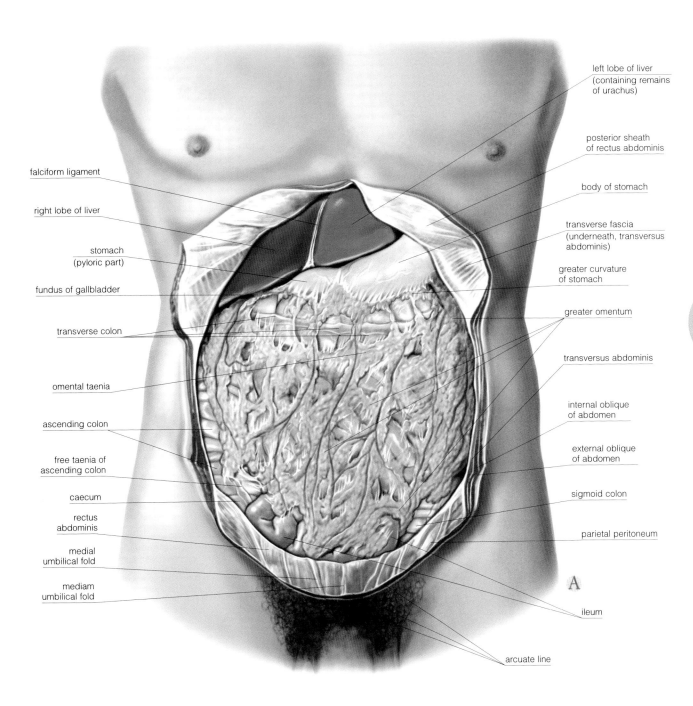

left lobe of liver
(containing remains
of urachus)

posterior sheath
of rectus abdominis

falciform ligament

body of stomach

right lobe of liver

transverse fascia
(underneath, transversus
abdominis)

stomach
(pyloric part)

greater curvature
of stomach

fundus of gallbladder

greater omentum

transverse colon

423

transversus abdominis

omental taenia

internal oblique
of abdomen

ascending colon

external oblique
of abdomen

free taenia of
ascending colon

sigmoid colon

caecum

rectus
abdominis

parietal peritoneum

medial
umbilical fold

mediam
umbilical fold

A

ileum

arcuate line

STOMACH (I). MORPHOLOGY and MUSCULATURE
GENERAL VIEW

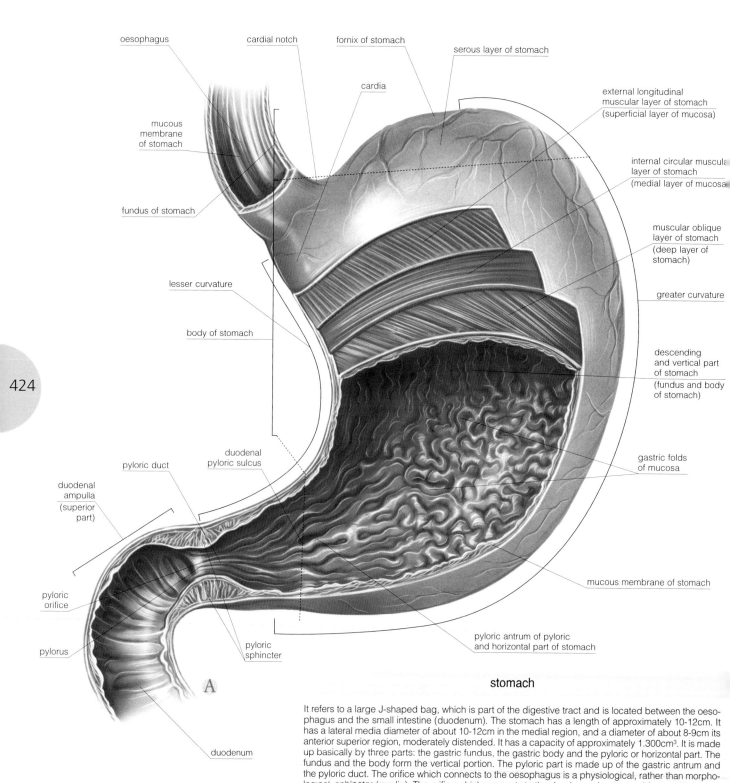

oesophagus

cardial notch

fornix of stomach

serous layer of stomach

cardia

external longitudinal muscular layer of stomach (superficial layer of mucosa)

mucous membrane of stomach

internal circular muscula layer of stomach (medial layer of mucosa

fundus of stomach

muscular oblique layer of stomach (deep layer of stomach)

lesser curvature

greater curvature

body of stomach

descending and vertical part of stomach (fundus and body of stomach)

duodenal pyloric sulcus

gastric folds of mucosa

duodenal ampulla (superior part)

pyloric duct

pyloric orifice

mucous membrane of stomach

pylorus

pyloric sphincter

pyloric antrum of pyloric and horizontal part of stomach

duodenum

A

424

stomach

It refers to a large J-shaped bag, which is part of the digestive tract and is located between the oesophagus and the small intestine (duodenum). The stomach has a length of approximately 10-12cm. It has a lateral media diameter of about 10-12cm in the medial region, and a diameter of about 8-9cm its anterior superior region, moderately distended. It has a capacity of approximately 1.300cm³. It is made up basically by three parts: the gastric fundus, the gastric body and the pyloric or horizontal part. The fundus and the body form the vertical portion. The pyloric part is made up of the gastric antrum and the pyloric duct. The orifice which connects to the oesophagus is a physiological, rather than morphological, sphincter (cardia). The orifice which connects to the duodenum is a true sphincter with its own musculature (pylorus). It is mainly projected on the superior central region of the abdomen wall, or epigastrium. However, it is also projected in the left superior region, or the left hypochondrium. The stomach receives food which has already been ground down and insalivated in the mouth. There, food is mixed with the gastric juices, thus finalizing fragmentation and starting gastric digestion. Once gastric digestion has been performed, the liquid substance passes on to the small intestine, initially the duodenum, where gastric digestion finalizes and absorption, or digestion proper, starts.

STOMACH (II). WALL

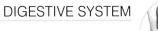

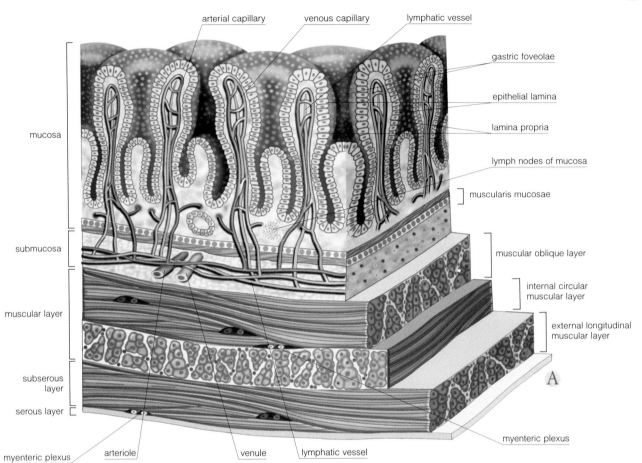

arterial capillary
venous capillary
lymphatic vessel

gastric foveolae

epithelial lamina

lamina propria

lymph nodes of mucosa

muscularis mucosae

muscular oblique layer

internal circular muscular layer

external longitudinal muscular layer

mucosa

submucosa

muscular layer

subserous layer

serous layer

myenteric plexus
arteriole
venule
lymphatic vessel

myenteric plexus

GASTRIC WALL. HISTOLOGICAL SECTION

425

cardial notch
fornix of stomach

muscular layer of oesophagus

oesophagus (abdominal part)

muscular layer of stomach

fundus of stomach

GASTRIC WALL LAYERS

external longitudinal muscular layer

body of stomach

gastric folds of mucosa

pyloric sphincter
angular notch

circular muscular layer

internal circular muscular layer

duodenum (superior part)

duodenal ampulla

duodenum (descending part)

pyloric antrum

A

STOMACH (III). VASCULARIZATION and RELATIONS
ANTERIOR VIEW

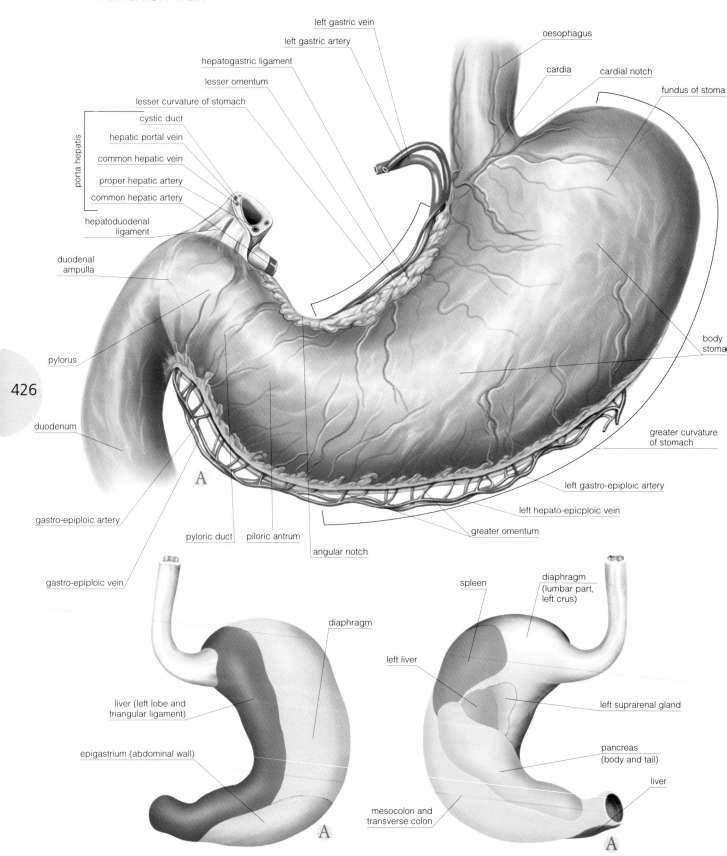

left gastric vein

left gastric artery

hepatogastric ligament

lesser omentum

lesser curvature of stomach

cystic duct

hepatic portal vein

common hepatic vein

proper hepatic artery

common hepatic artery

porta hepatis

hepatoduodenal ligament

duodenal ampulla

pylorus

426

duodenum

gastro-epiploic artery

gastro-epiploic vein

A

pyloric duct

piloric antrum

angular notch

oesophagus

cardia

cardial notch

fundus of stoma

body stoma

greater curvature of stomach

left gastro-epiploic artery

left hepato-epicploic vein

greater omentum

diaphragm

liver (left lobe and triangular ligament)

epigastrium (abdominal wall)

A

RELATIONS. ANTERIOR VIEW

spleen

diaphragm (lumbar part, left crus)

left liver

left suprarenal gland

pancreas (body and tail)

liver

mesocolon and transverse colon

A

RELATIONS. POSTERIOR VIEW

SMALL INTESTINE (I)

small intestine

The small intestine is a long tract, approximately 6m long, which starts in the stomach and curls inside the anterior central region of the abdominal cavity. Its lumen from 15 to 30mm. It forms several creases and U-shaped curves, which allows it to perfectly adapt to a very small space. The duodenum has four parts which mainly surround the head of the pancreas in an almost complete circle. Its total length is 25cm. The duodenum is secondarily retroperitoneal. Its anterior side is coated with peritoneum. The duodenojejunal flexure is the point where the intestine becomes intraperitoneal and is called jejunum. It is approximately 2.5m long. The limit between the jejunum and the ileum is hard to define macroscopically. The jejunum is usually in the left superior region of the colic framework. The ileum, which is the last portion of the small intestine, is usually in the inferior right portion. The ileum is approximately 3.5m long. The terminal ileum communicates with the colon in the ileocecal joint, where the ileocecal valve is located. The pancreatic juices are poured into the small intestine, as well as bile and the secretions of the intestine proper. This finalizes digestion. The digestion in the intestine can be luminal, that is to say, in lumen, or from the membrane, in the mucous surface. Fundamentally, the pancreatic enzymes and the bile break up food in basic absorbable substances. On the other hand, the enzymes associate with food and prepare the nutrients to be absorbed. Basically, the pancreatic enzymes split the proteins are into minor peptic fragments. The membrane enzymes split the proteins into aminoacids. Carbohydrates are split by the action of pancreatic amylase. Lipids are digested by biliary acids and the pancreatic lipase. In this region, the mucous cells absorb the nutritious substances of food, which subsequently pass to the blood and the lymph.

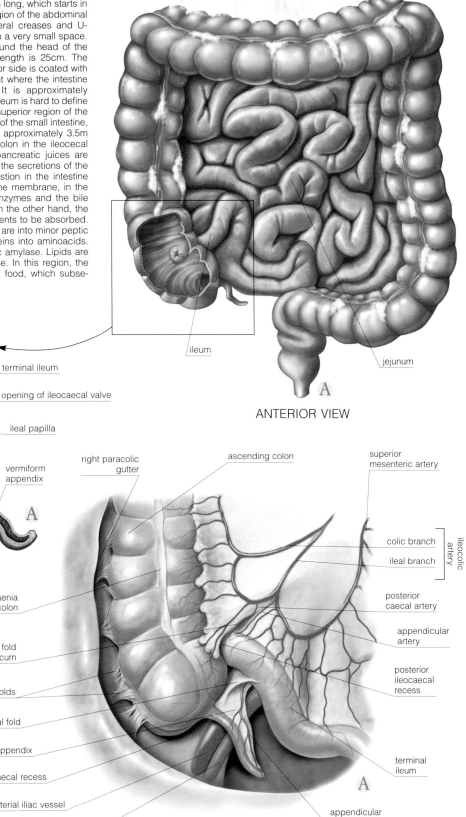

ileum

jejunum

ANTERIOR VIEW

terminal ileum

opening of ileocaecal valve

ileal papilla

vermiform appendix

cecum

orifice of vermiform appendix

free taenia of colon

CAECUM

right paracolic gutter

ascending colon

superior mesenteric artery

free taenia of colon

vascular fold of caecum

caecal folds

ileocaecal fold

meso-appendix

retrocaecal recess

external arterial iliac vessel

external venous iliac vessel

colic branch

ileal branch

ileocolic artery

posterior caecal artery

appendicular artery

posterior ileocaecal recess

terminal ileum

appendicular artery

SMALL INTESTINE (II). DUODENUM

ANTERIOR VIEW and RELATIONS with PANCREAS

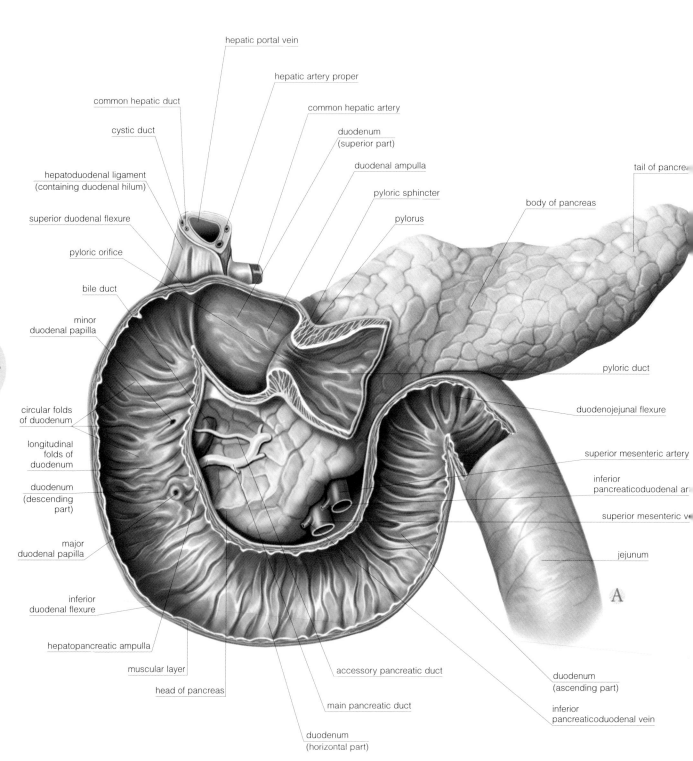

hepatic portal vein

hepatic artery proper

common hepatic duct

common hepatic artery

cystic duct

duodenum
(superior part)

duodenal ampulla

tail of pancreas

hepatoduodenal ligament
(containing duodenal hilum)

pyloric sphincter

body of pancreas

superior duodenal flexure

pylorus

pyloric orifice

bile duct

minor
duodenal papilla

pyloric duct

circular folds
of duodenum

duodenojejunal flexure

longitudinal
folds of
duodenum

superior mesenteric artery

duodenum
(descending
part)

inferior
pancreaticoduodenal artery

superior mesenteric vein

major
duodenal papilla

jejunum

inferior
duodenal flexure

A

hepatopancreatic ampulla

muscular layer

accessory pancreatic duct

duodenum
(ascending part)

head of pancreas

inferior
pancreaticoduodenal vein

main pancreatic duct

duodenum
(horizontal part)

SMALL INTESTINE (III). JEJUNUM. ILEUM

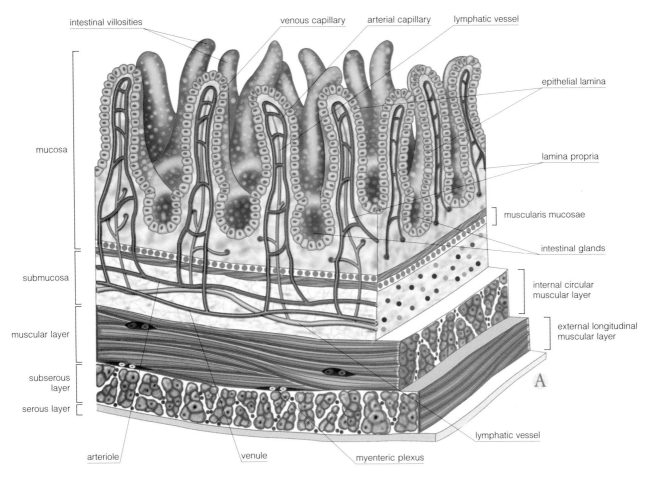

intestinal villosities

venous capillary

arterial capillary

lymphatic vessel

epithelial lamina

lamina propria

muscularis mucosae

intestinal glands

internal circular muscular layer

external longitudinal muscular layer

mucosa

submucosa

muscular layer

subserous layer

serous layer

arteriole

venule

myenteric plexus

lymphatic vessel

SMALL INTESTINE WALL
HISTOLOGICAL SECTION

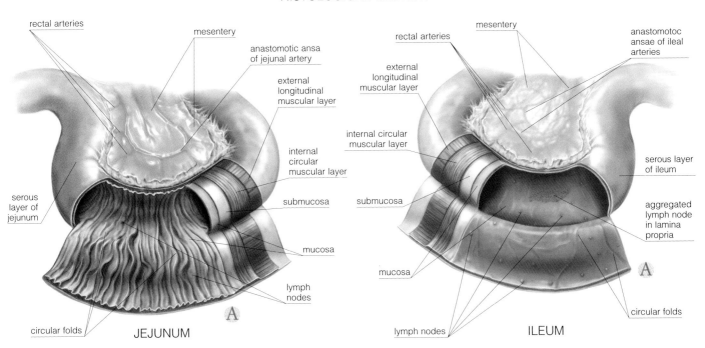

rectal arteries

mesentery

anastomotic ansa of jejunal artery

external longitudinal muscular layer

internal circular muscular layer

submucosa

mucosa

lymph nodes

serous layer of jejunum

circular folds

JEJUNUM

mesentery

rectal arteries

anastomotoc ansae of ileal arteries

external longitudinal muscular layer

internal circular muscular layer

submucosa

mucosa

lymph nodes

serous layer of ileum

aggregated lymph node in lamina propria

circular folds

ILEUM

SMALL INTESTINE (IV). ELEMENTS

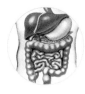

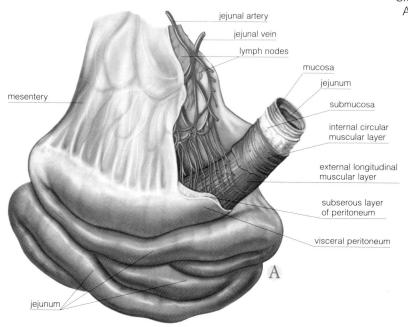

jejunal artery

jejunal vein

lymph nodes

mucosa

jejunum

submucosa

internal circular muscular layer

external longitudinal muscular layer

subserous layer of peritoneum

visceral peritoneum

mesentery

jejunum

ANATOMIC ELEMENTS of JEJUNAL ANSA

SMALL INTESTINAL WALL SECTIONS
ASCENDING WALL of DUODENUM

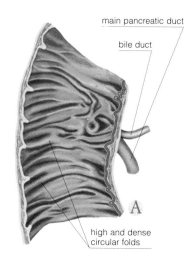

main pancreatic duct

bile duct

high and dense circular folds

DUODENAL MUCOSA RELIEF

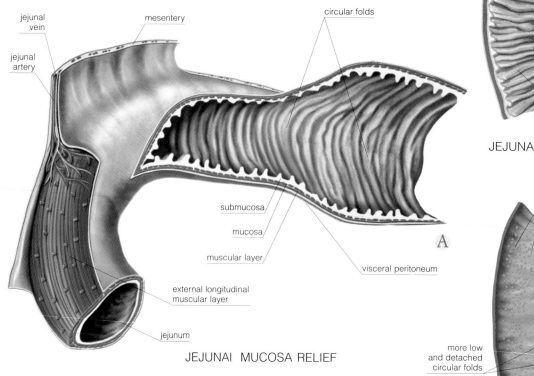

jejunal vein

jejunal artery

mesentery

circular folds

submucosa

mucosa

muscular layer

external longitudinal muscular layer

visceral peritoneum

jejunum

JEJUNAL MUCOSA RELIEF

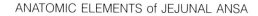

high and dense circular folds

JEJUNAL LAYERS DETAIL

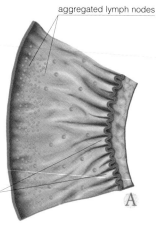

aggregated lymph nodes

more low and detached circular folds

ILEAL MUCOSA RELIEF

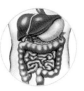

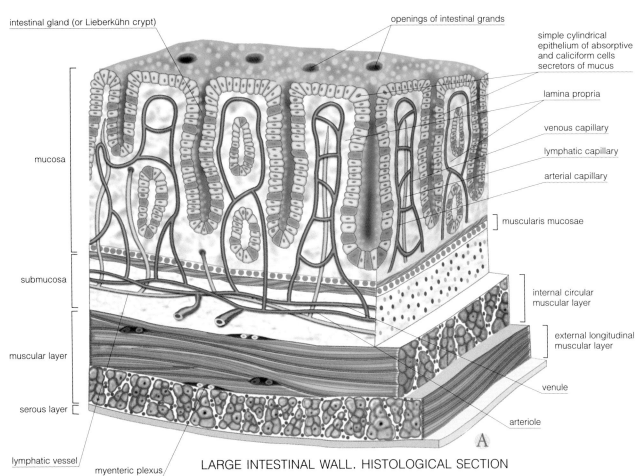

intestinal gland (or Lieberkühn crypt)

openings of intestinal grands

simple cylindrical epithelium of absorptive and caliciform cells secretors of mucus

lamina propria

venous capillary

lymphatic capillary

arterial capillary

muscularis mucosae

internal circular muscular layer

external longitudinal muscular layer

venule

arteriole

mucosa

submucosa

muscular layer

serous layer

lymphatic vessel

myenteric plexus

431

LARGE INTESTINAL WALL. HISTOLOGICAL SECTION

A

large intestine

Corresponds to the final part of the digestive tract. It is a tract, approximately 150cm long, and wider than the small intestine. Its diameter varies from 6-8cm in the caecum of the ascending colon, 5cm in the transverse colon and 3-5cm in the descending colon. The large intestine dilates slightly once again in the sigmoid colon and it initially presents a dilatation in the rectum called rectal ampulla, and from there, it reduces to 2-3cm in the anal duct. It is the continuation of the small intestine, and is joined to it through the ileal orifice. The ileocaecal valve is the separation between them, and the large intestine surrounds it like a frame. The large intestine has different parts: the caecum, ascending colon, transverse colon, descending colon, rectum and anus. The large intestine absorbs water from the remaining food. With the residue of undigested food, feces are formed, which are stored and later expelled through the process of defecation.

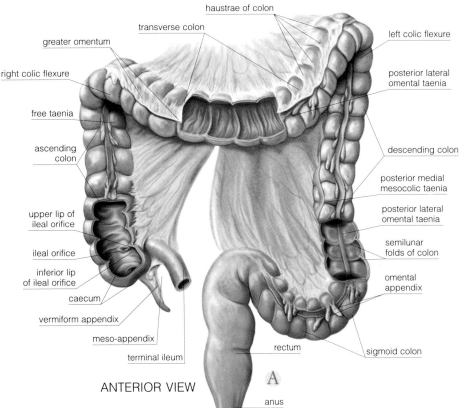

haustrae of colon

transverse colon

greater omentum

right colic flexure

free taenia

ascending colon

upper lip of ileal orifice

ileal orifice

inferior lip of ileal orifice

caecum

vermiform appendix

meso-appendix

terminal ileum

left colic flexure

posterior lateral omental taenia

descending colon

posterior medial mesocolic taenia

posterior lateral omental taenia

semilunar folds of colon

omental appendix

rectum

sigmoid colon

anus

ANTERIOR VIEW

A

LARGE INTESTINE (II)

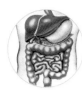

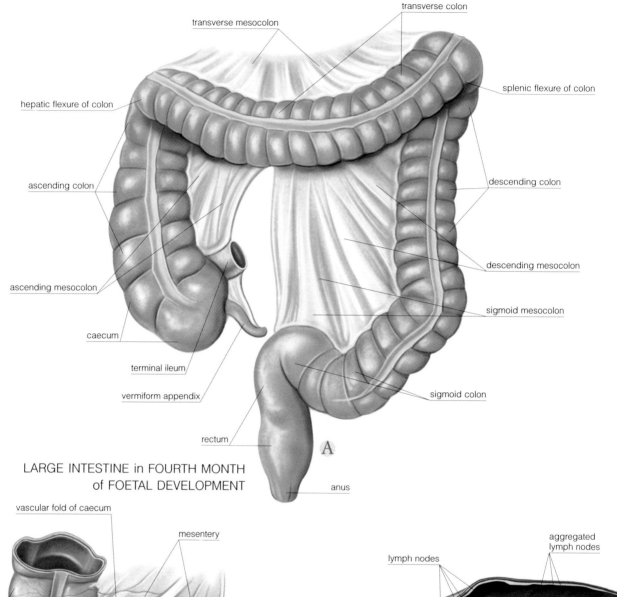

transverse mesocolon

transverse colon

hepatic flexure of colon

splenic flexure of colon

ascending colon

descending colon

descending mesocolon

ascending mesocolon

sigmoid mesocolon

caecum

terminal ileum

sigmoid colon

vermiform appendix

rectum

anus

432

LARGE INTESTINE in FOURTH MONTH of FOETAL DEVELOPMENT

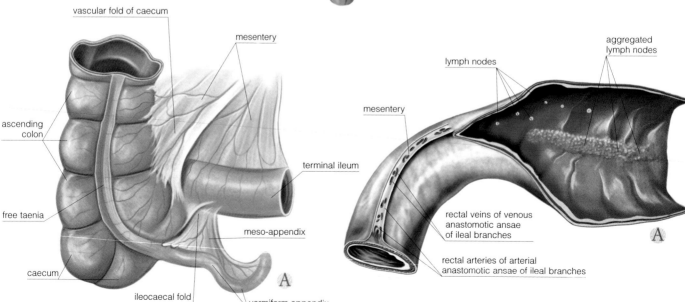

vascular fold of caecum

mesentery

aggregated lymph nodes

lymph nodes

mesentery

ascending colon

terminal ileum

free taenia

meso-appendix

rectal veins of venous anastomotic ansae of ileal branches

caecum

ileocaecal fold

rectal arteries of arterial anastomotic ansae of ileal branches

vermiform appendix

TERMINAL ILEUM

VERMIFORM APPENDIX and ADJACENT STRUCTURES

LARGE INTESTINE (III)

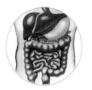

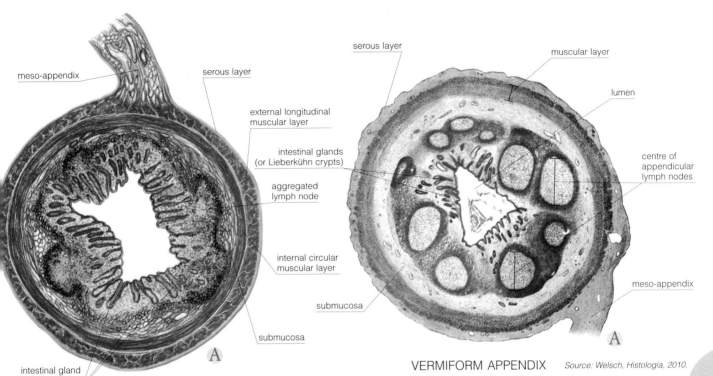

meso-appendix

serous layer

external longitudinal
muscular layer

intestinal glands
(or Lieberkühn crypts)

aggregated
lymph node

internal circular
muscular layer

submucosa

intestinal gland
Lieberkühn crypts)

**LARGE INTESTINE
TRANSVERSE SECTION**

serous layer

muscular layer

lumen

centre of
appendicular
lymph nodes

meso-appendix

submucosa

VERMIFORM APPENDIX   *Source: Welsch, Histología, 2010.*

433

*Refers to a transverse section system, where a great number of follicles are distributed
throughout the sheet proper and the submucosa. In addition to reaching the mucosa, they
can push the crypts and the muscular of the mucosa in a more or less intense manner.
These follicles are coated with a simple cell epithelium, which eases the processing
of the appendicular light antigen, as is the case with aggregate lymph follicles.*

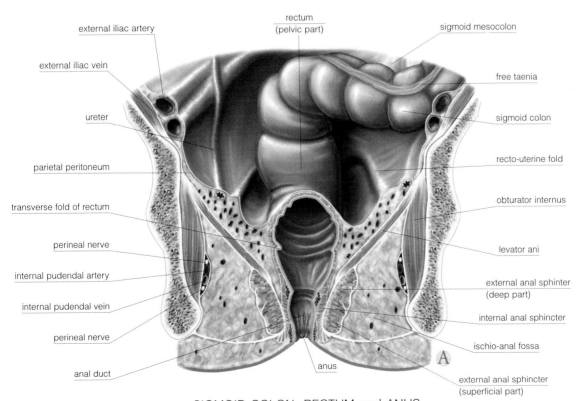

external iliac artery

external iliac vein

ureter

parietal peritoneum

transverse fold of rectum

perineal nerve

internal pudendal artery

internal pudendal vein

perineal nerve

anal duct

rectum
(pelvic part)

sigmoid mesocolon

free taenia

sigmoid colon

recto-uterine fold

obturator internus

levator ani

external anal sphincter
(deep part)

internal anal sphincter

ischio-anal fossa

external anal sphincter
(superficial part)

anus

**SIGMOID COLON, RECTUM and ANUS
FRONTAL SECTION and ANTERIOR VIEW**

LARGE INTESTINE (IV). RECTUM and ANUS

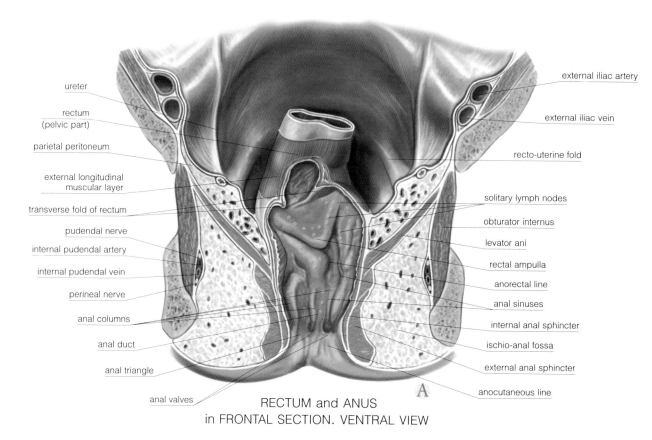

ureter

rectum
(pelvic part)

parietal peritoneum

external longitudinal
muscular layer

transverse fold of rectum

pudendal nerve

internal pudendal artery

internal pudendal vein

perineal nerve

anal columns

anal duct

anal triangle

anal valves

external iliac artery

external iliac vein

recto-uterine fold

solitary lymph nodes

obturator internus

levator ani

rectal ampulla

anorectal line

anal sinuses

internal anal sphincter

ischio-anal fossa

external anal sphincter

anocutaneous line

A

RECTUM and ANUS
in FRONTAL SECTION. VENTRAL VIEW

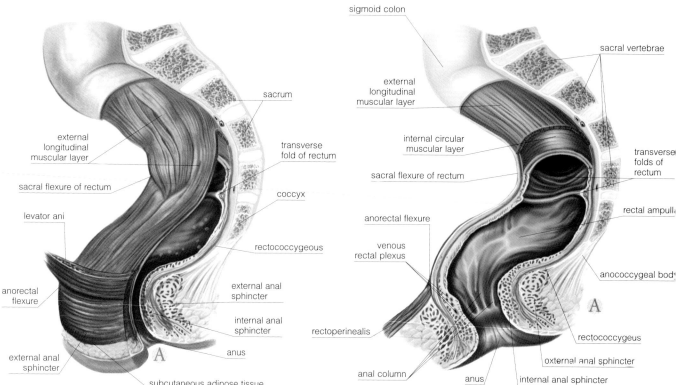

external
longitudinal
muscular layer

sacral flexure of rectum

levator ani

anorectal
flexure

external anal
sphincter

subcutaneous adipose tissue

sacrum

transverse
fold of rectum

coccyx

rectococcygeous

external anal
sphincter

internal anal
sphincter

anus

RIGHT LATERAL VIEW

sigmoid colon

external
longitudinal
muscular layer

internal circular
muscular layer

sacral flexure of rectum

anorectal flexure

venous
rectal plexus

rectoperinealis

anal column

sacral vertebrae

transverse
folds of
rectum

rectal ampulla

anococcygeal body

rectococcygeus

external anal sphincter

internal anal sphincter

anus

A

SAGITTAL SECTION

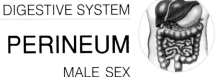

LARGE INTESTINE (V). PERINEUM

MALE SEX

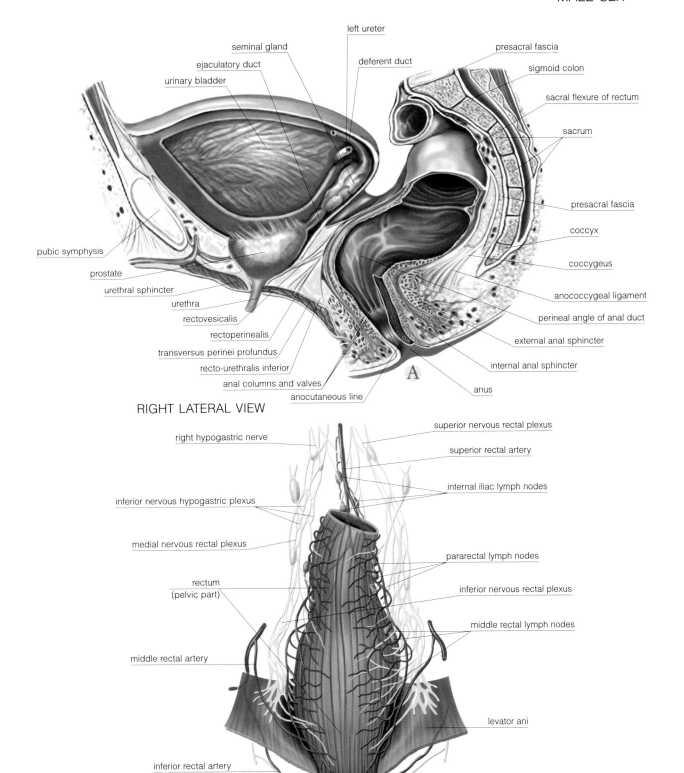

left ureter

seminal gland

ejaculatory duct

deferent duct

urinary bladder

presacral fascia

sigmoid colon

sacral flexure of rectum

sacrum

presacral fascia

coccyx

pubic symphysis

coccygeus

prostate

anococcygeal ligament

urethral sphincter

perineal angle of anal duct

urethra

external anal sphincter

rectovesicalis

internal anal sphincter

rectoperinealis

transversus perinei profundus

recto-urethralis inferior

anal columns and valves

anocutaneous line

anus

RIGHT LATERAL VIEW

435

superior nervous rectal plexus

right hypogastric nerve

superior rectal artery

internal iliac lymph nodes

inferior nervous hypogastric plexus

medial nervous rectal plexus

pararectal lymph nodes

rectum
(pelvic part)

inferior nervous rectal plexus

middle rectal lymph nodes

middle rectal artery

levator ani

inferior rectal artery

anal duct

external anal sphincter

internal anal sphincter

RECTUM and ANAL DUCT. ARTERIES, NERVES and LYMPH NODES

LIVER (I)

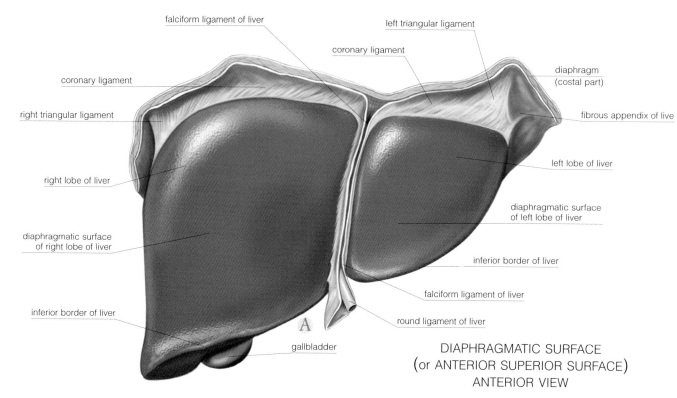

falciform ligament of liver

left triangular ligament

coronary ligament

coronary ligament

diaphragm
(costal part)

right triangular ligament

fibrous appendix of live

right lobe of liver

left lobe of liver

diaphragmatic surface
of right lobe of liver

diaphragmatic surface
of left lobe of liver

inferior border of liver

inferior border of liver

falciform ligament of liver

round ligament of liver

gallbladder

A

DIAPHRAGMATIC SURFACE
(or ANTERIOR SUPERIOR SURFACE)
ANTERIOR VIEW

436

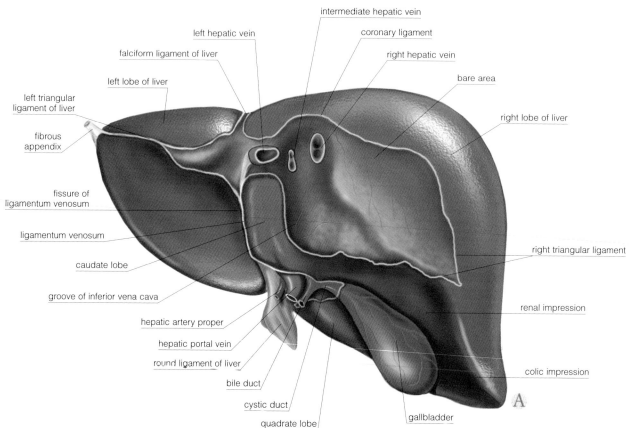

intermediate hepatic vein

left hepatic vein

coronary ligament

falciform ligament of liver

right hepatic vein

left lobe of liver

bare area

left triangular
ligament of liver

right lobe of liver

fibrous
appendix

fissure of
ligamentum venosum

ligamentum venosum

caudate lobe

right triangular ligament

groove of inferior vena cava

renal impression

hepatic artery proper

hepatic portal vein

round ligament of liver

colic impression

bile duct

cystic duct

quadrate lobe

gallbladder

A

VISCERAL SURFACE (or POSTERIOR INFERIOR SURFACE)
POSTERIOR VIEW

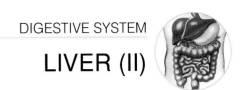

LIVER (II)

liver

The liver is a solid organ. Most of it is found in the left hypochondrium, that is to say, the right superior region of the abdominal cavity, under the diaphragm. However, the liver overtakes the right hypochondrium, also occupying part of the epigastrium and the left hypochondrium. It is the largest viscera in the human body. Its weight is approximately 1,500g in the corpse, to which approximately 800-900g of blood must be added. The liver has a hard consistency and its color is dark red. Its transversal size is approximately 28cm, 16cm in its posterior anterior direction, and 8cm crown-to-rump in the bulkiest region of the left hepatic lobule. Its main digestive function is to produce bile. The bile subsequently is poured into the duodenum through the biliary tracts. Bile is funda-

mental to digest fats of certain foods. It also has very important metabolic functions. It stores glucose, converts galactose and fructose into glucose, and also produces energy reserves (glycogen) from glucose. It also extracts energy from aminoacids, forms lipoproteins, synthesizes cholesterol and phospholipids and converts carbohydrates and proteins into fats. It also forms proteins, processes aminoacids and forms urea. Lastly, it also stores vitamins, forms substances for blood coagulation, stores iron or metabolizes and eliminates substances, medications or hormones. Filtration of venous blood from the portal vein is also performed in the inside of the liver. It is coated by the visceral peritoneum, which is organized to form a set of ligaments which attach the liver to the diaphragm.

437

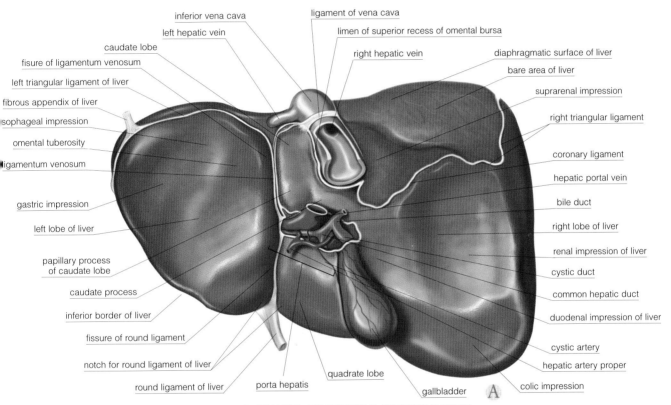

VISCERAL SURFACE. POSTERIOR INFERIOR VIEW

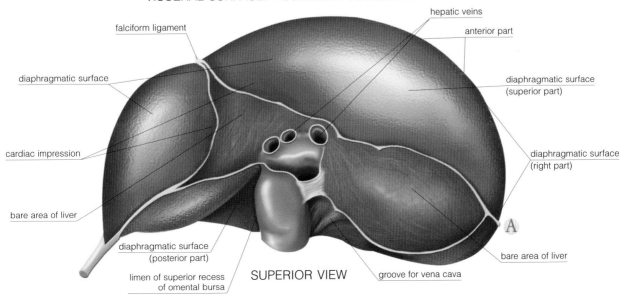

SUPERIOR VIEW

LIVER (III). HEPATIC SEGMENTS

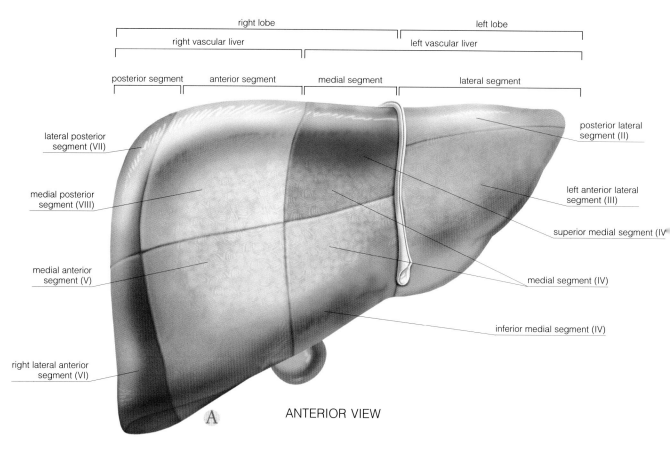

right lobe

right vascular liver

left lobe

left vascular liver

posterior segment   anterior segment   medial segment   lateral segment

lateral posterior
segment (VII)

medial posterior
segment (VIII)

medial anterior
segment (V)

right lateral anterior
segment (VI)

posterior lateral
segment (II)

left anterior lateral
segment (III)

superior medial segment (IV)

medial segment (IV)

inferior medial segment (IV)

ANTERIOR VIEW

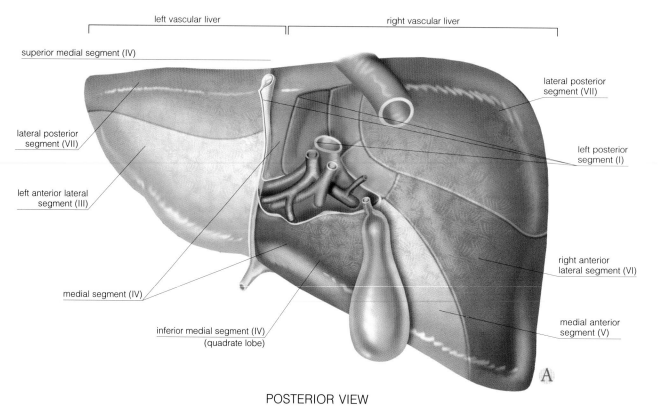

left vascular liver

right vascular liver

superior medial segment (IV)

lateral posterior
segment (VII)

lateral posterior
segment (VII)

left anterior lateral
segment (III)

left posterior
segment (I)

medial segment (IV)

inferior medial segment (IV)
(quadrate lobe)

right anterior
lateral segment (VI)

medial anterior
segment (V)

POSTERIOR VIEW

438

LIVER (IV). ARTERIAL and VENOUS VASCULARIZATION and INTRAHEPATIC BILE DUCTS

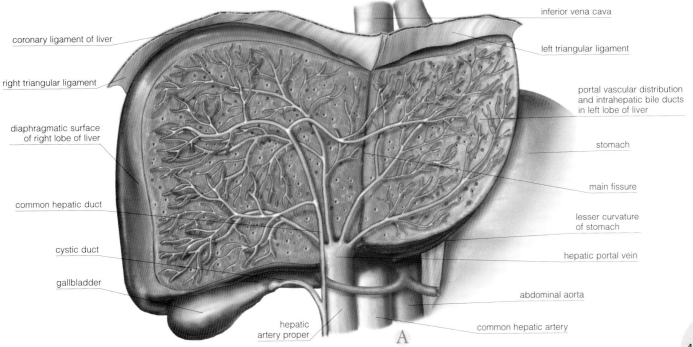

coronary ligament of liver

right triangular ligament

diaphragmatic surface of right lobe of liver

common hepatic duct

cystic duct

gallbladder

hepatic artery proper

inferior vena cava

left triangular ligament

portal vascular distribution and intrahepatic bile ducts in left lobe of liver

stomach

main fissure

lesser curvature of stomach

hepatic portal vein

abdominal aorta

common hepatic artery

A

SCHEMA of VENOUS PORTAL DISTRIBUTION and INTRAHEPATIC BILE DUCTS
FRONTAL SECTION. ANTERIOR VIEW

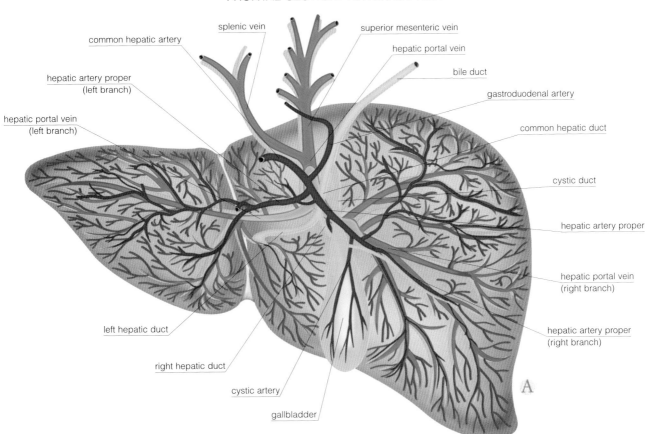

common hepatic artery

hepatic artery proper (left branch)

hepatic portal vein (left branch)

left hepatic duct

right hepatic duct

cystic artery

gallbladder

splenic vein

superior mesenteric vein

hepatic portal vein

bile duct

gastroduodenal artery

common hepatic duct

cystic duct

hepatic artery proper

hepatic portal vein (right branch)

hepatic artery proper (right branch)

A

GALLBLADDER

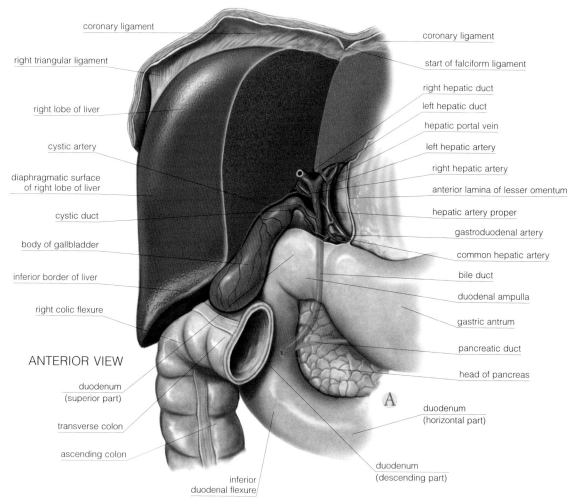

ANTERIOR VIEW

coronary ligament

right triangular ligament

right lobe of liver

cystic artery

diaphragmatic surface
of right lobe of liver

cystic duct

body of gallbladder

inferior border of liver

right colic flexure

duodenum
(superior part)

transverse colon

ascending colon

inferior
duodenal flexure

coronary ligament

start of falciform ligament

right hepatic duct

left hepatic duct

hepatic portal vein

left hepatic artery

right hepatic artery

anterior lamina of lesser omentum

hepatic artery proper

gastroduodenal artery

common hepatic artery

bile duct

duodenal ampulla

gastric antrum

pancreatic duct

head of pancreas

duodenum
(horizontal part)

duodenum
(descending part)

BILE DUCTS

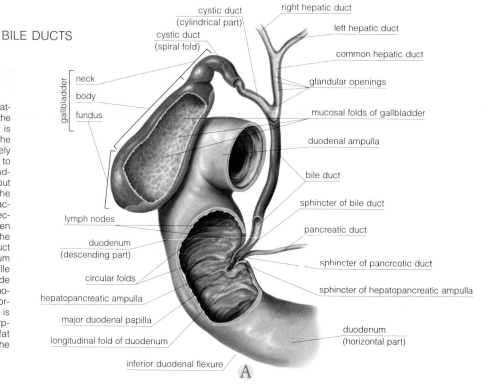

cystic duct
(cylindrical part)

cystic duct
(spiral fold)

right hepatic duct

left hepatic duct

common hepatic duct

glandular openings

mucosal folds of gallbladder

duodenal ampulla

bile duct

sphincter of bile duct

pancreatic duct

sphincter of pancreatic duct

sphincter of hepatopancreatic ampulla

duodenum
(horizontal part)

gallbladder {
neck
body
fundus
}

lymph nodes

duodenum
(descending part)

circular folds

hepatopancreatic ampulla

major duodenal papilla

longitudinal fold of duodenum

inferior duodenal flexure

gallbladder

Refers to a pear-shaped bag which is located in the inferior part of the right lobule of the liver. The gallbladder stores the bile that is poured by the hepatic biliary ducts. The capacity of the gallbladder is approximately 30-60ml. However, a quantity equivalent to 450ml of bile can be stored in the gallbladder, equivalent to 12 hours of production, but concentrated. While the bile remains in the gallbladder, it concentrates due to the extraction of water, sodium, chlorine and other electrolytes. An adult person secretes between 600 and 1.200ml of bile a day. Through the cystic duct, bile is poured into the biliary duct and from it, it pours into the duodenum through the hepatopancreatic ampulla. Bile contains 82% water. Its components include bilirubin and biliary salts, in addition to cholesterol, lecithin and other organic and inorganic substances. Its function in digestion is to emulsify fats and cooperate in the absorption of the products which result from fat digestion, through the cell membrane of the enterocytes of the small intestine.

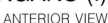

PANCREAS (I). LOCATION and ADJACENT ORGANS (I)

ANTERIOR VIEW

pancreas

Gland which is located in the peritoneum, behind the abdominal cavity and fundamentally at the same height of the supracolic or supramesocolic space, between the LI and LIV vertebrae. It is surrounded by the duodenum, and is located under the liver and behind the stomach. It plays an important exocrine role, since it segregates a set of liquids, the pancreatic juices, which are poured into the duodenum through a major duodenal papillary. Thanks to these alkaline fluids, which are rich in enzymes, proteins, carbohydrates, fats and nucleic acids can be broken down to basic components, which allows the organism to absorb them. Trypsin, chymotrypsin, and carboxypolypeptidase, which are pancreatic juices, are secreted inactively once they reach the duodenum through the action of a duodenal enzyme called enterokinase.

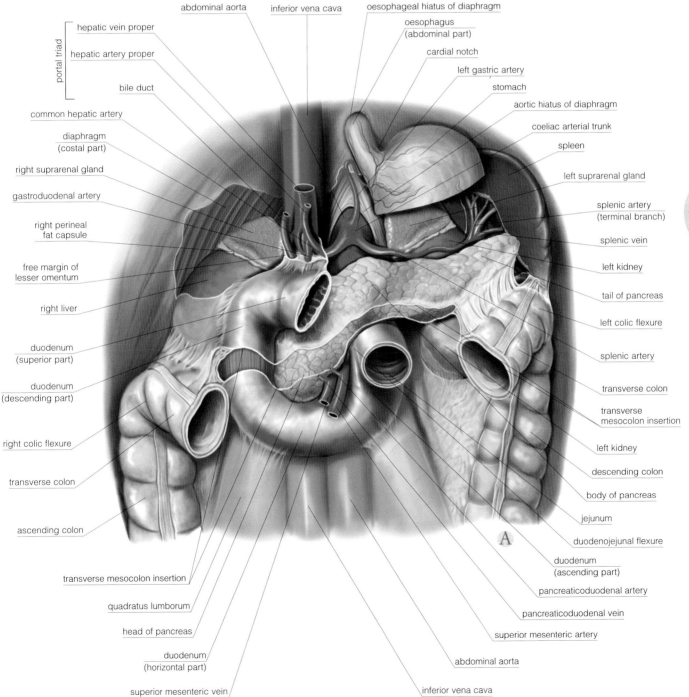

441

PANCREAS (II). LOCATION and ADJACENT ORGANS (II)
ANTERIOR VIEW

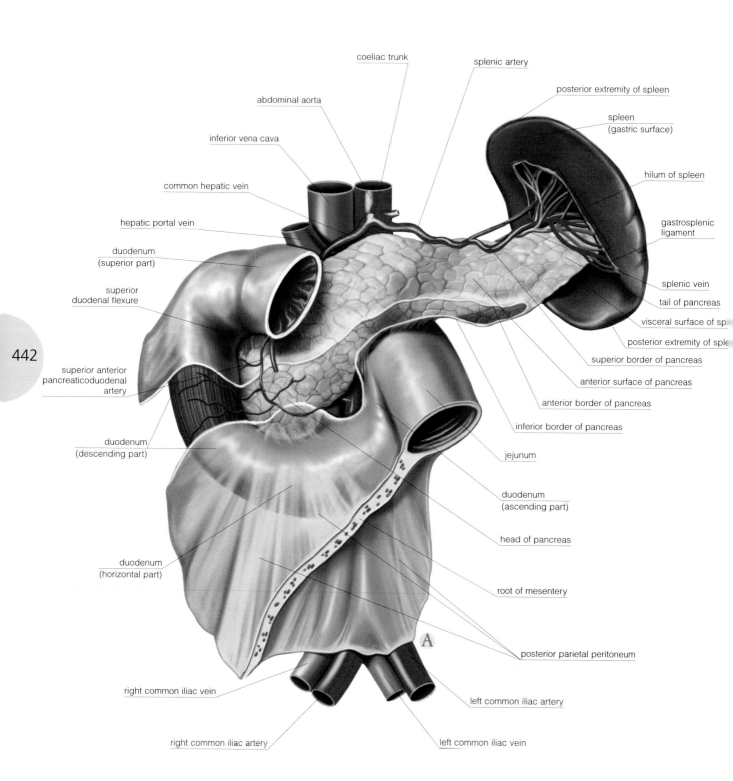

coeliac trunk

splenic artery

abdominal aorta

posterior extremity of spleen

spleen
(gastric surface)

inferior vena cava

hilum of spleen

common hepatic vein

hepatic portal vein

gastrosplenic
ligament

duodenum
(superior part)

splenic vein

superior
duodenal flexure

tail of pancreas

visceral surface of sp

442

posterior extremity of sple

superior border of pancreas

superior anterior
pancreaticoduodenal
artery

anterior surface of pancreas

anterior border of pancreas

inferior border of pancreas

duodenum
(descending part)

jejunum

duodenum
(ascending part)

head of pancreas

duodenum
(horizontal part)

root of mesentery

A

posterior parietal peritoneum

right common iliac vein

left common iliac artery

right common iliac artery

left common iliac vein

PANCREAS (III)

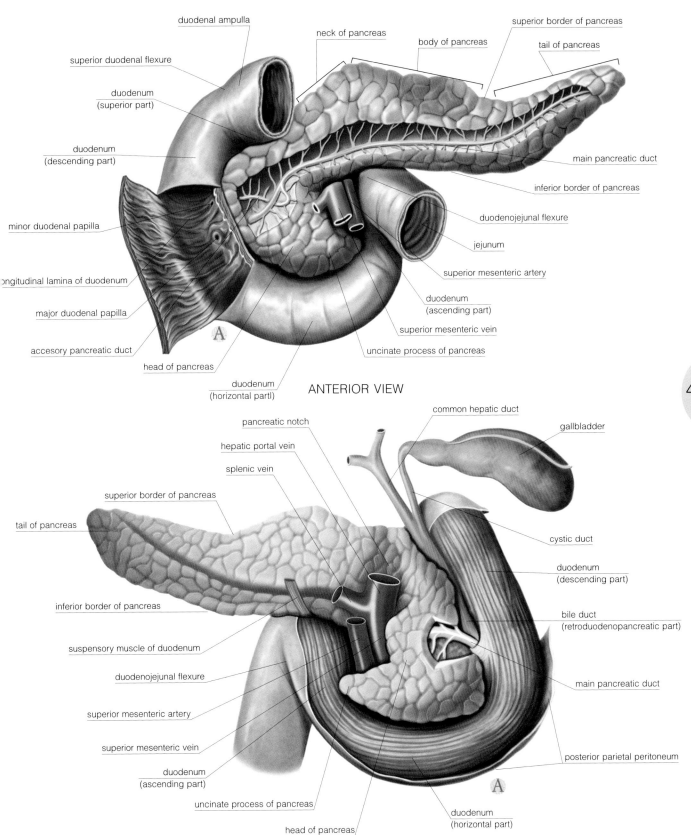

duodenal ampulla

neck of pancreas

body of pancreas

superior border of pancreas

tail of pancreas

superior duodenal flexure

duodenum
(superior part)

duodenum
(descending part)

main pancreatic duct

inferior border of pancreas

duodenojejunal flexure

minor duodenal papilla

jejunum

ongitudinal lamina of duodenum

superior mesenteric artery

duodenum
(ascending part)

major duodenal papilla

superior mesenteric vein

accesory pancreatic duct

uncinate process of pancreas

head of pancreas

duodenum
(horizontal partl)

ANTERIOR VIEW

443

pancreatic notch

common hepatic duct

gallbladder

hepatic portal vein

splenic vein

superior border of pancreas

tail of pancreas

cystic duct

duodenum
(descending part)

inferior border of pancreas

bile duct
(retroduodenopancreatic part)

suspensory muscle of duodenum

duodenojejunal flexure

main pancreatic duct

superior mesenteric artery

superior mesenteric vein

duodenum
(ascending part)

posterior parietal peritoneum

uncinate process of pancreas

duodenum
(horizontal part)

head of pancreas

POSTERIOR VIEW

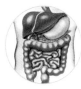

SPLEEN (I)

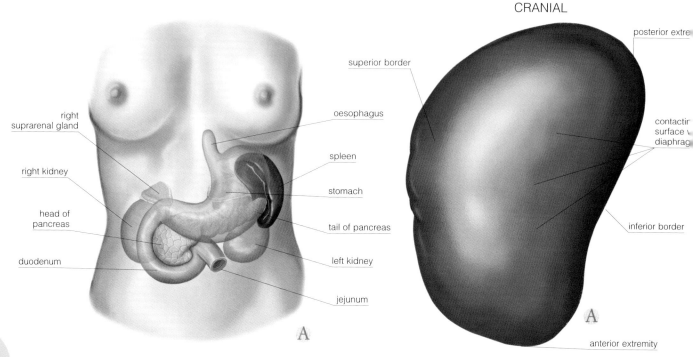

LOCATION and PROJECTION

right suprarenal gland
right kidney
head of pancreas
duodenum

oesophagus
spleen
stomach
tail of pancreas
left kidney
jejunum

A

DIAPHRAGMATIC SURFACE

CRANIAL

superior border
posterior extre
contactir surface v diaphrag
inferior border
anterior extremity
CAUDAL

A

444

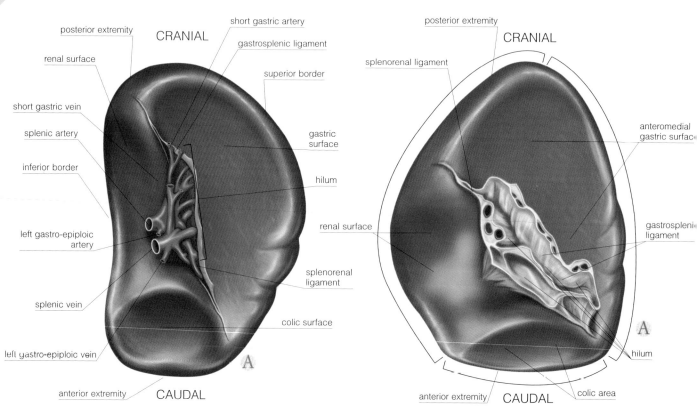

CRANIAL

posterior extremity
renal surface
short gastric vein
splenic artery
inferior border
left gastro-epiploic artery
splenic vein
left gastro-epiploic vein

short gastric artery
gastrosplenic ligament
superior border
gastric surface
hilum
splenorenal ligament
colic surface

A

CAUDAL

VISCERAL SURFACE

CRANIAL

posterior extremity
splenorenal ligament
renal surface

anteromedial gastric surfac
gastrospleni ligament
hilum

A

anterior extremity
colic area
CAUDAL

VISCERAL SURFACE

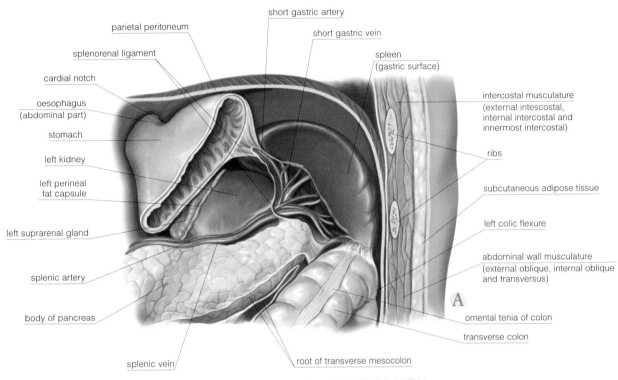

parietal peritoneum
splenorenal ligament
cardial notch
oesophagus
(abdominal part)
stomach
left kidney
left perineal
fat capsule
left suprarenal gland
splenic artery
body of pancreas
splenic vein

short gastric artery
short gastric vein
spleen
(gastric surface)

intercostal musculature
(external intescostal,
internal intercostal and
innermost intercostal)
ribs
subcutaneous adipose tissue
left colic flexure
abdominal wall musculature
(external oblique, internal oblique
and transversus)
omental tenia of colon
transverse colon
root of transverse mesocolon

LEFT SUBPHRENIC REGION. ANTERIOR VIEW

445

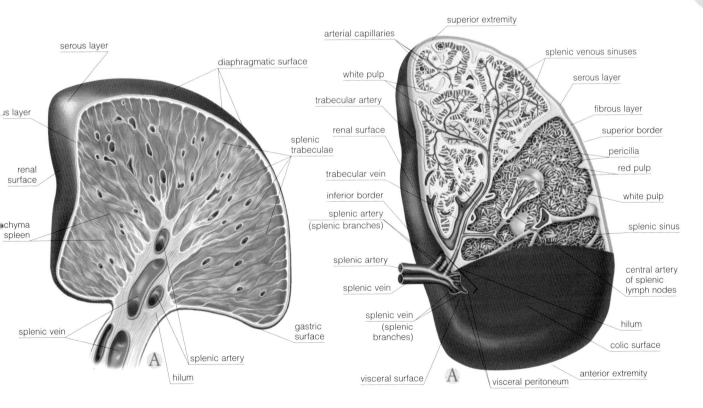

serous layer
diaphragmatic surface
...us layer
splenic
trabeculae
renal
surface
...chyma
spleen
splenic vein
splenic artery
hilum
gastric
surface

TRANSVERSE SECTION. CAUDAL VIEW

superior extremity
arterial capillaries
white pulp
trabecular artery
renal surface
trabecular vein
inferior border
splenic artery
(splenic branches)
splenic artery
splenic vein
splenic vein
(splenic
branches)
visceral surface

splenic venous sinuses
serous layer
fibrous layer
superior border
pericilia
red pulp
white pulp
splenic sinus
central artery
of splenic
lymph nodes
hilum
colic surface
anterior extremity
visceral peritoneum

HISTOLOGICAL STRUCTURE

ABDOMEN (I)
TRANSVERSE SECTION at LEVEL to INTERVERTEBRAL DISK
BETWEEN TXII and LI VERTEBRAE. CAUDAL VIEW

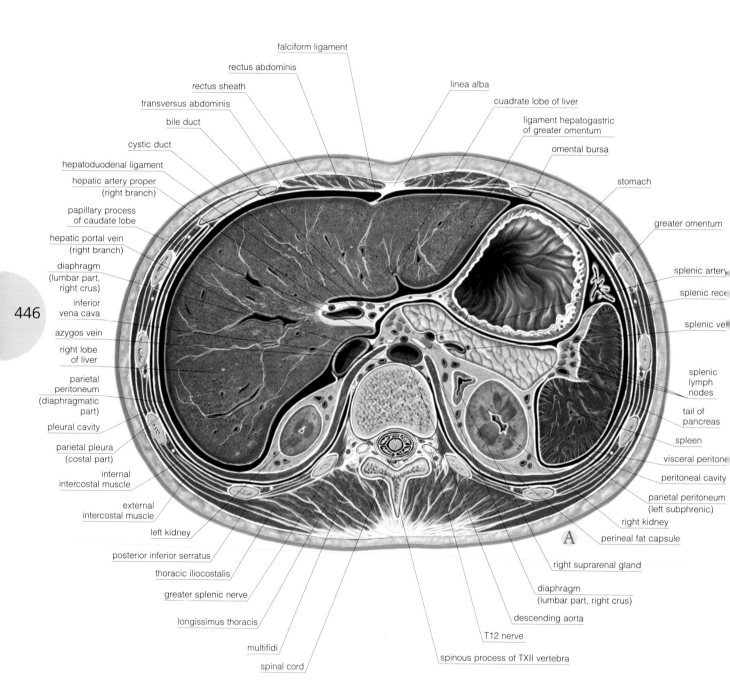

falciform ligament

rectus abdominis

rectus sheath

transversus abdominis

bile duct

cystic duct

hepatoduodenal ligament

hepatic artery proper
(right branch)

papillary process
of caudate lobe

hepatic portal vein
(right branch)

diaphragm
(lumbar part,
right crus)

inferior
vena cava

azygos vein

right lobe
of liver

parietal
peritoneum
(diaphragmatic
part)

pleural cavity

parietal pleura
(costal part)

internal
intercostal muscle

external
intercostal muscle

left kidney

posterior inferior serratus

thoracic iliocostalis

greater splenic nerve

longissimus thoracis

multifidi

spinal cord

linea alba

cuadrate lobe of liver

ligament hepatogastric
of greater omentum

omental bursa

stomach

greater omentum

splenic artery

splenic rece

splenic ve

splenic
lymph
nodes

tail of
pancreas

spleen

visceral periton

peritoneal cavity

parietal peritoneum
(left subphrenic)

right kidney

perineal fat capsule

right suprarenal gland

diaphragm
(lumbar part, right crus)

descending aorta

T12 nerve

spinous process of TXII vertebra

A

446

ABDOMEN (II)

TRANSVERSE SECTION at LEVEL to LI VERTEBRA. CAUDAL VIEW

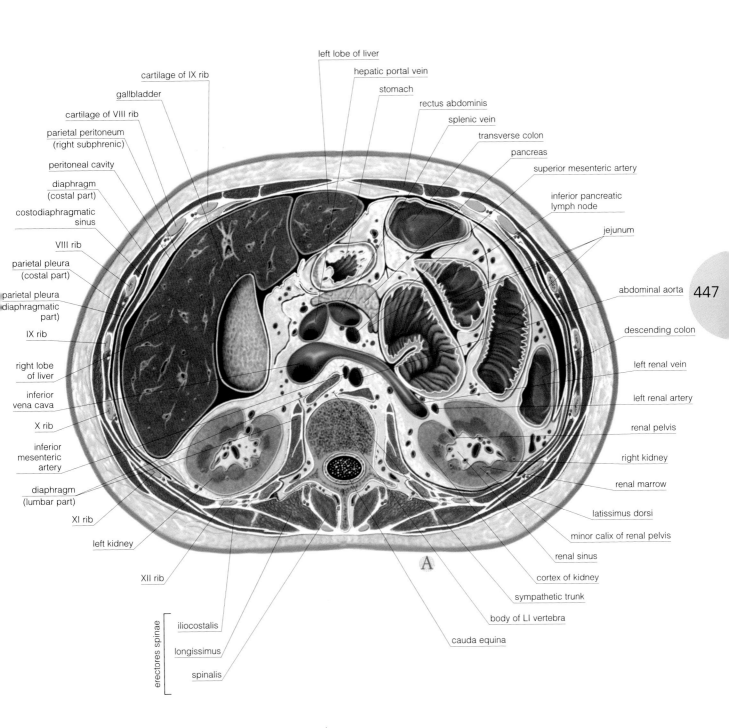

left lobe of liver

hepatic portal vein

stomach

cartilage of IX rib

rectus abdominis

gallbladder

splenic vein

cartilage of VIII rib

transverse colon

parietal peritoneum
(right subphrenic)

pancreas

peritoneal cavity

superior mesenteric artery

diaphragm
(costal part)

inferior pancreatic
lymph node

costodiaphragmatic
sinus

jejunum

VIII rib

parietal pleura
(costal part)

abdominal aorta   447

parietal pleura
(diaphragmatic
part)

descending colon

IX rib

left renal vein

right lobe
of liver

left renal artery

inferior
vena cava

renal pelvis

X rib

right kidney

inferior
mesenteric
artery

renal marrow

diaphragm
(lumbar part)

latissimus dorsi

XI rib

minor calix of renal pelvis

left kidney

renal sinus

cortex of kidney

XII rib

sympathetic trunk

body of LI vertebra

erectores spinae

iliocostalis

cauda equina

longissimus

spinalis

A

ABDOMEN (III)

MALE SEX. CORONAL SECTION at LEVEL to PUBIC SYMPHYSIS. ANTERIOR VIEW

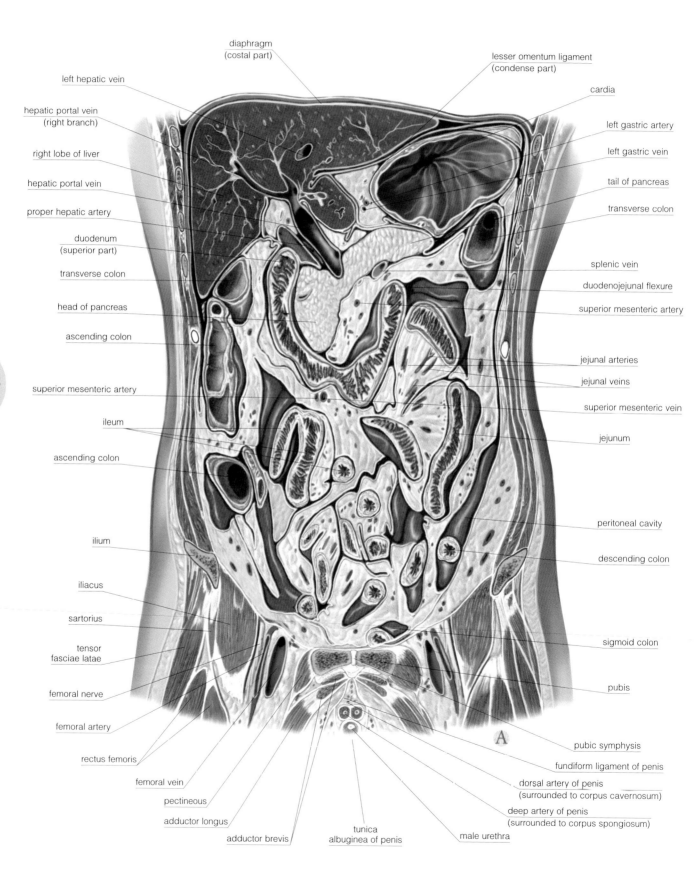

diaphragm
(costal part)

lesser omentum ligament
(condense part)

cardia

left hepatic vein

hepatic portal vein
(right branch)

left gastric artery

left gastric vein

right lobe of liver

tail of pancreas

hepatic portal vein

transverse colon

proper hepatic artery

duodenum
(superior part)

splenic vein

transverse colon

duodenojejunal flexure

head of pancreas

superior mesenteric artery

ascending colon

jejunal arteries

jejunal veins

superior mesenteric artery

superior mesenteric vein

ileum

jejunum

ascending colon

peritoneal cavity

ilium

descending colon

iliacus

sartorius

tensor
fasciae latae

sigmoid colon

femoral nerve

pubis

femoral artery

pubic symphysis

rectus femoris

fundiform ligament of penis

femoral vein

dorsal artery of penis
(surrounded to corpus cavernosum)

pectineous

deep artery of penis
(surrounded to corpus spongiosum)

adductor longus

adductor brevis

tunica
albuginea of penis

male urethra

A

RESPIRATORY SYSTEM

The respiratory system is formed by a set of organs and tubular structures and few cavernous, which function is the pulmonary ventilation and the exchange of gases between the internal medium and the environment. These organs may be classified in upper tracts (mouth, nasal cavities, pharynx and upper portion of the larynx) and lower tracts (trachea, bronchial tree and lung, where alveolus are housed). In the lungs takes place the exchange of gases. The rest of organs are conducts in which pass the air that gets in (inhalation) and gets out (exhalation) from the lungs. Before gets in the air is conveniently prepared while goes through the upper aerial tracts.

An individual can survive several days without taking food and many hours without drinking, but is just capable of tolerate few minutes without breathe. And is that the millions of cells that form the human body need of a constant supply of oxygen, not only to survive but also to be able to develop its functions and expel the carbon dioxide that produces. This make us tell that the respiratory system has a double function: nutritious (through the supply of oxygen from the air inhaled to all the cells) and purifying (expelling the residual carbon dioxide, product of the cellular metabolism).

The respiration involves four phases:

- Pulmonary ventilation: Circulation of the inhaled air by the lungs in order to renovate the carbon dioxide that contains the alveolus.

- External respiration: Exchange of gases into the blood (that liberate the carbon dioxide contained and collects the oxygen from the alveolus) and the alveolus (that liberate oxygen of the inhaled air to the blood and collect the carbon dioxide that contains).

- Transport of gases: Through the heart and the vascular net the oxygen collected by the blood reaches all the cells of the body.

- Internal respiration: Exchange of gases between the arteriovenous capillary net and the cells: the arterial capillaries provide oxygen to the cells and the venous capillaries collect from them the carbon dioxide to be expelled.

In a healthy individual, the respiratory process that includes inhalation and exhalation is repeated automatically about fifteen times per minute and in that take part the muscles of respiration.

The respiratory system has also another important function, the phonation thanks of which the individual is able to communicate verbally with his similars.

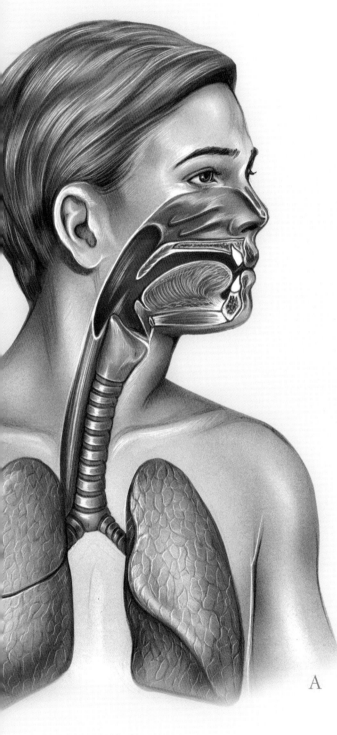

A

RESPIRATORY SYSTEM

GENERAL VIEW

respiratory system

The respiratory system consists of organs and structures which allow the capture of oxygen -which is necessary to revitalize cells, and with them, the organs of the human body- and the elimination of carbon dioxide -which is damaging to the perfect functioning of the structures and mechanisms of the body-.This is carried out through complementary processes: inhaling and exhaling, as well as the oxygenation of venous blood which reaches the lungs from all corners of the body through the pulmonary arteries. The respiratory system has a nutritive and purifying purpose, as it fulfills two objectives: to enable oxygen to reach the blood, which is fundamental for human cell metabolism, as well as to ease the expulsion of carbon dioxide, which is a residual product of said metabolism. The respiratory system consists of respiratory tracts and of two terminal structures, the lungs. Its functioning is closely related to the heart.

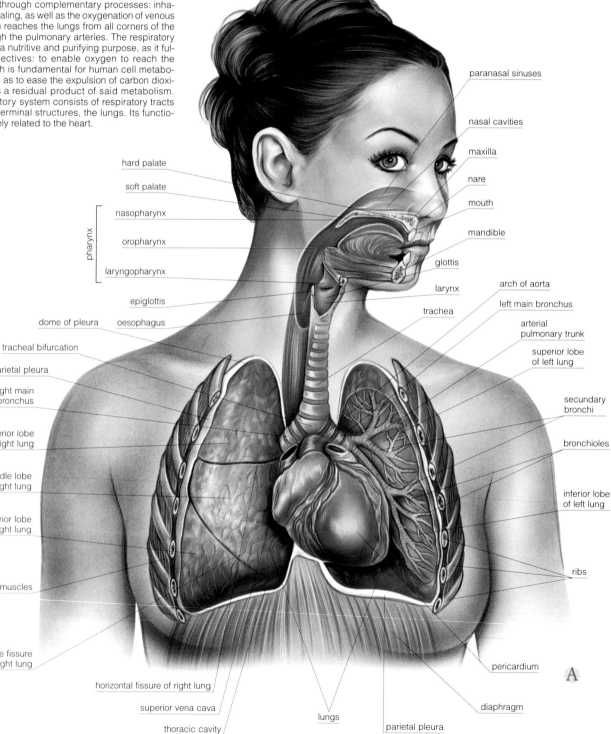

paranasal sinuses

nasal cavities

maxilla

nare

mouth

mandible

glottis

hard palate

soft palate

nasopharynx

oropharynx

pharynx

laryngopharynx

epiglottis

dome of pleura   oesophagus

tracheal bifurcation

parietal pleura

right main bronchus

superior lobe of right lung

middle lobe of right lung

inferior lobe of right lung

intercostal muscles

oblique fissure of right lung

horizontal fissure of right lung

superior vena cava

thoracic cavity

larynx

trachea

arch of aorta

left main bronchus

arterial pulmonary trunk

superior lobe of left lung

secundary bronchi

bronchioles

inferior lobe of left lung

ribs

pericardium

diaphragm

parietal pleura

lungs

A

UPPER RESPIRATORY TRACT (I)
LATERAL VIEW

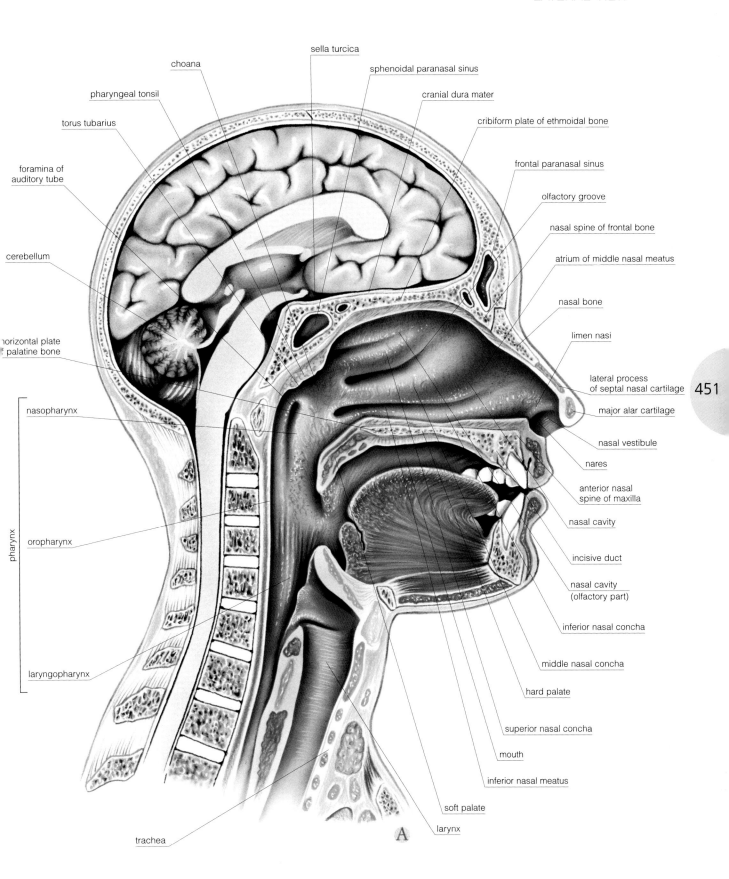

sella turcica

choana

sphenoidal paranasal sinus

pharyngeal tonsil

cranial dura mater

torus tubarius

cribiform plate of ethmoidal bone

foramina of
auditory tube

frontal paranasal sinus

olfactory groove

nasal spine of frontal bone

cerebellum

atrium of middle nasal meatus

nasal bone

limen nasi

horizontal plate
of palatine bone

lateral process
of septal nasal cartilage

451

nasopharynx

major alar cartilage

nasal vestibule

nares

anterior nasal
spine of maxilla

nasal cavity

oropharynx

incisive duct

nasal cavity
(olfactory part)

inferior nasal concha

middle nasal concha

laryngopharynx

hard palate

pharynx

superior nasal concha

mouth

inferior nasal meatus

soft palate

larynx

trachea

A

UPPER RESPIRATORY TRACT (II). NOSE

LATERAL WALL

respiration and upper respiratory tract

Picks up oxygen from the atmosphere or dissolve in the water to transport it to the lungs, in order to oxygenate the blood and then, for the same way, expel to the outside the carbon dioxide. Consist of three phases: pulmonary respiration (passing of air through the upper air tracts from the nose or the mouth until the pulmonary alveolus and vice verse) transport of the oxygen to the cells of the blood (is done through the red blood cells, or dissolve in the plasma) and also of the carbon dioxide from these (already combined with the hemoglobin or as bicarbonate) and internal respiration (in which the necessary energy is generated for the functional units to carry out their mission in the organism). The upper air tracts, besides of containing the openings of communication with the outside to inhale and exhale the air, have the function of filter and warm such air, before is introduced into the trachea to avoid the passing of harmful elements or that an excessive cold may damage the respiratory tracts. It takes part of the upper aerial tracts the nasal and oral cavities, the paranasal sinuses and the ethmoid cells, etc.

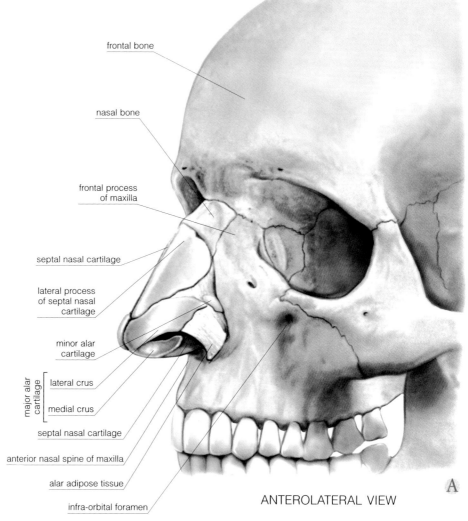

frontal bone

nasal bone

frontal process of maxilla

septal nasal cartilage

lateral process of septal nasal cartilage

minor alar cartilage

major alar cartilage
- lateral crus
- medial crus

septal nasal cartilage

anterior nasal spine of maxilla

alar adipose tissue

infra-orbital foramen

ANTEROLATERAL VIEW

A

nose

Is a protuberance found in the middle part of the face and constitute the beginning of the respiratory system. Consist of one external part (nasal pyramid, or nose in strict sense) and of some upholstered cavities of pituitary mucosa (nasal pits). Its external portion is formed specially by cartilages. The reverse extends since the upper angle to the vortex. In the lower face are found the nostrils that limits on the sides with the wings of the nose and are separated one another by a fleshy portion of skin that covers the nasal septum. The external portion of the nose is covered by skin that in the upper portion is fine, while the one that covers the cartilaginous portion is thicker, due to the sebaceous glands that contains. The respiratory function of the nose consists in receive the external air, warm it up, moisten and purify it in order to reach the pulmonary alveolus in the best conditions.

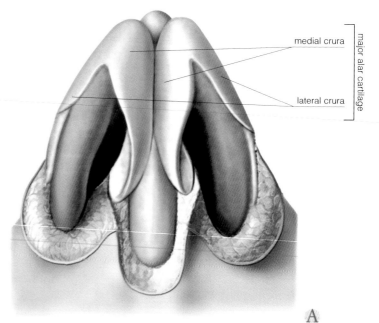

medial crura

major alar cartilage

lateral crura

INFERIOR VIEW

A

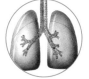

UPPER RESPIRATORY TRACT (III). NASAL CAVITY (I)
LATERAL WALL

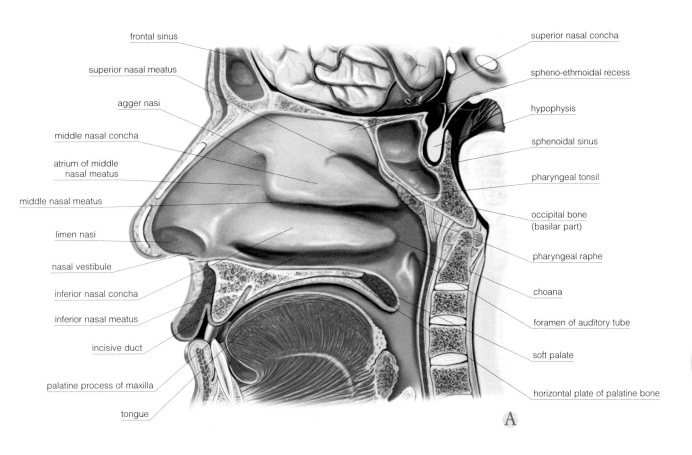

frontal sinus

superior nasal meatus

agger nasi

middle nasal concha

atrium of middle nasal meatus

middle nasal meatus

limen nasi

nasal vestibule

inferior nasal concha

inferior nasal meatus

incisive duct

palatine process of maxilla

tongue

superior nasal concha

spheno-ethmoidal recess

hypophysis

sphenoidal sinus

pharyngeal tonsil

occipital bone (basilar part)

pharyngeal raphe

choana

foramen of auditory tube

soft palate

horizontal plate of palatine bone

A

453

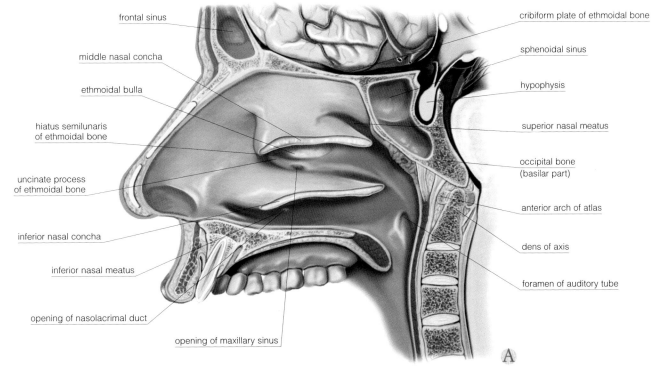

frontal sinus

middle nasal concha

ethmoidal bulla

hiatus semilunaris of ethmoidal bone

uncinate process of ethmoidal bone

inferior nasal concha

inferior nasal meatus

opening of nasolacrimal duct

opening of maxillary sinus

cribiform plate of ethmoidal bone

sphenoidal sinus

hypophysis

superior nasal meatus

occipital bone (basilar part)

anterior arch of atlas

dens of axis

foramen of auditory tube

A

UPPER RESPIRATORY TRACT (IV). NASAL CAVITY (II)

MEDIAL WALL

nasal cavities

The nasal cavities are two and are found between the floor of the cranium and the roof of the mouth. Is possible to get inside them through the nostrils, but these opens to the back to the nasopharynx by the choanae, are bounded laterally by the maxillary bone, palatines, lower cornet and lacrimal and medially by the ethmoidal and vomer bones. Each cavity is divided into two halves (right and left), also divided by the nasal septum. Its floor is formed by the hard palate that separates it from the oral cavity. Its lateral walls contain the cornets and the nasal meati. The mucus is strongly adhered to the periosteum of the bones and cartilages that hold the nose and continues with the coating of all the cavities in which communicates the nose: the nasofarynx for the back, the paranasal sinuses for above and the sides and the lacrimal sac and the conjunctive for above. With the nasal cavities begins (inhalation) and ends (exhalation) the respiratory cycle. Its function is to filter, warm and moisten the inhaled air before enteres the lower respiratory tracts.

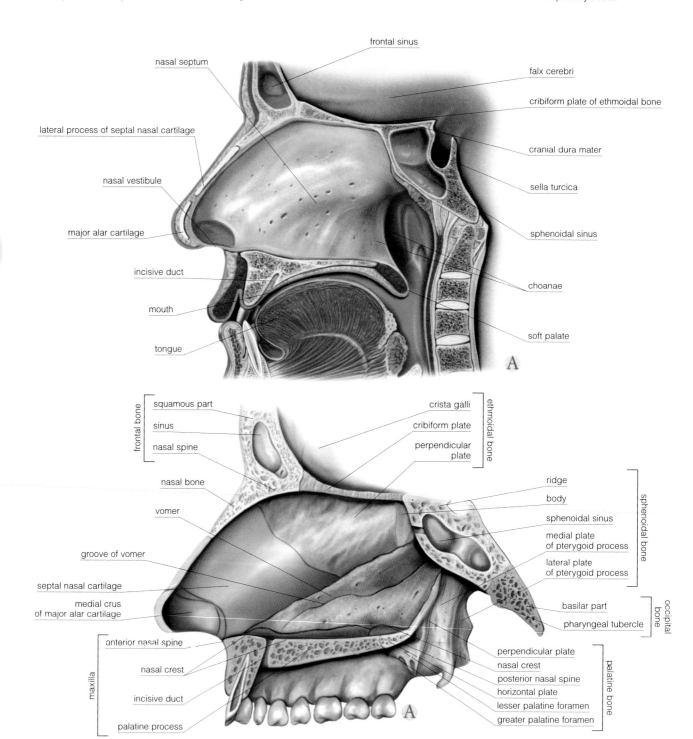

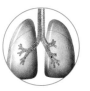

UPPER RESPIRATORY TRACT (V). NASAL CAVITY (III)

MEDIAL WALL

nasal conchae (or nasal cornets)

The cornets are independent bones under which lies the lower meatus, or nasolacrimal duct mouth, lower nasal (or lower nasal conch). Consist in an osseous prominence covered by mucus, which function is to create turbulence in the inhaled air in order to warm it up and moisten before reaches the farynx.

The cornets divide the nasal cavity in four passing scopes:
- Sphenoidal sinus: Is located posterior in relation to the upper cornet and in there is found the orifice of the sphenoid sinus.
- Upper nasal meatus: Narrow passage between the upper cornet and the medium in which the ethmoid sinuses flow through one or more orifices.

- Medium meatus: Contains the ethmoidal infundibulum, through of which communicates with the frontal sinus. The frontonasal infundibulum is the passage of lower way that leads downwardds, from each one of the frontal sinus and goes to the infundibulum. The semilunar hiatus is a semilunar furrow in which the frontal sinus opens. The ethmoidal blister is a rounded elevation founded above the hiatus that appears when the medium cornet is extracted. The maxillary sinus also flows in the extreme of the medium meatus.
- Lower meatus: Horizontal passage, to the lower nasal cornet. The conduct nasolacrimal that drains the tears of the lacrimal sac, it opens in the anterior portion of this meatus.

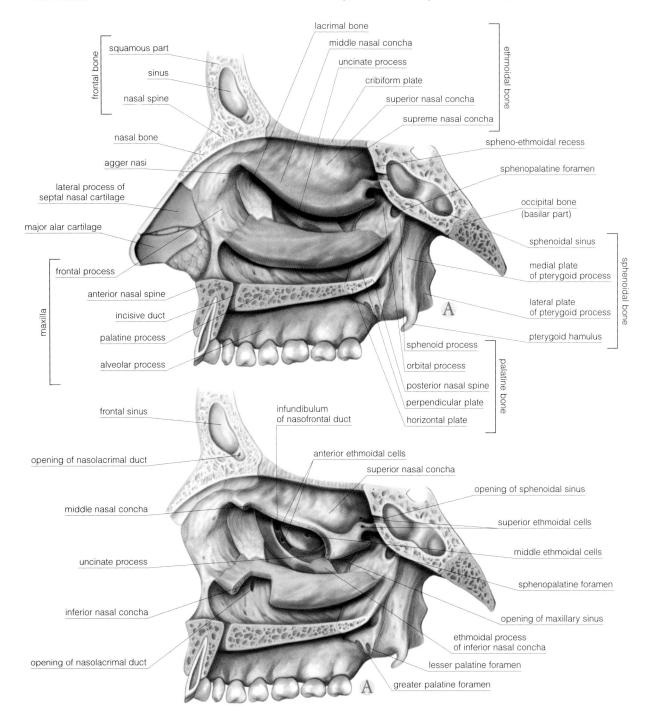

UPPER RESPIRATORY TRACT (VI)
PARANASAL SINUSES (I)

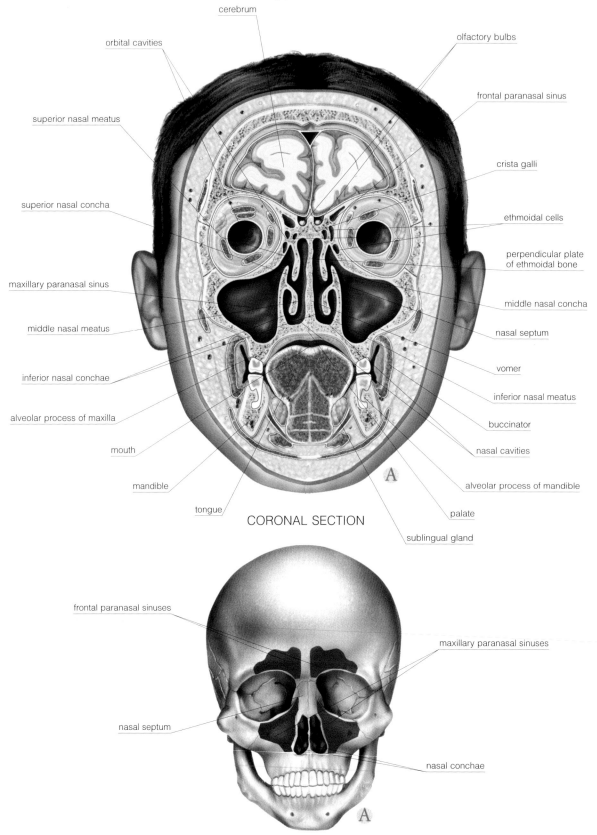

cerebrum

orbital cavities

olfactory bulbs

frontal paranasal sinus

superior nasal meatus

crista galli

superior nasal concha

ethmoidal cells

perpendicular plate
of ethmoidal bone

maxillary paranasal sinus

middle nasal concha

middle nasal meatus

nasal septum

inferior nasal conchae

vomer

inferior nasal meatus

alveolar process of maxilla

buccinator

mouth

nasal cavities

mandible

alveolar process of mandible

tongue

palate

CORONAL SECTION

sublingual gland

frontal paranasal sinuses

maxillary paranasal sinuses

nasal septum

nasal conchae

FRONTAL VIEW

UPPER RESPIRATORY TRACT (VII)
PARANASAL SINUSES (II)

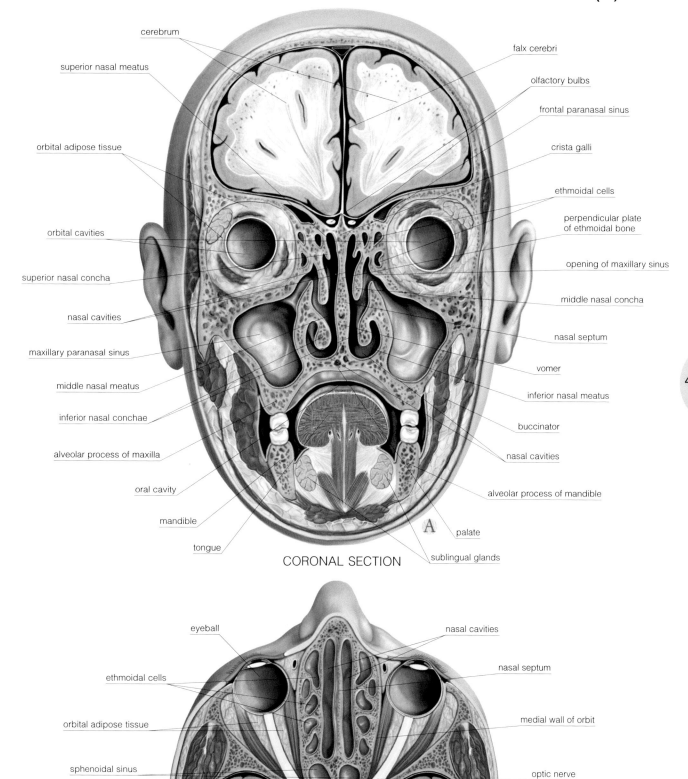

cerebrum

falx cerebri

superior nasal meatus

olfactory bulbs

frontal paranasal sinus

orbital adipose tissue

crista galli

ethmoidal cells

perpendicular plate
of ethmoidal bone

orbital cavities

opening of maxillary sinus

superior nasal concha

middle nasal concha

nasal cavities

nasal septum

maxillary paranasal sinus

vomer

middle nasal meatus

inferior nasal meatus

inferior nasal conchae

buccinator

alveolar process of maxilla

nasal cavities

oral cavity

alveolar process of mandible

mandible

tongue

palate

CORONAL SECTION

sublingual glands

A

eyeball

nasal cavities

ethmoidal cells

nasal septum

orbital adipose tissue

medial wall of orbit

sphenoidal sinus

optic nerve

optic chiasm

cerebrum

HORIZONTAL SECTION

A

457

VASCULAR SYSTEM (I). SUPERIOR MEDIASTINUM
ANTERIOR VIEW

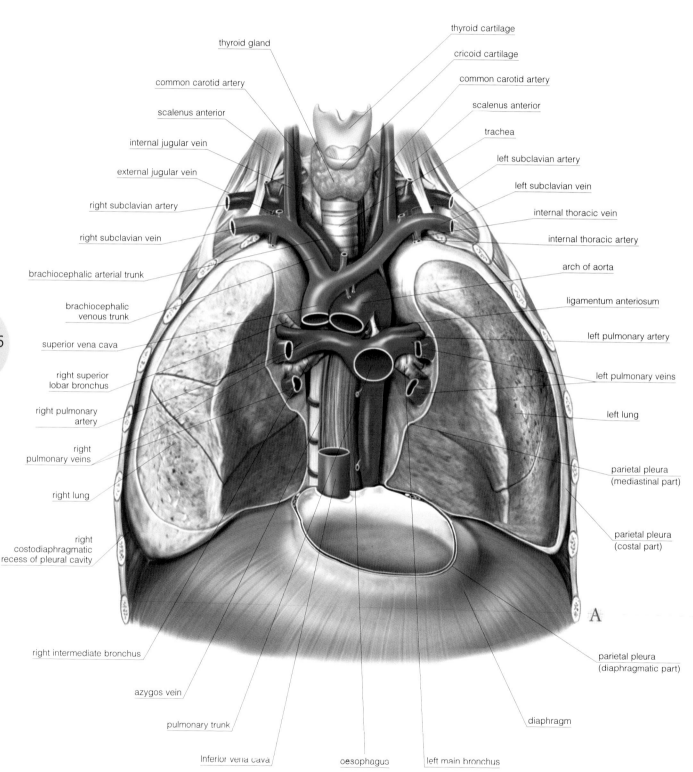

thyroid gland

thyroid cartilage

cricoid cartilage

common carotid artery

common carotid artery

scalenus anterior

scalenus anterior

internal jugular vein

trachea

external jugular vein

left subclavian artery

right subclavian artery

left subclavian vein

right subclavian vein

internal thoracic vein

brachiocephalic arterial trunk

internal thoracic artery

brachiocephalic
venous trunk

arch of aorta

ligamentum anteriosum

superior vena cava

left pulmonary artery

right superior
lobar bronchus

left pulmonary veins

right pulmonary
artery

left lung

right
pulmonary veins

parietal pleura
(mediastinal part)

right lung

parietal pleura
(costal part)

right
costodiaphragmatic
recess of pleural cavity

parietal pleura
(diaphragmatic part)

right intermediate bronchus

azygos vein

pulmonary trunk

diaphragm

Inferior vena cava

oesophagus

left main bronchus

A

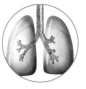

VASCULAR SYSTEM (II). TRACHEA and BRONCHI
ANTERIOR VIEW

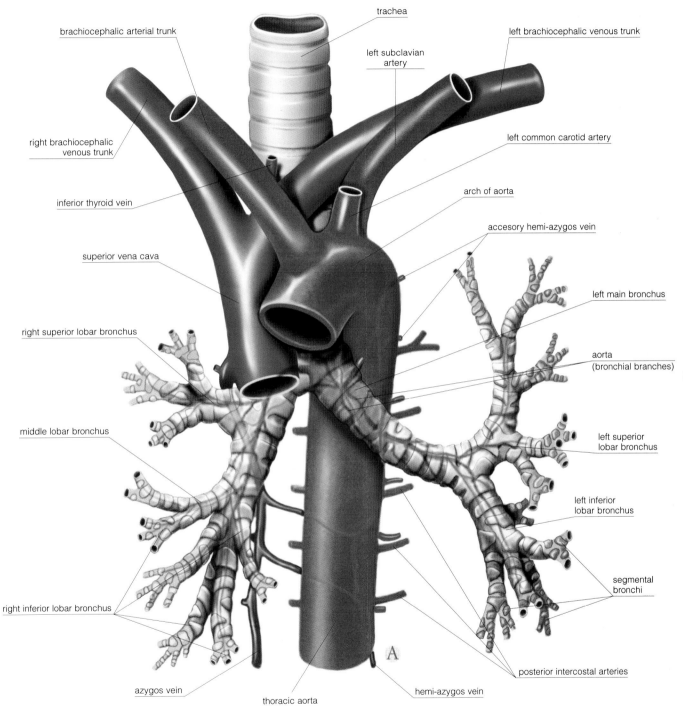

trachea

brachiocephalic arterial trunk

left brachiocephalic venous trunk

left subclavian artery

right brachiocephalic venous trunk

left common carotid artery

inferior thyroid vein

arch of aorta

accesory hemi-azygos vein

superior vena cava

left main bronchus

right superior lobar bronchus

aorta (bronchial branches)

467

middle lobar bronchus

left superior lobar bronchus

left inferior lobar bronchus

segmental bronchi

right inferior lobar bronchus

azygos vein

posterior intercostal arteries

thoracic aorta

hemi-azygos vein

bronchial arteries and veins

The bronchial arteries and veins are in charge to provide the blood to the pulmonary tissue. The irrigation of the pulmonary takes place through the bronchial arteries, branches of the thoracic aorta, or the right posterior intercostals artery, in some cases. Due to the location of bronchus in respect to the thoracic aorta, the bronchial arteries generally penetrate in the bronchus for the posterior part. The venous drainage of the bronchus is carried out by bronchial veins. The left bronchial vein drains in the hemi-azygos accessory, and the right in the vein azygos. Is not rare that exists shocks or anastomosis, that communicate the bronchial veins with the pulmonary veins, causing with that a mix, always not very significant, of oxygenated blood with blood poor in oxygen.

VASCULAR SYSTEM (III). LUNGS (I)
POSTERIOR VIEW

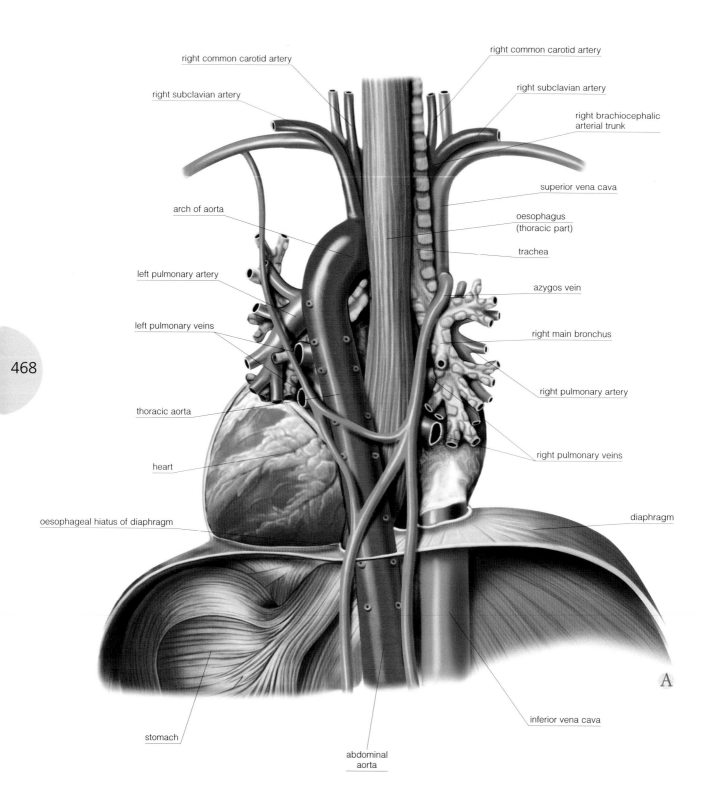

right common carotid artery

right subclavian artery

arch of aorta

left pulmonary artery

left pulmonary veins

thoracic aorta

heart

oesophageal hiatus of diaphragm

stomach

abdominal
aorta

right common carotid artery

right subclavian artery

right brachiocephalic
arterial trunk

superior vena cava

oesophagus
(thoracic part)

trachea

azygos vein

right main bronchus

right pulmonary artery

right pulmonary veins

diaphragm

inferior vena cava

A

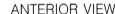

VASCULAR SYSTEM (IV). LUNGS (II)
ANTERIOR VIEW

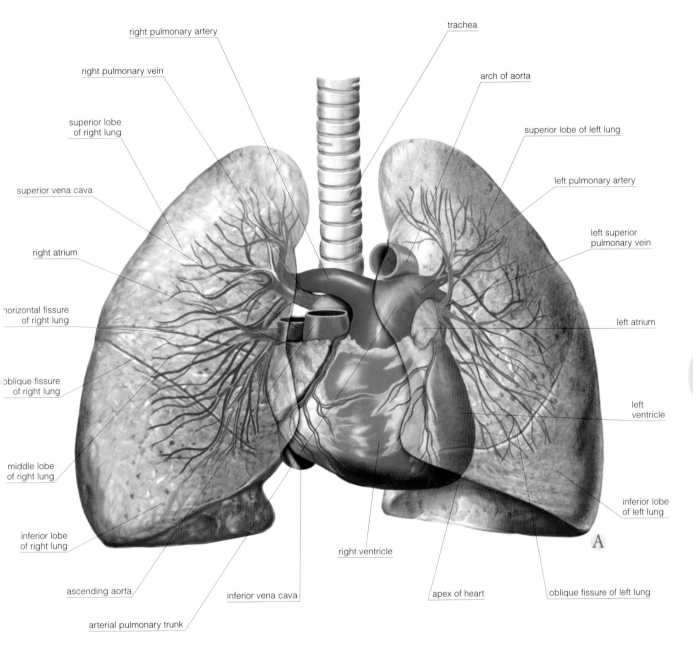

right pulmonary artery

right pulmonary vein

superior lobe
of right lung

superior vena cava

right atrium

horizontal fissure
of right lung

oblique fissure
of right lung

middle lobe
of right lung

inferior lobe
of right lung

ascending aorta

arterial pulmonary trunk

inferior vena cava

right ventricle

apex of heart

trachea

arch of aorta

superior lobe of left lung

left pulmonary artery

left superior
pulmonary vein

left atrium

left
ventricle

inferior lobe
of left lung

oblique fissure of left lung

A

469

pulmonary arteries and veins

The pulmonary arteries and veins are in charge of the gaseous exchange that is carried out in the pulmonary alveolus.

The pulmonary arteries are the only arteries of the organism that transport blood poor in oxygen. Are born from the division of the arterial trunk that originate in the right ventricle and carry blood poorly oxygenated from this to the lungs to be purified, the division of the pulmonary arteries follows the ramification of the bronchial tree. Together with the lobar bronchus, ramify and extend the arterial trunks (lobar arteries) to the interior of the lung, in which level the arteries are bigger than the bronchus. The lobar arteries continue ramifying to give origin to the segmental arteries. Both the arteries and the bronchus are located in the center of the respective pulmonary unit, forming the bronchopulmonary and broncho-arterial segments.

The venous vessels don't follow the bronchial ramification, as they run between the pulmonary segments and collects the blood of each segment (intrasegmentary portion) or of two neighbor segments (intersegmentary portion) to afterwards form the four pulmonary veins (two right ones and two left ones) that end in the left atrium. In contrast, therefore, to what occurs to the pulmonary arteries, the pulmonary veins are also the only veins of the human body that transport oxygenated blood, that means, which has been purified in the exchange of gases done in the alveolus.

LUNGS (I)
INTERNAL VIEW

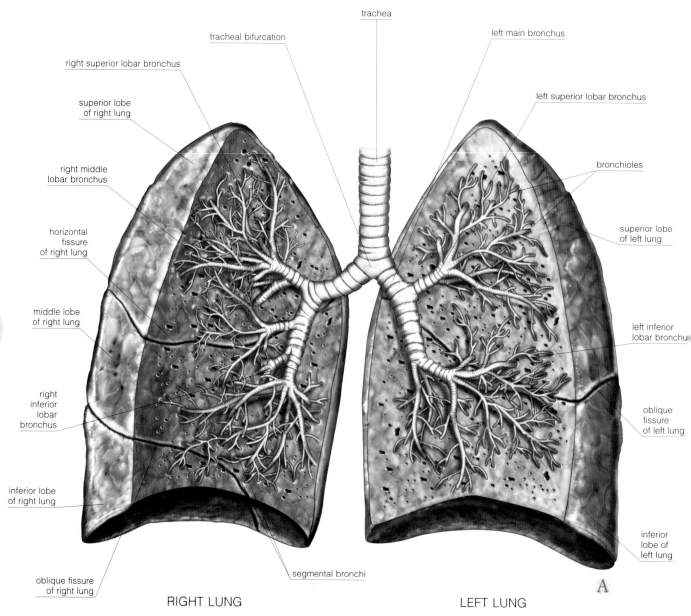

trachea

tracheal bifurcation

left main bronchus

right superior lobar bronchus

left superior lobar bronchus

superior lobe
of right lung

right middle
lobar bronchus

bronchioles

horizontal
fissure
of right lung

superior lobe
of left lung

middle lobe
of right lung

left inferior
lobar bronchu

right
inferior
lobar
bronchus

oblique
fissure
of left lung

inferior lobe
of right lung

inferior
lobe of
left lung

oblique fissure
of right lung

segmental bronchi

RIGHT LUNG

LEFT LUNG

A

lungs

The lungs are two (right and left) and constitute essential organs of the respiratory system. Are of spongy consistence, located inside the thoracic cavity, one of each side of the thorax and separate one from the other for the heart and the organs of the mediastinum. Also are separated of the abdominal viscera by the diaphragm. Are covered by the visceral pleura and are divided in lobes (the right one has three and the left one has two). In the interior are found the bronchus, that are divided in bronchioles these are divided in several ramifications each time of smaller caliber until derived in the alveolus, in which interior takes place the hematosis. Arteries, veins and bronchi penetrate in the lung in order to oxygenate the venous blood that comes from the heart. In the man, the right lung weighs about 625g and the left one about 570g. The lungs have around 300 millions of alveoli, with a respiratory surface of about 70m². In the adult every minute is produced about 12-20 respirations and its total capacity vary between 3.6 and 9.4l in men and 2.5 and 6.9 in women.

470

LUNGS (II). MEDIASTINAL SURFACES and HILA

MEDIASTINAL SURFACES

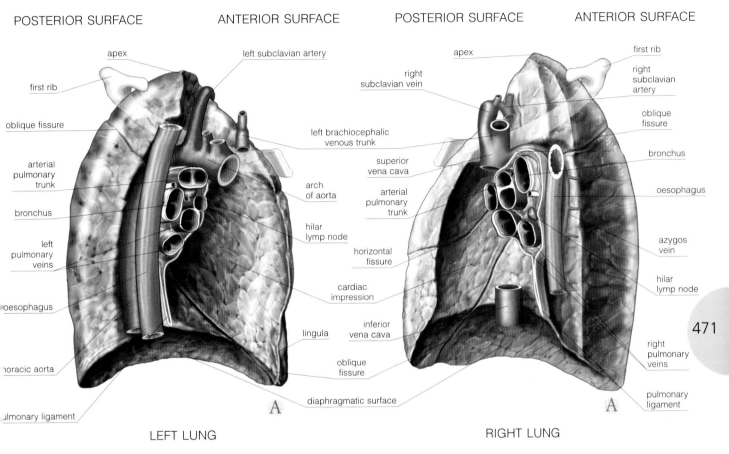

POSTERIOR SURFACE   ANTERIOR SURFACE   POSTERIOR SURFACE   ANTERIOR SURFACE

LEFT LUNG   RIGHT LUNG

471

HILA of LUNG

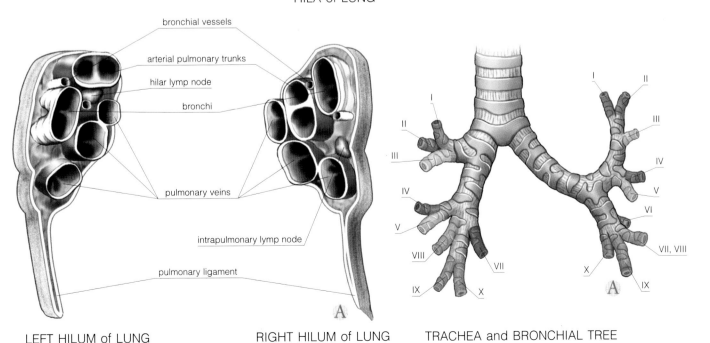

LEFT HILUM of LUNG   RIGHT HILUM of LUNG   TRACHEA and BRONCHIAL TREE

LUNGS (III). LOBES and SEGMENTS (I)

ANTERIOR VIEW

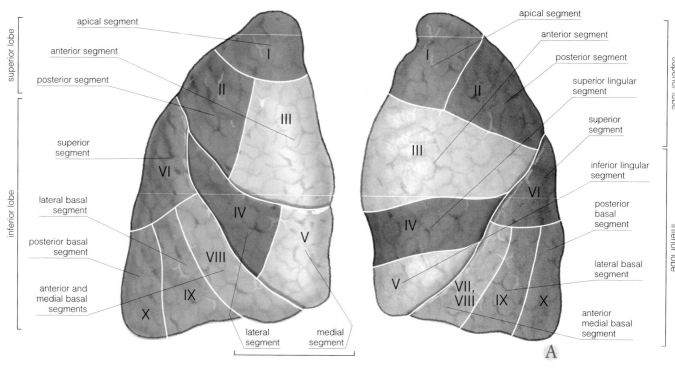

LATERAL VIEW

RIGHT LUNG   LEFT LUNG

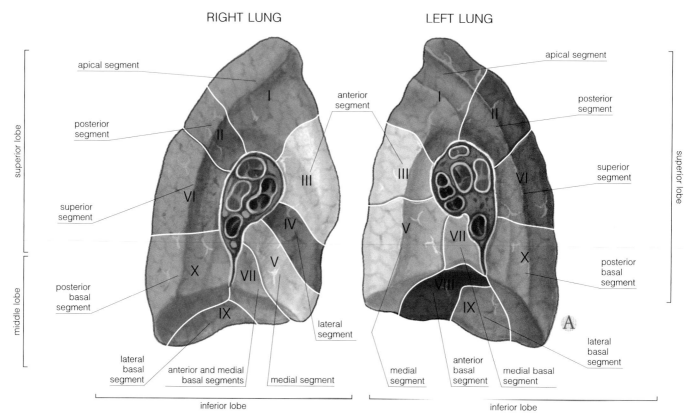

MEDIAL VIEW

RIGHT LUNG   LEFT LUNG

472

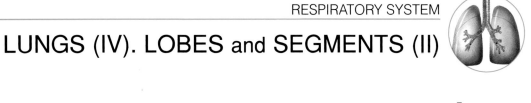

LUNGS (IV). LOBES and SEGMENTS (II)

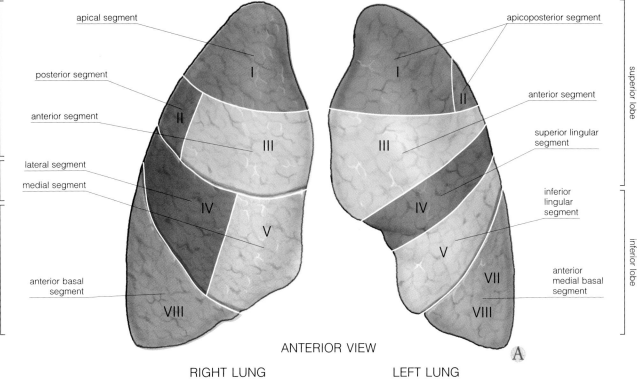

superior lobe

apical segment

posterior segment

anterior segment

lateral segment

medial segment

anterior basal segment

inferior lobe

I

II

III

IV

V

VIII

apicoposterior segment

anterior segment

superior lingular segment

inferior lingular segment

anterior medial basal segment

I

II

III

IV

V

VII

VIII

superior lobe

inferior lobe

ANTERIOR VIEW

RIGHT LUNG   LEFT LUNG

473

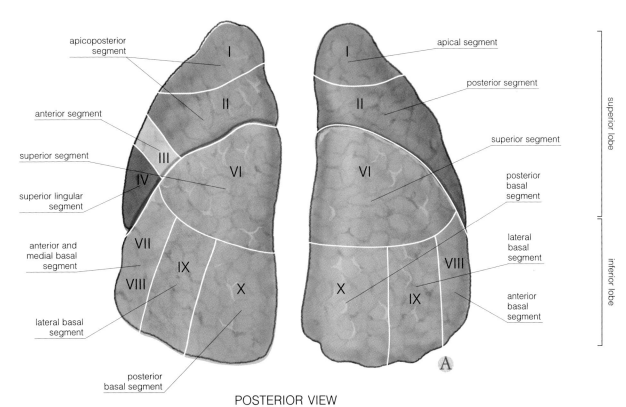

superior lobe

apicoposterior segment

anterior segment

superior segment

superior lingular segment

anterior and medial basal segment

lateral basal segment

posterior basal segment

inferior lobe

I

II

III

IV

VI

VII

VIII

IX

X

apical segment

posterior segment

superior segment

posterior basal segment

lateral basal segment

anterior basal segment

I

II

VI

X

IX

VIII

superior lobe

inferior lobe

POSTERIOR VIEW

LEFT LUNG   RIGHT LUNG

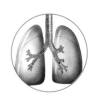

LUNGS (V). PULMONARY SEGMENTS

PULMONARY SEGMENTATION in THORACIC CT

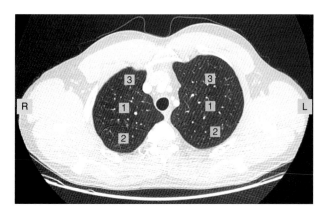
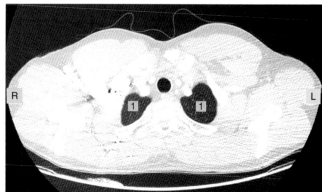

474

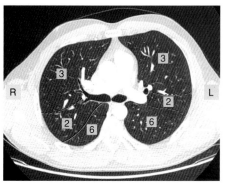
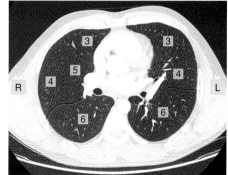
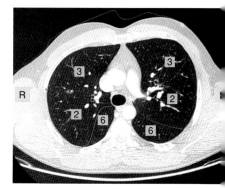

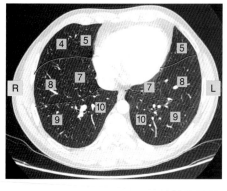
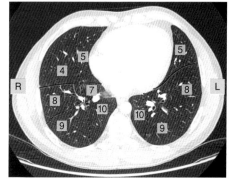
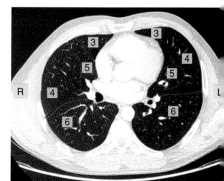

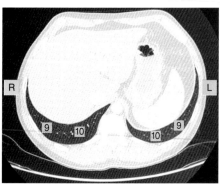
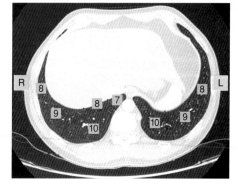
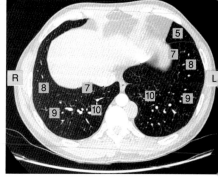

A

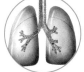

BRONCHIAL TREE (I)
ANTERIOR VIEW

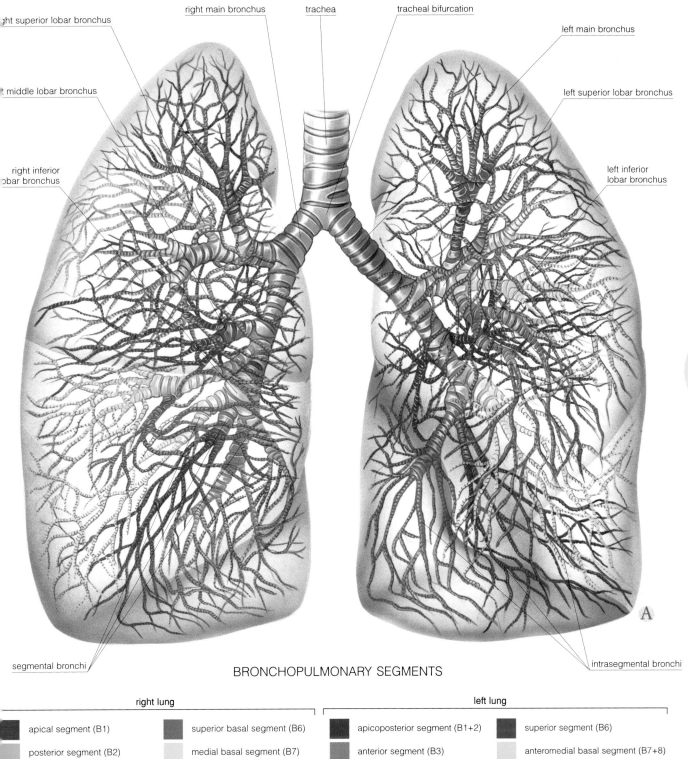

right superior lobar bronchus — right main bronchus — trachea — tracheal bifurcation — left main bronchus

middle lobar bronchus — left superior lobar bronchus

right inferior lobar bronchus — left inferior lobar bronchus

segmental bronchi — intrasegmental bronchi

BRONCHOPULMONARY SEGMENTS

475

right lung		left lung	
apical segment (B1)	superior basal segment (B6)	apicoposterior segment (B1+2)	superior segment (B6)
posterior segment (B2)	medial basal segment (B7)	anterior segment (B3)	anteromedial basal segment (B7+8)
anterior segment (B3)	anterior basal segment (B8)	superior segment (B4) } lingular segment	lateral basal segment (B9)
lateral segment (B4)	lateral basal segment (B9)	inferior segment (B5) } lingular segment	posterior basal segment (B10)
medial segment (B5)	posterior basal segment (B10)		

BRONCHIAL TREE (II). INTERNAL STRUCTURE

internal structure of the lung

In the lungs we can distinguish two nets. One of them is the bronchiolar, in which circulate the inhaled air (loaded of oxygen) or exhaled (that contains carbon dioxide), is constituted by the trachea, the bronchus, and the derivatives of them (bronchioles and alveolus, etc.). The other is the sanguineous net that is formed by the set of venous and arterial vessels that are in charge of make reach until the lungs the blood poor in oxygen that have come to the heart from all the body and once oxygenated return it to the heart to be boosted again to all the organism. These two nets are perfectly synchronized and conjoined in order to accomplish their main function: purify the blood.

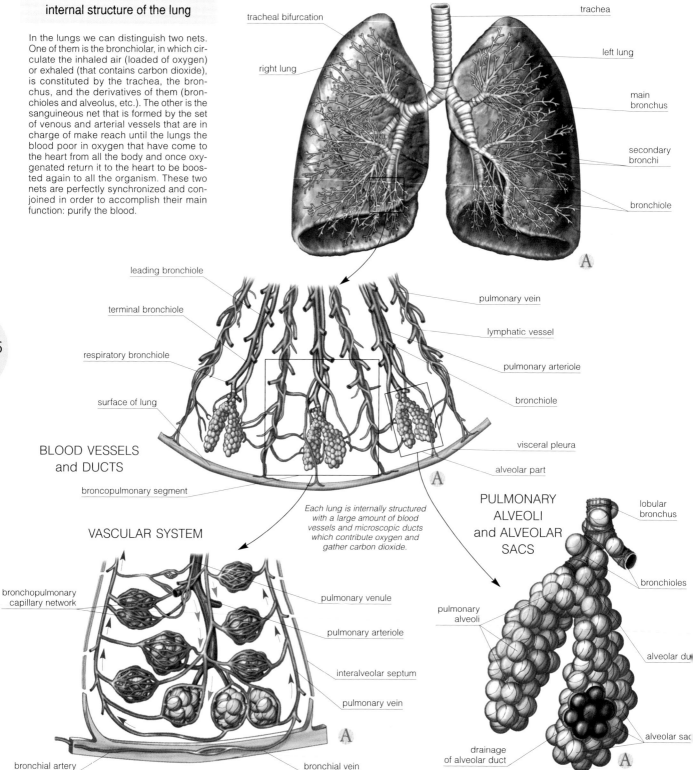

tracheal bifurcation

right lung

trachea

left lung

main bronchus

secondary bronchi

bronchiole

A

leading bronchiole

terminal bronchiole

respiratory bronchiole

surface of lung

pulmonary vein

lymphatic vessel

pulmonary arteriole

bronchiole

visceral pleura

alveolar part

BLOOD VESSELS and DUCTS

broncopulmonary segment

A

Each lung is internally structured with a large amount of blood vessels and microscopic ducts which contribute oxygen and gather carbon dioxide.

VASCULAR SYSTEM

bronchopulmonary capillary network

pulmonary venule

pulmonary arteriole

interalveolar septum

pulmonary vein

bronchial artery

bronchial vein

A

The arrows indicate the path the blood takes ever since it enters the bronchopulmonary area in order to be purified (blue arrows), until it returns to the heart, once it has been oxygenated (red arrows).

PULMONARY ALVEOLI and ALVEOLAR SACS

lobular bronchus

bronchioles

pulmonary alveoli

alveolar du

alveolar sac

drainage of alveolar duct

A

The pulmonary arteries wind up in the alveolar sacs and in the alveoli. The exchange of carbon dioxide occurs in that area. The carbon dioxide carried by the blood is exchanged by the oxygen contributed by the inspired air. Each lung has hundreds of millions of bronchial alveoli.

RESPIRATORY FUNCTION

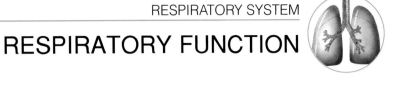

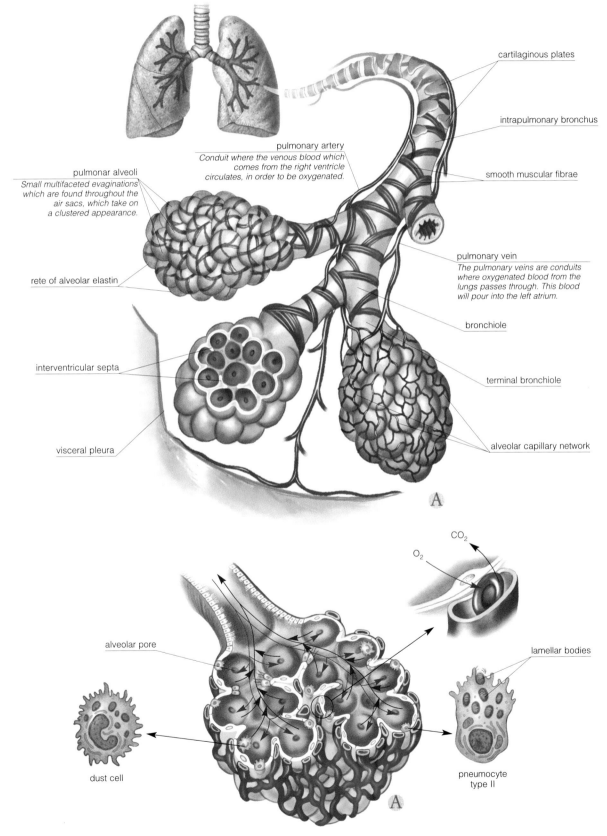

cartilaginous plates

intrapulmonary bronchus

smooth muscular fibrae

pulmonary artery
Conduit where the venous blood which comes from the right ventricle circulates, in order to be oxygenated.

pulmonar alveoli
Small multifaceted evaginations which are found throughout the air sacs, which take on a clustered appearance.

rete of alveolar elastin

pulmonary vein
The pulmonary veins are conduits where oxygenated blood from the lungs passes through. This blood will pour into the left atrium.

bronchiole

interventricular septa

terminal bronchiole

visceral pleura

alveolar capillary network

A

477

alveolar pore

CO_2

O_2

lamellar bodies

dust cell

pneumocyte type II

A

INTRAPULMONARY TRACT (I)
PULMONARY ALVEOLUS (I)

gas exchange

In respiration, the lungs facilitate the exchange of carbon dioxide (CO_2) coming from the pulmonary capillaries with oxygen (O_2). This, occurs in the alveoli by diffusion through the respiratory membrane, a thin tissue barrier that lies between the alveoli pulmonary and the adjacent capillaries and is composed of the alveolar and capillary walls. This membrane consists of four layers: alveolar wall (formed by alveolar cells type I and type II and alveolar macrophage associated) epithelial basement membrane (located just below the alveolar wall), capillary basement membrane (often fused with the epithelial basement membrane) and capillary endothelium. This membrane has a thickness of 0.2mm, allowing the rapid spread of gas. For the exchange of gases, the lungs have about 300 million alveoli, which add up to an area of 70m².

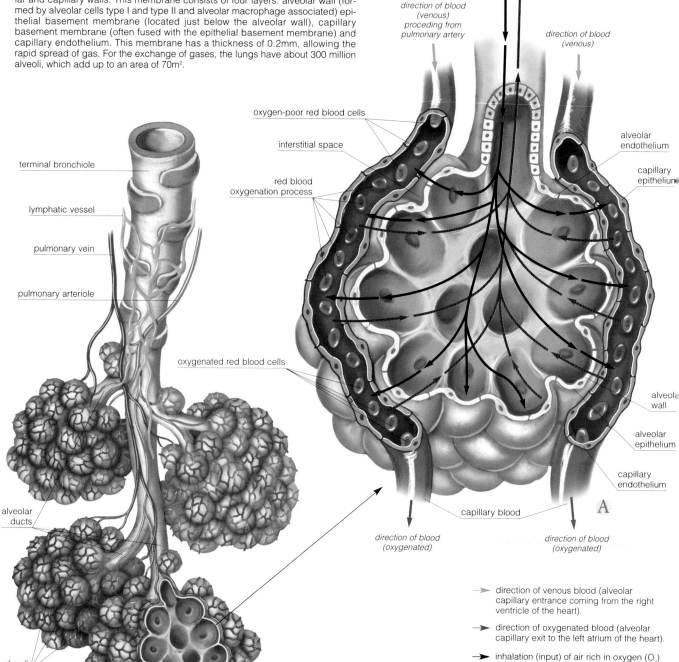

inhalation exhalation

direction of blood (venous) proceding from pulmonary artery

direction of blood (venous)

oxygen-poor red blood cells

interstitial space

red blood oxygenation process

terminal bronchiole

lymphatic vessel

pulmonary vein

pulmonary arteriole

oxygenated red blood cells

alveolar ducts

alveoli

pulmonary alveolar capillaries

alveolar endothelium

capillary epithelium

alveolar wall

alveolar epithelium

capillary endothelium

capillary blood

direction of blood (oxygenated)

direction of blood (oxygenated)

A

direction of venous blood (alveolar capillary entrance coming from the right ventricle of the heart).

direction of oxygenated blood (alveolar capillary exit to the left atrium of the heart).

inhalation (input) of air rich in oxygen (O_2) into the alveoli.

exhalation (output) of air laden with carbon dioxide (CO_2) to the outside of the alveoli.

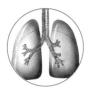

INTRAPULMONARY TRACT (II)
PULMONARY ALVEOLUS (II)

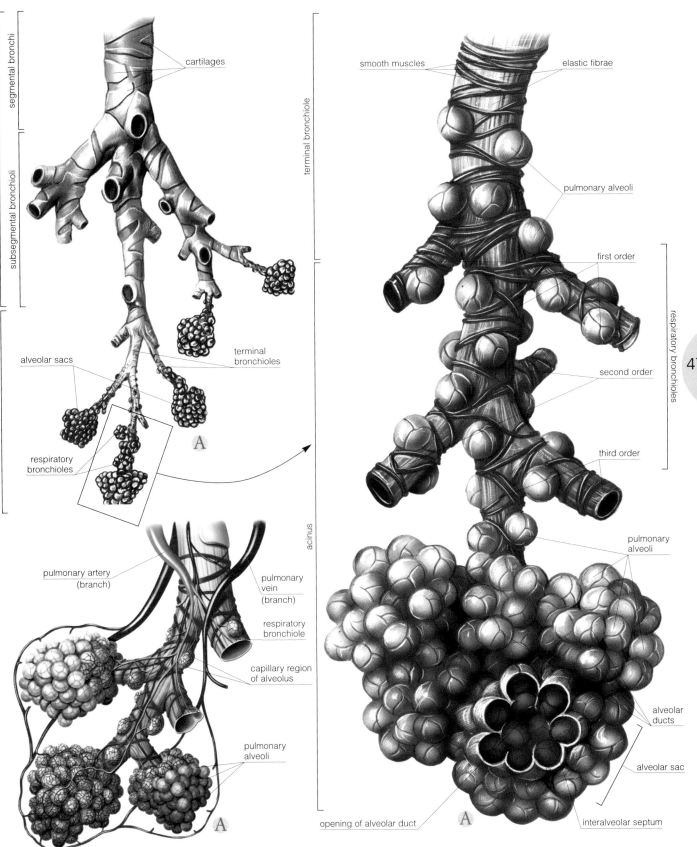

segmental bronchi

subsegmental bronchioli

cartilages

terminal bronchiole

terminal bronchioles

alveolar sacs

respiratory bronchioles

A

acinus

pulmonary artery (branch)

pulmonary vein (branch)

respiratory bronchiole

capillary region of alveolus

pulmonary alveoli

A

smooth muscles

elastic fibrae

pulmonary alveoli

first order

second order

respiratory bronchioles

third order

pulmonary alveoli

alveolar ducts

alveolar sac

opening of alveolar duct

interalveolar septum

A

479

INTRAPULMONARY TRACT (III)
PULMONARY ALVEOLUS (III)

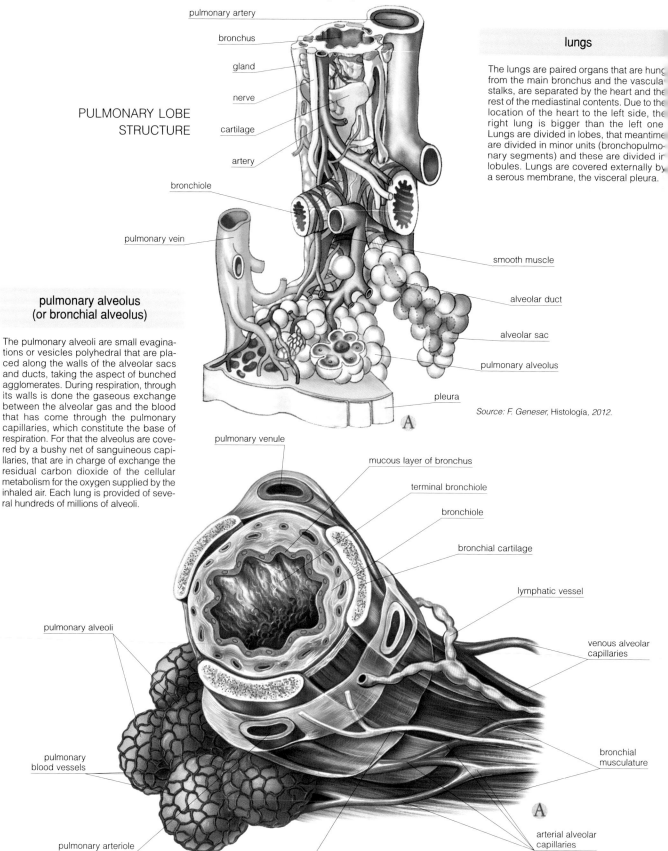

PULMONARY LOBE
STRUCTURE

pulmonary artery

bronchus

gland

nerve

cartilage

artery

bronchiole

pulmonary vein

smooth muscle

alveolar duct

alveolar sac

pulmonary alveolus

pleura

Source: F. Geneser, Histología, *2012.*

lungs

The lungs are paired organs that are hung from the main bronchus and the vascula[r] stalks, are separated by the heart and the rest of the mediastinal contents. Due to the location of the heart to the left side, the right lung is bigger than the left one. Lungs are divided in lobes, that meantime are divided in minor units (bronchopulmonary segments) and these are divided in lobules. Lungs are covered externally by a serous membrane, the visceral pleura.

pulmonary alveolus
(or bronchial alveolus)

The pulmonary alveoli are small evaginations or vesicles polyhedral that are placed along the walls of the alveolar sacs and ducts, taking the aspect of bunched agglomerates. During respiration, through its walls is done the gaseous exchange between the alveolar gas and the blood that has come through the pulmonary capillaries, which constitute the base of respiration. For that the alveolus are covered by a bushy net of sanguineous capillaries, that are in charge of exchange the residual carbon dioxide of the cellular metabolism for the oxygen supplied by the inhaled air. Each lung is provided of several hundreds of millions of alveoli.

480

pulmonary venule

mucous layer of bronchus

terminal bronchiole

bronchiole

bronchial cartilage

lymphatic vessel

venous alveolar capillaries

pulmonary alveoli

pulmonary blood vessels

bronchial musculature

pulmonary arteriole

nerve

arterial alveolar capillaries

LUNGS and PLEURA

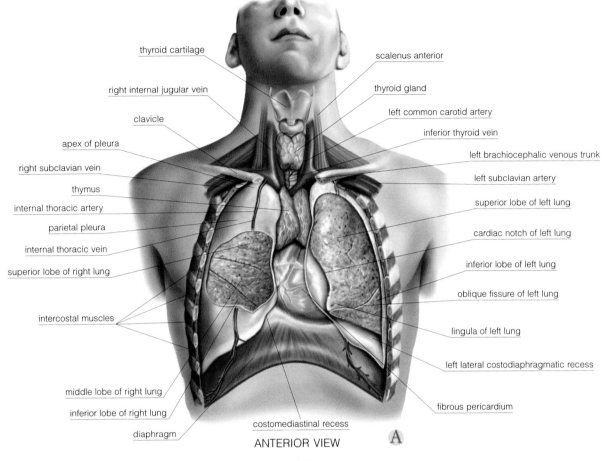

thyroid cartilage

scalenus anterior

right internal jugular vein

thyroid gland

clavicle

left common carotid artery

inferior thyroid vein

apex of pleura

left brachiocephalic venous trunk

right subclavian vein

left subclavian artery

thymus

superior lobe of left lung

internal thoracic artery

cardiac notch of left lung

parietal pleura

internal thoracic vein

inferior lobe of left lung

superior lobe of right lung

oblique fissure of left lung

intercostal muscles

lingula of left lung

left lateral costodiaphragmatic recess

middle lobe of right lung

inferior lobe of right lung

fibrous pericardium

diaphragm

costomediastinal recess

ANTERIOR VIEW Ⓐ

481

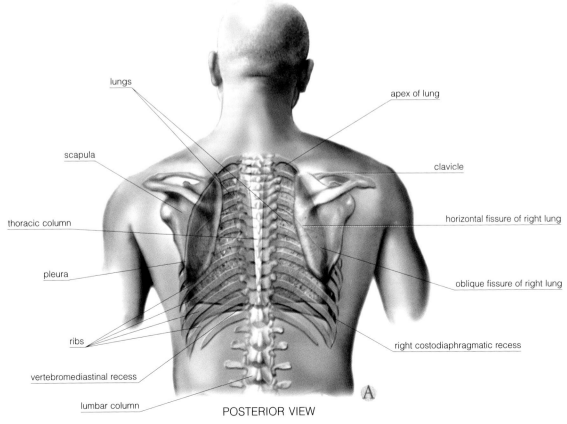

lungs

apex of lung

scapula

clavicle

thoracic column

horizontal fissure of right lung

pleura

oblique fissure of right lung

ribs

right costodiaphragmatic recess

vertebromediastinal recess

lumbar column

POSTERIOR VIEW Ⓐ

RESPIRATORY MUSCLES
ANTERIOR VIEW

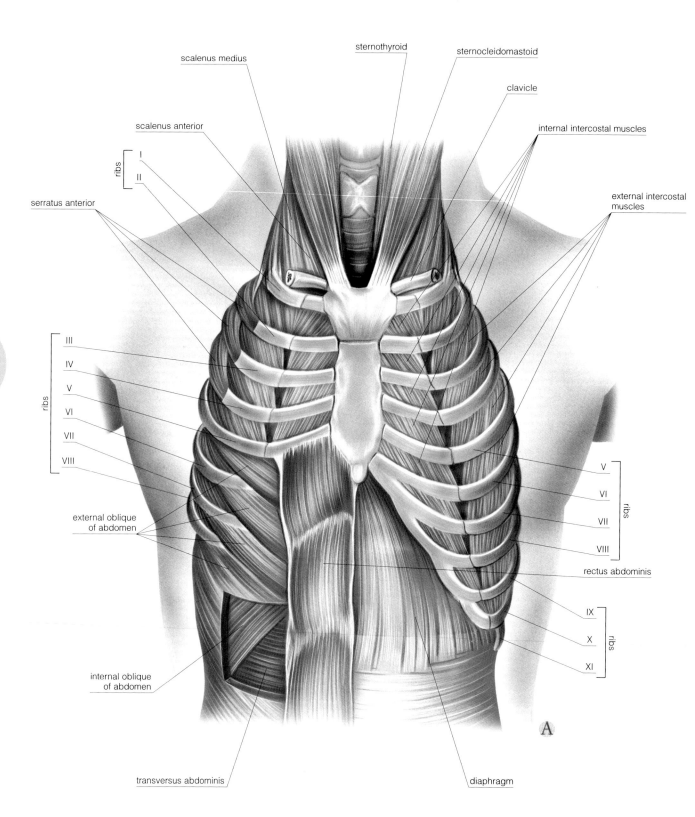

scalenus medius

sternothyroid

sternocleidomastoid

clavicle

internal intercostal muscles

scalenus anterior

ribs
I
II

external intercostal muscles

serratus anterior

ribs
III
IV
V
VI
VII
VIII

V
VI
VII
VIII
ribs

external oblique of abdomen

rectus abdominis

IX
X
XI
ribs

internal oblique of abdomen

transversus abdominis

diaphragm

A

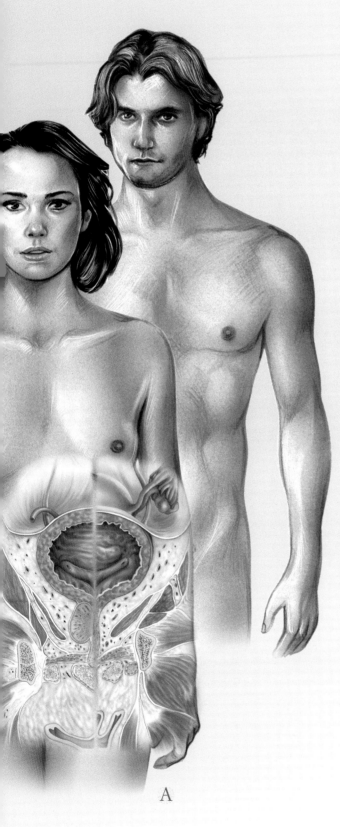

A

NEPHRO-URINARY SYSTEM

T he nephro-urinary system is formed by a set of organs and structures, which primordial function is the filtering of the blood, the extraction of it from the harmful products or not usable and its expulsion to the exterior of the organism through the urine in the micturition.

The human body it maintains and develops through a permanent work of the cells. This work and the vital circle of these cells generate constantly multitude of waste that are poured into the blood to be depurated or eliminated. An excessive accumulation of waste in the blood is pernicious, because apart from altering the composition (which would deprive this to accomplish its function) these waste can be toxic, which would favor the appearance of pathologies of diverse typology and gravity. The nephrourinary system has the depurator function by nature.

Among all the organs of this system, for the quantity and quality of its functions, the kidneys are the most important, thus these performs a role of filter, thanks of which the corporal liquid are depurated and equilibrated. In this way and in an interrupted form, filter the plasma, excrete in the urine the toxins coming from the liver and the metabolic residuals like the urea and the ions that are not interesting and return to the sanguineous torrent, those substances that are useful. Although the skin and the lungs also have this function of excretion of substances of waste, in the kidneys this function is more primordial.

The kidneys also take care of maintain steady the composition of liquids that circulate for the body, and guarantee all the time the balance between this liquids and the electrolytes and other compositional elements, that obligate them to be aware of the necessities that might arise as a consequence of the different variations that in this sense experience the organism in order to proceed to the kind of action adequate to each case, an action that is promoted and controlled by the hormones.

The kidneys secrete the rennin (enzyme that regulates the arterial pressure and renal function) and the erythropoietin (hormone that stimulate the production of erythrocytes in the red medulla of the bones. And the renal cells transform as well the vitamin D, responsible of the deposits of calcium in the bones, in its active form.

Other organs and structures complement and collaborate in one way or another to the action of the kidneys. Thus the ureters collaborate to the expulsion of the waste transporting the urine, from the kidneys until the urinary bladder where they are stored waiting for the moment to be expelled in the micturition. This is done through a sphincteric mechanism that functions voluntarily, through the urethra that communicates the bladder with the outside.

NEPHRO-URINARY SYSTEM
GENERAL ANTERIOR VIEW

MALE SEX

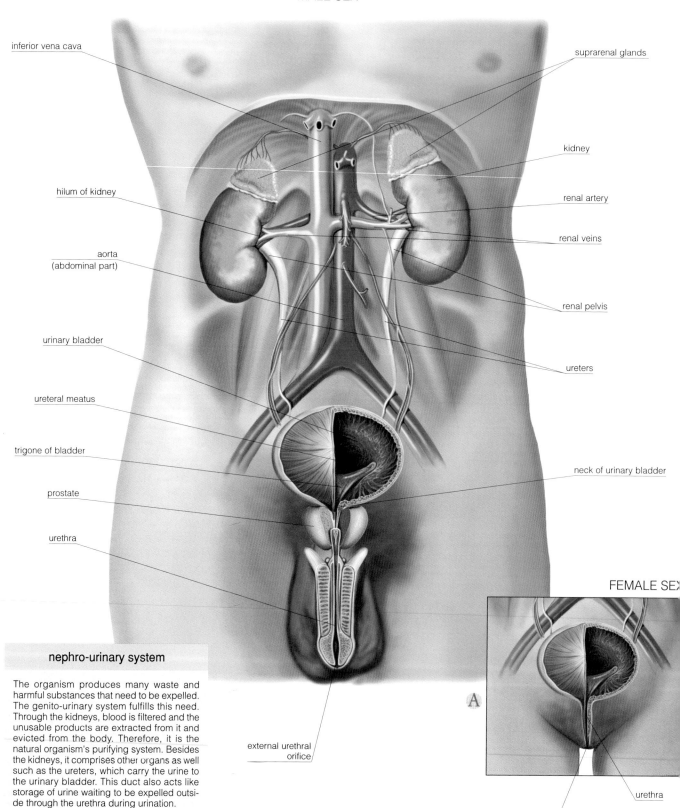

inferior vena cava

suprarenal glands

kidney

hilum of kidney

renal artery

renal veins

aorta
(abdominal part)

renal pelvis

urinary bladder

ureters

ureteral meatus

trigone of bladder

neck of urinary bladder

prostate

urethra

FEMALE SEX

A

external urethral
orifice

urethra

external urethral orifice

nephro-urinary system

The organism produces many waste and harmful substances that need to be expelled. The genito-urinary system fulfills this need. Through the kidneys, blood is filtered and the unusable products are extracted from it and evicted from the body. Therefore, it is the natural organism's purifying system. Besides the kidneys, it comprises other organs as well such as the ureters, which carry the urine to the urinary bladder. This duct also acts like storage of urine waiting to be expelled outside through the urethra during urination.

484

KIDNEY (I)

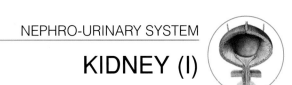

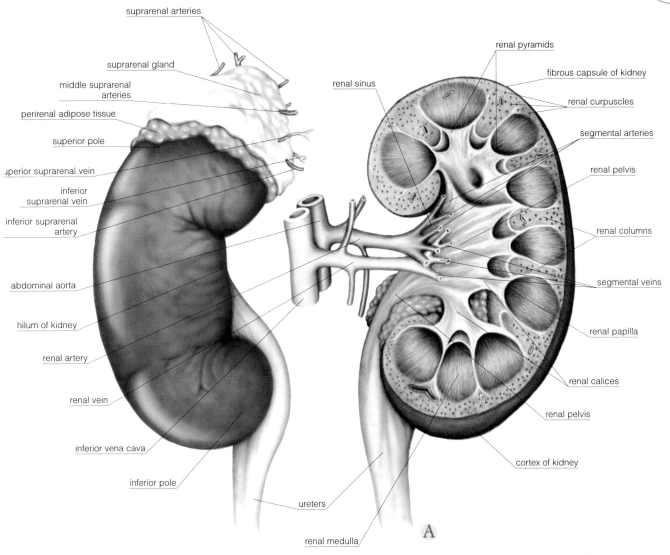

suprarenal arteries

suprarenal gland

middle suprarenal
arteries

perirenal adipose tissue

superior pole

uperior suprarenal vein

inferior
suprarenal vein

inferior suprarenal
artery

abdominal aorta

hilum of kidney

renal artery

renal vein

inferior vena cava

inferior pole

ureters

renal medulla

renal sinus

renal pyramids

fibrous capsule of kidney

renal curpuscles

segmental arteries

renal pelvis

renal columns

segmental veins

renal papilla

renal calices

renal pelvis

cortex of kidney

ANTERIOR VIEW

**MIDDLE LONGITUDINAL SECTION
POSTERIOR VIEW**

kidneys

Are two organs located in the back of the abdominal cavity, one to each side of the spine, they project in the media and posterior zones of the trunk, in the lumbar region. Have the form of a bean and are provided of a concavity in which is found the renal thread. Each kidney weights 130-170g and measures about 11.4cm of length, 5-7cm of width and 2.5cm of thickness. Generally the left kidney is found to a higher level than the right one. In the backside, the kidneys are covered by a robust musculature and for the last ribs that form the lower part of the thoracic cavity. Its upper part is covered by the suprarenal glands that are located above as a hood. Kidneys are in charge of regulating the water, the electrolytes and the acid-base of the blood. In its interior are done the operations of filtering and depuration of blood from the harmful substances that contains, which will form the urine, that after will be expelled from the body through the urethra in the micturition.

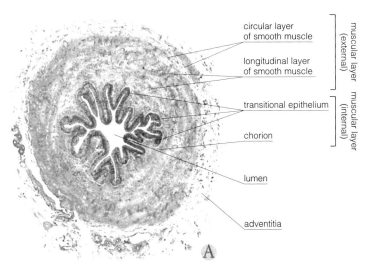

circular layer
of smooth muscle

longitudinal layer
of smooth muscle

muscular layer
(external)

transitional epithelium

chorion

muscular layer
(internal)

lumen

adventitia

URETER. TRANSVERSE SECTION

KIDNEY (II)

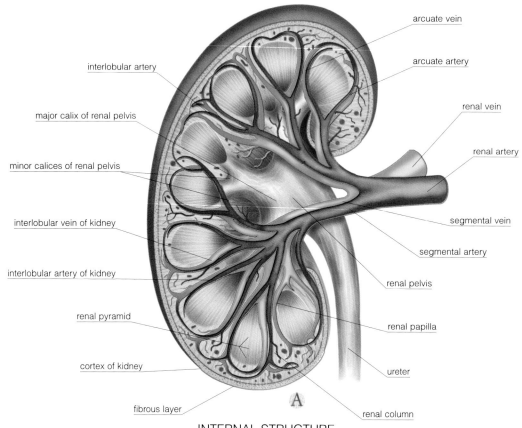

arcuate vein

arcuate artery

interlobular artery

renal vein

major calix of renal pelvis

renal artery

minor calices of renal pelvis

interlobular vein of kidney

segmental vein

interlobular artery of kidney

segmental artery

renal pelvis

renal pyramid

renal papilla

cortex of kidney

ureter

fibrous layer

renal column

INTERNAL STRUCTURE

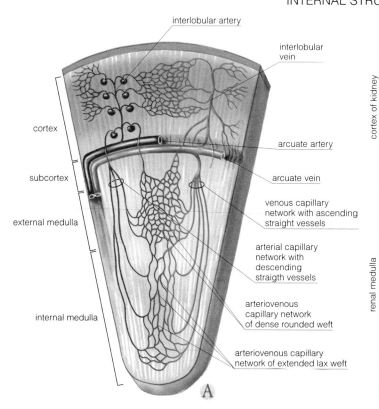

interlobular artery

interlobular vein

cortex

arcuate artery

subcortex

arcuate vein

external medulla

venous capillary network with ascending straight vessels

arterial capillary network with descending straight vessels

internal medulla

arteriovenous capillary network of dense rounded weft

arteriovenous capillary network of extended lax weft

BLOOD VESSELS

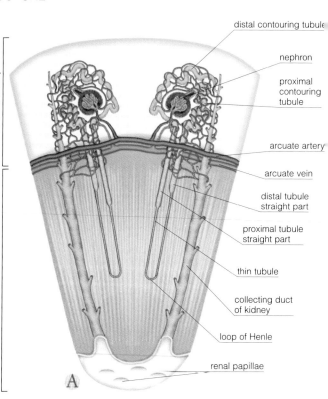

distal contouring tubule

nephron

proximal contouring tubule

cortex of kidney

arcuate artery

arcuate vein

distal tubule straight part

proximal tubule straight part

renal medulla

thin tubule

collecting duct of kidney

loop of Henle

renal papillae

CONICAL TISSUE SECTION

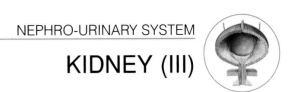

KIDNEY (III)

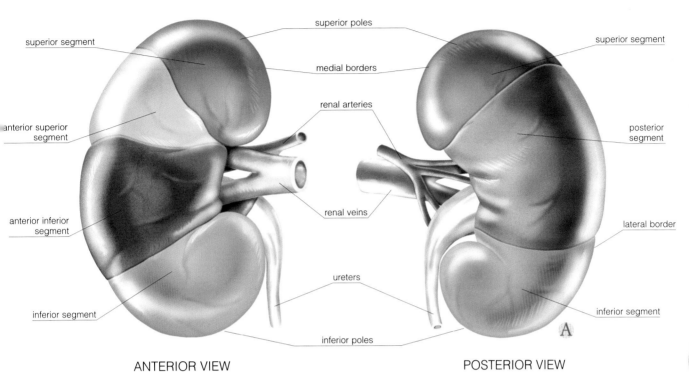

superior poles

superior segment

medial borders

superior segment

anterior superior segment

renal arteries

posterior segment

anterior inferior segment

renal veins

lateral border

inferior segment

ureters

inferior segment

inferior poles

ANTERIOR VIEW

POSTERIOR VIEW

RENAL SEGMENTS

487

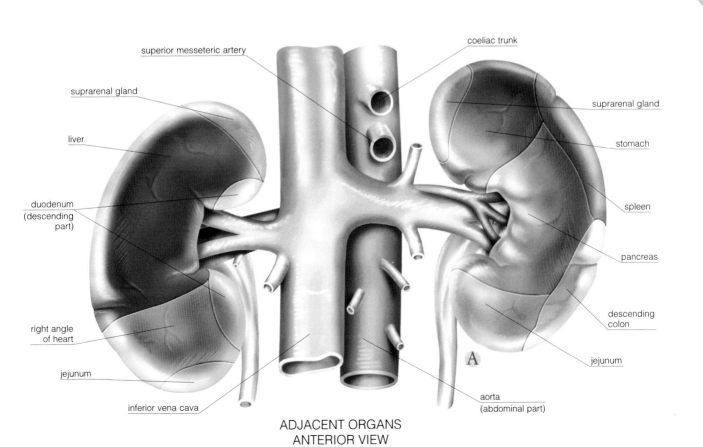

superior messeteric artery

coeliac trunk

suprarenal gland

suprarenal gland

liver

stomach

duodenum (descending part)

spleen

right angle of heart

pancreas

jejunum

descending colon

inferior vena cava

jejunum

aorta (abdominal part)

ADJACENT ORGANS
ANTERIOR VIEW

RENAL CORPUSCLE. HISTOLOGIC CHARACTERISTICS

renal corpuscle

The parietal layer of Bowman's capsule is composed by a flat, simple epithelium. The visceral layer, instead, is modified to form podocytes.

The ultrafiltrate enters in the urinary space and abandon the renal corpuscle to the high of its urinary pole, through the maximal contouring tubule.

The glomerular afferent arteriole enters in the renal corpuscle and the glomerular efferent arteriole abandons to the high of its vascular pole. The first irrigate the glomerulus, while the second drains it.

The component of dense macule of the distal tubule is found very close of the yuxtaglomerular cells of the glomerular arterioles.

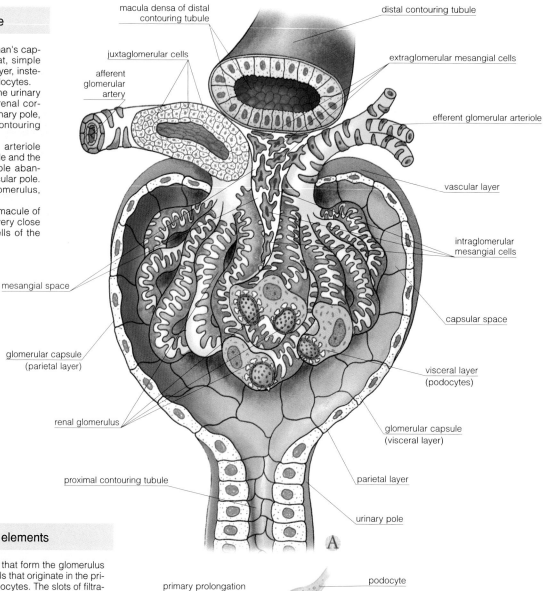

macula densa of distal contouring tubule

distal contouring tubule

juxtaglomerular cells

extraglomerular mesangial cells

afferent glomerular artery

efferent glomerular arteriole

vascular layer

intraglomerular mesangial cells

mesangial space

capsular space

glomerular capsule (parietal layer)

visceral layer (podocytes)

renal glomerulus

glomerular capsule (visceral layer)

parietal layer

proximal contouring tubule

urinary pole

A

glomerular elements

The fenestrated capillaries that form the glomerulus are wrapped by the pedicels that originate in the primary extensions of the podocytes. The slots of filtration between the adjacent pedicels are closed by thin diaphragms that, together with the basal laminas fused of the podocytes and of the capillary endothelium, contribute to form the barrier of filtration.

primary prolongation of podocyte

podocyte

endothelium

basal lamina

secondary prolongation of podocyte

spillways of filtration

primary prolongation of podocyte

body of podocyte

A

488

URINARY BLADDER and URETHRA (I)

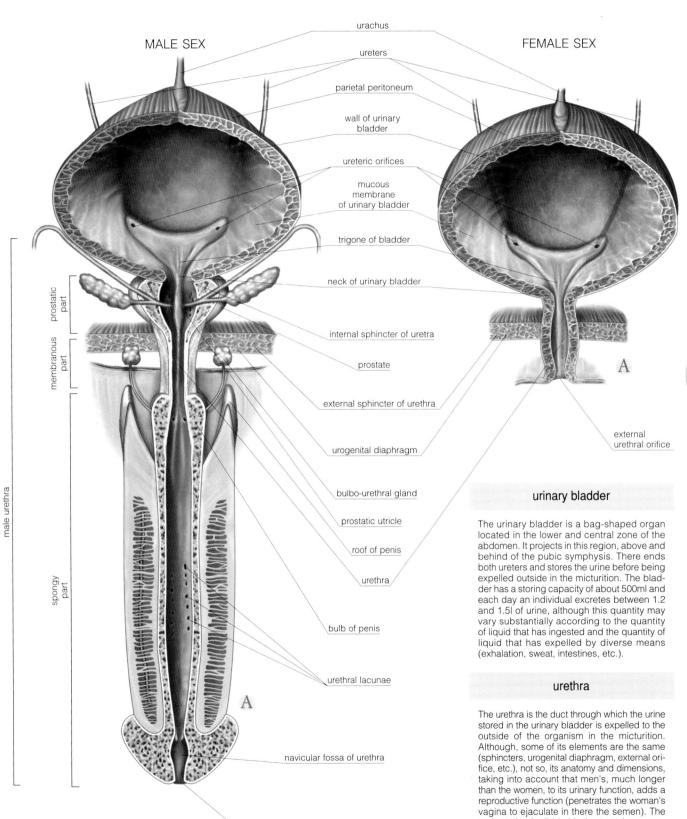

MALE SEX

FEMALE SEX

urachus

ureters

parietal peritoneum

wall of urinary bladder

ureteric orifices

mucous membrane of urinary bladder

trigone of bladder

neck of urinary bladder

internal sphincter of uretra

prostate

external sphincter of urethra

urogenital diaphragm

bulbo-urethral gland

prostatic utricle

roof of penis

urethra

bulb of penis

urethral lacunae

navicular fossa of urethra

external urethral orifice

external urethral orifice

prostatic part

membranous part

spongy part

male urethra

A

A

489

urinary bladder

The urinary bladder is a bag-shaped organ located in the lower and central zone of the abdomen. It projects in this region, above and behind of the pubic symphysis. There ends both ureters and stores the urine before being expelled outside in the micturition. The bladder has a storing capacity of about 500ml and each day an individual excretes between 1.2 and 1.5l of urine, although this quantity may vary substantially according to the quantity of liquid that has ingested and the quantity of liquid that has expelled by diverse means (exhalation, sweat, intestines, etc.).

urethra

The urethra is the duct through which the urine stored in the urinary bladder is expelled to the outside of the organism in the micturition. Although, some of its elements are the same (sphincters, urogenital diaphragm, external orifice, etc.), not so, its anatomy and dimensions, taking into account that men's, much longer than the women, to its urinary function, adds a reproductive function (penetrates the woman's vagina to ejaculate in there the semen). The male urethra is divided in three portions: prostatic, membranous and penile.

URINARY BLADDER and URETHRA (II)

MALE SEX. FRONTAL SECTION

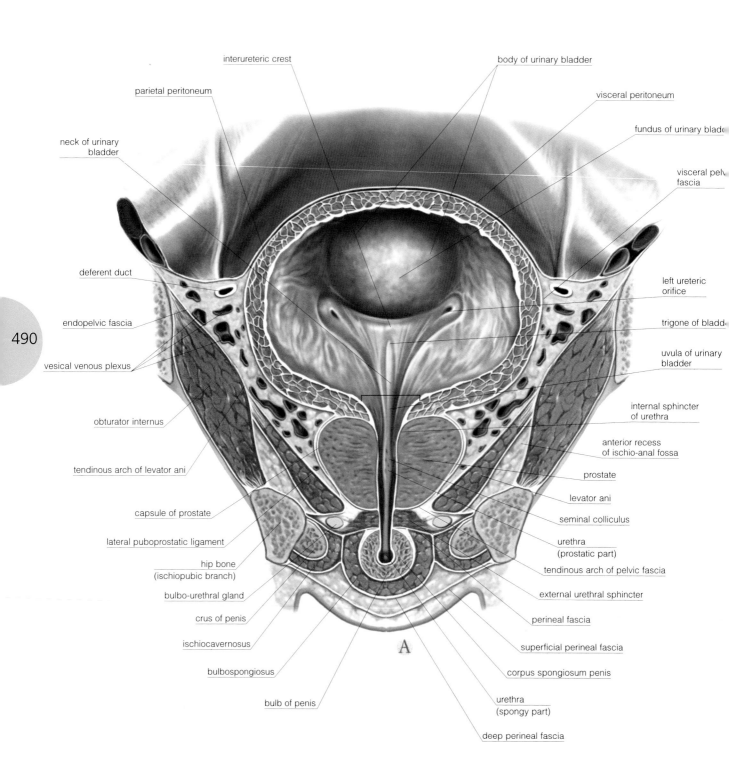

interureteric crest

body of urinary bladder

parietal peritoneum

visceral peritoneum

neck of urinary bladder

fundus of urinary blad

visceral pel\ fascia

deferent duct

left ureteric orifice

endopelvic fascia

trigone of bladd

vesical venous plexus

uvula of urinary bladder

obturator internus

internal sphincter of urethra

tendinous arch of levator ani

anterior recess of ischio-anal fossa

capsule of prostate

prostate

lateral puboprostatic ligament

levator ani

hip bone (ischiopubic branch)

seminal colliculus

bulbo-urethral gland

urethra (prostatic part)

crus of penis

tendinous arch of pelvic fascia

ischiocavernosus

external urethral sphincter

bulbospongiosus

perineal fascia

bulb of penis

superficial perineal fascia

corpus spongiosum penis

urethra (spongy part)

deep perineal fascia

490

A

URINARY BLADDER and URETHRA (III)
FEMALE SEX. FRONTAL SECTION

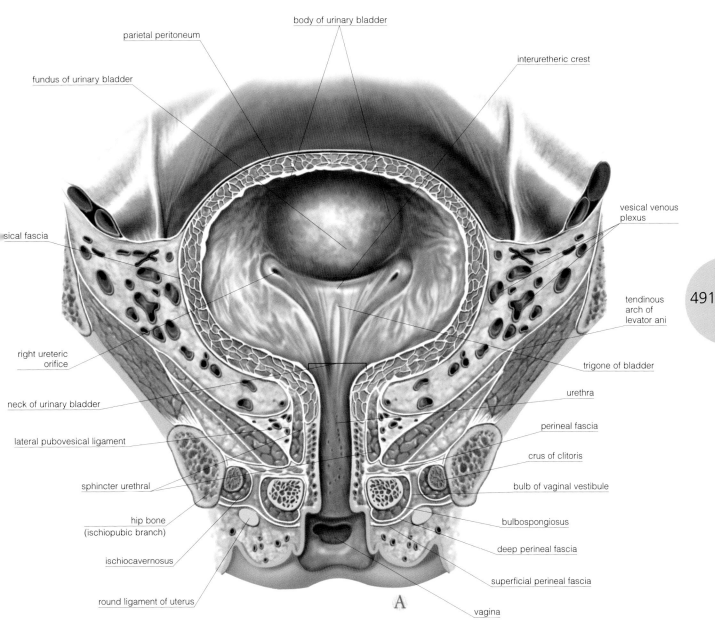

parietal peritoneum

body of urinary bladder

interuretheric crest

fundus of urinary bladder

vesical venous plexus

sical fascia

tendinous arch of levator ani

491

right ureteric orifice

trigone of bladder

neck of urinary bladder

urethra

lateral pubovesical ligament

perineal fascia

crus of clitoris

sphincter urethral

bulb of vaginal vestibule

hip bone (ischiopubic branch)

bulbospongiosus

ischiocavernosus

deep perineal fascia

superficial perineal fascia

round ligament of uterus

A

vagina

URINARY BLADDER and URETHRA (IV)

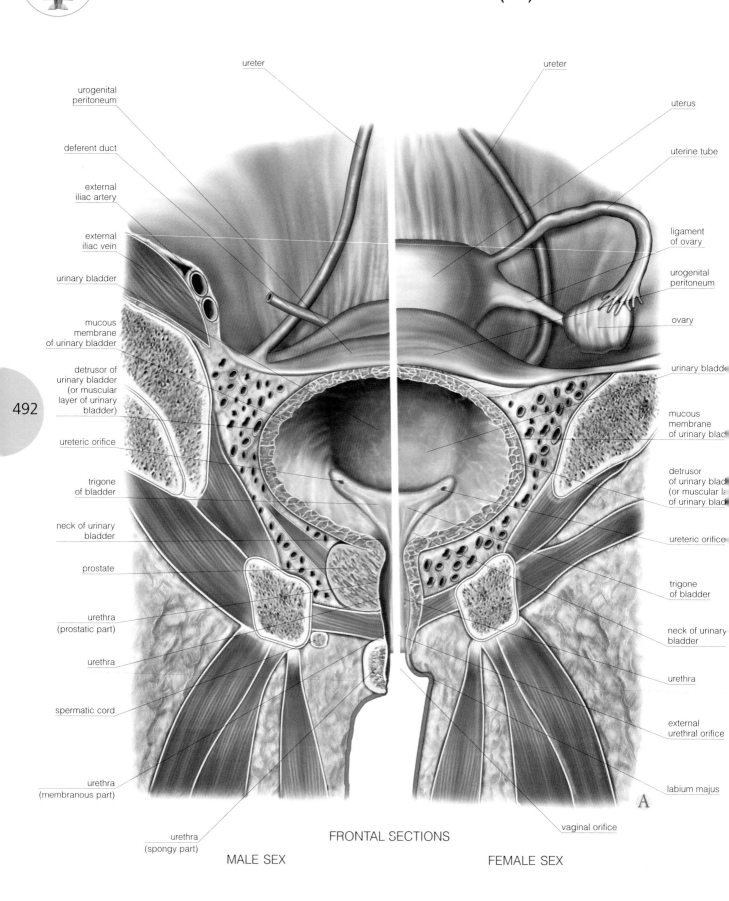

ureter

urogenital
peritoneum

deferent duct

external
iliac artery

external
iliac vein

urinary bladder

mucous
membrane
of urinary bladder

detrusor of
urinary bladder
(or muscular
layer of urinary
bladder)

ureteric orifice

trigone
of bladder

neck of urinary
bladder

prostate

urethra
(prostatic part)

urethra

spermatic cord

urethra
(membranous part)

urethra
(spongy part)

492

ureter

uterus

uterine tube

ligament
of ovary

urogenital
peritoneum

ovary

urinary bladd

mucous
membrane
of urinary blad

detrusor
of urinary blad
(or muscular la
of urinary blad

ureteric orifice

trigone
of bladder

neck of urinary
bladder

urethra

external
urethral orifice

labium majus

vaginal orifice

FRONTAL SECTIONS

MALE SEX

FEMALE SEX

A

URINARY STRUCTURES

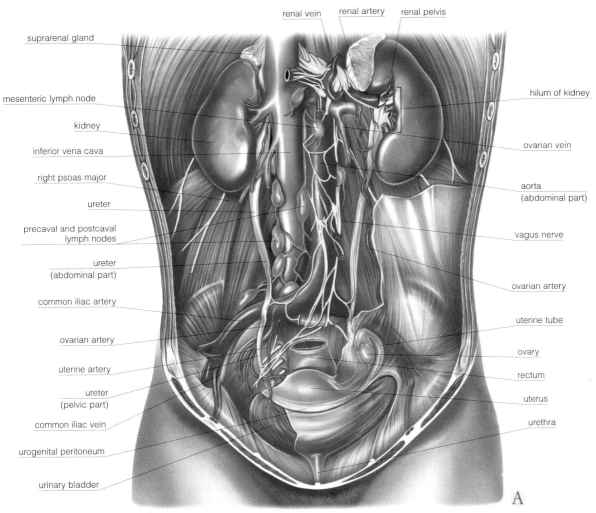

renal vein   renal artery   renal pelvis

suprarenal gland

mesenteric lymph node

kidney

inferior vena cava

right psoas major

ureter

precaval and postcaval
lymph nodes

ureter
(abdominal part)

common iliac artery

ovarian artery

uterine artery

ureter
(pelvic part)

common iliac vein

urogenital peritoneum

urinary bladder

hilum of kidney

ovarian vein

aorta
(abdominal part)

vagus nerve

ovarian artery

uterine tube

ovary

rectum

uterus

urethra

A

FEMALE SEX. ANTERIOR VIEW

493

MALE SEX. PROSTATE
and ATTACHED ORGANS

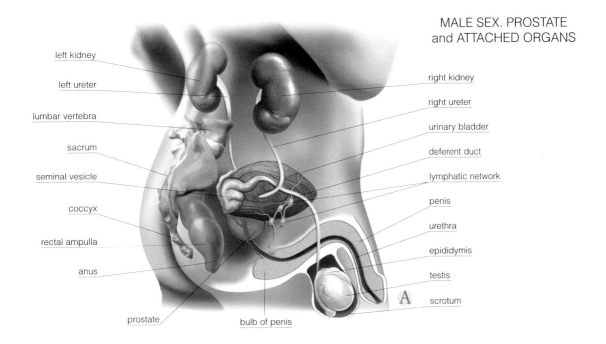

left kidney

left ureter

lumbar vertebra

sacrum

seminal vesicle

coccyx

rectal ampulla

anus

prostate

bulb of penis

right kidney

right ureter

urinary bladder

deferent duct

lymphatic network

penis

urethra

epididymis

testis

scrotum

A

PELVIS. VISCERAE

MALE SEX. ABDOMINAL WALL. SECTION and CRANIAL VIEW

494

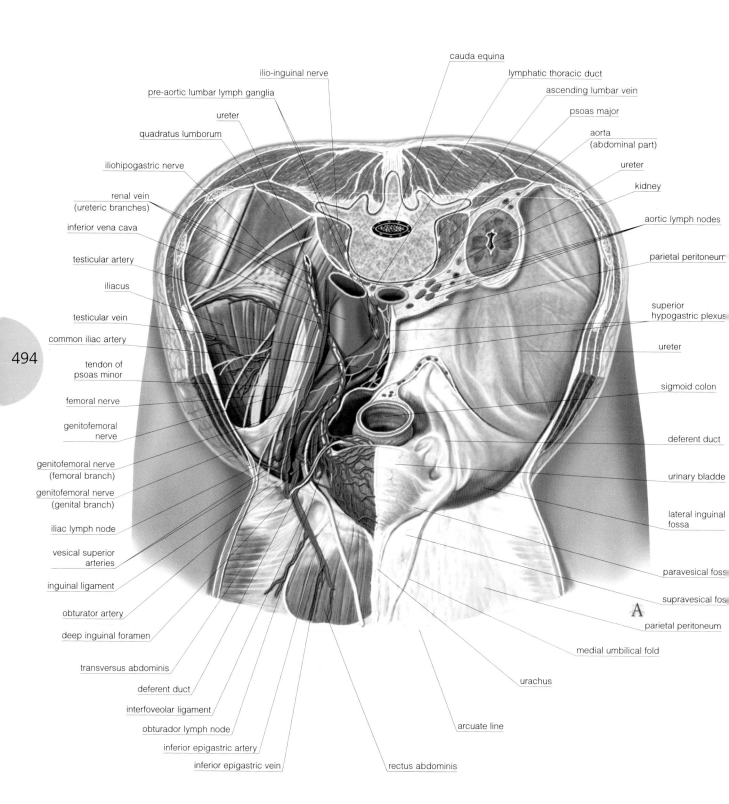

cauda equina

ilio-inguinal nerve

lymphatic thoracic duct

pre-aortic lumbar lymph ganglia

ascending lumbar vein

ureter

psoas major

quadratus lumborum

aorta
(abdominal part)

iliohipogastric nerve

ureter

renal vein
(ureteric branches)

kidney

inferior vena cava

aortic lymph nodes

testicular artery

parietal peritoneum

iliacus

superior
hypogastric plexus

testicular vein

common iliac artery

ureter

tendon of
psoas minor

sigmoid colon

femoral nerve

genitofemoral
nerve

deferent duct

genitofemoral nerve
(femoral branch)

urinary bladde

genitofemoral nerve
(genital branch)

lateral inguinal
fossa

iliac lymph node

vesical superior
arteries

paravesical foss

inguinal ligament

supravesical fos

obturator artery

A

deep inguinal foramen

parietal peritoneum

transversus abdominis

medial umbilical fold

deferent duct

urachus

interfoveolar ligament

obturador lymph node

inferior epigastric artery

arcuate line

inferior epigastric vein

rectus abdominis

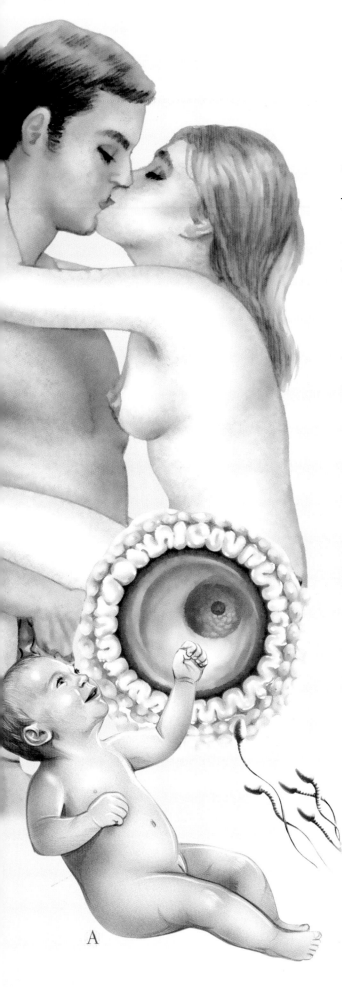

GENITAL SYSTEM

Among the essential functions of all living beings, besides the processes of birth and growth, is reproduction. The term genital apparatus is given to the set of organs used by the individual to naturally perpetuate the species. For this to occur, sexual coupling of a man and a woman through intercourse is essential. But a more complete view of the human person, which includes among other factors sensations, feelings, personal relationships, certain drives, etc. necessarily leads one to assign additional important functions to the genital apparatus, that have much to do with love, pleasure and the emotional balance of the human being.

Set of organs allowing reproduction between a man and a woman. However, seen from a more complete perspective of the human species to include feelings, sensations, relationships, etc., it can also have important roles related to love, pleasure and emotional equilibrium. The reproductive function is the determinant factor in the establishment of specific genital characteristics of males and females. Even though the mechanics of reproduction requires in both cases the intervention of the gonads, adjoining structures and ducts, in each sex there are characteristic organs with unique roles. Thus, in order for the male to produce semen (which is then introduced in the female vagina to allow fertilization), the combined function of the testes, the vas deferens, the epididymis, the efferent ductules, the ejaculatory duct, the urethra, the prostatic, seminal and bulbourethral glands, as well as the penis is necessary. And in order for the female to produce a mature egg cell, as well as to collect semen (which contains the spermatozoa that fertilizes the egg, leading to an ulterior pregnancy and delivery), the combined action of the ovaries, fallopian tubes, uterus, vagina and vulva is essential. In the process of giving birth to a new being, both men and women have critical and complementary roles.

The genital system of the baby remains dormant until puberty, when the gonads become active, leading to the production of sperm (or male gametes) in men and egg cells (or female gametes) in women. The testes and the ovaries release a series of hormones that are essential not only for the development and function of the genital organs, but also to trigger a sexual impulse between the sexes, leading to sexual intercourse and natural fertilization. Once a spermatozoon is able to penetrate a mature egg and fertilize it, a zygote (which is the first cell of the new individual) is formed. In a series of events that occur in the uterus, other cells are gradually formed from this zygote, leading to the formation of a new human being. This process, which can be considered the culmination of reproduction, takes nine months for completion from the moment of fertilization.

MALE GENITAL SYSTEM (I)

RIGHT LATERAL GENERAL VIEW

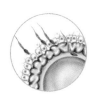

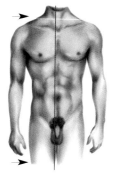

male genital system

Set of organs and structures belonging to the male, allowing him to fulfill his reproductive role. They are constituted basically by the penis, the prostate, the spermatic cords and the testicles. In order for a new human being to be born in a natural way, the participation of a man is essential. His body must contribute male cells (spermatozoa) which are produced in the testes. From the testicles, the spermatozoa travel to the seminiferous tubules and, before entering the urethra, they receive the liquid that is secreted by the prostate gland, forming semen. During sexual intercourse, by ejaculation through the penis, the male releases his semen inside the vagina of the female. In order for fertilization to occur, one of the spermatozoa present in the semen -on its way through the interior of the female genital apparatus (vagina, uterus, fallopian tubes)- must find an ovocyte that can be fertilized. This sperm must then penetrate and combine with the ovocyte, giving rise to the formation of an embryo that nests in the uterus, where it will later undergo the process of gestation. Fertilization occurs in the distal third of the fallopian tube.

496

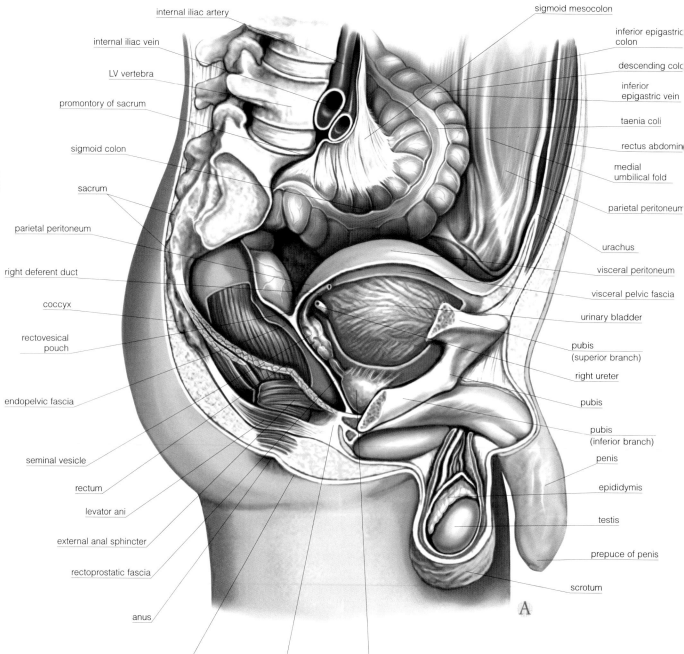

internal iliac artery
internal iliac vein
LV vertebra
promontory of sacrum
sigmoid colon
sacrum
parietal peritoneum
right deferent duct
coccyx
rectovesical pouch
endopelvic fascia
seminal vesicle
rectum
levator ani
external anal sphincter
rectoprostatic fascia
anus

sigmoid mesocolon
inferior epigastric colon
descending colon
inferior epigastric vein
taenia coli
rectus abdomin
medial umbilical fold
parietal peritoneum
urachus
visceral peritoneum
visceral pelvic fascia
urinary bladder
pubis (superior branch)
right ureter
pubis
pubis (inferior branch)
penis
epididymis
testis
prepuce of penis
scrotum

perineum   perineal body   prostate

A

MALE GENITAL SYSTEM (II)
RIGHT LATERAL GENERAL VIEW

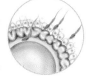

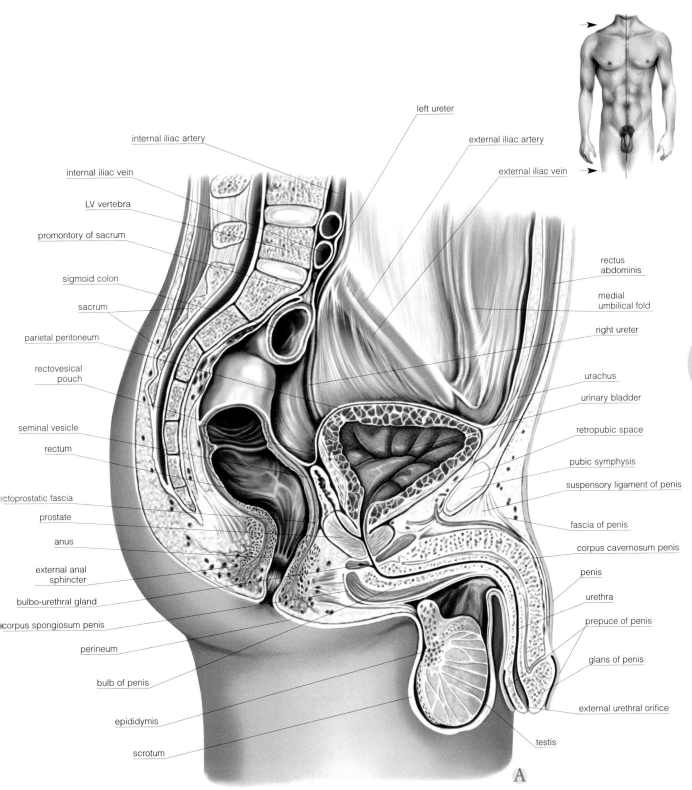

left ureter

internal iliac artery

external iliac artery

internal iliac vein

external iliac vein

LV vertebra

promontory of sacrum

rectus abdominis

sigmoid colon

medial umbilical fold

sacrum

right ureter

parietal peritoneum

rectovesical pouch

urachus

urinary bladder

seminal vesicle

retropubic space

rectum

pubic symphysis

suspensory ligament of penis

ctoprostatic fascia

prostate

fascia of penis

anus

corpus cavernosum penis

external anal sphincter

penis

bulbo-urethral gland

urethra

corpus spongiosum penis

prepuce of penis

perineum

glans of penis

bulb of penis

external urethral orifice

epididymis

testis

scrotum

497

A

MALE GENITAL SYSTEM (III)

ANTERIOR GENERAL VIEW

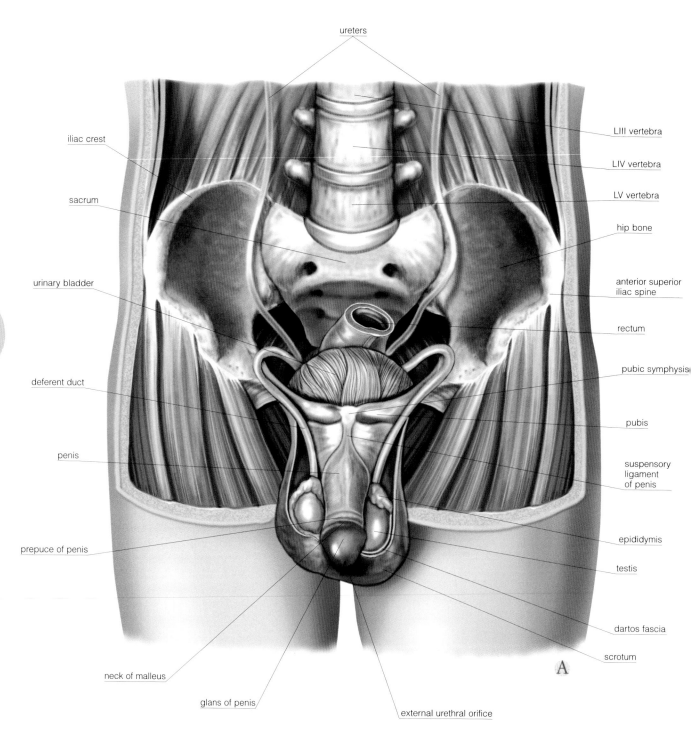

ureters

LIII vertebra

LIV vertebra

LV vertebra

hip bone

anterior superior iliac spine

rectum

pubic symphysis

pubis

suspensory ligament of penis

epididymis

testis

dartos fascia

scrotum

iliac crest

sacrum

urinary bladder

deferent duct

penis

prepuce of penis

neck of malleus

glans of penis

external urethral orifice

A

MALE GENITAL SYSTEM (IV). PENIS and SCROTUM
ANTERIOR VIEW

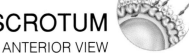

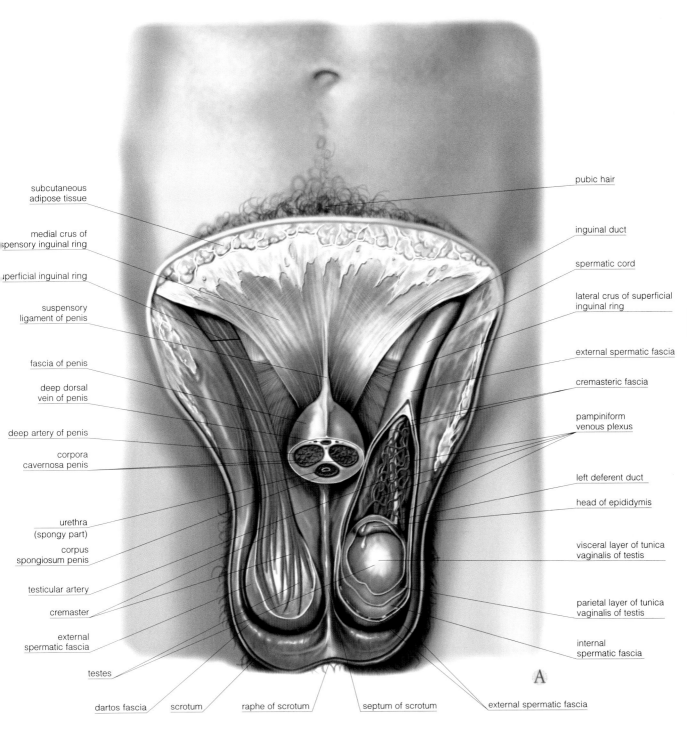

subcutaneous adipose tissue

medial crus of spensory inguinal ring

uperficial inguinal ring

suspensory ligament of penis

fascia of penis

deep dorsal vein of penis

deep artery of penis

corpora cavernosa penis

urethra (spongy part)

corpus spongiosum penis

testicular artery

cremaster

external spermatic fascia

testes

dartos fascia

scrotum

raphe of scrotum

septum of scrotum

pubic hair

inguinal duct

spermatic cord

lateral crus of superficial inguinal ring

external spermatic fascia

cremasteric fascia

pampiniform venous plexus

left deferent duct

head of epididymis

visceral layer of tunica vaginalis of testis

parietal layer of tunica vaginalis of testis

internal spermatic fascia

external spermatic fascia

A

MALE GENITAL SYSTEM (V). SPERMATIC DUCTS
POSTERIOR VIEW

500

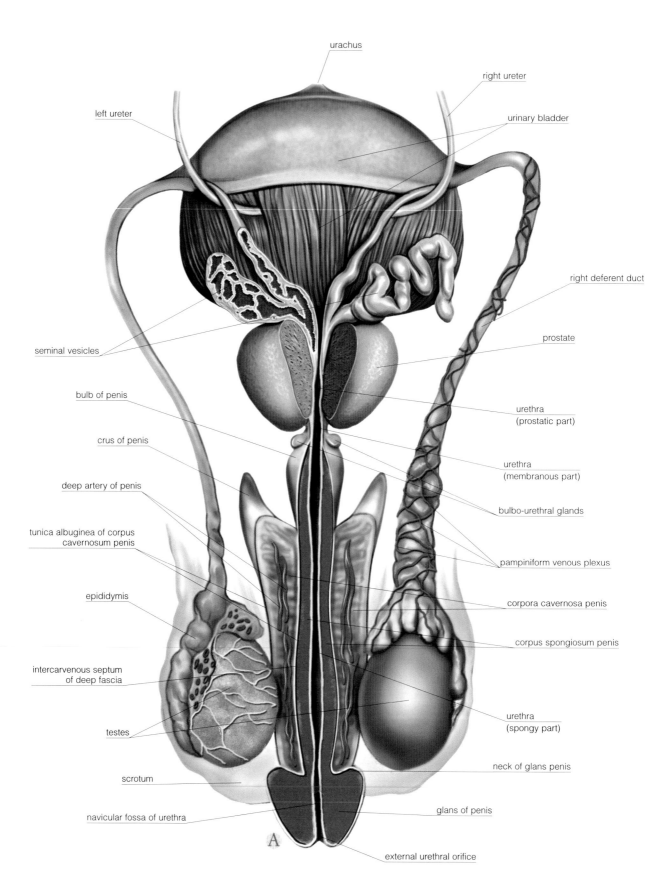

urachus

right ureter

left ureter

urinary bladder

right deferent duct

prostate

seminal vesicles

urethra
(prostatic part)

bulb of penis

urethra
(membranous part)

crus of penis

bulbo-urethral glands

deep artery of penis

tunica albuginea of corpus
cavernosum penis

pampiniform venous plexus

epididymis

corpora cavernosa penis

intercarvenous septum
of deep fascia

corpus spongiosum penis

testes

urethra
(spongy part)

scrotum

neck of glans penis

navicular fossa of urethra

glans of penis

A

external urethral orifice

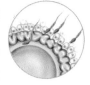

MALE GENITAL SYSTEM (VI). PELVIS and PERINEUM (I)

SAGITTAL SECTION

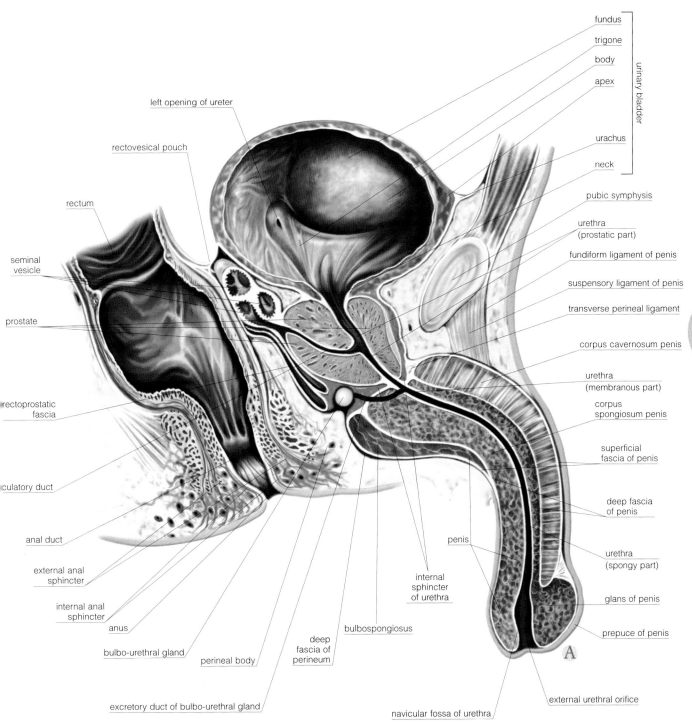

fundus

trigone

body

apex

urachus

neck

urinary bladder

left opening of ureter

rectovesical pouch

pubic symphysis

urethra
(prostatic part)

fundiform ligament of penis

suspensory ligament of penis

transverse perineal ligament

rectum

seminal
vesicle

prostate

501

corpus cavernosum penis

urethra
(membranous part)

corpus
spongiosum penis

rectoprostatic
fascia

superficial
fascia of penis

deep fascia
of penis

ejaculatory duct

anal duct

urethra
(spongy part)

penis

external anal
sphincter

internal
sphincter
of urethra

glans of penis

internal anal
sphincter

anus

bulbospongiosus

prepuce of penis

bulbo-urethral gland

perineal body

deep
fascia of
perineum

A

excretory duct of bulbo-urethral gland

navicular fossa of urethra

external urethral orifice

MALE GENITAL SYSTEM (VII)
PELVIS and PERINEUM (II)

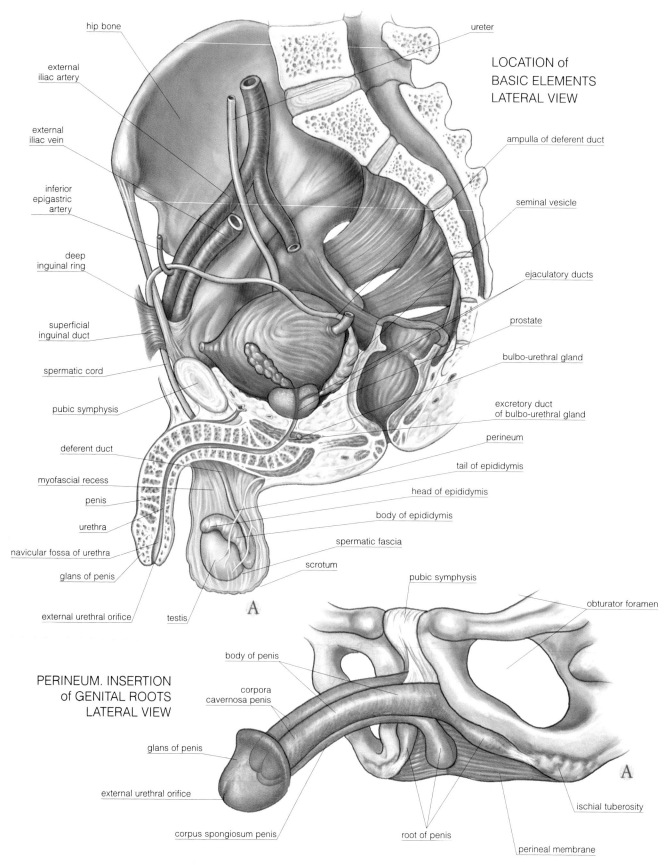

hip bone

external
iliac artery

external
iliac vein

inferior
epigastric
artery

deep
inguinal ring

superficial
inguinal duct

spermatic cord

pubic symphysis

deferent duct

myofascial recess

penis

urethra

navicular fossa of urethra

glans of penis

external urethral orifice

testis

A

ureter

LOCATION of
BASIC ELEMENTS
LATERAL VIEW

ampulla of deferent duct

seminal vesicle

ejaculatory ducts

prostate

bulbo-urethral gland

excretory duct
of bulbo-urethral gland

perineum

tail of epididymis

head of epididymis

body of epididymis

spermatic fascia

scrotum

PERINEUM. INSERTION
of GENITAL ROOTS
LATERAL VIEW

body of penis

corpora
cavernosa penis

glans of penis

external urethral orifice

corpus spongiosum penis

pubic symphysis

obturator foramen

root of penis

ischial tuberosity

perineal membrane

A

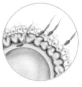

MALE GENITAL SYSTEM (VIII)
PELVIS and PERINEUM (III)

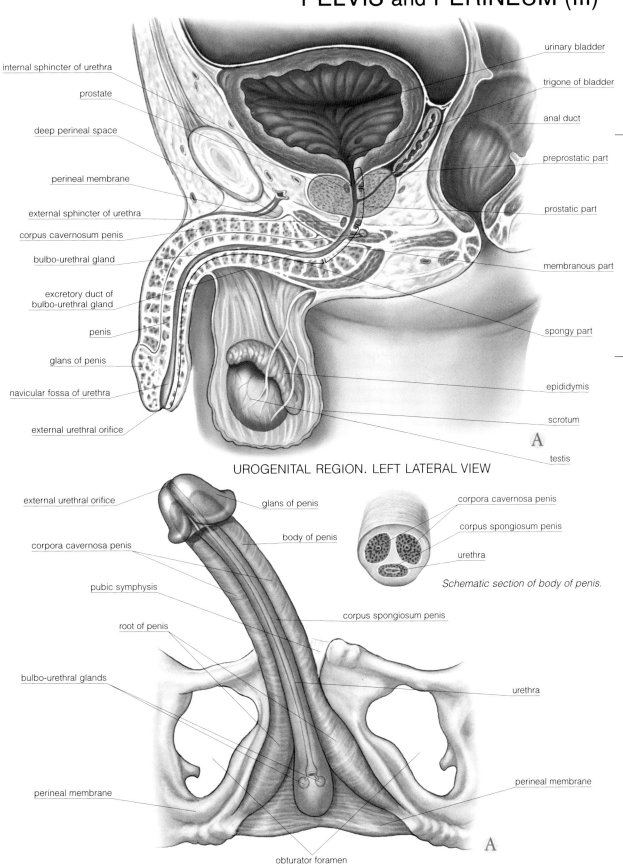

internal sphincter of urethra

prostate

deep perineal space

perineal membrane

external sphincter of urethra

corpus cavernosum penis

bulbo-urethral gland

excretory duct of
bulbo-urethral gland

penis

glans of penis

navicular fossa of urethra

external urethral orifice

urinary bladder

trigone of bladder

anal duct

preprostatic part

prostatic part

membranous part

spongy part

epididymis

scrotum

testis

urethra

A

UROGENITAL REGION. LEFT LATERAL VIEW

external urethral orifice

glans of penis

corpora cavernosa penis

pubic symphysis

body of penis

corpora cavernosa penis

corpus spongiosum penis

urethra

Schematic section of body of penis.

root of penis

corpus spongiosum penis

bulbo-urethral glands

urethra

perineal membrane

perineal membrane

obturator foramen

A

503

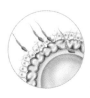

MALE GENITAL SYSTEM (IX)
UROGENITAL REGION. WALL LAYERS

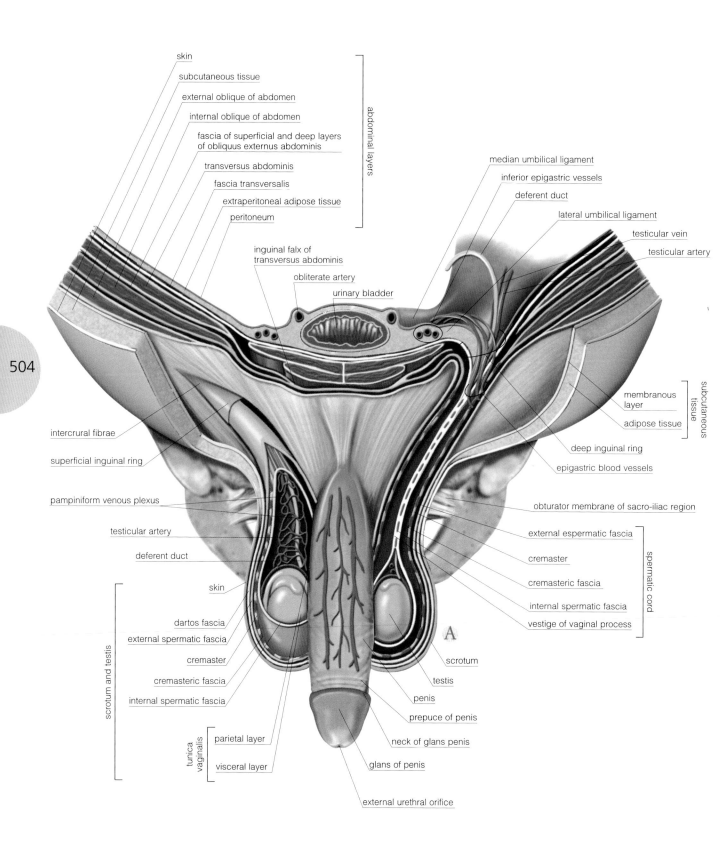

skin

subcutaneous tissue

external oblique of abdomen

internal oblique of abdomen

fascia of superficial and deep layers
of obliquus externus abdominis

transversus abdominis

fascia transversalis

extraperitoneal adipose tissue

peritoneum

abdominal layers

median umbilical ligament

inferior epigastric vessels

deferent duct

lateral umbilical ligament

testicular vein

testicular artery

inguinal falx of
transversus abdominis

obliterate artery

urinary bladder

504

subcutaneous tissue

membranous
layer

adipose tissue

deep inguinal ring

epigastric blood vessels

intercrural fibrae

superficial inguinal ring

pampiniform venous plexus

testicular artery

deferent duct

obturator membrane of sacro-iliac region

external espermatic fascia

cremaster

cremasteric fascia

internal spermatic fascia

vestige of vaginal process

spermatic cord

skin

dartos fascia

external spermatic fascia

cremaster

cremasteric fascia

internal spermatic fascia

scrotum and testis

tunica vaginalis

parietal layer

visceral layer

scrotum

testis

penis

prepuce of penis

neck of glans penis

glans of penis

A

external urethral orifice

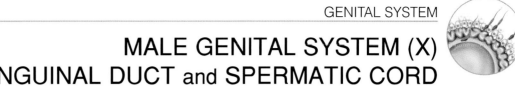

MALE GENITAL SYSTEM (X)
INGUINAL DUCT and SPERMATIC CORD

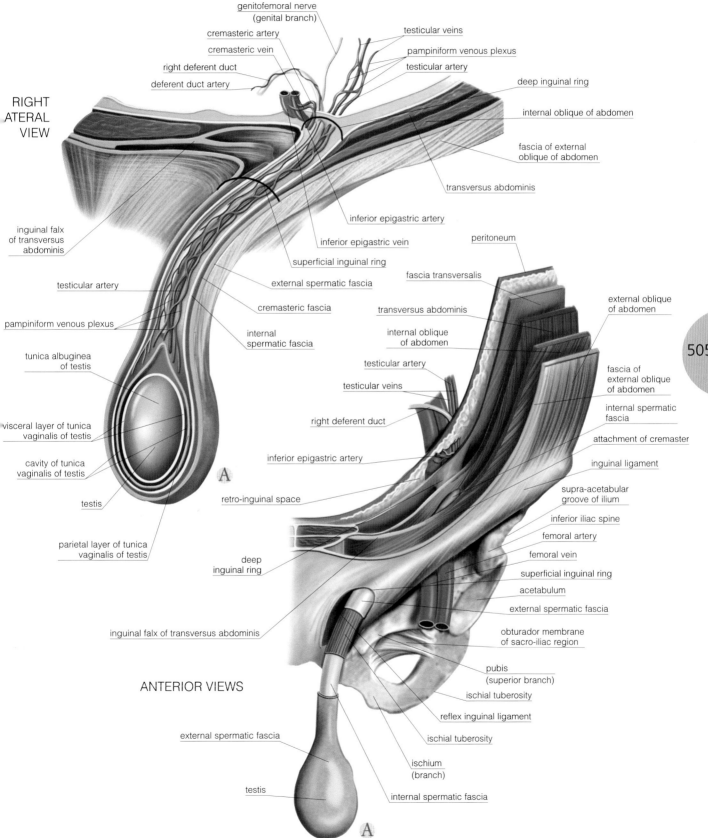

RIGHT
LATERAL
VIEW

genitofemoral nerve
(genital branch)

cremasteric artery

cremasteric vein

right deferent duct

deferent duct artery

testicular veins

pampiniform venous plexus

testicular artery

deep inguinal ring

internal oblique of abdomen

fascia of external
oblique of abdomen

transversus abdominis

inferior epigastric artery

inferior epigastric vein

superficial inguinal ring

external spermatic fascia

cremasteric fascia

internal
spermatic fascia

peritoneum

fascia transversalis

transversus abdominis

internal oblique
of abdomen

testicular artery

testicular veins

right deferent duct

inferior epigastric artery

inguinal falx
of transversus
abdominis

testicular artery

pampiniform venous plexus

tunica albuginea
of testis

visceral layer of tunica
vaginalis of testis

cavity of tunica
vaginalis of testis

testis

parietal layer of tunica
vaginalis of testis

external oblique
of abdomen

fascia of
external oblique
of abdomen

internal spermatic
fascia

attachment of cremaster

inguinal ligament

supra-acetabular
groove of ilium

inferior iliac spine

femoral artery

femoral vein

superficial inguinal ring

acetabulum

external spermatic fascia

obturador membrane
of sacro-iliac region

pubis
(superior branch)

ischial tuberosity

reflex inguinal ligament

ischial tuberosity

ischium
(branch)

internal spermatic fascia

retro-inguinal space

deep
inguinal ring

inguinal falx of transversus abdominis

A

ANTERIOR VIEWS

external spermatic fascia

testis

A

505

MALE GENITAL SYSTEM (XI). PELVIS
TRANSVERSE SECTION. SUPERIOR VIEW at the LEVEL of the LIII VERTEBRA

506

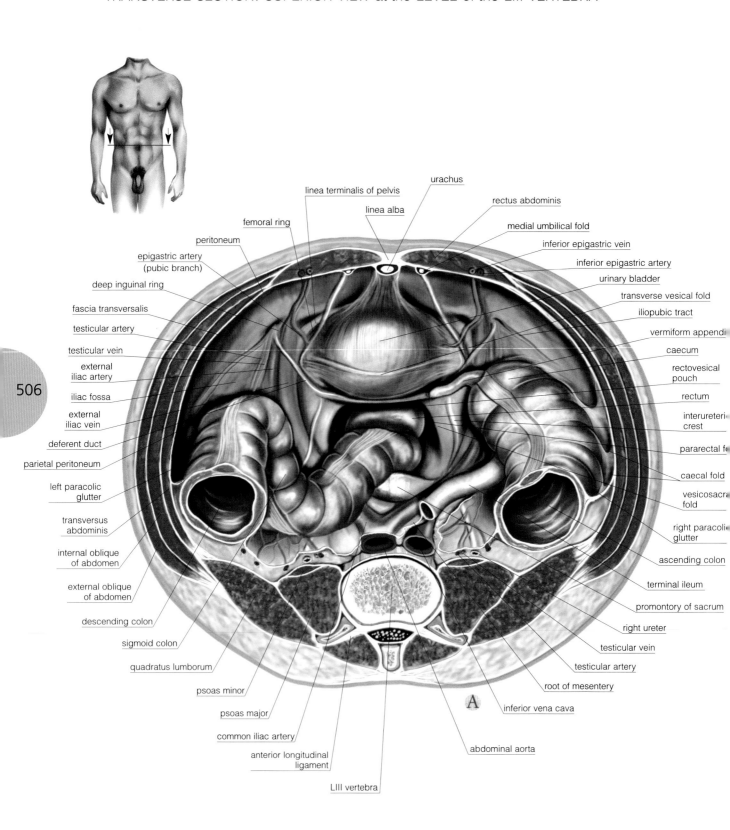

urachus

linea terminalis of pelvis

rectus abdominis

linea alba

femoral ring

medial umbilical fold

peritoneum

inferior epigastric vein

epigastric artery
(pubic branch)

inferior epigastric artery

deep inguinal ring

urinary bladder

fascia transversalis

transverse vesical fold

testicular artery

iliopubic tract

testicular vein

vermiform appendi

external
iliac artery

caecum

iliac fossa

rectovesical
pouch

external
iliac vein

rectum

deferent duct

interureteri
crest

parietal peritoneum

pararectal f

left paracolic
glutter

caecal fold

transversus
abdominis

vesicosacra
fold

internal oblique
of abdomen

right paracoli
glutter

external oblique
of abdomen

ascending colon

descending colon

terminal ileum

sigmoid colon

promontory of sacrum

quadratus lumborum

right ureter

psoas minor

testicular vein

psoas major

testicular artery

common iliac artery

root of mesentery

anterior longitudinal
ligament

inferior vena cava

abdominal aorta

LIII vertebra

A

MALE GENITAL SYSTEM (XII). PENIS (I)

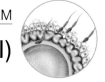

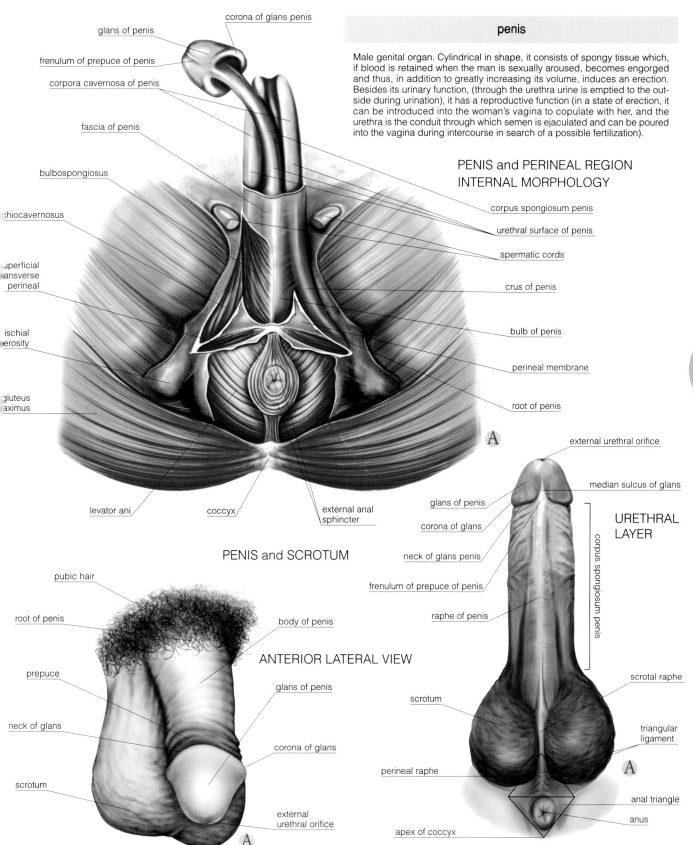

penis

Male genital organ. Cylindrical in shape, it consists of spongy tissue which, if blood is retained when the man is sexually aroused, becomes engorged and thus, in addition to greatly increasing its volume, induces an erection. Besides its urinary function, (through the urethra urine is emptied to the outside during urination), it has a reproductive function (in a state of erection, it can be introduced into the woman's vagina to copulate with her, and the urethra is the conduit through which semen is ejaculated and can be poured into the vagina during intercourse in search of a possible fertilization).

PENIS and PERINEAL REGION
INTERNAL MORPHOLOGY

corona of glans penis
glans of penis
frenulum of prepuce of penis
corpora cavernosa of penis
fascia of penis
bulbospongiosus
ischiocavernosus
superficial transverse perineal
ischial tuberosity
gluteus maximus
corpus spongiosum penis
urethral surface of penis
spermatic cords
crus of penis
bulb of penis
perineal membrane
root of penis
levator ani
coccyx
external anal sphincter

A

507

PENIS and SCROTUM

ANTERIOR LATERAL VIEW

pubic hair
root of penis
body of penis
glans of penis
prepuce
neck of glans
corona of glans
scrotum
external urethral orifice

A

external urethral orifice
glans of penis
median sulcus of glans
corona of glans
neck of glans penis
frenulum of prepuce of penis
raphe of penis
URETHRAL LAYER
corpus spongiosum penis
scrotum
scrotal raphe
triangular ligament
perineal raphe
anal triangle
anus
apex of coccyx

A

MALE GENITAL SYSTEM (XIII). PENIS (II)
SECTIONS

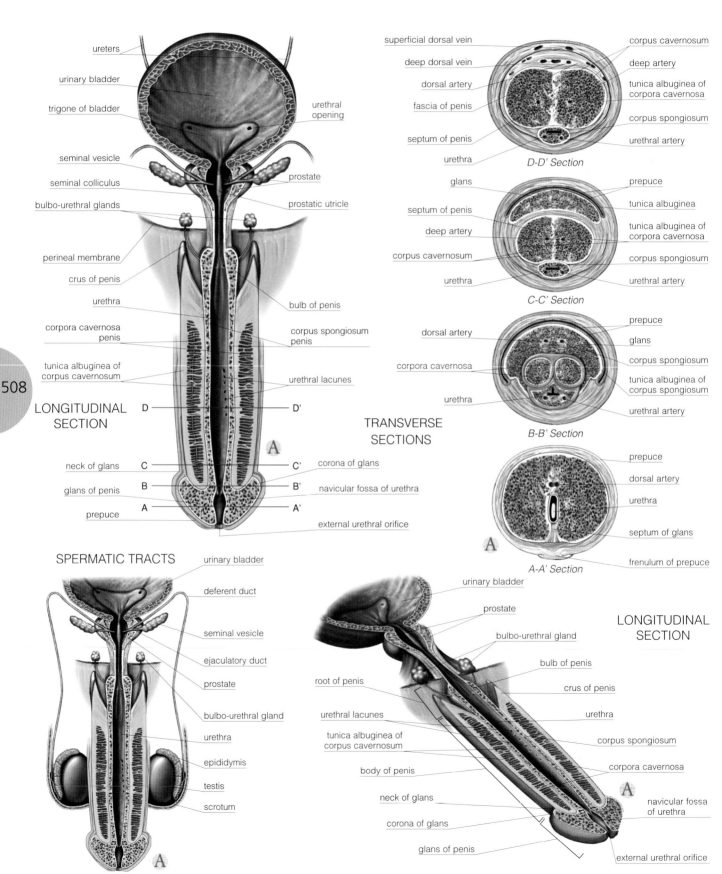

ureters

urinary bladder

trigone of bladder

urethral opening

seminal vesicle

seminal colliculus

prostate

bulbo-urethral glands

prostatic utricle

perineal membrane

crus of penis

urethra

bulb of penis

corpora cavernosa penis

corpus spongiosum penis

tunica albuginea of corpus cavernosum

urethral lacunes

508

LONGITUDINAL SECTION

D — D'

neck of glans C — C' corona of glans

glans of penis B — B' navicular fossa of urethra

prepuce A — A'

external urethral orifice

superficial dorsal vein

corpus cavernosum

deep dorsal vein

deep artery

dorsal artery

tunica albuginea of corpora cavernosa

fascia of penis

corpus spongiosum

septum of penis

urethral artery

urethra

D-D' Section

glans

prepuce

septum of penis

tunica albuginea

deep artery

tunica albuginea of corpora cavernosa

corpus cavernosum

corpus spongiosum

urethra

urethral artery

C-C' Section

prepuce

dorsal artery

glans

corpora cavernosa

corpus spongiosum

tunica albuginea of corpus spongiosum

urethra

urethral artery

B-B' Section

TRANSVERSE SECTIONS

prepuce

dorsal artery

urethra

septum of glans

frenulum of prepuce

A-A' Section

SPERMATIC TRACTS

urinary bladder

deferent duct

seminal vesicle

ejaculatory duct

prostate

bulbo-urethral gland

urethra

epididymis

testis

scrotum

urinary bladder

prostate

bulbo-urethral gland

bulb of penis

crus of penis

root of penis

urethral lacunes

urethra

tunica albuginea of corpus cavernosum

corpus spongiosum

body of penis

corpora cavernosa

neck of glans

navicular fossa of urethra

corona of glans

glans of penis

external urethral orifice

LONGITUDINAL SECTION

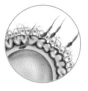

MALE GENITAL SYSTEM (XIV). TESTES

TESTIS

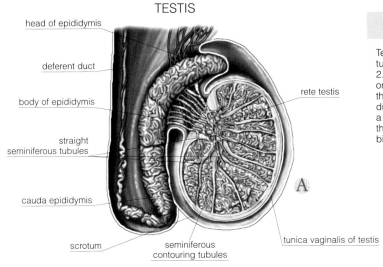

- head of epididymis
- deferent duct
- body of epididymis
- straight seminiferous tubules
- cauda epididymis
- scrotum
- seminiferous contouring tubules
- rete testis
- tunica vaginalis of testis

testes

Testes are two glandular, ovoid organs that are contained in the scrotum. Each testicle is about 4cm long, about 2.5cm wide and about 2.5cm thick. Testes communicate with the remainder of the genital organs using different conduits. Alongside their posteromedial edge is the epididymis, from where the vas deferens exits. Its function is to produce spermatozoa (or male sex cells, through which men can fertilize a female egg) and the male hormones testosterone (responsible for the growth and development of male sexual characteristics) and inhibin (it inhibits the secretion of gonadotropin releasing hormone).

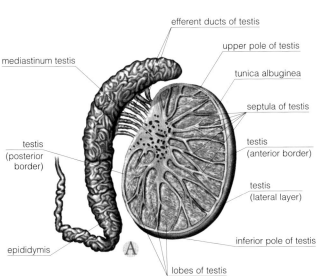

- efferent ducts of testis
- mediastinum testis
- testis (posterior border)
- epididymis
- lobes of testis
- upper pole of testis
- tunica albuginea
- septula of testis
- testis (anterior border)
- testis (lateral layer)
- inferior pole of testis

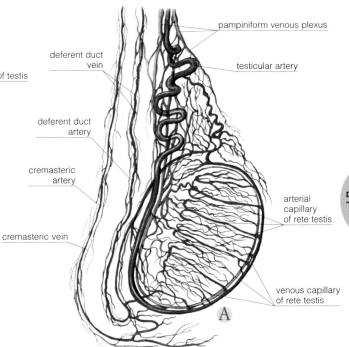

- deferent duct vein
- deferent duct artery
- cremasteric artery
- cremasteric vein
- pampiniform venous plexus
- testicular artery
- arterial capillary of rete testis
- venous capillary of rete testis

509

TESTIS, EPIDIDYMIS and SPERMATIC CORD BLOOD VESSELS. LATERAL VIEW

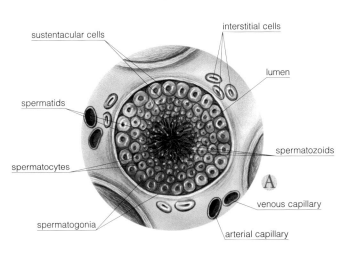

- sustentacular cells
- spermatids
- spermatocytes
- spermatogonia
- interstitial cells
- lumen
- spermatozoids
- venous capillary
- arterial capillary

TUBULUS SEMINIFEROUS. TRANSVERSE SECTION

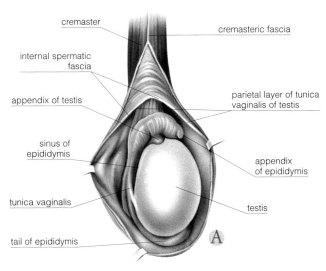

- cremaster
- internal spermatic fascia
- appendix of testis
- sinus of epididymis
- tunica vaginalis
- tail of epididymis
- cremasteric fascia
- parietal layer of tunica vaginalis of testis
- appendix of epididymis
- testis

TESTIS and EDIPIDYMIS. SECTION

MALE GENITAL SYSTEM (XV)
SPERMATOGENESIS and SPERMIOGENESIS

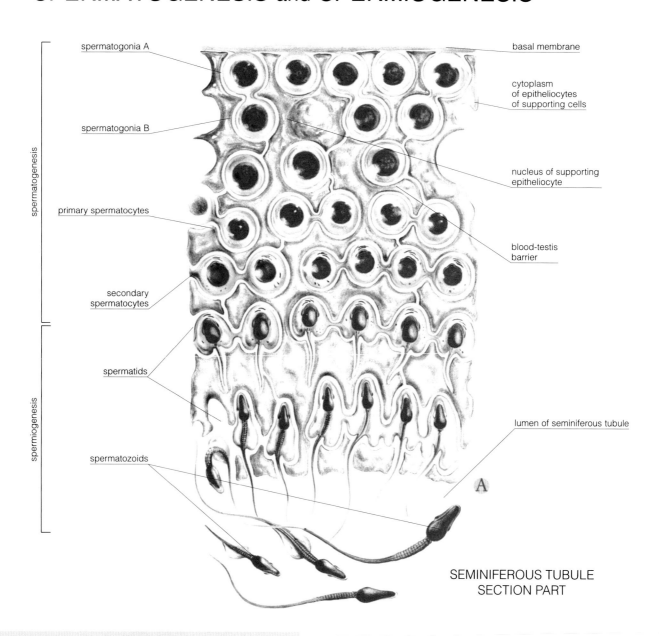

spermatogonia A

spermatogonia B

primary spermatocytes

secondary spermatocytes

spermatids

spermatozoids

spermatogenesis

spermiogenesis

basal membrane

cytoplasm
of epitheliocytes
of supporting cells

nucleus of supporting
epitheliocyte

blood-testis
barrier

lumen of seminiferous tubule

A

SEMINIFEROUS TUBULE
SECTION PART

510

spermatogenesis

Process followed by the germ cells that are found inside the testicle to become spermatozoa. This process begins in men approximately by age 13, and remains active continuously from then on and for life, although the quantity and quality of sperm cells produced by men per day is much higher at youth and, as the years pass, will gradually abate. In a male human body in the prime of life, each day around 300 million sperm cells complete their process of spermatogenesis.

spermiogenesis

Second phase of sperm formation, during which spermatids, thanks to the action of Sertoli cells, become spermatozoa. During this stage, the acrosome (Essentials for the sperm cell to fertilize the egg cell) and the flagellum (necessary for the sperm cell to move in search of an egg to fertilize) form.

SCHEMA of SPERMATOGENESIS

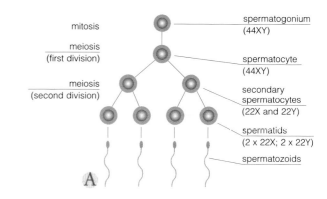

mitosis

meiosis
(first division)

meiosis
(second division)

spermatogonium
(44XY)

spermatocyte
(44XY)

secondary
spermatocytes
(22X and 22Y)

spermatids
(2 x 22X; 2 x 22Y)

spermatozoids

A

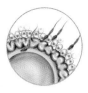

MALE GENITAL SYSTEM (XVI). SPERMATOGENESIS

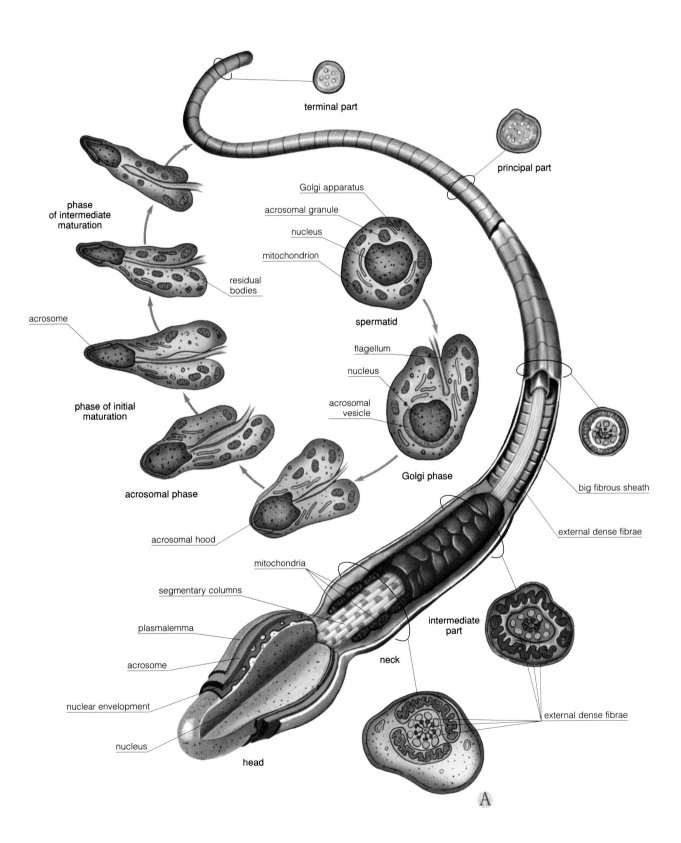

terminal part

principal part

Golgi apparatus

acrosomal granule

nucleus

mitochondrion

spermatid

phase
of intermediate
maturation

residual
bodies

flagellum

nucleus

acrosomal
vesicle

Golgi phase

acrosome

phase of initial
maturation

acrosomal phase

acrosomal hood

mitochondria

segmentary columns

plasmalemma

acrosome

nuclear envelopment

nucleus

head

neck

intermediate
part

big fibrous sheath

external dense fibrae

external dense fibrae

A

MALE GENITAL SYSTEM (XVII)
URINARY BLADDER, PROSTATE and URETHRA (I)
POSTERIOR VIEW

512

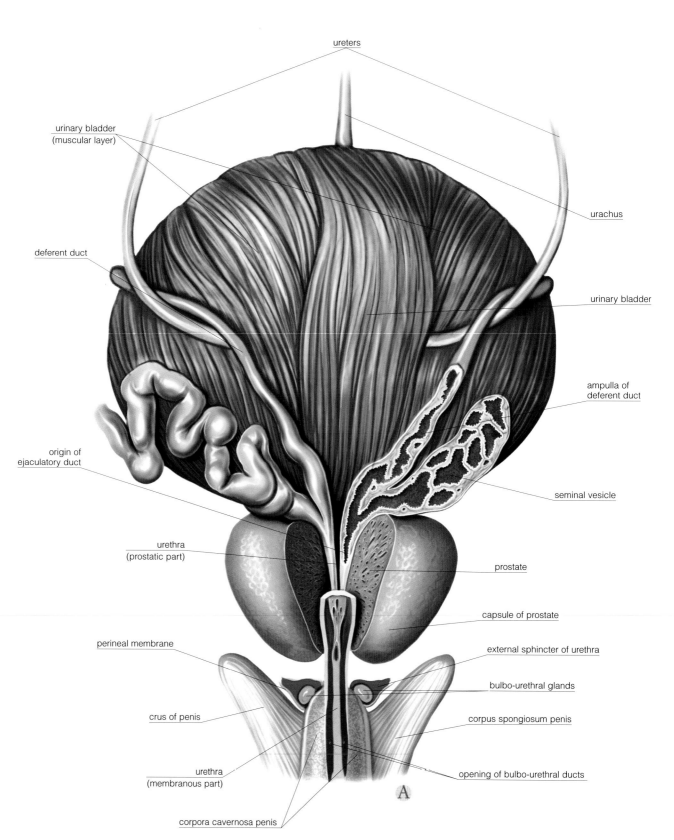

ureters

urinary bladder
(muscular layer)

urachus

deferent duct

urinary bladder

ampulla of
deferent duct

origin of
ejaculatory duct

seminal vesicle

urethra
(prostatic part)

prostate

capsule of prostate

perineal membrane

external sphincter of urethra

bulbo-urethral glands

crus of penis

corpus spongiosum penis

urethra
(membranous part)

opening of bulbo-urethral ducts

A

corpora cavernosa penis

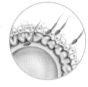

MALE GENITAL SYSTEM (XVIII)
URINARY BLADDER, PROSTATE and URETHRA (II)
ANTERIOR VIEW

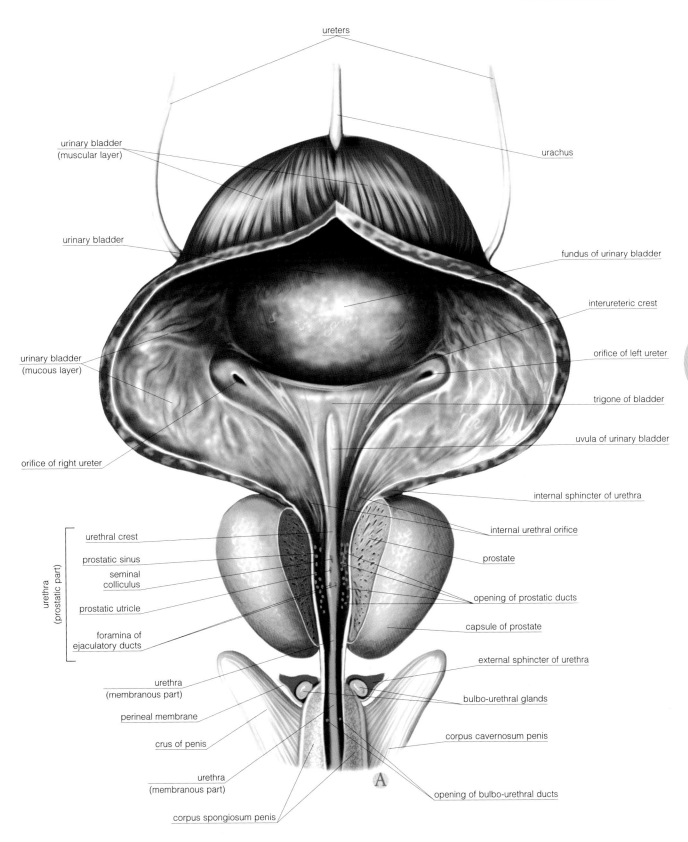

ureters

urinary bladder
(muscular layer)

urachus

urinary bladder

fundus of urinary bladder

interureteric crest

orifice of left ureter

urinary bladder
(mucous layer)

trigone of bladder

uvula of urinary bladder

orifice of right ureter

internal sphincter of urethra

internal urethral orifice

urethral crest

prostatic sinus

seminal
colliculus

prostate

prostatic utricle

opening of prostatic ducts

foramina of
ejaculatory ducts

capsule of prostate

urethra
(prostatic part)

urethra
(membranous part)

external sphincter of urethra

perineal membrane

bulbo-urethral glands

crus of penis

corpus cavernosum penis

urethra
(membranous part)

A

corpus spongiosum penis

opening of bulbo-urethral ducts

513

MALE GENITAL SYSTEM (XIX). PROSTATE (I)

URETHRA. PROSTATIC PART

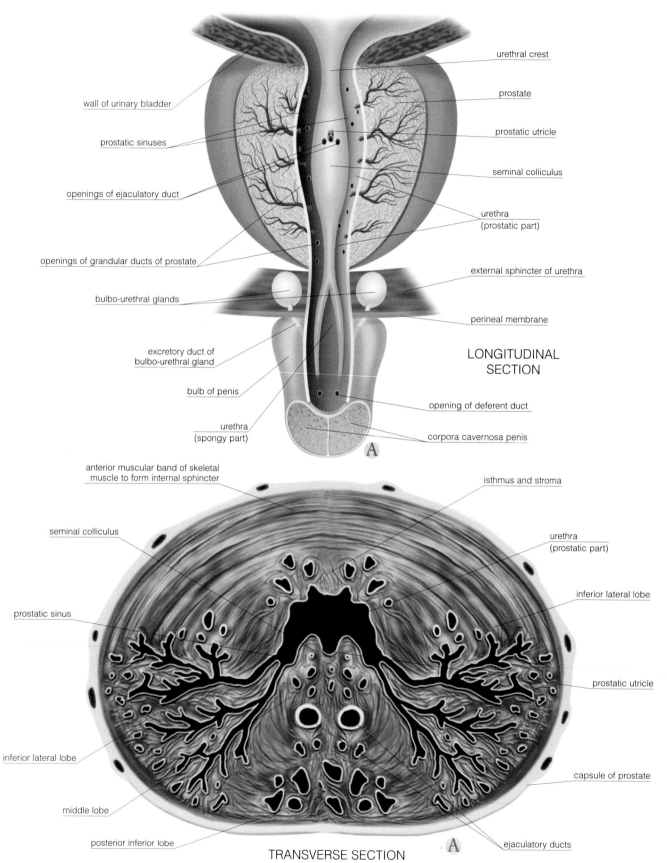

urethral crest

prostate

wall of urinary bladder

prostatic utricle

prostatic sinuses

seminal colliculus

openings of ejaculatory duct

urethra
(prostatic part)

openings of grandular ducts of prostate

external sphincter of urethra

bulbo-urethral glands

perineal membrane

excretory duct of
bulbo-urethral gland

LONGITUDINAL
SECTION

bulb of penis

opening of deferent duct

urethra
(spongy part)

corpora cavernosa penis

514

anterior muscular band of skeletal
muscle to form internal sphincter

isthmus and stroma

seminal colliculus

urethra
(prostatic part)

prostatic sinus

inferior lateral lobe

prostatic utricle

inferior lateral lobe

capsule of prostate

middle lobe

posterior inferior lobe

ejaculatory ducts

TRANSVERSE SECTION

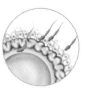

MALE GENITAL SYSTEM (XX). PROSTATE (II)

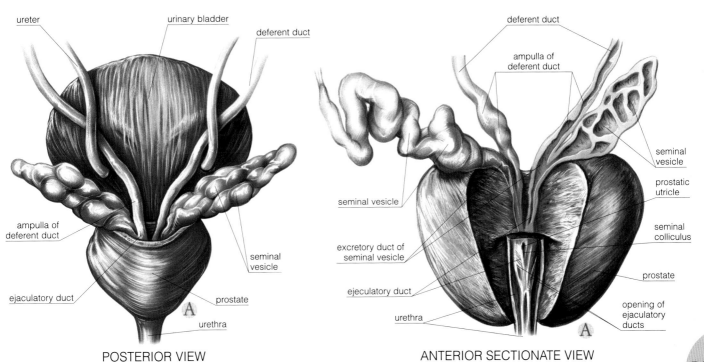

POSTERIOR VIEW

ANTERIOR SECTIONATE VIEW

prostate

Gland characterictic of male individuals, that is shaped like a cone flattened from front to back and its surface is smooth. Three lobes can be distinguished (one middle and two lateral) and it is located behind the symphysis pubis, under the neck of the urinary bladder, which it surrounds together with the urethra, and in front of the rectal ampoule. It measures about 2cm x 4cm x 3cm and weights about 20g. It is covered by a fibrous membrane that contains muscle fibers in its inner layer. It secretes a not very dense, opalescent and slightly alkaline liquid that forms part of semen. It is crossed obliquely by the urethra, in which the spermatic ducts empty, at the level of the prominence of the seminal colliculus.

seminal vesicle

Each of the two saccular glands, left and right, where the vas deferens discharge the seminal fluid. They are located in the pelvic cavity, behind the urinary bladder, in front of the rectum and immediately over the base of the prostate. They are pear-shaped with a thick superior and external end, and another, internal and pointed, inferior end, which joins the corresponding vas deferens to form the ejaculatory duct. They produce an alkaline secretion, rich in fructose, which promotes sperm motility and enhances the quality of semen.

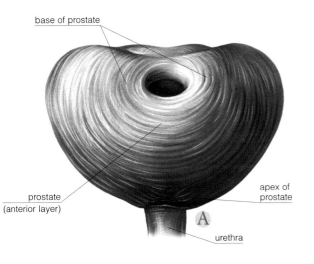

POSTERIOR VIEW

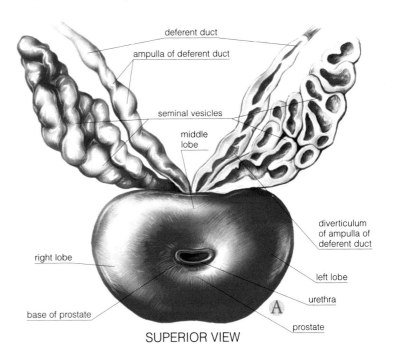

SUPERIOR VIEW

FEMALE GENITAL SYSTEM (I)

RIGHT GENERAL VIEW

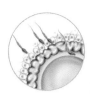

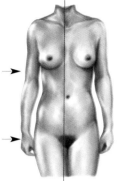

female genital system

Set of organs and structures belonging to the woman, allowing her to fulfill her reproductive role. They include basically the vulva, the vagina, the uterus, the fallopian tubes and the ovaries. For a new human being to be born in a natural way, the participation of the woman is essential. Her body must contribute an egg cell (ovocyte) which is produced alternatively in one of the ovaries, once approximately every 28 days, corresponding to the duration of the menstrual cycle. Once mature and expelled from the ovary, the ovocyte must wait for a spermatozoo (deposited in the vagina of the woman during sex by the penis to penetrate and fertilize it. If this event takes place, an embry will form and nest in the uterine endometrium. Later it will becom a foetus and, once pregnancy has concluded, it will give rise t a new individual. If the ovocyte is not fertilized, it will be expelle to the outside through the vagina during menstruation, accom panied by other residual uterine elements and blood.

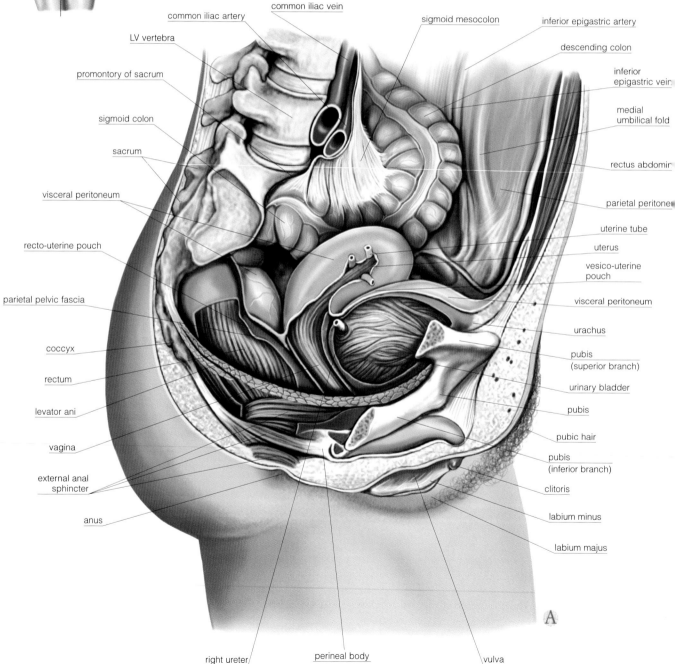

common iliac artery
common iliac vein
sigmoid mesocolon
inferior epigastric artery
LV vertebra
descending colon
promontory of sacrum
inferior epigastric vein
sigmoid colon
medial umbilical fold
sacrum
rectus abdomin
visceral peritoneum
parietal peritone
recto-uterine pouch
uterine tube
uterus
vesico-uterine pouch
parietal pelvic fascia
visceral peritoneum
urachus
coccyx
pubis (superior branch)
rectum
urinary bladder
levator ani
pubis
vagina
pubic hair
external anal sphincter
pubis (inferior branch)
clitoris
anus
labium minus
labium majus
right ureter
perineal body
vulva
A

FEMALE GENITAL SYSTEM (II)
RIGHT GENERAL VIEW

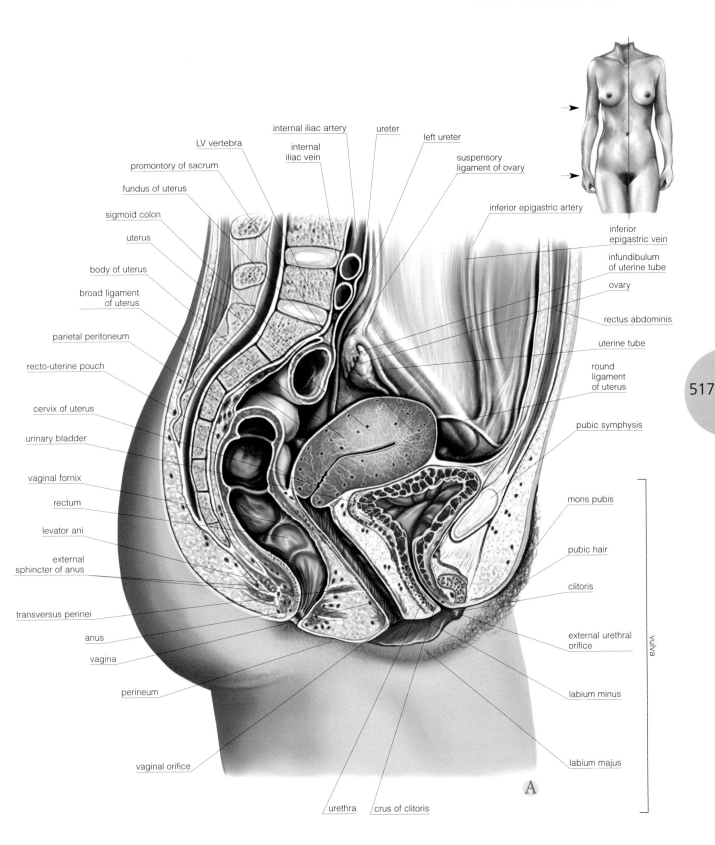

internal iliac artery

LV vertebra

internal iliac vein

ureter

left ureter

promontory of sacrum

suspensory ligament of ovary

fundus of uterus

sigmoid colon

inferior epigastric artery

uterus

inferior epigastric vein

body of uterus

infundibulum of uterine tube

broad ligament of uterus

ovary

parietal peritoneum

rectus abdominis

recto-uterine pouch

uterine tube

cervix of uterus

round ligament of uterus

urinary bladder

pubic symphysis

vaginal fornix

mons pubis

rectum

pubic hair

levator ani

clitoris

external sphincter of anus

transversus perinei

external urethral orifice

anus

vagina

labium minus

perineum

labium majus

vaginal orifice

urethra

crus of clitoris

vulva

517

FEMALE GENITAL SYSTEM (III)
ANTERIOR VIEW

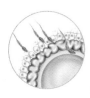

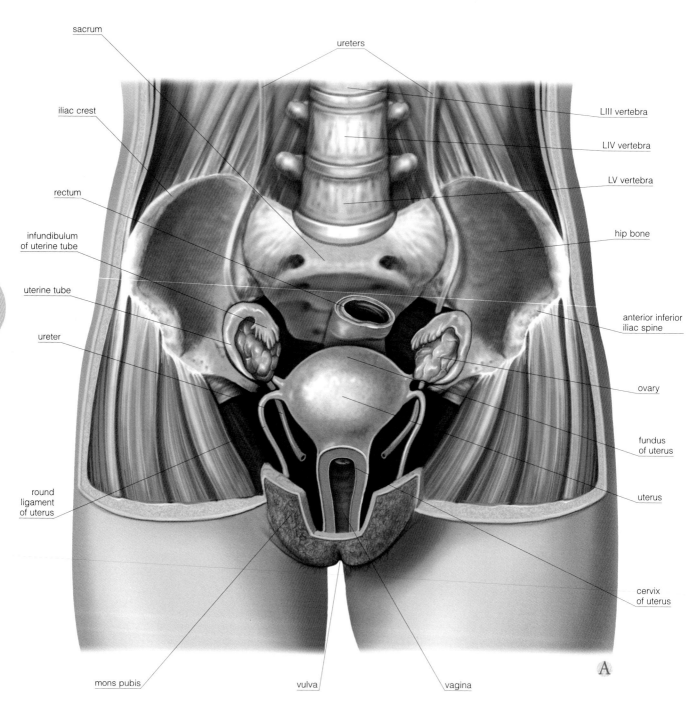

sacrum

iliac crest

rectum

infundibulum
of uterine tube

uterine tube

ureter

round
ligament
of uterus

mons pubis

ureters

LIII vertebra

LIV vertebra

LV vertebra

hip bone

anterior inferior
iliac spine

ovary

fundus
of uterus

uterus

cervix
of uterus

vulva

vagina

518

A

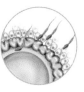

FEMALE GENITAL SYSTEM (IV). VULVA and PERINEUM

vulva

Set of external sexual organs in women. Situated below the mons pubis, in the lower abdominal region, and between the medial sides of both thighs, it is the externally visible part of the female genital apparatus. It contains, among others, the labia majora and minora, the clitoris, and the external orifices of the urethra and the vagina.

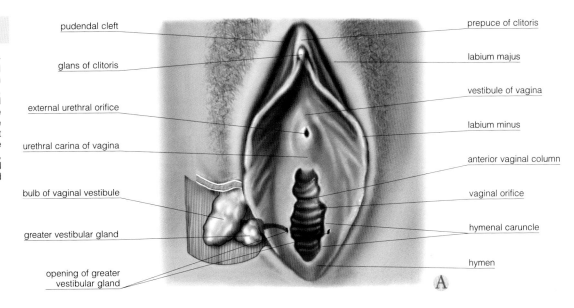

pudendal cleft

glans of clitoris

external urethral orifice

urethral carina of vagina

bulb of vaginal vestibule

greater vestibular gland

opening of greater vestibular gland

prepuce of clitoris

labium majus

vestibule of vagina

labium minus

anterior vaginal column

vaginal orifice

hymenal caruncle

hymen

A

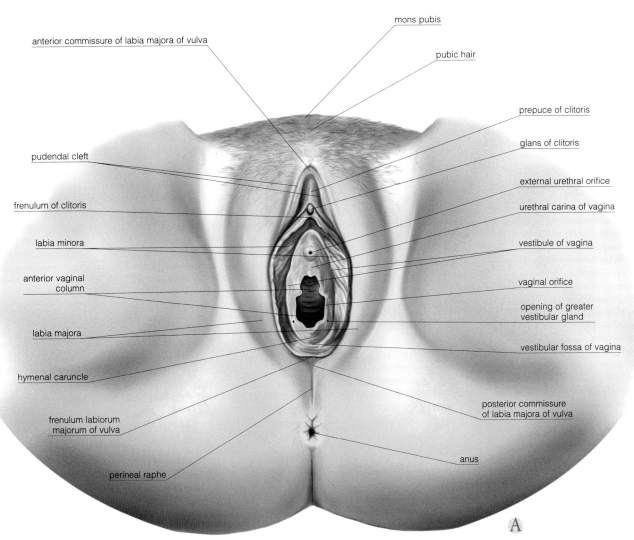

mons pubis

pubic hair

anterior commissure of labia majora of vulva

prepuce of clitoris

glans of clitoris

pudendal cleft

external urethral orifice

frenulum of clitoris

urethral carina of vagina

labia minora

vestibule of vagina

anterior vaginal column

vaginal orifice

opening of greater vestibular gland

labia majora

vestibular fossa of vagina

hymenal caruncle

posterior commissure of labia majora of vulva

frenulum labiorum majorum of vulva

anus

perineal raphe

A

FEMALE GENITAL SYSTEM (V)
UTERUS, UTERINE TUBE, OVARIES and VAGINA (I)

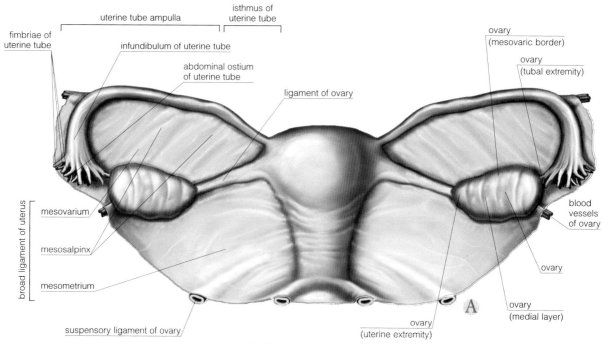

uterine tube ampulla

isthmus of
uterine tube

fimbriae of
uterine tube

infundibulum of uterine tube

abdominal ostium
of uterine tube

ligament of ovary

ovary
(mesovaric border)

ovary
(tubal extremity)

mesovarium

mesosalpinx

mesometrium

broad ligament of uterus

blood
vessels
of ovary

ovary

ovary
(medial layer)

suspensory ligament of ovary

ovary
(uterine extremity)

FRONTAL GENERAL VIEW

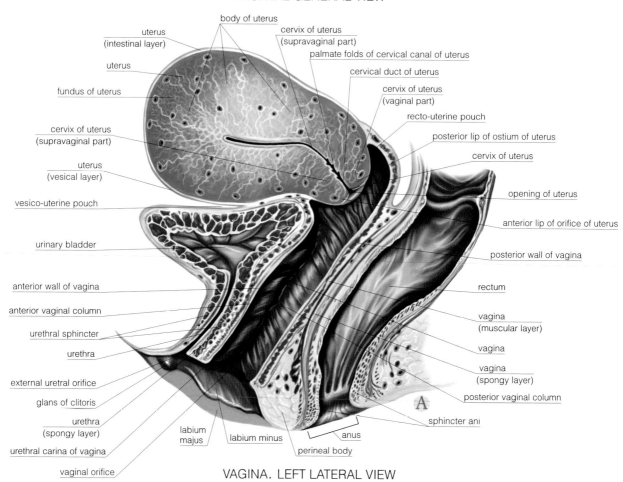

body of uterus

uterus
(intestinal layer)

cervix of uterus
(supravaginal part)

palmate folds of cervical canal of uterus

uterus

cervical duct of uterus

fundus of uterus

cervix of uterus
(vaginal part)

recto-uterine pouch

cervix of uterus
(supravaginal part)

posterior lip of ostium of uterus

cervix of uterus

uterus
(vesical layer)

opening of uterus

vesico-uterine pouch

anterior lip of orifice of uterus

urinary bladder

posterior wall of vagina

anterior wall of vagina

rectum

anterior vaginal column

vagina
(muscular layer)

urethral sphincter

vagina

urethra

vagina
(spongy layer)

external uretral orifice

posterior vaginal column

glans of clitoris

urethra
(spongy layer)

sphincter ani

urethral carina of vagina

labium
majus

labium minus

anus

vaginal orifice

perineal body

VAGINA. LEFT LATERAL VIEW

520

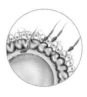

FEMALE GENITAL SYSTEM (VI)
UTERUS, UTERINE TUBE, OVARIES and VAGINA (II)

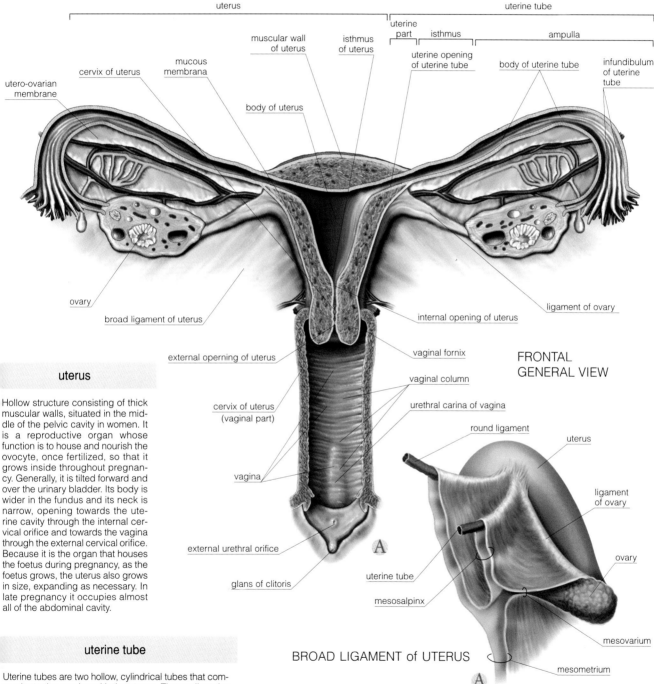

FRONTAL GENERAL VIEW

521

BROAD LIGAMENT of UTERUS

uterus

Hollow structure consisting of thick muscular walls, situated in the middle of the pelvic cavity in women. It is a reproductive organ whose function is to house and nourish the ovocyte, once fertilized, so that it grows inside throughout pregnancy. Generally, it is tilted forward and over the urinary bladder. Its body is wider in the fundus and its neck is narrow, opening towards the uterine cavity through the internal cervical orifice and towards the vagina through the external cervical orifice. Because it is the organ that houses the foetus during pregnancy, as the foetus grows, the uterus also grows in size, expanding as necessary. In late pregnancy it occupies almost all of the abdominal cavity.

uterine tube

Uterine tubes are two hollow, cylindrical tubes that communicate the ovaries with the uterus. They collect the ovocyte, once released from the ovary, and transport it to the uterus, and they are the way that spermatozoa follow from the uterus in search of the egg to fertilize it, an event which, if it does occur, takes place in the area of the ampoule. Each tube is placed at the upper end of the broad ligament of the uterus, and its measures are about 11.4cm long and 6mm in diameter. Its walls consist of three layers: mucosa, muscularis and serosa. Four parts can be distinguished: infundibulum, ampullary region, isthmus and uterine portion.

broad ligament of uterus

Prolongation of the peritoneal layer separating the pelvic from the abdominal cavity. It is positioned in front, above and behind the uterus, and up to the fallopian tubes. Three parts can be defined in it: anterior, from the neck and the lower half of the body of the uterus to the round ligament, middle, from the round ligament to the tubes, and superior, covering the tubes posteriorly and, in this part, projecting into the uterus.

FEMALE GENITAL SYSTEM (VII)
PELVIS and PERINEUM (I)
LOCATION of BASIC ELEMENTS. LATERAL VIEW

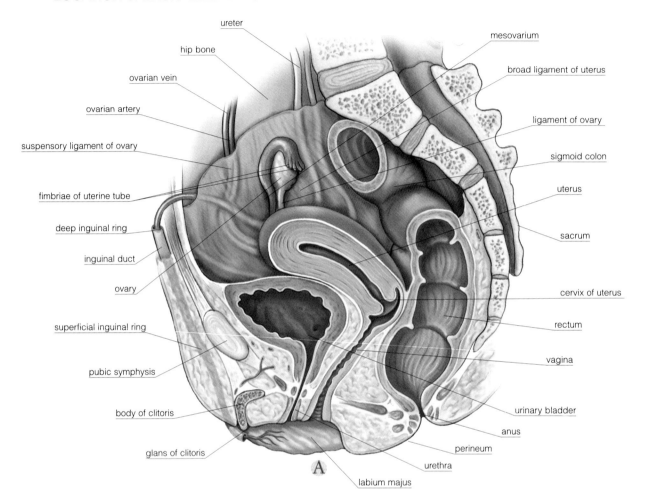

ureter
hip bone
ovarian vein
ovarian artery
suspensory ligament of ovary
fimbriae of uterine tube
deep inguinal ring
inguinal duct
ovary
superficial inguinal ring
pubic symphysis
body of clitoris
glans of clitoris

mesovarium
broad ligament of uterus
ligament of ovary
sigmoid colon
uterus
sacrum
cervix of uterus
rectum
vagina
urinary bladder
anus
perineum
urethra
labium majus

A

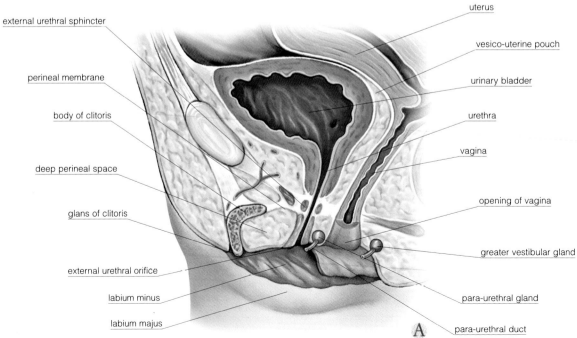

external urethral sphincter
perineal membrane
body of clitoris
deep perineal space
glans of clitoris
external urethral orifice
labium minus
labium majus

uterus
vesico-uterine pouch
urinary bladder
urethra
vagina
opening of vagina
greater vestibular gland
para-urethral gland
para-urethral duct

A

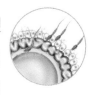

FEMALE GENITAL SYSTEM (VIII)
PELVIS and PERINEUM (II)

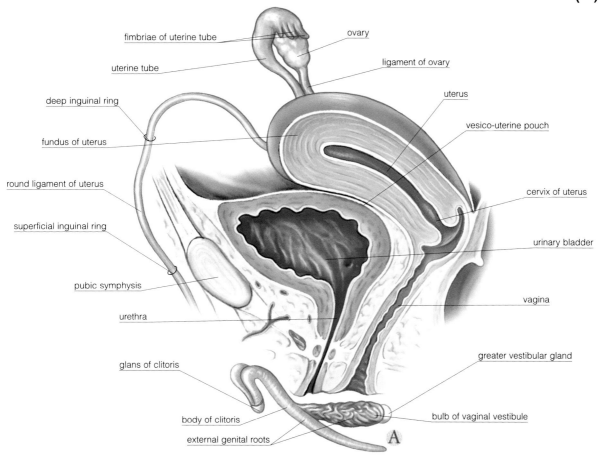

fimbriae of uterine tube

ovary

uterine tube

ligament of ovary

deep inguinal ring

uterus

fundus of uterus

vesico-uterine pouch

round ligament of uterus

cervix of uterus

superficial inguinal ring

urinary bladder

pubic symphysis

urethra

vagina

glans of clitoris

greater vestibular gland

body of clitoris

external genital roots

bulb of vaginal vestibule

UROGENITAL REGION. LEFT LATERAL VIEW

523

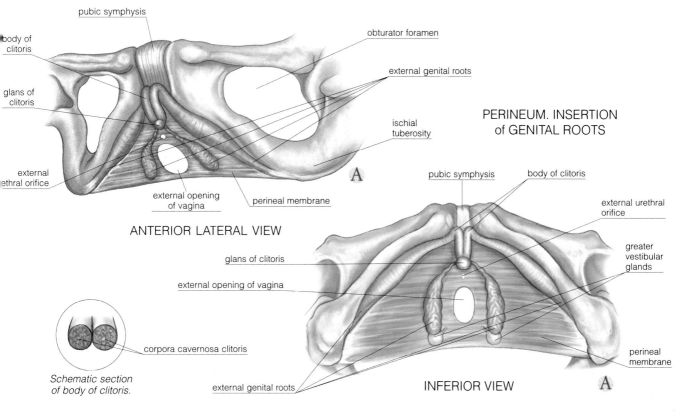

pubic symphysis

obturator foramen

body of clitoris

external genital roots

glans of clitoris

PERINEUM. INSERTION of GENITAL ROOTS

ischial tuberosity

external urethral orifice

pubic symphysis

body of clitoris

external opening of vagina

perineal membrane

external urethral orifice

ANTERIOR LATERAL VIEW

glans of clitoris

greater vestibular glands

external opening of vagina

corpora cavernosa clitoris

perineal membrane

Schematic section of body of clitoris.

external genital roots

INFERIOR VIEW

FEMALE GENITAL SYSTEM (IX)
PELVIS and PERINEUM (III)

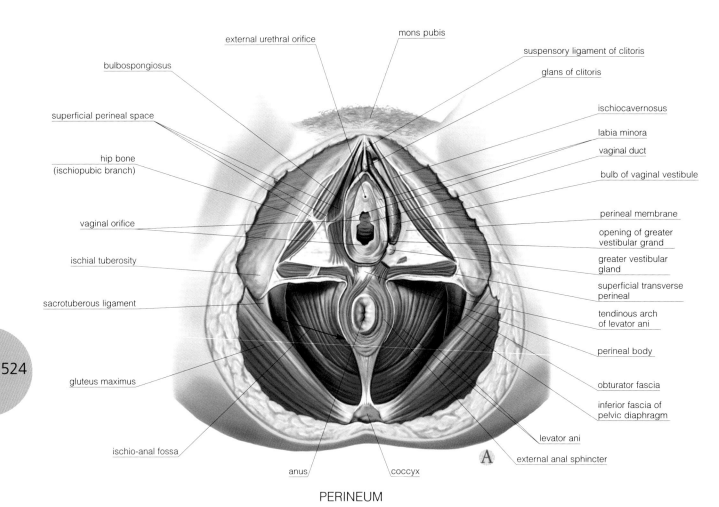

external urethral orifice

mons pubis

suspensory ligament of clitoris

glans of clitoris

bulbospongiosus

ischiocavernosus

superficial perineal space

labia minora

vaginal duct

hip bone
(ischiopubic branch)

bulb of vaginal vestibule

perineal membrane

vaginal orifice

opening of greater
vestibular grand

greater vestibular
gland

ischial tuberosity

superficial transverse
perineal

sacrotuberous ligament

tendinous arch
of levator ani

perineal body

gluteus maximus

obturator fascia

inferior fascia of
pelvic diaphragm

levator ani

external anal sphincter

ischio-anal fossa

anus

coccyx

PERINEUM

suspensory ligament of clitoris

sphincter urethral

body of clitoris

glans of clitoris

crus of clitoris

perineal membrane

urethra

compressor urethrae

hip bone
(ischiopubic branch)

bulb of vaginal vestibule

vagina

perineal membrane

sphincter urethrovaginalis

duct of greater vestibular gland

transversus perinei profundus

greater vestibular gland

VAGINA and CLITORIS

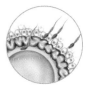

FEMALE GENITAL SYSTEM (X)
VAGINA, UTERUS and ADJACENT STRUCTURES
ANTERIOR VIEW

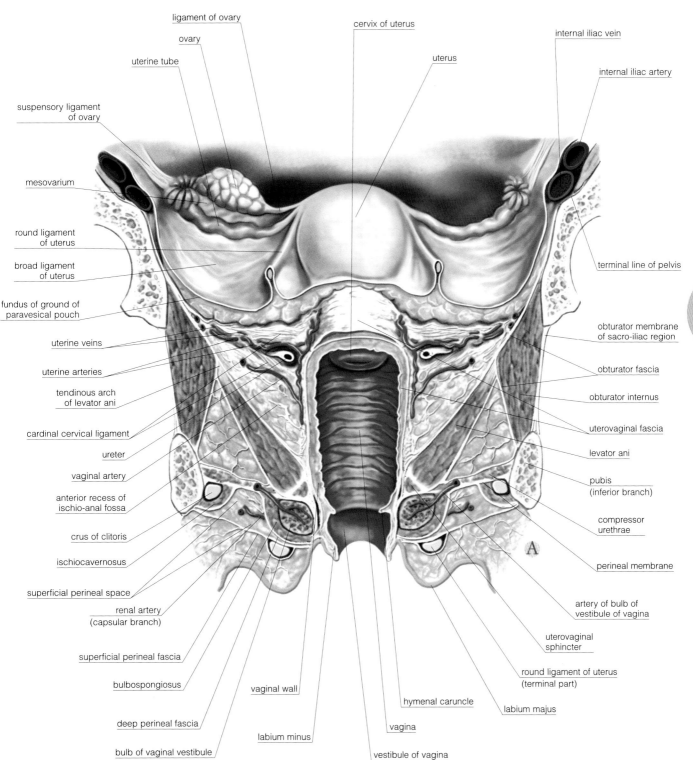

ligament of ovary

ovary

uterine tube

cervix of uterus

uterus

internal iliac vein

internal iliac artery

suspensory ligament of ovary

mesovarium

round ligament of uterus

broad ligament of uterus

fundus of ground of paravesical pouch

uterine veins

uterine arteries

tendinous arch of levator ani

cardinal cervical ligament

ureter

vaginal artery

anterior recess of ischio-anal fossa

crus of clitoris

ischiocavernosus

superficial perineal space

renal artery (capsular branch)

superficial perineal fascia

bulbospongiosus

deep perineal fascia

bulb of vaginal vestibule

labium minus

vaginal wall

vestibule of vagina

vagina

hymenal caruncle

labium majus

round ligament of uterus (terminal part)

uterovaginal sphincter

artery of bulb of vestibule of vagina

perineal membrane

compressor urethrae

pubis (inferior branch)

levator ani

uterovaginal fascia

obturator internus

obturator fascia

obturator membrane of sacro-iliac region

terminal line of pelvis

525

A

FEMALE GENITAL SYSTEM (XIII)

TRANSVERSE SECTION. SUPERIOR VIEW at the LEVEL of the LIII VERTEBRA

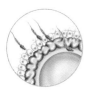

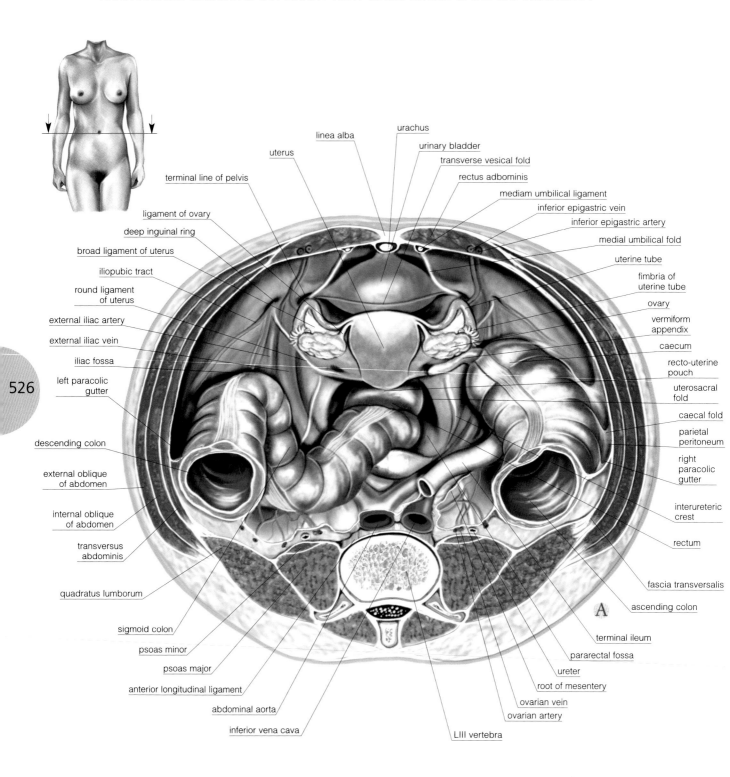

linea alba

urachus

uterus

urinary bladder

transverse vesical fold

terminal line of pelvis

rectus abdominis

mediam umbilical ligament

inferior epigastric vein

ligament of ovary

inferior epigastric artery

deep inguinal ring

medial umbilical fold

broad ligament of uterus

uterine tube

iliopubic tract

fimbria of uterine tube

round ligament of uterus

ovary

external iliac artery

vermiform appendix

external iliac vein

caecum

iliac fossa

recto-uterine pouch

left paracolic gutter

uterosacral fold

526

caecal fold

descending colon

parietal peritoneum

external oblique of abdomen

right paracolic gutter

internal oblique of abdomen

interureteric crest

transversus abdominis

rectum

quadratus lumborum

fascia transversalis

ascending colon

sigmoid colon

A

psoas minor

terminal ileum

psoas major

pararectal fossa

anterior longitudinal ligament

ureter

root of mesentery

abdominal aorta

ovarian vein

inferior vena cava

ovarian artery

LIII vertebra

FEMALE GENITAL SYSTEM (XIV). PELVIC FLOOR

TRANSVERSE SECTION. SUPERIOR VIEW at the LEVEL of the SI VERTEBRA

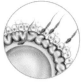

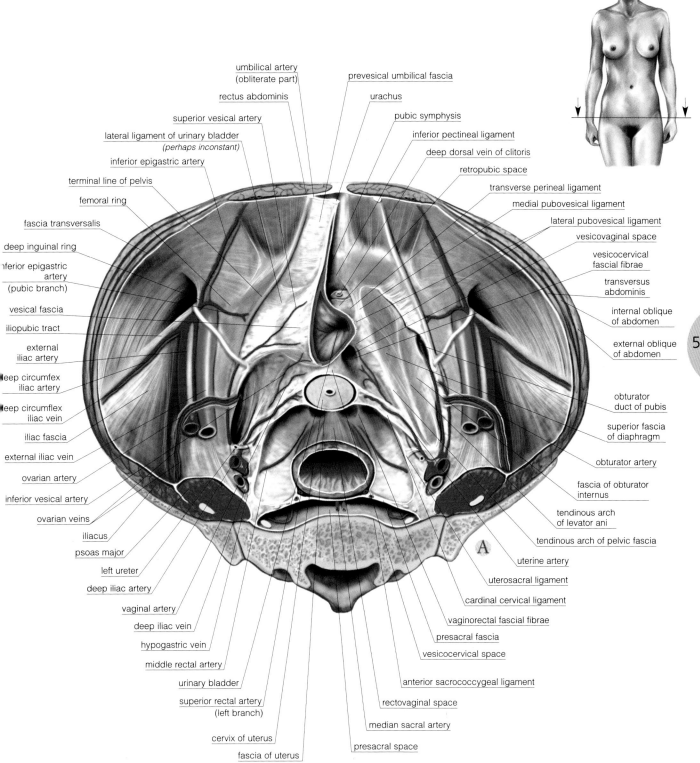

umbilical artery
(obliterate part)

rectus abdominis

superior vesical artery

lateral ligament of urinary bladder
(perhaps inconstant)

inferior epigastric artery

terminal line of pelvis

femoral ring

fascia transversalis

deep inguinal ring

inferior epigastric
artery
(pubic branch)

vesical fascia

iliopubic tract

external
iliac artery

deep circumfex
iliac artery

deep circumflex
iliac vein

iliac fascia

external iliac vein

ovarian artery

inferior vesical artery

ovarian veins

iliacus

psoas major

left ureter

deep iliac artery

vaginal artery

deep iliac vein

hypogastric vein

middle rectal artery

urinary bladder

superior rectal artery
(left branch)

cervix of uterus

fascia of uterus

prevesical umbilical fascia

urachus

pubic symphysis

inferior pectineal ligament

deep dorsal vein of clitoris

retropubic space

transverse perineal ligament

medial pubovesical ligament

lateral pubovesical ligament

vesicovaginal space

vesicocervical
fascial fibrae

transversus
abdominis

internal oblique
of abdomen

external oblique
of abdomen

527

obturator
duct of pubis

superior fascia
of diaphragm

obturator artery

fascia of obturator
internus

tendinous arch
of levator ani

tendinous arch of pelvic fascia

uterine artery

uterosacral ligament

cardinal cervical ligament

vaginorectal fascial fibrae

presacral fascia

vesicocervical space

anterior sacrococcygeal ligament

rectovaginal space

median sacral artery

presacral space

Ⓐ

FEMALE GENITAL SYSTEM (XV). VAGINA and UTERUS

vagina

Musculocutaneous conduit that runs from the neck of the uterus to the vulva, and is located between the bladder and the urethra (anteriorly) or rectum (posteriorly). Its primary function is to receive the male penis during intercourse, in order for it to deposit semen inside. It has a large distention capacity, to the point of expanding to let the foetus through during delivery. It also secretes a fluid (vaginal discharge) for lubrication, and is the passageway through which menstrual fluid is expelled in the final stage of each cycle, as well as the foetus during labor.

uterus

Hollow structure consisting of thick muscular walls, situated in the middle of the pelvic cavity in women. It is a reproductive organ whose function is to house and nourish the ovocyte, once fertilized, so that it grows inside throughout pregnancy. Before pregnancy it measures about 7.5cm long, 5cm wide and 2.5cm thick. Generally, it is tilted forward and over the urinary bladder. Its body is wider in the fundus and its neck is narrow, opening towards the uterine cavity through the internal cervical orifice and towards the vagina through the external cervical orifice. Because it is the organ that houses the foetus during pregnancy, as the foetus grows, the uterus also grows in size, expanding as necessary. In late pregnancy it occupies almost all of the abdominal cavity.

528

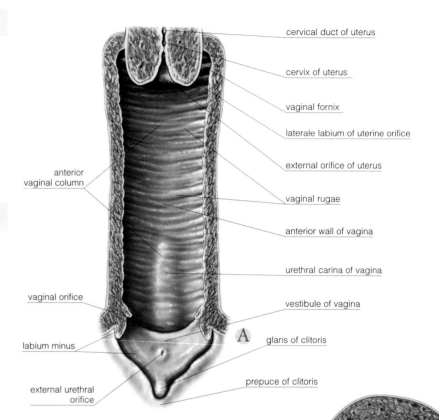

cervical duct of uterus
cervix of uterus
vaginal fornix
laterale labium of uterine orifice
external orifice of uterus
vaginal rugae
anterior wall of vagina
urethral carina of vagina
vestibule of vagina
glans of clitoris
prepuce of clitoris

anterior vaginal column
vaginal orifice
labium minus
external urethral orifice

VAGINAL DUCT. POSTERIOR VIEW

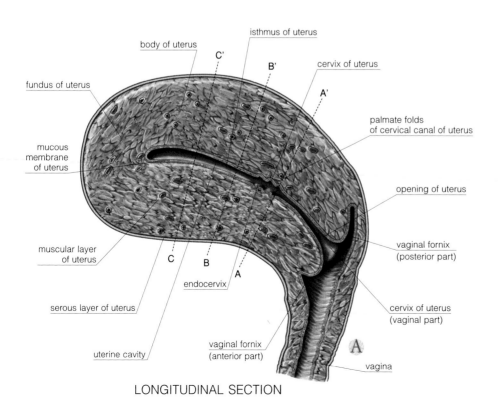

body of uterus
isthmus of uterus
C'
B'
cervix of uterus
A'
palmate folds of cervical canal of uterus
opening of uterus
vaginal fornix (posterior part)
cervix of uterus (vaginal part)
vagina

fundus of uterus
mucous membrane of uterus
muscular layer of uterus
serous layer of uterus
C
B
A
endocervix
uterine cavity
vaginal fornix (anterior part)

LONGITUDINAL SECTION

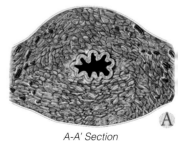

C-C' Section

B-B' Section

A-A' Section

TRANSVERSE SECTIONS

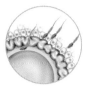

FEMALE GENITAL SYSTEM (XVI). OVARIAN CYCLE

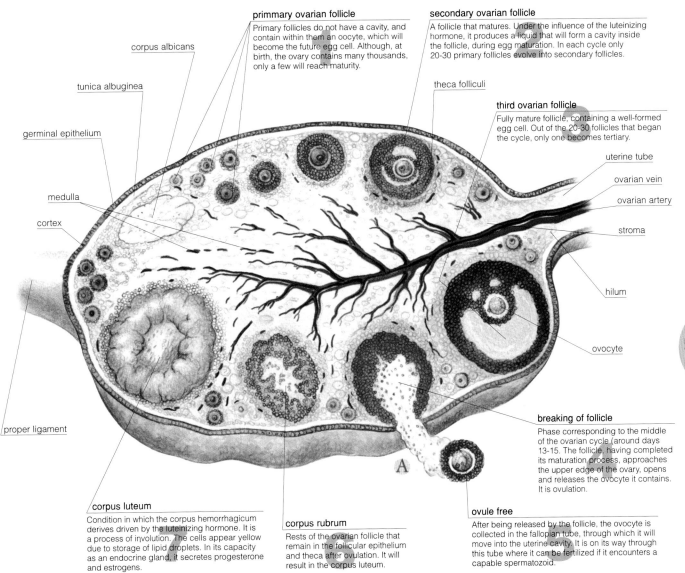

primmary ovarian follicle
Primary follicles do not have a cavity, and contain within them an oocyte, which will become the future egg cell. Although, at birth, the ovary contains many thousands, only a few will reach maturity.

secondary ovarian follicle
A follicle that matures. Under the influence of the luteinizing hormone, it produces a liquid that will form a cavity inside the follicle, during egg maturation. In each cycle only 20-30 primary follicles evolve into secondary follicles.

third ovarian follicle
Fully mature follicle, containing a well-formed egg cell. Out of the 20-30 follicles that began the cycle, only one becomes tertiary.

corpus albicans

tunica albuginea

germinal epithelium

medulla

cortex

proper ligament

theca folliculi

uterine tube

ovarian vein

ovarian artery

stroma

hilum

ovocyte

529

breaking of follicle
Phase corresponding to the middle of the ovarian cycle (around days 13-15. The follicle, having completed its maturation process, approaches the upper edge of the ovary, opens and releases the ovocyte it contains. It is ovulation.

corpus luteum
Condition in which the corpus hemorrhagicum derives driven by the luteinizing hormone. It is a process of involution. The cells appear yellow due to storage of lipid droplets. In its capacity as an endocrine gland, it secretes progesterone and estrogens.

corpus rubrum
Rests of the ovarian follicle that remain in the follicular epithelium and theca after ovulation. It will result in the corpus luteum.

ovule free
After being released by the follicle, the ovocyte is collected in the fallopian tube, through which it will move into the uterine cavity. It is on its way through this tube where it can be fertilized if it encounters a capable spermatozoid.

ovary

The ovaries are two pearly, glandular organs with an ovoid shape that are located within the peritoneum, on either side of the pelvic cavity, in the wall of the minor pelvis, in the ovarian fossa. They are bound to the uterus by the utero-ovarian ligament and are next to the uterine horn. They measure 2.5 to 4,4cm long, 2cm wide and 0.51cm thick. They remain inactive until puberty, when they begin to be stimulated by hormonal action. Their role is twofold: to produce ova (or female sex cells) and female hormones (estrogen and progesterone), which determine the female sexual characteristics and the menstrual cycle. They remain inactive until puberty, when they enter into a period of intense activity resulting in menarche (which may appear between 9 and 17 years of age), indicating the start of the ovarian cycle. Thus, approximately every 28 days, the period which one cycle normally lasts, and alternatively, one of the ovaries will release a mature egg, capable of being fertilized by a spermatozoid. In case fecundation is not produced, this egg will be expelled outside (it is menstruation) and the ovary will begin a new cycle. The succession of ovarian cycles goes from puberty until the woman enters into menopause (around age 50).

SCHEMA of OVOGENESIS

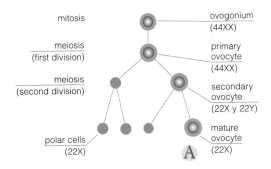

mitosis	ovogonium (44XX)
meiosis (first division)	primary ovocyte (44XX)
meiosis (second division)	secondary ovocyte (22X y 22Y)
polar cells (22X)	mature ovocyte (22X)

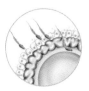
POSTPARTUM (I). BREAST (or MAMMARY GLAND) (I)

breast (or mammary gland)

Breasts are each of the glandular structures found in female mammals and whose main function is to secrete the milk that naturally nourishes the infant during the first months of life. In humans, the breasts are two structures with a hemispherical shape, located on the anterior superior and lateral regions of the trunk in women. Externally, they are formed by integumentary tissue, and in their frontal region they exhibit an areola, or circular area, having a darker pigmentation. In the center stands the nipple, a small erectile protrusion with a free end, or tip, where the galactophorous ducts pour their secretion outside. Internally, the breast is composed of 15-20 lobes of glandular tissue, separated by divisions called interlobular septa, each of which drains into a galactophorous duct, as well as subcutaneous adipose tissue, which sorrounds all sides of the mammary gland itself. Beyond the strictly anatomical aspects, the breast is extremely important for women due to its multiple implications: as a secondary sexual characteristic, an attraction element for males, an erogenous zone and an instrument for pleasure, as an element of corporal aesthetics, various psychological aspects (self-esteem, emotional balance, etc.) social aspects (beauty, success, etc.), etc. As a result of the growth of the mammary glands that occurs during adolescence, the breasts in women are much more voluminous than in men, because in women, after childbirth, they will secrete milk with which to feed the infant. During pregnancy they increase in size and may become more sensitive, and the areola and nipple acquire a darker color, features which can also often appear in many women during the ovulation phase of their menstrual cycle.

530

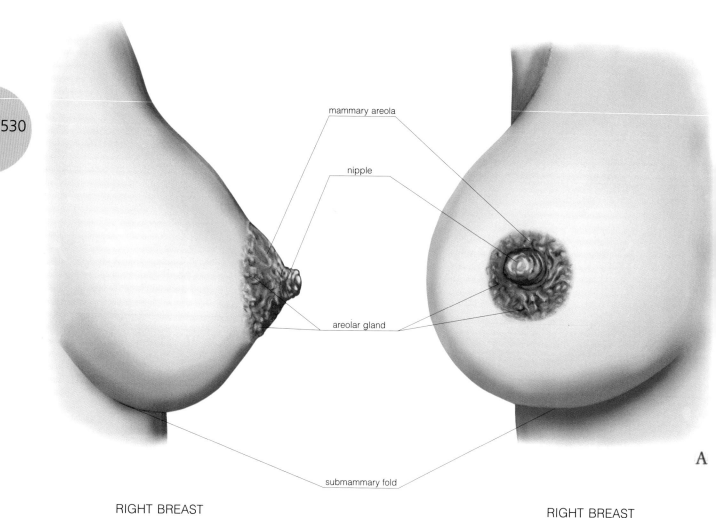

mammary areola

nipple

areolar gland

submammary fold

RIGHT BREAST
LATERAL VIEW

RIGHT BREAST
FRONTAL VIEW, LIGHTLY OBLIQUE

A

POSTPARTUM (II). BREAST (or MAMMARY GLAND) (II)

PARTIAL SECTION. ANTERIOR VIEW

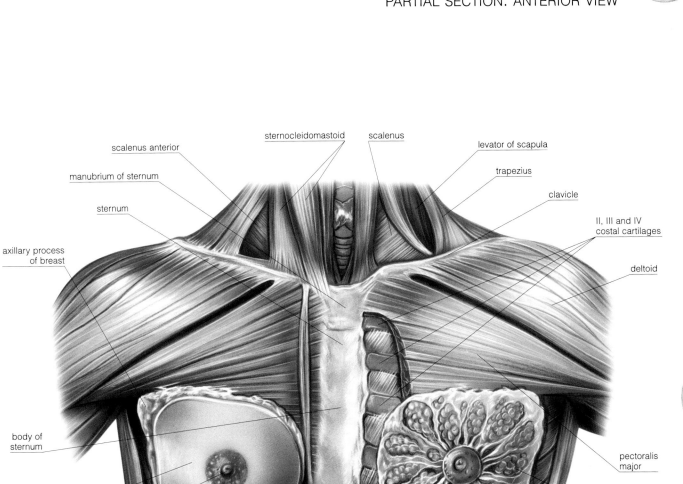

531

A

POSTPARTUM (III). BREAST (or MAMMARY GLAND) (III)

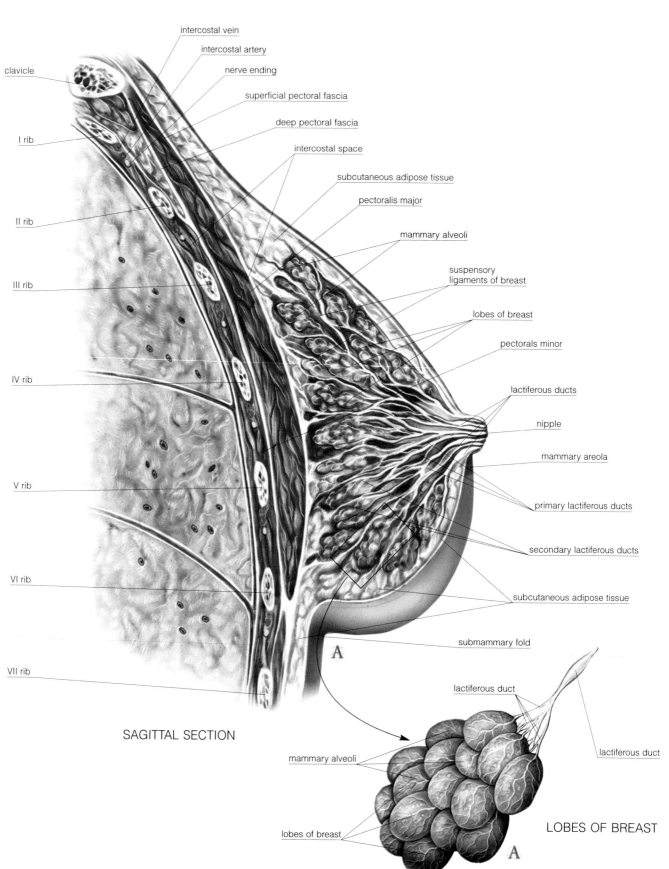

intercostal vein

intercostal artery

clavicle

nerve ending

superficial pectoral fascia

deep pectoral fascia

I rib

intercostal space

subcutaneous adipose tissue

pectoralis major

II rib

mammary alveoli

suspensory
ligaments of breast

III rib

lobes of breast

pectorals minor

IV rib

lactiferous ducts

nipple

mammary areola

V rib

primary lactiferous ducts

secondary lactiferous ducts

subcutaneous adipose tissue

VI rib

submammary fold

VII rib

SAGITTAL SECTION

lactiferous duct

lactiferous duct

mammary alveoli

lobes of breast

LOBES OF BREAST

A

IMMUNE SYSTEM

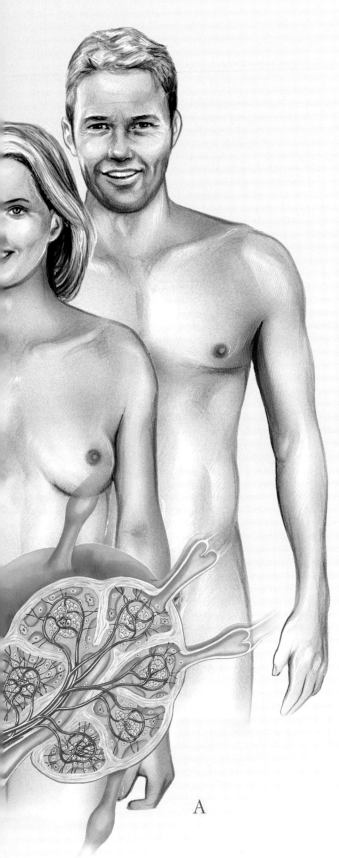

The life of a human being runs in a surrounding, an environment, an atmosphere, in which constantly appear thousands of external agents that can damage it. The air that breath, the climate, the solar rays, accidents caused by falls, labor, incidental, domestic, epidemics, etc. anyway, the virus, bacteria or microbes, constitute a constant threat, against which we must fight. For all this the organism is endowed with a defense system that forms a barrier of resistant against these agents.

Therefore, the immunitary system is formed by a set of organs and functions which object is the production of antibodies and activated cells capable of fight and neutralize any estrange intruder that can damage the human body or any of its organs and systems.

There is a nonspecific resistance that involves a series of mechanisms that confers to the human body an immediate protection against multiple pathogens. Thus, the skin and mucous form a first barrier and the acids of the gastric juice also eliminate part of the bacteria that food ingested contains. Also constitute a barrier the antimicrobial proteins, the phagocytes, the cytolytic natural cells, immflamation and fever.

Also there is a specific resistant that means the one that triggers when occurs the invasion of a determinate agent, Is a slower answer and involves the activation of specialized cells in the fight against a concrete intruder, which they neutralized. The system that takes care of the specific resistant is the lymphatic and in it are implied the cardiovascular apparatus with the oxygen that provides the blood that circulates through it. And the digestive apparatus (that absorbs the fat contained in the food ingested).

Are two the types of immunitary answer that can be activated: the humoral (in which is fundamental the role of the lymphocytes of type B, that produce antibodies, which means substances that attach to the antigen and block it.) and the cellular (that is linked to the lymphocytes type T, which besides stimulate the lymphocytes B, go on the search of the antigen and get rid of it). The neutralized agent through the lymph is transported to the lymphatic nodes that will be in charge of expelling it. With that the danger will have been eliminated.

A

IMMUNE SYSTEM
ANTERIOR GENERAL VIEW

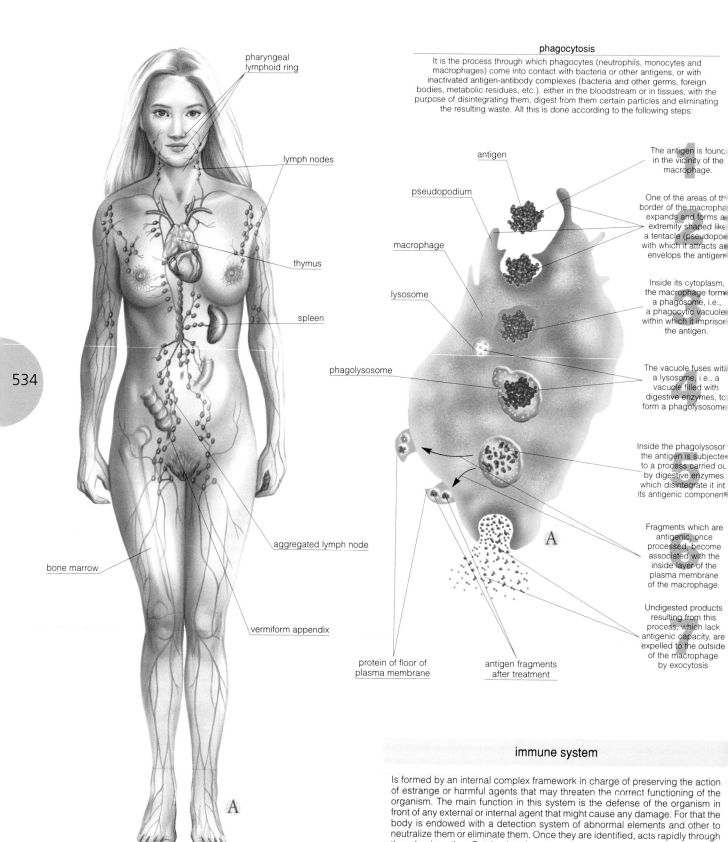

pharyngeal lymphoid ring

lymph nodes

thymus

spleen

aggregated lymph node

bone marrow

vermiform appendix

phagocytosis

It is the process through which phagocytes (neutrophils, monocytes and macrophages) come into contact with bacteria or other antigens, or with inactivated antigen-antibody complexes (bacteria and other germs, foreign bodies, metabolic residues, etc.). either in the bloodstream or in tissues, with the purpose of disintegrating them, digest from them certain particles and eliminating the resulting waste. All this is done according to the following steps:

antigen

pseudopodium

macrophage

lysosome

phagolysosome

The antigen is found in the vicinity of the macrophage.

One of the areas of the border of the macrophage expands and forms an extremity shaped like a tentacle (pseudopod with which it attracts and envelops the antigen.

Inside its cytoplasm, the macrophage forms a phagosome, i.e., a phagocytic vacuole within which it imprison the antigen.

The vacuole fuses with a lysosome, i.e., a vacuole filled with digestive enzymes, to form a phagolysosome.

Inside the phagolysosome the antigen is subjected to a process carried out by digestive enzymes, which disintegrate it into its antigenic component.

Fragments which are antigenic, once processed, become associated with the inside layer of the plasma membrane of the macrophage.

Undigested products resulting from this process, which lack antigenic capacity, are expelled to the outside of the macrophage by exocytosis.

protein of floor of plasma membrane

antigen fragments after treatment

immune system

Is formed by an internal complex framework in charge of preserving the action of estrange or harmful agents that may threaten the correct functioning of the organism. The main function in this system is the defense of the organism in front of any external or internal agent that might cause any damage. For that the body is endowed with a detection system of abnormal elements and other to neutralize them or eliminate them. Once they are identified, acts rapidly through three basic action: Catch, absorb and expel.

IMMUNE ORGANS (I). SPLEEN

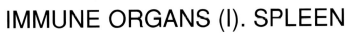

spleen

s a lymphoid organ that projects in the left upper zone of the abdomen, known as left hypochondrium, is oval shaped, color purple, glandular aspect and measures about 25mm of length. It consists of a capsule of connective tissue that covers it and the splenetic pulp or interior tissue. Its consistency is flexible. The splenetic pulp contains at the same time the red pulp (formed by vascular sinus in which circulates the blood, separated from the pulp by macrophages cords that phagocytose the erythrocytes and the strange antigen) and the white pulp (formed by lymphocytes T and B, plays a defensive function as they phagocytose the strange agents and form the sheaths around the arteries). The red pulp acts as a blood warehouse and collaborates to its renovation destroying the old erythrocytes. The white pulp meantime contributes to the elaboration of antibodies. The spleen, then, disintegrate the red cells (RBCs) and forms free hemoglobin that, then the liver will transform in Bilirubin. Also acts as a reservoir of the blood and produces lymphocytes and plasmatic cells. It has a vascular capacity of about 100 and 300ml, that constitute the 4% out of the total of blood of the body and contains about 30% out of the total of thrombocytes. Is a primary immunitary organ.

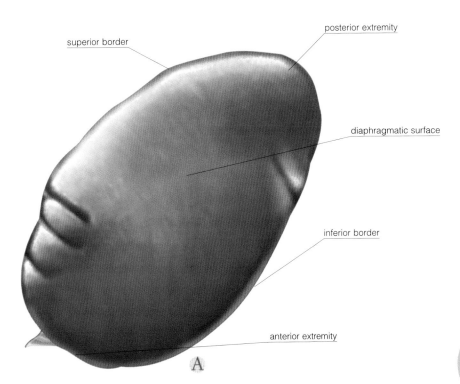

superior border

posterior extremity

diaphragmatic surface

inferior border

anterior extremity

A

SUPERIOR VIEW

535

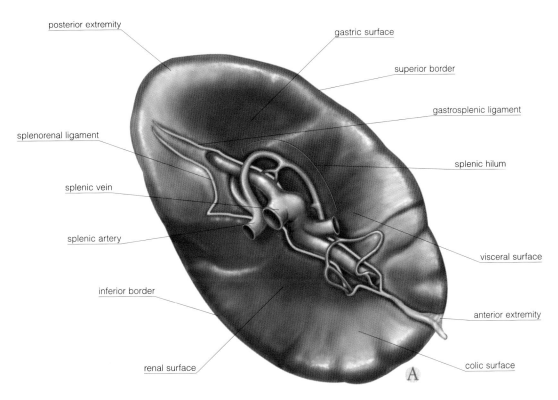

posterior extremity

gastric surface

superior border

gastrosplenic ligament

splenorenal ligament

splenic hilum

splenic vein

splenic artery

visceral surface

inferior border

anterior extremity

renal surface

colic surface

A

INFERIOR VIEW

IMMUNE ORGANS (II). LYMPH NODE. STRUCTURE

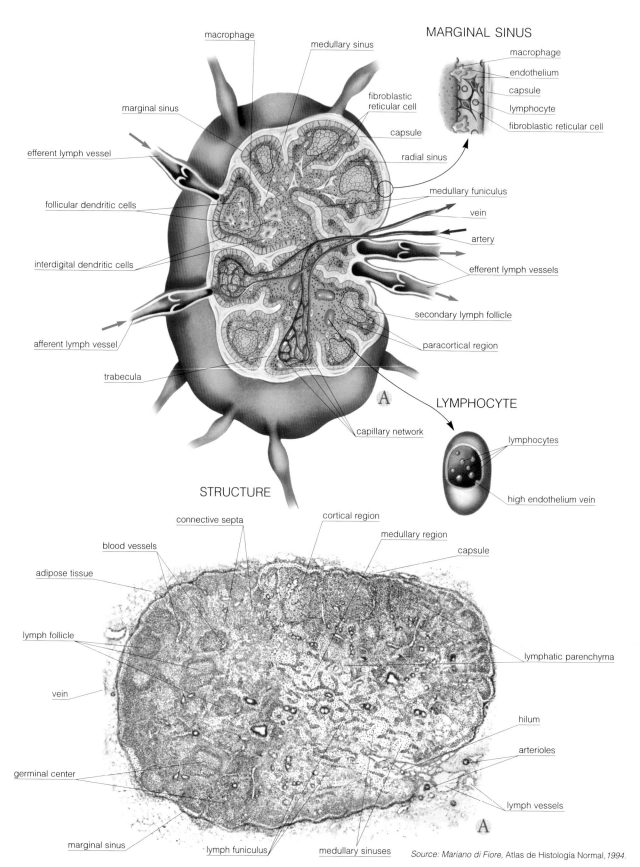

MARGINAL SINUS

macrophage
endothelium
capsule
lymphocyte
fibroblastic reticular cell

macrophage
medullary sinus
fibroblastic reticular cell
capsule
radial sinus

marginal sinus
efferent lymph vessel
follicular dendritic cells
interdigital dendritic cells
afferent lymph vessel
trabecula

medullary funiculus
vein
artery
efferent lymph vessels
secondary lymph follicle
paracortical region

A

capillary network

LYMPHOCYTE

lymphocytes
high endothelium vein

STRUCTURE

connective septa
blood vessels
adipose tissue
lymph follicle
vein
germinal center
marginal sinus

cortical region
medullary region
capsule

lymphatic parenchyma

hilum
arterioles
lymph vessels

A

lymph funiculus
medullary sinuses

Source: Mariano di Fiore, Atlas de Histología Normal, 1994.

LONGITUDINAL HISTOLOGIC SECTION

536

IMMUNE ORGANS (III). LYMPH NODE.
BONE MARROW. AGGREGATED LYMPH NODES

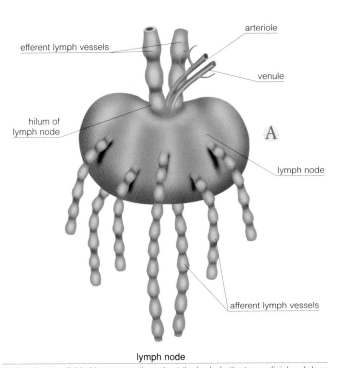

A

efferent lymph vessels

arteriole

venule

hilum of lymph node

lymph node

afferent lymph vessels

lymph node

...mph nodes are divided into groups throughout the body, both at superficial and deep ...atomical planes, interspersed between the lymphatic network. There are about 600 ...roughout the body, their shape resembles that of a bean and their size varies substan-...lly (from 1 to 25mm in length) according to their level of activity. Near the mammary ...ands, armpits and inguinal regions, large clusters of lymph nodes concentrate. Lymph ...ains into them. Their function is to act as a filter. Thus, as lymph enters one end of the ...mph node through the afferent vessels, the foreign substances it carries gets trapped by ...e reticular fibers of the sinusoids. Macrophages eliminate certain substances by pha-...ocytosis, while lymphocytes are responsible for destroying other substances by immuno-...gic mechanisms. Lymph, once filtered, exits the lymph node through efferent vessels to join the lymphatic network.

articular cartilage

spongy substance

epiphysial line

red bone marrow

compact bone

articular cartilage

yellow bone marrow

hypophysial line

Femur. **A**

537

bone marrow

It is a spongy tissue located in the medullary cavities of bones. It consists of a rich vascular network and a series of cells that produce all the cells that can be found in the blood (red marrow or hematogenous marrow) or a large array of adipose cells and connective tissue (yellow marrow, or adipose marrow). Nervous pathways flow through its interior and the spinal nerves that will innervate the whole body arise from it. Besides being an energy reserve, its key role is twofold: to produce blood cells and to play an important immune role, since it is where the precursors of B and T lymphocytes originate, which are crucial during most of the defensive processes of the body.

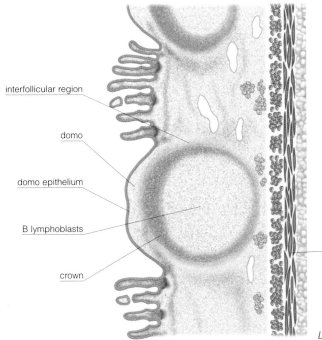

interfollicular region

domo

domo epithelium

B lymphoblasts

crown

muscularis mucosae

A

aggregated lymph node

Aggregated lymph nodes are formed by densely grouped follicles situated in the lamina propria of the mucosa and submucosa of the vermiform appendix and ileum to filter the lymph coming from the intestinal tube (second half of the duodenum and ileum). Here a series of plaques form, 1-4cm in length, containing 10-14 follicles and forming a protrusion in the mucosa in an area that has no villi. In the regions occupied by these nodules, antigens are trapped and phagocytosed. They are then poured into the lymphatic duct to be expelled.

Longitudinal section of ileum.

IMMUNE ORGANS (IV). THYMUS. PHARYNGEAL LYMPHOID RING. VERMIFORM APPEND

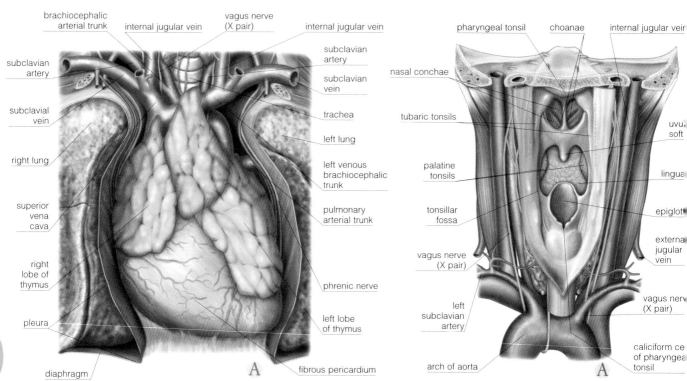

brachiocephalic arterial trunk
internal jugular vein
vagus nerve (X pair)
internal jugular vein
subclavian artery
subclavian artery
subclavian vein
subclavial vein
trachea
left lung
right lung
left venous brachiocephalic trunk
pulmonary arterial trunk
superior vena cava
right lobe of thymus
phrenic nerve
pleura
left lobe of thymus
diaphragm
fibrous pericardium

A

pharyngeal tonsil
choanae
internal jugular vein
nasal conchae
tubaric tonsils
uvu..
soft
palatine tonsils
lingua
tonsillar fossa
epiglott
vagus nerve (X pair)
externa jugular vein
left subclavian artery
vagus ner (X pair)
arch of aorta
caliciform ce of pharyngea tonsil

A

thymus

Lymphoid organ situated in the thoracic cavity, in the upper mediastinum, in front and above the heart and behind the sternum. It consists of two lobes, usually of different size, which in turn contain many lobules. In the newborn it is about 5cm long and 1,5cm wide, and weighs about 25g. It develops gradually to reach a weight of between 35 and 50g at puberty, at which point it starts its involution. In adults, thymic tissue weighs only about 5g and occupies a small space behind the manubrium of the sternum. The lobes consist of an outer cortex and an inner medulla, which contain the thymocytes or immature T lymphocytes. It is one of the primary organs of the immune system. In order to fulfill its role (producing T cells, specialized in defending the body against foreign substances or elements), it secretes thymosin, thymostimulin, thymuline, etc., substances having hormonal activity and which promote the development and differentiation of T lymphocytes.

pharyngeal lymphoid ring

It is one of secondary lymphoid organs, or lymphoepithelial organs, which form the tonsil that surround the outlet orifices of the buccal and nasal cavities (pharyngeal-or adenoid palatine, lingual). These tonsils contain lymphatic tissue arranged as very dense clusters o follicles that are located under the mucosal epithelium, whose surface is covered by crypt (or deep grooves) which extend toward the bottom of the tonsil, in such a way that it can b considered as an organ. Its function is to trap, phagocytose and expel antigens and othe foreign or harmful elements.

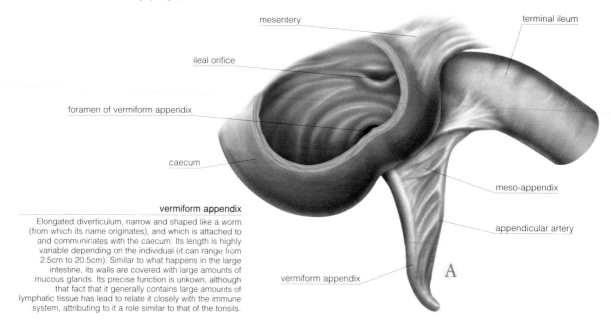

mesentery
terminal ileum
ileal orifice
foramen of vermiform appendix
caecum
meso-appendix
appendicular artery
vermiform appendix

A

vermiform appendix

Elongated diverticulum, narrow and shaped like a worm (from which its name originates), and which is attached to and communicates with the caecum. Its length is highly variable depending on the individual (it can range from 2.5cm to 20.5cm). Similar to what happens in the large intestine, its walls are covered with large amounts of mucous glands. Its precise function is unkown, although that fact that it generally contains large amounts of lymphatic tissue has lead to relate it closely with the immune system, attributing to it a role similar to that of the tonsils.

ENDOCRINE SYSTEM

The endocrine system, formed by glands and structures that produce hormones, is the second system of regulation and organization of the human body, after the nervous system, with which works synergistically to coordinate the cellular control and the homeostasis. But while the nervous regulates the activity of the muscles and glands through impulses produce by the neurons that provokes an immediate answer, the endocrine system influence over the metabolic activity of the cells through the hormones that generates a slower answer.

The hormones, product of secretion of the endocrine glands, are chemical substances that stimulate, inhibit or regulate the functioning of different organs that sometimes are far away from the origin point of those. When reach the organ the receptor of the membranes of the cells join to such hormones and activate allowing the pass to the inside, so that the hormone acts. The function of the hormones is to produce specific effects over one or more tissues or over processes (cellular division, protein synthesis, energy production, pubertal development, sexual characters, libido activation, etc.). The answer of the tissues and muscles to the action of the hormones, equal to most of the cells, use to be of more lasting effects than those of neurons.

Different to other organs the glands of the endocrine system are very small and of discrete appearance and are found dispersed all over the body. There are two kinds: exocrine (that through its ducts secretes its non hormonal secretions to a tubular structure or to a cavity) and endocrine (that pour to the blood or the lymph the hormones that produce and are endowed of a wide vascular drainage).

The common disposition of the hormonopoietic cells in hoods or like a dense net favors the contact with the sanguineous and lymphatic capillaries and the perfect reception of secretions from such glands.

Besides the endocrine glands (pituitary, thyroid, parathyroid, adrenal, pineal and thymus) there are some organs that, apart from their exocrine secretions, also produce hormones; is the case of the pancreas and the sexual glands. The hypothalamus belongs to the nervous system but produces and liberate hormones; that s why can be considered a neuroendocrine organ. There are tissues and organs that also produce hormones, even though is not their main function; is the case of the stomach, the small intestine, the heart, the kidneys, the placenta, certain tumor cells, etc.

The action of hormones is decisive, in the reproduction, the growth and development of the body, the activation of the immunitary defense, the balance of electrolytes, the regulation of cellular metabolism and a long etcetera.

The secretion of the endocrine glands can be affected, by the nervous system, because of the level of nutrients and minerals in the blood and for the action of other hormones.

A

ENDOCRINE SYSTEM

hormonal control of hypothalamus

Hormones can reach any part or organ of the body, but the cell membranes of these organs have specific receptors that select a determined set of hormones, ushering in those that are going to be useful in developing the role that these organs have assigned. Hormones are controlled by brain centers specialized in each one of them and the hypothalamus is the gland that regulates their production. Through special blood vessels and nerve endings, the hormones produced move into the pituitary gland. While some of these hormones stimulate certain glands to produce and release other hormones, others act directly on certain glands to activate their function.

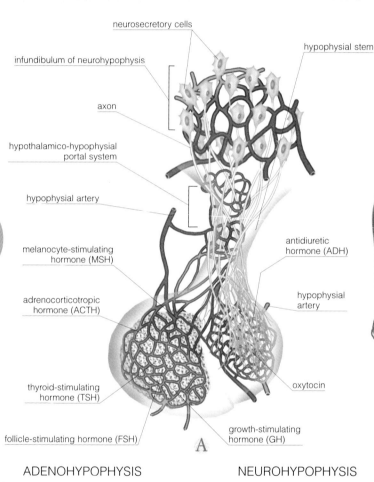

neurosecretory cells

hypophysial stem

infundibulum of neurohypophysis

axon

hypothalamico-hypophysial portal system

hypophysial artery

melanocyte-stimulating hormone (MSH)

adrenocorticotropic hormone (ACTH)

antidiuretic hormone (ADH)

hypophysial artery

thyroid-stimulating hormone (TSH)

oxytocin

follicle-stimulating hormone (FSH)

growth-stimulating hormone (GH)

A

ADENOHYPOPHYSIS   NEUROHYPOPHYSIS

pineal gland

hypophysis

parathyroid gland

thyroid gland

thymus

suprarenal glands

pancreas

ovaries (women)

testes (men)

A

endocrine system

Is constituted by a set of glands that relate each other, that segregate hormones which function may go from stimulate the functioning of different organs or even stop it, according to the situation in which the organism is found, and with certain stages of the life of the individual. These glands are structures that act through the hormones that segregate, to regulate the corporal functioning. It can be affirm, then that together with the nervous system, the endocrine is a control system. The hormones are chemical substances which function is to produce specific effects over one o more tissues or over processes (cellular division, synthesis of proteins, energy production, sexual characters, libido activation etc.). Its action is directly related with the chemical activity of cells. The main endocrine glands are: the pineal, pituitary, thyroid, parathyroid, thymus, suprarenal, the pancreas, the testicles, -in men- and ovaries -in women-. The secretion of the endocrine glands might be affected by the nervous system, because of the level of nutrients and minerals in the blood and for the action of other hormones.

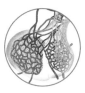

HYPOPHYSIS. PINEAL GLAND. THYMUS
SUPRARRENAL GLANDS

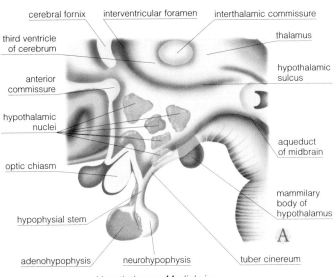

Hypothalamus. Medial view.

hypophysis

ngle structure, small and ovoid in shape, located inside the skull, in the sphenoid bone
avity known as the sella turcica. It consists of two parts or lobes: anterior (or adenohy-
ophysis), which originates from the pituitary diverticulum (or Rathke's pouch), and poste-
or (or neurohypophysis), formed by the nervous tissue of the infundibular stem. It is the
ze of a bean. It's size is approximately 1,3cm long, 1cm wide and 0,5cm thick, and it
eighs about 0,6g. It is called the master gland of the body due to the great variety of hor-
ones it secretes, and due to the influence these hormones have on the whole body. The
nterior pituitary secretes the hormones somatotropin (which regulates cell division and
rotein synthesis for growth) adrenocorticotropin (which regulates the function of the adre-
al cortex), thyrotropic (which regulates the function of the thyroid), prolactin (induces
ecretion of milk by the breast), and gonadotropins (FSH and LH, which affect the gonads).
ne neurohypophysis secretes the hormones oxytocin (which acts on the uterine smooth
uscle) and antidiuretic (which increases water reabsorption by the renal tubules).

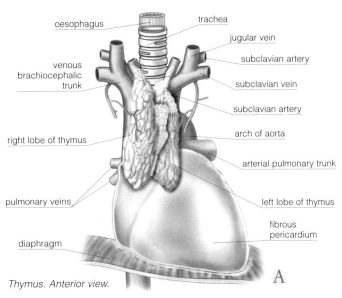

Thymus. Anterior view.

thymus

Lymphoid organ situated in the thoracic cavity, in the upper mediastinum, in front and above
the heart, and behind the sternum. It consists of two lobes which typically have a different
size, and which in turn contain many lobules. In the newborn, its size is about 5cm long and
1,5cm wide, and it weighs about 25g. It gradually develops to reach a weight of 35 - 50g at
puberty, after which it starts a process of involution. In adults, thymic tissue weighs only about
5g and occupies a small space behind the manubrium of the sternum. The lobes consist of
an outer cortex and an inner medulla, containing the thymocytes or immature T lymphocytes.
It is the primary organ of the immune system. In order to carry out its function (producing
T cells, specialized in defending the body against foreign substances and elements), it secretes thymostimulin, thymulin, etc., substances having hormonal activity that promote the development and differentiation of T lymphocytes.

541

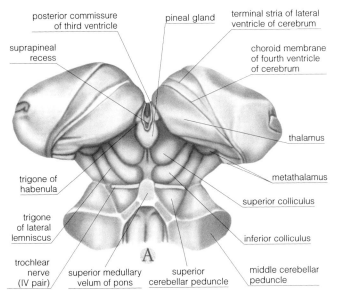

Mesencephalon. Posterior view.

pineal gland

Very small structure with a flattened, conical shape, located inside the brain, in the epitha-
amus, in a pouch situated above the superior colliculus and below the splenium of the
corpus callosum. While its precise function is not known, it is formed by glandular and nervous cells which, in response to norepinephrine, perform the synthesis and release of
melatonin, a hormone that influences sleep-wake cycles and other circadian rhythms.

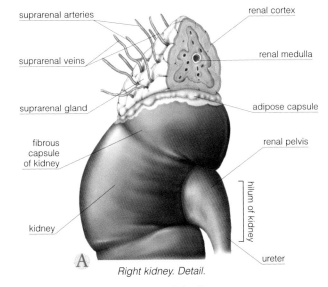

Right kidney. Detail.

suprarenal gland

The adrenal glands are two, they have a pyramidal shape and, like a cap, they cover the
top of both kidneys. They are grayish in color, are encased within a connective tissue capsule, and adapt to the convexity of the upper poles of the kidney. In adults they weigh between 4 and 14g (generally those in men outweigh that of women). They consist of two
areas: a peripheral area (or cortex) and a central one (or medulla). The first area synthesizes three groups of steroid hormones from cholesterol: glucocorticoids (cortisol, corticos-
terone), which regulate glucose metabolism, mineralocorticoids (aldosterone, dehydroe-
piandrosterone), which maintain the fluid and mineral balance, and androgens and estrogens (estradiol), which stimulate the changes of the body during puberty. The second area
synthesizes and stores three catecholamines: dopamine, norepinephrine, and epinephrine, which influence specially the cardiovascular apparatus and the nervous system.

THYROID GLAND. PARATHYROID GLANDS

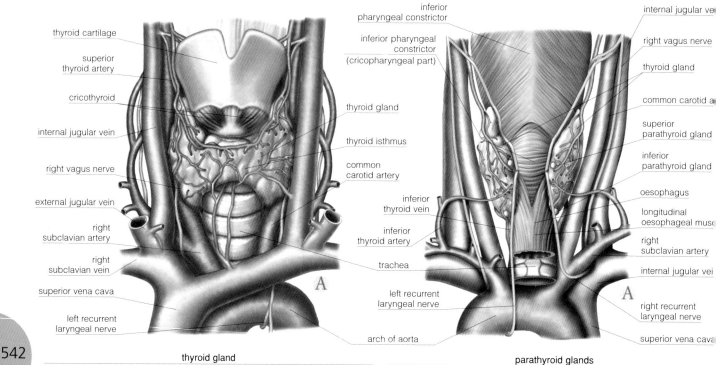

thyroid cartilage

superior thyroid artery

cricothyroid

internal jugular vein

right vagus nerve

external jugular vein

right subclavian artery

right subclavian vein

superior vena cava

left recurrent laryngeal nerve

thyroid gland

thyroid isthmus

common carotid artery

inferior thyroid vein

inferior thyroid artery

trachea

left recurrent laryngeal nerve

arch of aorta

A

inferior pharyngeal constrictor

inferior pharyngeal constrictor (cricopharyngeal part)

thyroid gland

internal jugular ve

right vagus nerve

thyroid gland

common carotid a

superior parathyroid gland

inferior parathyroid gland

oesophagus

longitudinal oesophageal musc

right subclavian artery

internal jugular vei

right recurrent laryngeal nerve

superior vena cava

A

thyroid gland

Single endocrine gland, pink in color, located at the base of the neck, at either side of the bottom part of the larynx and the upper trachea. It consists of two lateral lobes, right and left, which are joined by an isthmus (thyroid isthmus) and is covered by a membrane (thyroid capsule). It consists of microscopic vesicles and thyroid follicles, enveloped by a pasty substance (colloid), a mixture of thyroglobulin and iodine, from which two hormones are synthesized, thyroxine (decisive in the production of energy and for increasing the level of protein synthesis in tissues) and triiodothyronine (having superior biological activity and faster anabolic effects than thyroxine). Both contribute to the maturation of the nervous system.

parathyroid glands

Four very small glands found on the posterior part and lower edge of the thyroid gland, included within it. They originate from the endoderm of the branchial clefts and occur pairs of variable number, typically two. They measure about 6mm in length and 3-4mm width. Their external appearance is that of fatty tissue and their color is usually light brow They produce parathyroid hormone, one of the main regulators of the metabolism of ca cium and phosphorus; therefore, they control bone metabolism.

the thyroid tissue

The thyroid tissue is comprised of two types of cells: follicular and parafollicular cells. Most of the thyroid tissue is made up of follicular cells, which secrete thyroxine (Tf) and triiodothyronine (T3). Parafollicular cells, also called C cells, secrete the hormone calcitonin. The thyroid gland plays an important role in regulating metabolism and balancing calcium in the body. The T4 and T3 hormones stimulate each tissue of the body to generate proteins and increase the quantity of oxygen used by cells. As the work of cells becomes more intense, the organs will have to work more. Triiodothyronine has a superior biological activity and anabolic effects which are faster than thyroxine. They both contribute to the maturation of the nervous system. The hormone calcitonin works together with the hormone parathyroid to regulate calcium levels in the body.

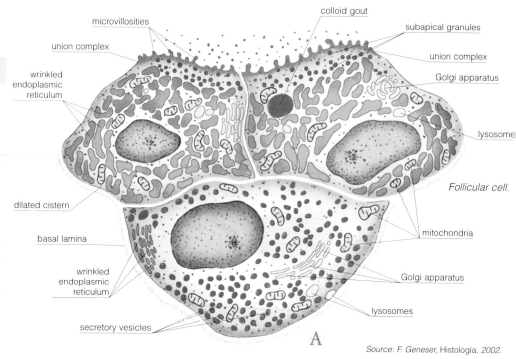

microvillosities

union complex

wrinkled endoplasmic reticulum

dilated cistern

basal lamina

wrinkled endoplasmic reticulum

secretory vesicles

colloid gout

subapical granules

union complex

Golgi apparatus

lysosome

Follicular cell.

mitochondria

Golgi apparatus

lysosomes

A

Source: F. Geneser, Histologia, *2002.*

C CELL STRUCTURE

PANCREAS. TESTES. OVARIES

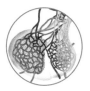

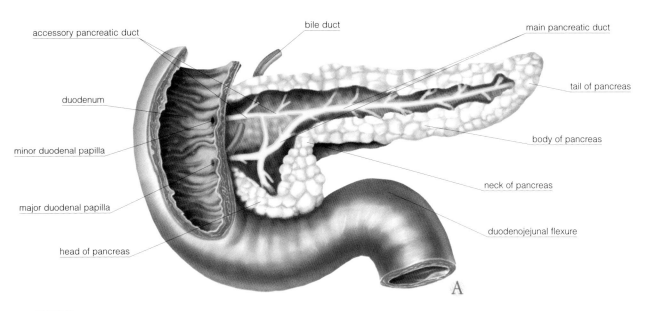

accessory pancreatic duct

bile duct

main pancreatic duct

tail of pancreas

duodenum

body of pancreas

minor duodenal papilla

neck of pancreas

major duodenal papilla

duodenojejunal flexure

head of pancreas

A

pancreas

Composite acinotubular gland situated in the upper part of the abdominal cavity, under the liver, behind the stomach and in front of the LI and LII lumbar vertebrae. It has two functions: exocrine (digestive) and endocrine (not digestive). In order to fulfill these roles it is equipped with multiple secretory units, or acini. During digestion it plays a major exocrine role, since it secretes a series of fluids, the pancreatic juices, which are discharged into the duodenum through the major duodenal papilla, thanks to which foods are broken up into basic components, which allows them to be absorbed by the body. The endocrine function is performed by masses of cells called islets of Langerhans, which are scattered throughout the exocrine glandular tissue. These cells secrete hormones that enter the blood and are crucial in the metabolism of carbohydrates: insulin (which lowers glucose levels in the blood), glucagon (which raises the levels of glucose in the blood), and somatostatin (which acts as an inhibitor of the two previous hormones as well as of the growth hormone and of gastrin of the stomach). Therefore, they regulate the transit of glucose, the main food of the cell, to the interior of the cell.

543

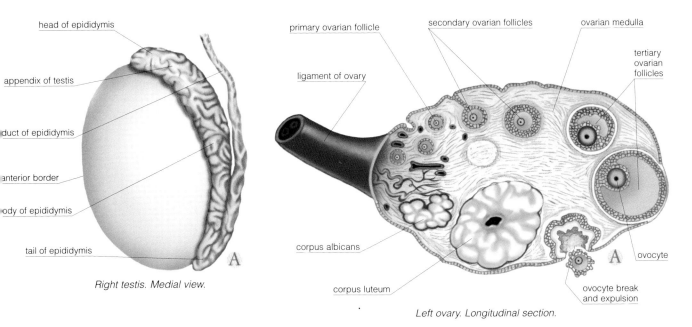

head of epididymis

primary ovarian follicle

secondary ovarian follicles

ovarian medulla

appendix of testis

ligament of ovary

tertiary ovarian follicles

duct of epididymis

anterior border

body of epididymis

tail of epididymis

A

corpus albicans

ovocyte

corpus luteum

ovocyte break and expulsion

Right testis. Medial view.

Left ovary. Longitudinal section.

testis

The testicles are the two male glandular organs, ovoid in shape, located inside the scrotum. Each testicle is about 4cm long, 2.5cm wide, and 2.5cm thick. Their function is the production of spermatozoa (male sexual cells, which allow men to fertilize a female ovum) and of the male hormones testosterone (responsible for growth and development of male sexual characteristics) and inhibin (which inhibits the secretion of gonadotropin-releasing hormone).

ovary

The ovaries are the female genital glands. They are two, almond-shaped. They are located one on each side of the pelvic cavity, and are connected to the uterus by the utero-ovarian ligament, close to the fallopian tubes. They are 2.5-4.4cm long, 2cm wide, and 1cm thick. Their role is to produce ova, or female sexual cells, as well as characteristic female hormones.

MAIN ENDOCRINE GLANDS (I)

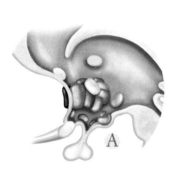

HYPOTHALAMUS

Thyrotropin-releasing hormone (TRH)
- Stimulates the synthesis and secretion of thyrotropin.
- Activates secretion by the thyroid gland.

Corticotropin-releasing hormone (CRH)
- Stimulates the action of corticotropin (ACTH).
- Stimulates the hormonal action of the adrenal glands.

Somatotropin-releasing hormone (GHRH)
- Stimulates the production and secretion of growth hormone (GH) in the adenohypophysis.

Somatotropin-inhibiting hormone (GHIH)
- Inhibits the production of growth hormone.

Gonadotropin-inhibiting hormone (GnRH)
- Promotes the production and secretion of hormones of the hypothalamic-pituitary-gonadal axis: follicle-stimulating hormone (FSH) and luteinizing hormone (LH).
- Participates in male and female genital development.

Prolactin inhibiting factors (PIF)
- They inhibit pituitary secretion of prolactin.

544

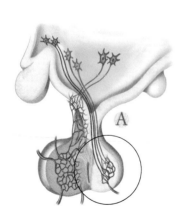

NEUROHYPOPHYSIS

Antidiuretic hormone (ADH)
- Stimulates water reabsorption in the kidney.
- Induces vasoconstriction and increased blood pressure.

Oxytocin (OXT)
- Stimulates contraction of uterine muscle fibers during delivery.
- Activates milk ejection during lactation.

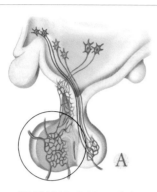

ADENOHYPOPHYSIS

Thyroid-stimulating hormone (TSH)
- Stimulates the production or secretion of thyroxine.
- Stimulates the activity of the thyroid gland (increase and absorption of O_2 and of protein synthesis, influences the metabolism of carbohydrates and lipids).

Adrenocorticotropic hormone (ACTH)
- Stimulates the hormonal productive capacity of the adrenal glands (glucocorticoids-fascicular zone-and androgens-reticular zone-).

- Influences the maintenance of the electrolitic equilibrium and the production of carbohydrates in the liver.

Growth hormone (GH)
- Stimulates the production and secretion of growth hormone by the adenohypophysis, which is important organism (liver, muscles, bones, cartileges, tissues, etc

Follicle-stimulating hormone (FSH)
- Acts on the gonads, stimulating spermatogenesis in the seminiferous tubules in men and follicular maturation in the ovary in women.
- Activates estradiol production during the first half of the menstrual cycle.

Luteinizing hormone (LH)
- Completes the action of the follicle-stimulating hormon activates ovulation, proliferation of the epithelial cells of the follicle and progesterone synthesis, and stimulates testosterone production by the interstitial cells (Leydig cells) in the testicle.
- It has a general anabolic effect in the organism.

Prolactin hormone (PRL)
- Its function is related to the female reproductive cycle and the maintenance of pregnancy.
- Mammary tissue proliferation and milk secretion.

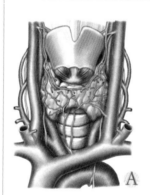

THYROID GLAND

Tyrosine (T_4)
- Stimulates metabolism of carbohydrates and fats.
- Activates oxygen consumption and protein degradation inside the cell, in addition to cell differentiation.

Triiodothyronine (T_3)
- Stimulates metabolism of carbohydrates and fats.
- Active oxygen consumption and protein degradation inside the cell, in addition to cell differentiation.

Calcitonin
- Decreases the concentration of calcium and phosphorus in plasma.
- Activates the deposition of calcium in bones, reducing calcium serum concentrations.
- Acts as an antagonist of parathyroid hormone.

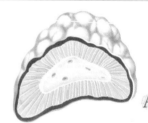

SUPRARENAL CORTEX

Cortisol (glucocorticoid)
- It is the main glucocorticoid that is synthesized in the fascicular zone of the adrenal cortex.
- Acts on the metabolism of glucose, proteins and fats, developing an important mineralocorticoid action.
- Regulates the immune system (inflammatory action).

Aldosterone (mineralocorticoid)
- Intervenes in the hydroelectrolitic balance of the organism through the control of sodium and potassium exchange in the convoluted distal tubule of the renal glomerulus: rsodium reabsorption with water retention and potassium and hydrogen ion excretion.

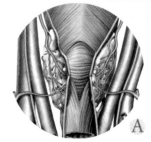

PARATHYROID GLANDS

Parotid hormone (PTH)
- It has a triple action: on the kidneys (increases excretion of phosphates), on bones (stimulates osteoclast activity) and on the intestine (increased calcium absorption).

MAIN ENDOCRINE GLANDS (II)

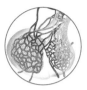

ENDOCRINE PANCREAS

Insulin
- In the liver it produces a stimulus to the synthesis of glycogen and an inhibition of glycogenolysis and gluconeogenesis.
- Decreases glycemia and promotes the use of glucose in muscle and adipose tissue.
- Promotes lipogenesis, is antilipolytic and anti-ketogenic and has an anabolic effect (stimulates protein synthesis and saves amino acids by inhibiting gluconeogenesis).

Glucagon
- Contrary to the action of insulin, it increases blood glucose levels.
- Induced by increased phosphorilase activity of the liver, it helps to mobilize liver glycogen reserves.
- Increases peripheral glucose utilization, reduces gastric motility and pancreatic secretions, and increases urinary excretion of nitrogen and potassium.

Somatostatin (SS)
- It has a paracrine action. Thus, it inhibits the release of growth hormone and many others: somatotropin, thyrotropin and corticotropin (by the adenohypophysis), insulin and glucagon (in the pancreas), gastrin (by the gastric mucosa), secretin (by the intestinal mucosa) and renin (by the kidney).

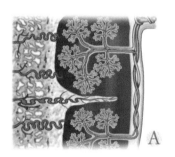

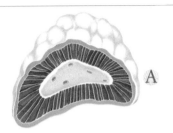

SUPRARENAL MEDULLA

Noradrenaline (NA)
- Neurotransmitter acting on adrenergic α and β receptors.
- It is secreted by the adrenal medulla as a response to splanchnic stimulation.
- Powerful vasoconstrictor that is activated in response to hypertension and stress situations

Adrenaline
- Powerful stimulator of the adrenergic receptors of the sympathetic nervous system
- Stimulant that increases heart rate and increases cardiac output.

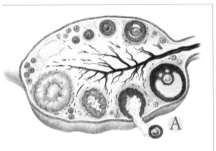

OVARIES

Estradiol
- It is the most potent natural ovarian and placental estrogen.
- Prepares the uterus so that the fertilized egg can be implanted in the endometrium.
- Promotes the maturation and maintenance of the complementary female reproductive organs and determines secondary sex characteristics (uterine tubes, uterus and vagina).

Progesterone
- It is considered the pregnancy hormone. Thus, it prepares the uterus for the reception and development of the fertilized egg, inducing a change in the endometrium from the proliferative to the secretory phase, and creates a more favorable uterine environment for pregnancy to develop in the best possible conditions.
- Promotes the development of the mammary gland for breastfeeding.

Relaxin
- It is secreted by the corpus luteum during pregnancy.
- Promotes relaxation of ligaments and pelvic cartilages, contributing to an increase in the diameters of the birth canal (symphysis pubis and cervix).

Inhibin
- Inhibits the activity of the pituitary, particularly the secretion of follicle stimulating hormone (FSH).
- Participates in the control of gametogenesis, in embryonic and fetal development, and in hematopoiesis.

Activin
- It stimulates the activity of the pituitary, especially the secretion of follicle stimulating hormone (FSH).
- In general, its action is the opposite of inhibin.

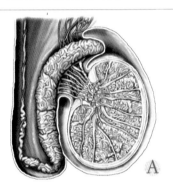

TESTES

Testosterone
- During the embryonic period, it regulates gonadotropic secretion and the differentiation of the mesonephric duct (formation of the epididymis, vas deferens and seminal vesicle) and stimulates skeletal muscle.
- Induces differentiation of secondary male sexual characteristics (penis, prostate, scrotum, etc.).
- It has protein anabolic properties (retention of nitrogen, calcium, phosphorus and potassium) and it is decisive for maintaining muscle mass and bone tissue in the male.

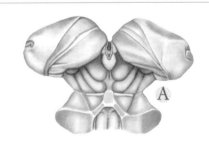

PINEAL GLAND

Melatonin
- Exerts an Influence over the hypothalamus and the anterior pituitary.
- Exerts an inhibitory action over different aspects related to gonadal, pituitary, thyroid, adrenal and parathyroid functions.
- Involved in the regulation of sleep, mood, puberty and ovarian cycles.

PLACENTA

Human chorionic gonadotrophin (HCG)
- Maintains corpus luteum function during the first weeks of pregnancy.
- Possibly favors steroidogenesis in the fetal-placental unit and stimulates testicular testosterone secretion.
- Its functions are similar to those of luteinizing hormone (LH).

Growth-stimulating hormone (GH)
- Enhances the functions of pituitary GH.
- From the viewpoint of the immune system, it is similar to somatotropin.
- Inhibits insulin activity of the mother during pregnancy.

Estrogen
- Its functions are similar to those of the ovarian estrogens.
- Responsible for the development of female secondary sexual characteristics.

Progestagen
- Its functions are similar to those of progesterone.

Relaxin
- Its functions are similar to relaxin secreted by the ovaries.

Somatomammotropin
- Its functions are similar to those of prolactin.

Leptin
- Is a part of the feedback loop and provides information to the brain about the state of nutrient reserves and bodily energy expenditure.

MAIN ENDOCRINE GLANDS (III)

GASTRO-INTESTINAL TRACT

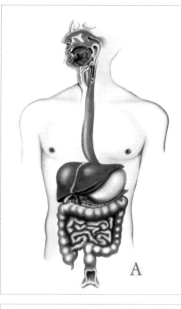

A

Gastrin
- Secreted by the mucosa of the pyloric antrum, it stimulates secretion of gastric juice and, more timidly, of pancreatic juice.

Secretin
- Secreted by the S-cells of the mucosa of the duodenum and jejunum, it stimulates secretion of the exocrine pancreas and, to a lesser extent, of bile in the liver, inhibits secretion of gastric acid, stimulates pepsin secretion, inhibits digestive tract motility, activates contraction of the gallbladder, etc. All this facilitates the action of digestive enzymes.

Cholecystokinin (CCK)
- Stimulates contraction of the gallbladder with consequent release of bile and pancreatic enzyme secretion.

Ghrelin
- Stimulates secretion of growth hormone (GH) and of appetite.

Motiline
- Increases the motor and electrical activity of the stomach and of the small intestine, increases internal esophageal sphincter tone and stimulates pepsin secretion.
- Stimulates the alkalinization of the duodenum.

Gastrin-inhibiting peptide (GIP)
- Inhibits intestinal motility and secretion and increases insulin release.

Vaso-active intestinal peptide (VIP)
- Promotes relaxation of the cardia, stomach and gallbladder.
- Stimulates the secretion of water into the bile and pancreatic juices.
- Inhibits hydrochloric acid secretion.

Enteroglucagon (GLP-1)
- Glucagon-like peptide having a hyperglycemic effect, released by the small intestinal mucosa in response to glucose ingestion.
- It has properties similar to those of pancreatic glucagon.

Glucagonoid peptide (GLP-2) and derived glucagon peptides
- Stimulate intestinal epithelial proliferation.

KIDNEYS

Renin
- One of the elements of the renin-angiotensin-aldosterone regulatory cycle, intended to maintain salt and water homeostasis and, therefore, the fundamental blood pressure mechanism.

D_3 vitamin
- Along with the skin and liver, it promotes intestinal absorption of dietary calcium and bone mineralization.

Erythropoietin
- Acts on the red blood cell precursors of the bone marrow, which, in turn, lead to, starting with the proerythroblast, to stimulate erythropoiesis (or formation of mature erythrocytes).

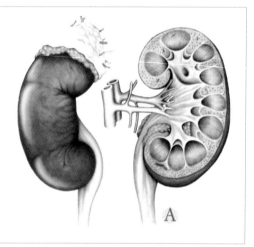

A

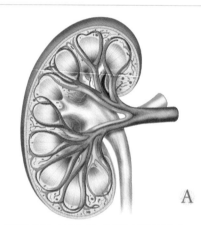

A

KIDNEY AND BLOOD VESSELS

Atrial natriuretic peptide (ANP)
- Acts on the kidney, increasing natriuresis and diuresis (renal sodium excretion), and in blood vessels, causing their dilation (decreasing blood pressure).

ADIPOSE TISSUE

Leptin
- Plays an important role in the regulation of nutrient intake and energy expenditure.
- Inhibits neuropeptide Y, which makes it anorexigenic.
- It has reproductive effects, since it acts on the secretion of gonadotropin-releasing hormone (GnRH).

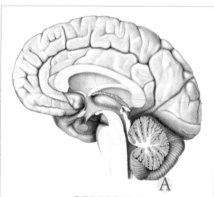

A

CEREBRUM

Neuropeptide Y (NPY)
- Located in the brain and in the gastrointestinal apparatus, it stimulates appetite.

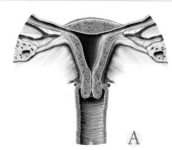

A

UTERUS

Prostaglandin F_{2a} (PGF_{2a})
- Stimulates bronchial and uterine smooth muscle contraction.
- Produces vasoconstriction in some vessels.
- Induces lysis of the corpus luteum.

NERVOUS SYSTEM

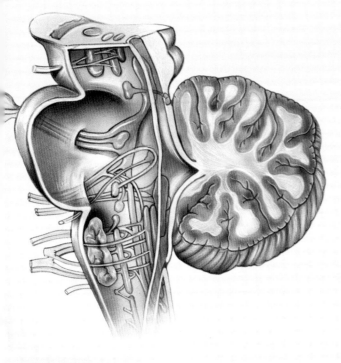

The nervous system is the set of elements that constitute the control center of the whole organism, which entails the function of regulate and organize everything that happens in it: thought, actions, emotions. with the endocrine system shares the function of ordering and keep the balance of the homeostasis. No doubt the nervous is the most complex of all the functional units of the organism and, in fact, being much, is still very little what it's known about it.

The functional unit of the nervous system, which function is to transport the bioelectric signals from the peripheral organs until the brain and transmit the pertinent response in each case from this to those, is the neuron.

In the nervous system we may consider different aspects:

- The nervous central system. Lead the voluntary corporal actions. Is constituted by the brain (is found in the interior of the cranial cavity and form part the brain and cerebellum), the trunk of the brain (formed by the midbrain, the bridge and the brainstem) and the spinal cord (that goes along the backbone).

- The peripheral nervous system. Is formed by the peripheral nerves, in which can be distinguished two types: cranial (that have its origin in the base of the brain and are usually known as cranial pairs, because form groups of two that go to one each sides of the body: (right and left) and spinals (have its origin in the spinal cord, extend all over the body and are able to transmit motor commands -in the case of the motor nerves- or sensitive stimuli -in the case of sensitive nerves-), and also the rachidian nodes (or groups of neural bodies that act as intermediate stations in the transmitter journey of the impulse until the cerebrum).

- The autonomous nervous system or vegetative. Is found in the base of the brain in the hypothalamus, and in the bulb. Controls the independent corporal functions of the will and the consciousness (respiration, heart rate, digestion, blood circulation, etc.). It consists of two components or antagonistic subsystems: the sympathetic or portion thoracolumbar, and the parasympathetic or portion bulbosacra.

The basic functions of the nervous system may be summarized in three:

- Receive the information of any change that takes place both inside and immediate outside of the organism, which is obtained through the intervention of the sensory receptors that transmit the stimuli or corresponding signals.

- Process the sensory information received and consequently decides the immediate answer pertinent in each case.

- Transmit such answer to activate a determinate action of the muscles or of the glands, which is denominated motor answer.

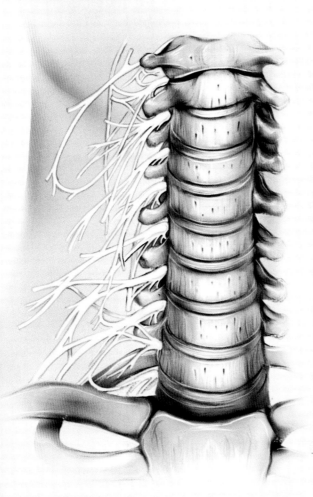

A

NERVOUS SYSTEM
POSTERIOR GENERAL VIEW

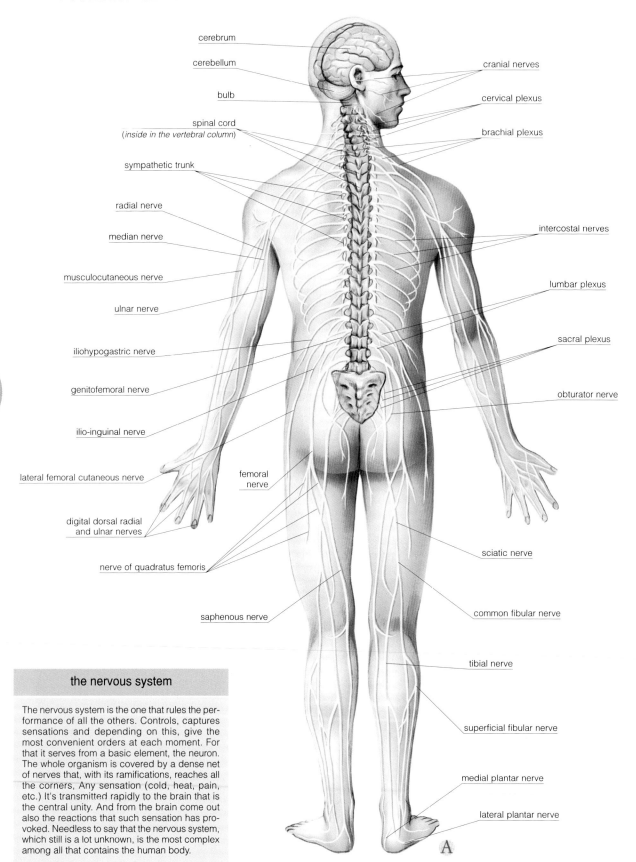

cerebrum

cerebellum

bulb

spinal cord
(*inside in the vertebral column*)

sympathetic trunk

radial nerve

median nerve

musculocutaneous nerve

ulnar nerve

iliohypogastric nerve

genitofemoral nerve

ilio-inguinal nerve

lateral femoral cutaneous nerve

digital dorsal radial
and ulnar nerves

nerve of quadratus femoris

saphenous nerve

femoral
nerve

cranial nerves

cervical plexus

brachial plexus

intercostal nerves

lumbar plexus

sacral plexus

obturator nerve

sciatic nerve

common fibular nerve

tibial nerve

superficial fibular nerve

medial plantar nerve

lateral plantar nerve

A

the nervous system

The nervous system is the one that rules the performance of all the others. Controls, captures sensations and depending on this, give the most convenient orders at each moment. For that it serves from a basic element, the neuron. The whole organism is covered by a dense net of nerves that, with its ramifications, reaches all the corners, Any sensation (cold, heat, pain, etc.) It's transmitted rapidly to the brain that is the central unity. And from the brain come out also the reactions that such sensation has provoked. Needless to say that the nervous system, which still is a lot unknown, is the most complex among all that contains the human body.

AUTONOMIC NERVOUS SYSTEM
GENERAL VIEW

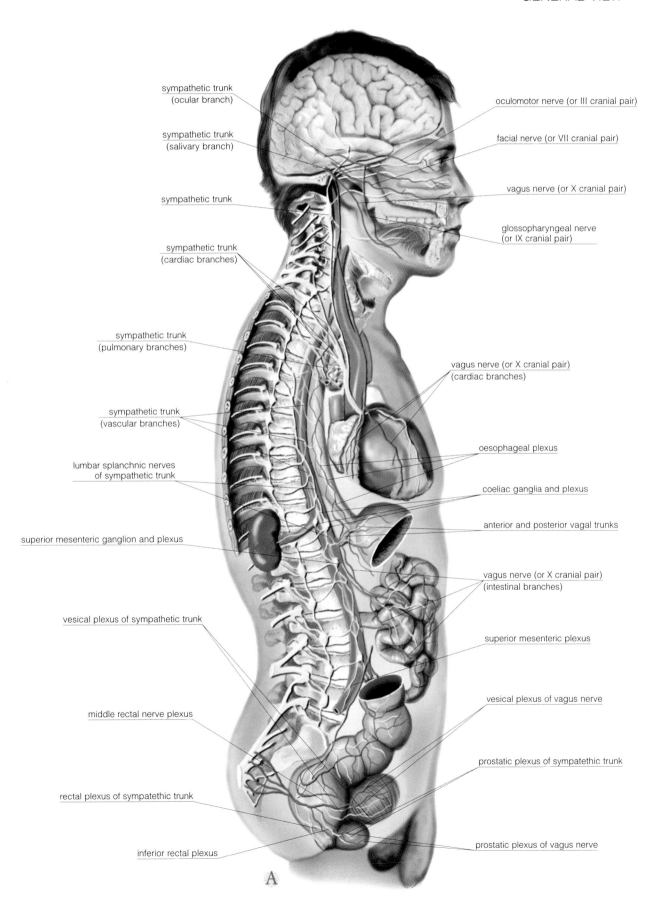

sympathetic trunk
(ocular branch)

sympathetic trunk
(salivary branch)

sympathetic trunk

sympathetic trunk
(cardiac branches)

sympathetic trunk
(pulmonary branches)

sympathetic trunk
(vascular branches)

lumbar splanchnic nerves
of sympathetic trunk

superior mesenteric ganglion and plexus

vesical plexus of sympathetic trunk

middle rectal nerve plexus

rectal plexus of sympatethic trunk

inferior rectal plexus

oculomotor nerve (or III cranial pair)

facial nerve (or VII cranial pair)

vagus nerve (or X cranial pair)

glossopharyngeal nerve
(or IX cranial pair)

vagus nerve (or X cranial pair)
(cardiac branches)

oesophageal plexus

coeliac ganglia and plexus

anterior and posterior vagal trunks

vagus nerve (or X cranial pair)
(intestinal branches)

superior mesenteric plexus

vesical plexus of vagus nerve

prostatic plexus of sympatethic trunk

prostatic plexus of vagus nerve

549

A

BASIC GENERAL ORGANIZATION

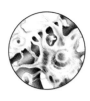

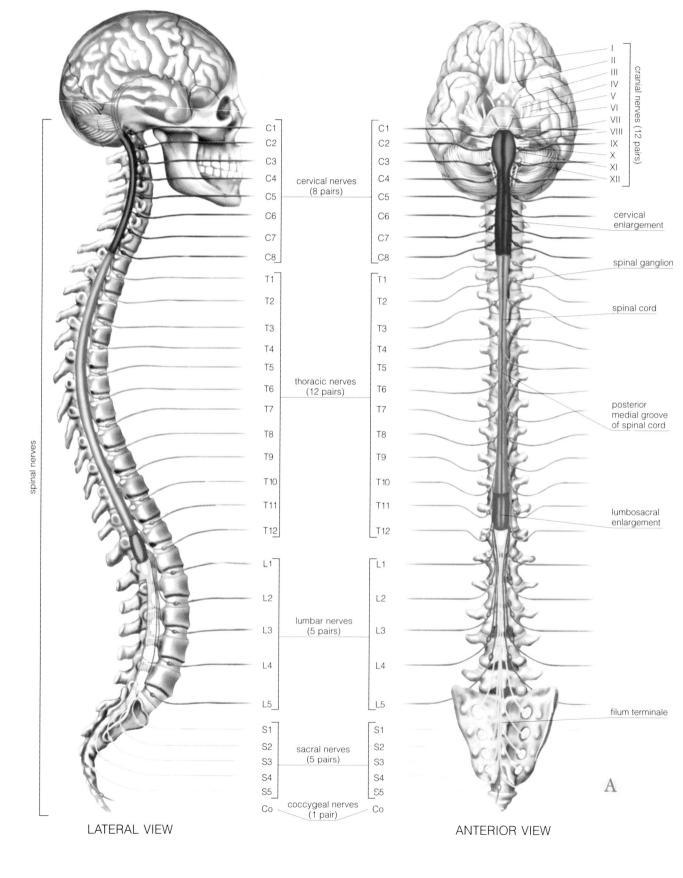

550

spinal nerves

C1
C2
C3
C4
C5   cervical nerves
C6   (8 pairs)
C7
C8

T1
T2
T3
T4
T5
T6   thoracic nerves
T7   (12 pairs)
T8
T9
T10
T11
T12

L1
L2
L3   lumbar nerves
L4   (5 pairs)
L5

S1
S2
S3   sacral nerves
S4   (5 pairs)
S5

Co   coccygeal nerves
            (1 pair)

cranial nerves (12 pairs)
I
II
III
IV
V
VI
VII
VIII
IX
X
XI
XII

cervical enlargement

spinal ganglion

spinal cord

posterior medial groove of spinal cord

lumbosacral enlargement

filum terminale

A

LATERAL VIEW

ANTERIOR VIEW

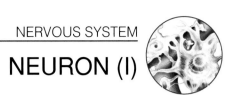

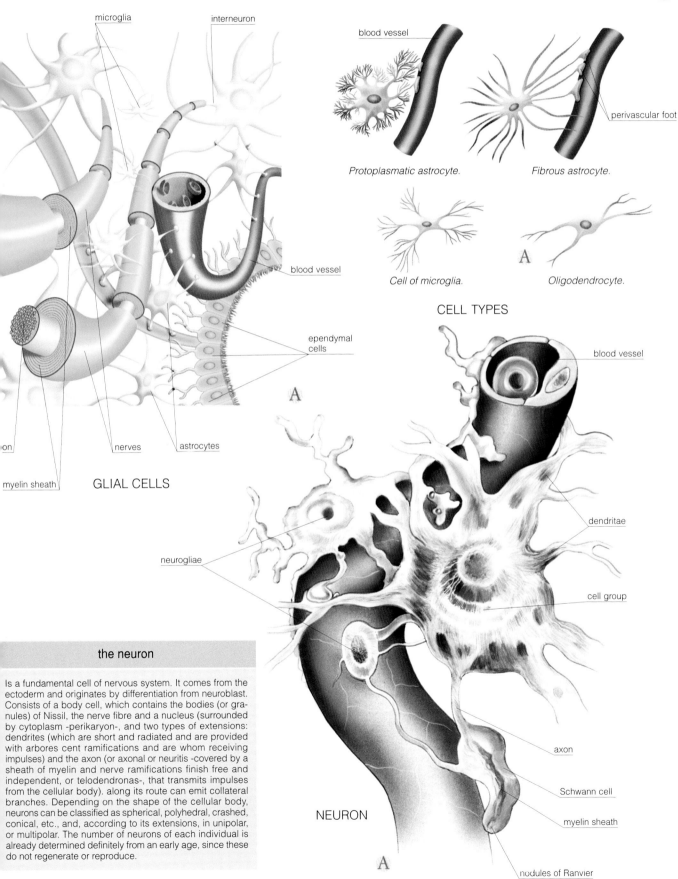

microglia

interneuron

blood vessel

blood vessel

ependymal cells

on

nerves

astrocytes

myelin sheath

GLIAL CELLS

Protoplasmatic astrocyte.

Fibrous astrocyte.

perivascular foot

Cell of microglia.

A

Oligodendrocyte.

CELL TYPES

blood vessel

551

dendritae

cell group

neurogliae

axon

Schwann cell

myelin sheath

NEURON

A

nodules of Ranvier

the neuron

Is a fundamental cell of nervous system. It comes from the ectoderm and originates by differentiation from neuroblast. Consists of a body cell, which contains the bodies (or granules) of Nissil, the nerve fibre and a nucleus (surrounded by cytoplasm -perikaryon-, and two types of extensions: dendrites (which are short and radiated and are provided with arbores cent ramifications and are whom receiving impulses) and the axon (or axonal or neuritis -covered by a sheath of myelin and nerve ramifications finish free and independent, or telodendronas-, that transmits impulses from the cellular body). along its route can emit collateral branches. Depending on the shape of the cellular body, neurons can be classified as spherical, polyhedral, crashed, conical, etc., and, according to its extensions, in unipolar, or multipolar. The number of neurons of each individual is already determined definitely from an early age, since these do not regenerate or reproduce.

NEURON (II). EFFERENT NEURON

motor neuron

The motor neuron also called efferent neurons are neurons with motor function, a kind of nervous cells efferent that transmit motor impulses from the brain or the spinal cord until the muscular tissue or glandular, this type of neurons are formed by multiple dendrites, a big central nucleus and a long axon. The bodies or corpuscles of Nissl are big granular and basophilic structures found in the cytoplasm of the nervous cells, are formed by endoplasmic reticulum rugous, and free polyribosomes. Constitute the place where the synthesis of protein is produced. Show changes in various psychological disorders and in pathologic conditions might dissolve or disappear (chromatolysis). They get dye with basic tints and contain ribonucleoproteins. The axon ramifies and ends in shape of terminal motor plates.

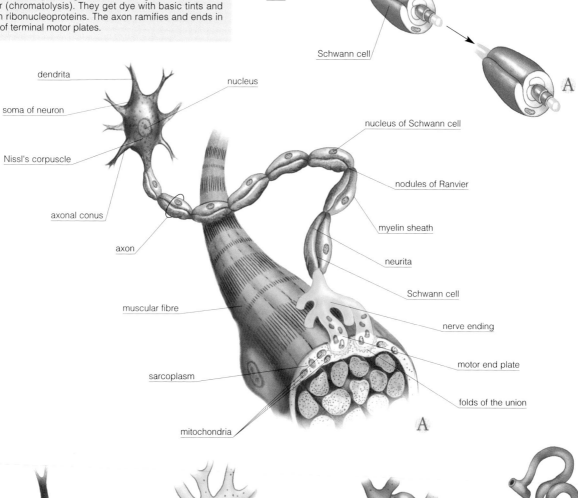

Schwann cell

amyelinic nerve fibre

axon

Schwann cell

axon

A

dendrita

nucleus

soma of neuron

nucleus of Schwann cell

Nissl's corpuscle

nodules of Ranvier

axonal conus

myelin sheath

axon

neurita

Schwann cell

muscular fibre

nerve ending

motor end plate

sarcoplasm

folds of the union

mitochondria

A

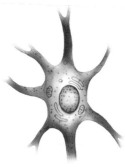

multipolar neuron
(spinal cord)

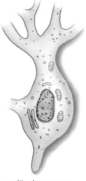

multipolar neuron
(cortex of cerebellum)

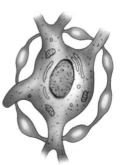

multipolar neuron
(autonomic ganglion)

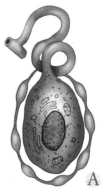

pseudomonopolar neuron
(spinal sensory ganglion)

552

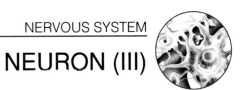

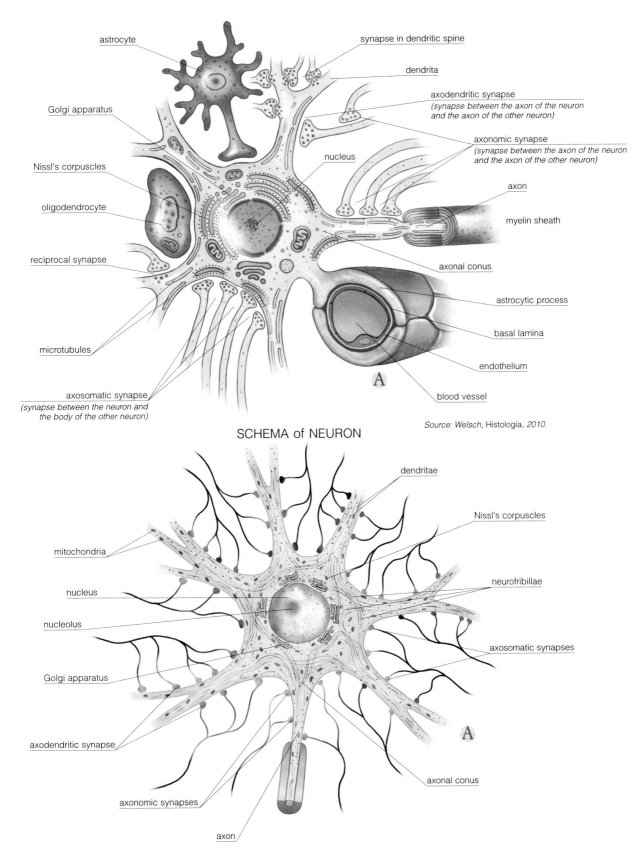

astrocyte

synapse in dendritic spine

dendrita

axodendritic synapse
(synapse between the axon of the neuron and the axon of the other neuron)

Golgi apparatus

axonomic synapse
(synapse between the axon of the neuron and the axon of the other neuron)

nucleus

axon

Nissl's corpuscles

myelin sheath

oligodendrocyte

reciprocal synapse

axonal conus

astrocytic process

basal lamina

microtubules

endothelium

A

axosomatic synapse
(synapse between the neuron and the body of the other neuron)

blood vessel

553

SCHEMA of NEURON

Source: Welsch, Histología, 2010.

dendritae

Nissl's corpuscles

mitochondria

neurofribillae

nucleus

nucleolus

axosomatic synapses

Golgi apparatus

A

axodendritic synapse

axonic conus

axonomic synapses

axon

NEURON COMPONENTS

NEURON (IV). NEURON TYPES

efferent neuron

Efferent neuron is the one that its function is to transmit motor impulses. This neuron supplies and controls organs and effectors tissue (endocrine and exocrine glands, muscle fibers).

sensory neurons

Neurons that its function is to transmit tactile stimulation in terms of environment as own organism.

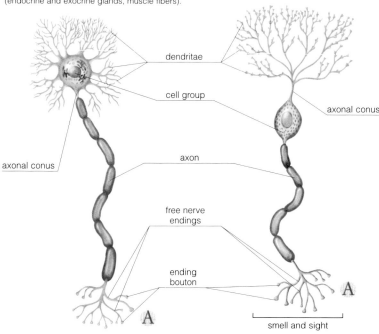

dendritae

cell group

axonal conus

axon

axonal conus

free nerve endings

ending bouton

smell and sight

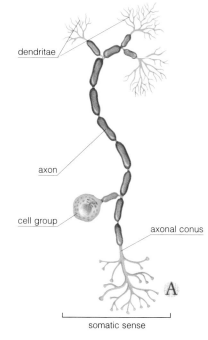

dendritae

axon

cell group

axonal conus

somatic sense

multipolar neuron

Neuron which presents more than two extensions cells, generally several dendrites and an axon. Its shape varies according to ramifications availability, while these neurons use to be pyramidal or vaults.

bipolar neuron

This neuron only has two extensions (a main dendrite and an axon, or two dendrites), one in each side of the cell body. It is found in inner ear (at the level of cochlear and vestibular nodes), in the retina of the eye and in cerebellum olfactory area.

psedo-unipolar neuron

Generally it is a primary sensitive neuron which was born as bipolar, b when developing, its extensions were functioned in only one that, rapic very near to the body cell that splits up into two branches, one that is directed to central system nervous and the other one is going to the periphery. For its structure and function, both correspond to axons supply of myelin sheath, that at level of its terminals spider veins, the behave as dendrites (it means, receive and process sensitive stimulu as stretching or friction). They are found in the spinal or sensitive ganglions of nerve roots of spinal nerves.

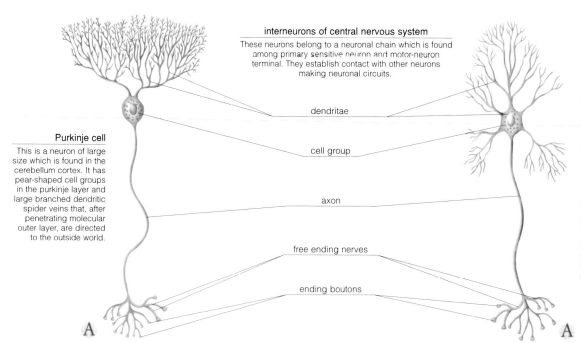

interneurons of central nervous system

These neurons belong to a neuronal chain which is found among primary sensitive neuron and motor-neuron terminal. They establish contact with other neurons making neuronal circuits.

dendritae

cell group

axon

free ending nerves

ending boutons

Purkinje cell

This is a neuron of large size which is found in the cerebellum cortex. It has pear-shaped cell groups in the purkinje layer and large branched dendritic spider veins that, after penetrating molecular outer layer, are directed to the outside world.

pyramidal cell

This is a very multipolar large cell that has pyram shape which is found in t brain cortex. It has a tail dendrite apical which is extended to the surface and several dendrites tha are expanding to inner part. Its size is variable. Its neurotransmitter looks to be glutamate and its effects over target cells are excitatory. From the pyramid cell are originate the big fibers that descer to the spinal cord and the sub cortical fascicles of association.

NEURON (V). STRUCTURE

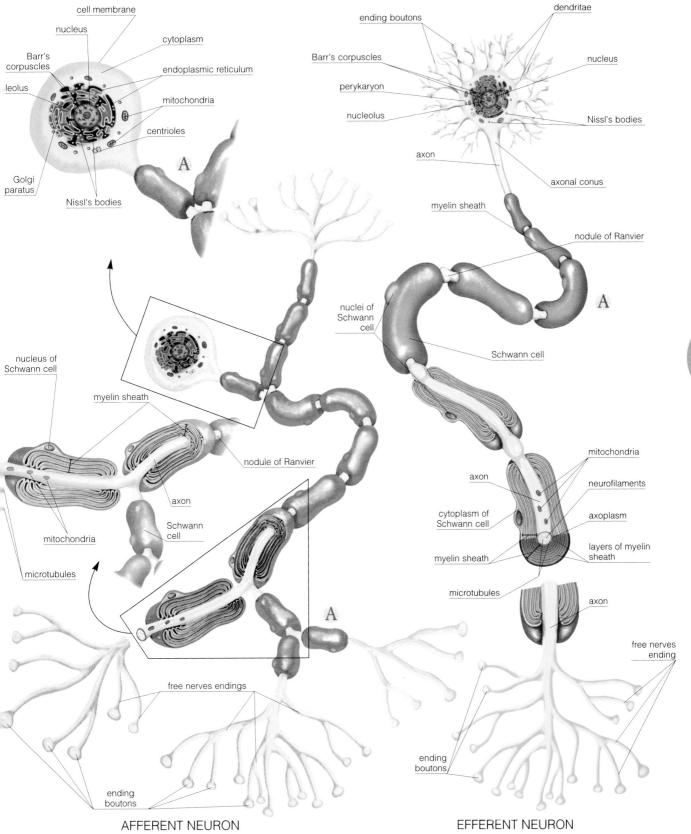

cell membrane

nucleus

cytoplasm

Barr's
corpuscles

endoplasmic reticulum

leolus

mitochondria

centrioles

Golgi
paratus

Nissl's bodies

A

ending boutons

dendritae

Barr's corpuscles

nucleus

perykaryon

nucleolus

Nissl's bodies

axon

axonal conus

myelin sheath

nodule of Ranvier

nuclei of
Schwann
cell

A

Schwann cell

nucleus of
Schwann cell

myelin sheath

nodule of Ranvier

axon

Schwann
cell

mitochondria

axon

neurofilaments

cytoplasm of
Schwann cell

axoplasm

mitochondria

layers of myelin
sheath

microtubules

myelin sheath

microtubules

axon

A

free nerves endings

free nerves
ending

ending
boutons

ending
boutons

AFFERENT NEURON

EFFERENT NEURON

NERVE (I)

nerve

Each one of the cord that relate the nervous centers or peripheral nodes with the different parts of the body, are formed by fascicles, or beams of axons, that project from several neurons. The majority of them come up to a point or determined area of the body and involves two types of fibers: sensorial or afferent (that transmit impulses from different receptors of the skin, from the sense's organs or from the internal until the brain and the spinal cord), and motors o efferent (that transmit signals from the brain and the spinal cord until a muscle or a gland). According to its constitution, nerves can be myelinics or amyelinics. In those the neuritis of the nervous cells are covered by a sheath of myelin, that is separated to certain intervals (nodules of Ranvier) and above of it there is a neurilemma (or sheath of Schwann). In the unmyelinic the neuritis are covered directly by the neurilemma. The difference between ones and the others lays in the fact that amyelinics have a minor speed of communication than myelinics. Traditionally nerves are classified in cranial, rachidian and organ-vegetatives (sympathetic and parasympathetic).

NERVE STRUCTURE

spinal sensory ganglion

A

epineurium

nerve

perineurium

endoneurium

blood vessels

nervous fasciculus

myelin sheath

axon

SYNAPSE

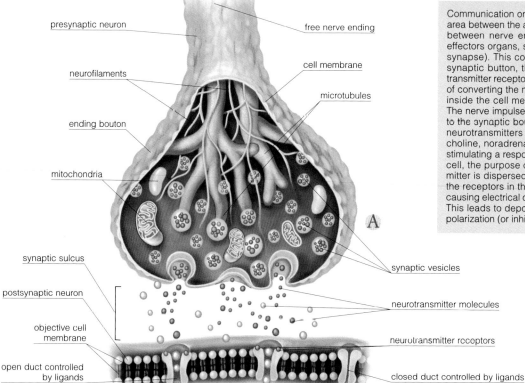

presynaptic neuron

free nerve ending

neurofilaments

cell membrane

microtubules

ending bouton

mitochondria

A

synaptic vesicles

synaptic sulcus

postsynaptic neuron

neurotransmitter molecules

objective cell membrane

neurotransmitter receptors

open duct controlled by ligands

closed duct controlled by ligands

synapse

Communication or transmission of nerve impulses area between the axon of one neuron and the den between nerve endings of a motor neuron and effectors organs, such as muscle (neuromuscular synapse). This communication area includes the synaptic button, the synaptic groove and neurotransmitter receptors. These impulses are in charge of converting the negative electric charge existing inside the cell membrane into a positive charge. The nerve impulse is transmitted through the axon to the synaptic boutons, releasing some chemical neurotransmitters (or substances, usually acetylcholine, noradrenalin, among others), capable of stimulating a response in the excited (presynaptic) cell, the purpose of the impulse. The neurotransmitter is dispersed along the synaptic cleft to join the receptors in the postsynaptic cell membrane, causing electrical changes in the postsynaptic cell. This leads to depolarization (excitation) or hyperpolarization (or inhibition).

NERVE (II). PERIPHERAL NERVE

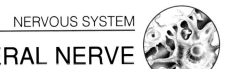

peripheral nerve

s called peripheral nerve to any nerve located out of the cen-
ral nervous system and connects with the brain to the spinal
cord through the receptors or peripheral effectors. The peripheral nerves are formed by beams of axons and dendrites.
Each peripheral nerve is wrapped by an epineurium that is a
ayer of connective tissue that surrounds it where are contained
the lymphatic sanguineous vessels. Each beam of axons and
dendrites is surrounded by the perineurium which means an
ntermediate layer of connective tissue. These layers establish
unions occluding each other.

The perineurium is isolated from elements of connective tissue
by nasal plaques, both in its internal and external surface.

The Schwann cells are big nucleated cells which cellular membrane surrounds in spiral the axons of peripheral myelinic neurons and are the origin of myelin. One only Schwann cell ela-
borates myelin between two nodules of Ranvier, besides of its
basal lamina these cells are surrounded by a net of thin reticular fibers that form the endoneurium.

The endoneurium is the most internal layer of the connective
tissue of the peripheral nerve and forms a layer interstitial
around each individual fiber outside the neurilemma.

The neurilemma is a fine membrane that wraps in spiral the
layers of myelin.

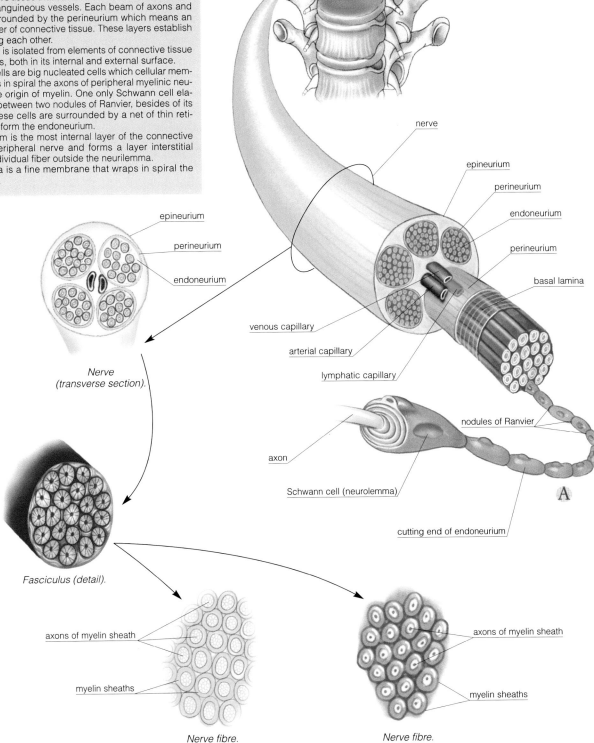

spinal cord

nerve

epineurium

perineurium

endoneurium

perineurium

basal lamina

venous capillary

arterial capillary

lymphatic capillary

nodules of Ranvier

axon

Schwann cell (neurolemma)

cutting end of endoneurium

A

557

epineurium

perineurium

endoneurium

*Nerve
(transverse section).*

Fasciculus (detail).

axons of myelin sheath

myelin sheaths

Nerve fibre.

axons of myelin sheath

myelin sheaths

Nerve fibre.

NERVE (III). NERVOUS TISSUE STRUCTURE

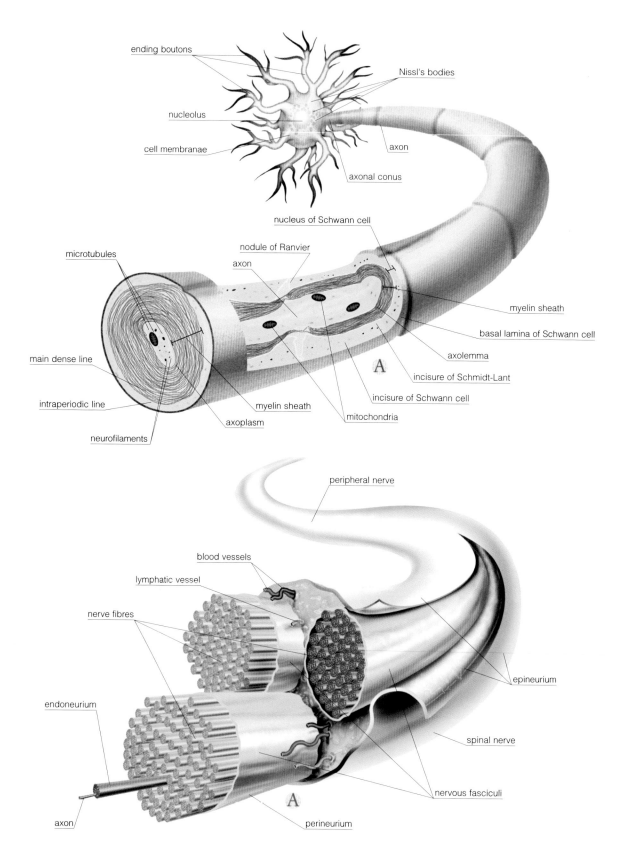

ending boutons

Nissl's bodies

nucleolus

cell membranae

axon

axonal conus

nucleus of Schwann cell

nodule of Ranvier

axon

microtubules

myelin sheath

basal lamina of Schwann cell

axolemma

incisure of Schmidt-Lant

incisure of Schwann cell

mitochondria

main dense line

intraperiodic line

myelin sheath

axoplasm

neurofilaments

A

558

peripheral nerve

blood vessels

lymphatic vessel

nerve fibres

epineurium

endoneurium

spinal nerve

nervous fasciculi

axon

perineurium

A

STRUCTURE of SPINAL NERVE

CENTRAL NERVOUS SYSTEM
CONSTITUENT PARTS of BRAIN

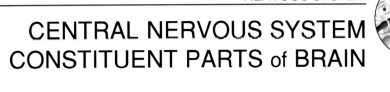

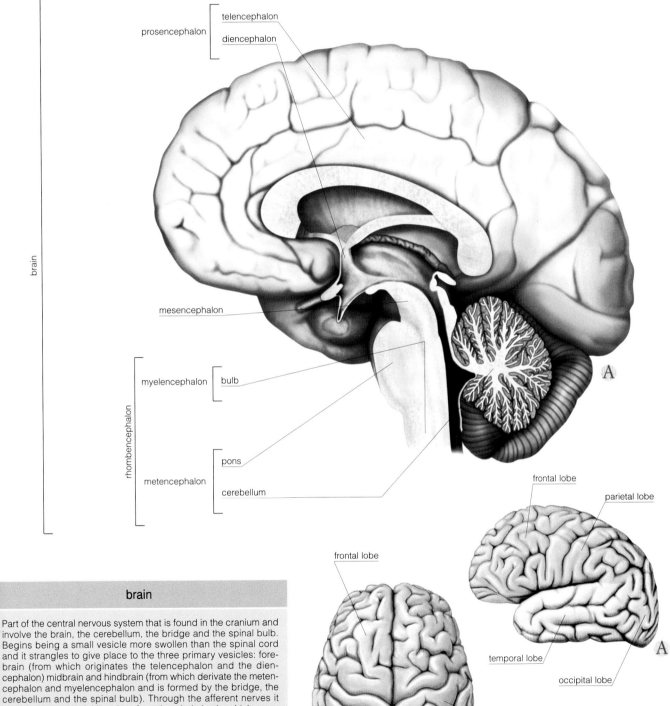

559

brain

Part of the central nervous system that is found in the cranium and involve the brain, the cerebellum, the bridge and the spinal bulb. Begins being a small vesicle more swollen than the spinal cord and it strangles to give place to the three primary vesicles: forebrain (from which originates the telencephalon and the diencephalon) midbrain and hindbrain (from which derivate the metencephalon and myelencephalon and is formed by the bridge, the cerebellum and the spinal bulb). Through the afferent nerves it receives the sensorial impulses from the whole body, which constitute the base of the perception. From here, its function is the control and coordination of the corporal activities through the reflex centers (cardiovascular, locomotive, respiratory system, etc.).The reception and sensitive integration, the production of language, the storing of the memory, the elaboration of thinking and the creation of emotions and feelings.

CEREBRUM (I)

SUPERIOR VIEW

cerebrum

Is the largest part of the encephalon, occupying almost the entire cranial cavity and resting upon the anterior and medial fossae of the base of the skull. It has a great longitudinal fissure that divides it into two hemispheres, or symmetrical halves, between which are the interhemispheric formations (corpus callosum, septum pellucidum, cerebral fornix and the sub thalamic region). Its outer surface presents a series of deep grooves (interlobular fissures) dividing it into four lobes (frontal, parietal, temporal, and occipital), which in turn are divided into other, less deep grooves (turns or circumvolutions). In sectional view, its surface presents the gray substance (composed by six cellular layers) and the deeper parts contain the white substance (formed by the axons of cortical cells, by those of the sensitive centripetal neurons, and by a group of axonomic connections). In the interior part of the hemispheres and the interhemispheric formations, there are intercommunicated cavities (ventricles) filled with cerebrospinal fluid. Although there is much that is unknown about the brain, it can be said that, in general, it is the center where motility and sensitivity of the human body are generated and where vegetative life is regulated; it is also the point of somatic insertion of everything related to the mind and feelings of human beings.

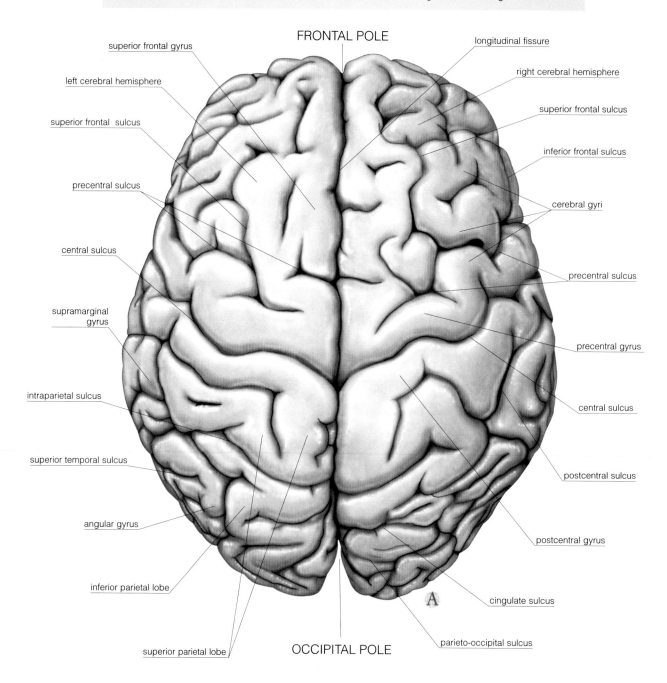

FRONTAL POLE

superior frontal gyrus

longitudinal fissure

left cerebral hemisphere

right cerebral hemisphere

superior frontal sulcus

superior frontal sulcus

inferior frontal sulcus

precentral sulcus

cerebral gyri

central sulcus

precentral sulcus

supramarginal gyrus

precentral gyrus

intraparietal sulcus

central sulcus

superior temporal sulcus

postcentral sulcus

angular gyrus

postcentral gyrus

inferior parietal lobe

cingulate sulcus

A

superior parietal lobe

OCCIPITAL POLE

parieto-occipital sulcus

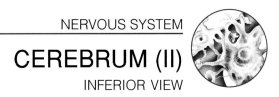

FRONTAL POLE

olfactory groove

longitudinal fissure

straight gyrus

olfactory bulb

orbital groove

olfactory nerve (or I cranial pair)

orbital gyri

optic nerve (or II cranial pair)

temporal pole

optic chiasm

uncus

anterior perforated substance

lateral sulcus

optic tract

inferior temporal sulcus

tuber cinereum

erior temporal gyrus

mammillary body
of hypothalamus

inferior border

posterior perforated
substance

rhinal sulcus

substantia nigra

ahippocampal gyrus

cerebral peduncle

inferior temporal gyrus

lateral geniculate body

occipitotemporal sulcus

red nucleus

eral occipitotemporal gyrus

medial geniculate body

pulvinar of thalamus

collateral sulcus

superior colliculus

medial occipitotemporal gyrus

cerebral aqueduct

splenium of corpus callosum

calcarine sulcus

apex of wedge

isthmus of cingulate gyrus

longitudinal fissure

OCCIPITAL POLE

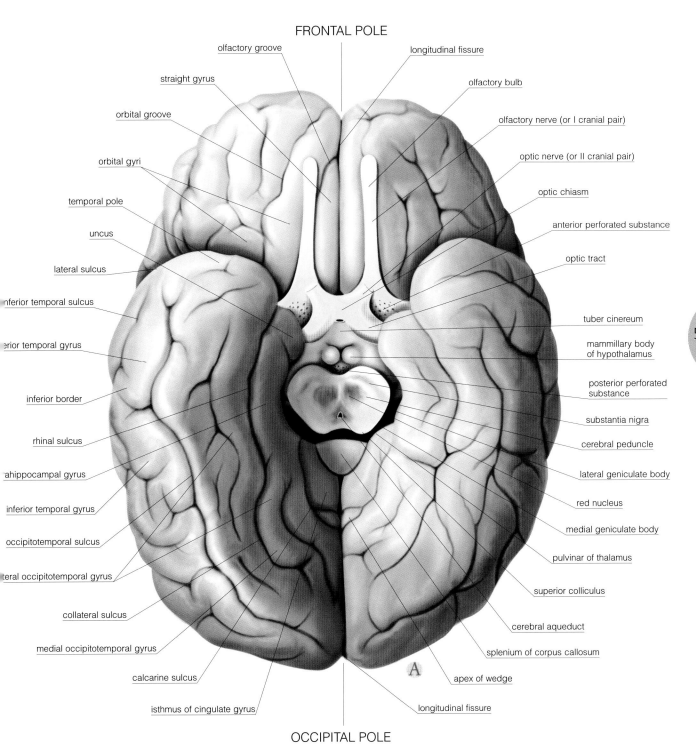

561

CEREBRUM (III)

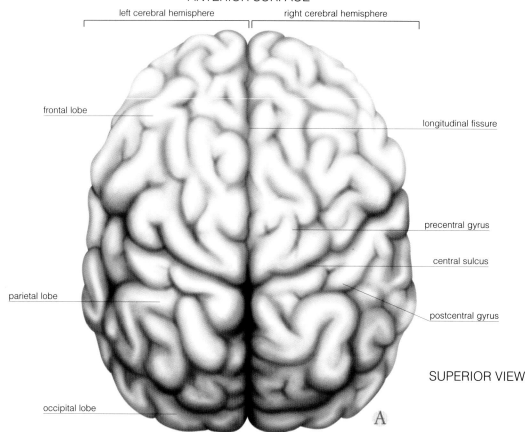

ANTERIOR SURFACE

left cerebral hemisphere   right cerebral hemisphere

frontal lobe

longitudinal fissure

precentral gyrus

central sulcus

parietal lobe

postcentral gyrus

SUPERIOR VIEW

occipital lobe

POSTERIOR SURFACE

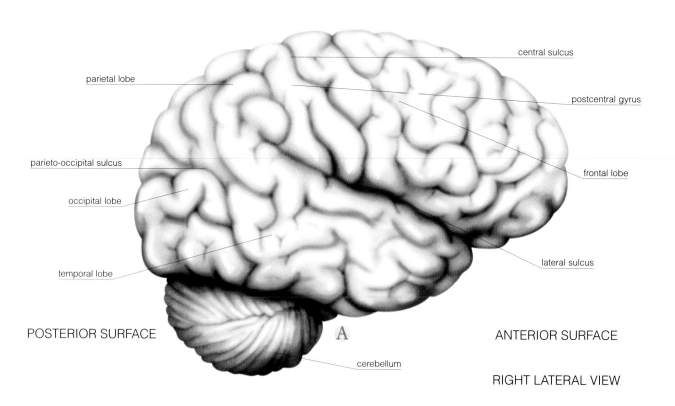

central sulcus

parietal lobe

postcentral gyrus

parieto-occipital sulcus

frontal lobe

occipital lobe

lateral sulcus

temporal lobe

POSTERIOR SURFACE

cerebellum

ANTERIOR SURFACE

RIGHT LATERAL VIEW

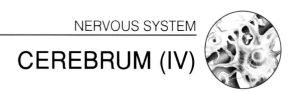

CEREBRUM (IV)

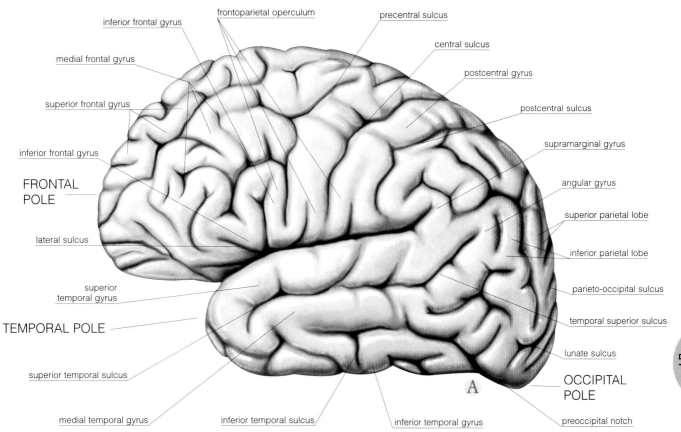

inferior frontal gyrus
frontoparietal operculum
precentral sulcus
central sulcus
medial frontal gyrus
postcentral gyrus
superior frontal gyrus
postcentral sulcus
inferior frontal gyrus
supramarginal gyrus
FRONTAL
POLE
angular gyrus
superior parietal lobe
lateral sulcus
inferior parietal lobe
superior
temporal gyrus
parieto-occipital sulcus
TEMPORAL POLE
temporal superior sulcus
superior temporal sulcus
lunate sulcus
OCCIPITAL
POLE
medial temporal gyrus
inferior temporal sulcus
inferior temporal gyrus
preoccipital notch

563

LATERAL VIEW

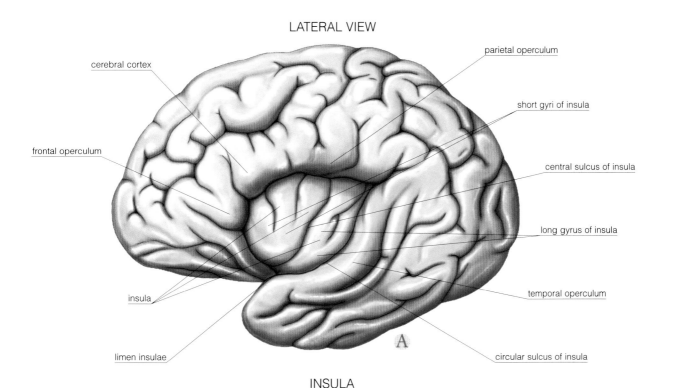

cerebral cortex
parietal operculum
short gyri of insula
frontal operculum
central sulcus of insula
long gyrus of insula
insula
temporal operculum
limen insulae
circular sulcus of insula

INSULA

CEREBRUM (V). VENTRICLES

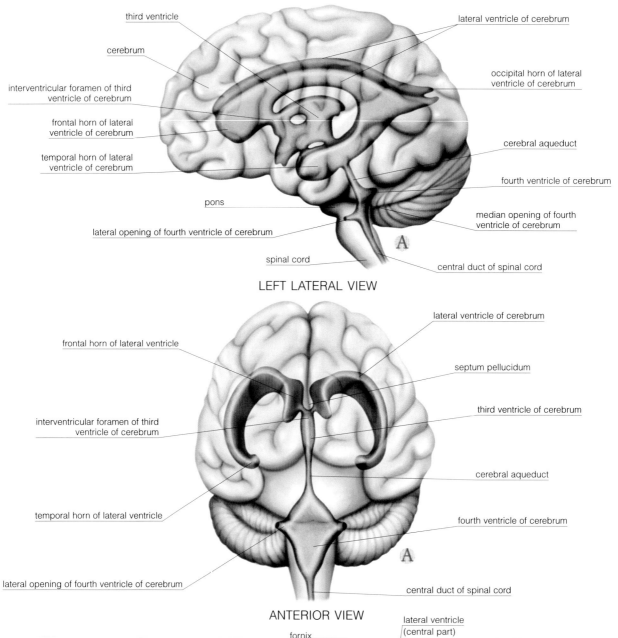

third ventricle

cerebrum

interventricular foramen of third ventricle of cerebrum

frontal horn of lateral ventricle of cerebrum

temporal horn of lateral ventricle of cerebrum

pons

lateral opening of fourth ventricle of cerebrum

spinal cord

lateral ventricle of cerebrum

occipital horn of lateral ventricle of cerebrum

cerebral aqueduct

fourth ventricle of cerebrum

median opening of fourth ventricle of cerebrum

central duct of spinal cord

LEFT LATERAL VIEW

frontal horn of lateral ventricle

interventricular foramen of third ventricle of cerebrum

temporal horn of lateral ventricle

lateral opening of fourth ventricle of cerebrum

lateral ventricle of cerebrum

septum pellucidum

third ventricle of cerebrum

cerebral aqueduct

fourth ventricle of cerebrum

central duct of spinal cord

ANTERIOR VIEW

564

VENTRICULAR SYSTEM

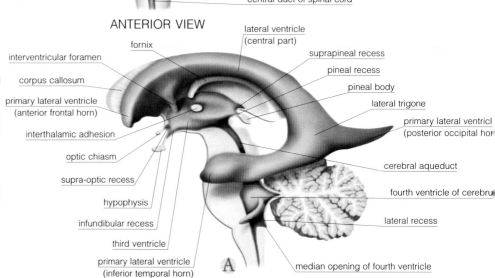

fornix

interventricular foramen

corpus callosum

primary lateral ventricle (anterior frontal horn)

interthalamic adhesion

optic chiasm

supra-optic recess

hypophysis

infundibular recess

third ventricle

primary lateral ventricle (inferior temporal horn)

lateral ventricle (central part)

suprapineal recess

pineal recess

pineal body

lateral trigone

primary lateral ventricl (posterior occipital hor

cerebral aqueduct

fourth ventricle of cerebru

lateral recess

median opening of fourth ventricle

cerebral ventricles

The ventricles of the cerebrum are cavities of the brain that contains cerebrospinal liquid. Have its origin in the widening that forms the light of the embryonic neural tube. They communicate each other and with the ependymal channel of the spinal cord, its internal face is covered by ependymal cells or cells of the neuroglia and contains the formations choroid (plexus and fabrics).

CEREBRUM (VI)

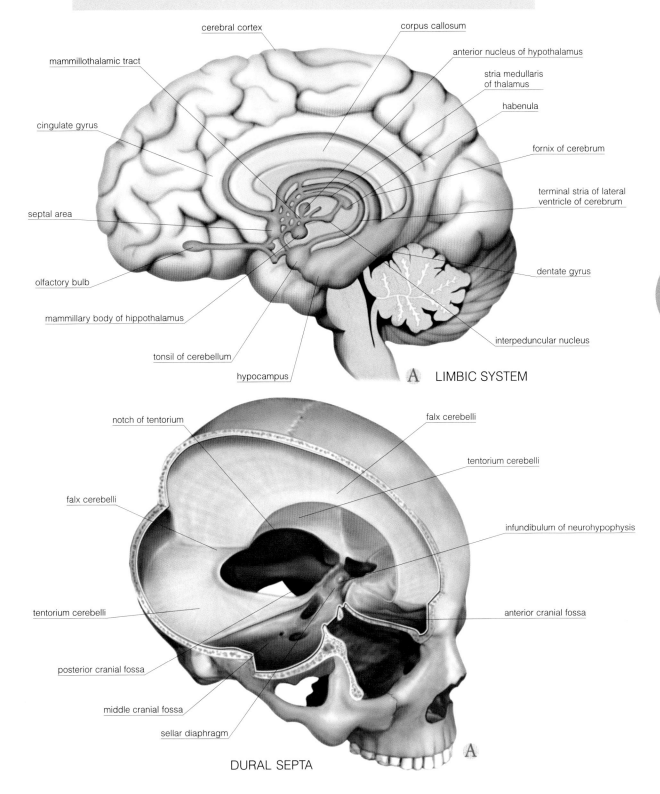

limbic system

Set of structures of the brain that is consists by the hippocampus, the tonsils, turner teeth, the cingulum and the fornix, septal region, etc. Involved in the olfactory sensations, in the autonomic nervous system and endocrine and is very important in other activities such as certain aspects of the emotion and the modulation of the affected relations of the behavior: thus, activated by felt motivation or sexual arousal.

cerebral cortex

corpus callosum

mammillothalamic tract

anterior nucleus of hypothalamus

stria medullaris of thalamus

habenula

cingulate gyrus

fornix of cerebrum

terminal stria of lateral ventricle of cerebrum

septal area

dentate gyrus

olfactory bulb

mammillary body of hippothalamus

interpeduncular nucleus

tonsil of cerebellum

hypocampus

A LIMBIC SYSTEM

notch of tentorium

falx cerebelli

falx cerebelli

tentorium cerebelli

infundibulum of neurohypophysis

tentorium cerebelli

anterior cranial fossa

posterior cranial fossa

middle cranial fossa

sellar diaphragm

A

DURAL SEPTA

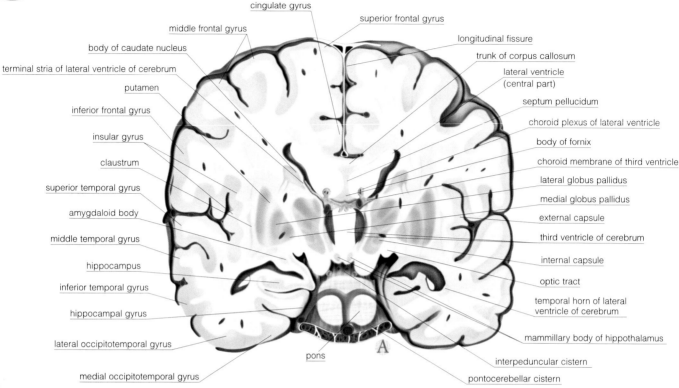

cingulate gyrus
superior frontal gyrus
middle frontal gyrus
longitudinal fissure
body of caudate nucleus
trunk of corpus callosum
terminal stria of lateral ventricle of cerebrum
lateral ventricle (central part)
putamen
septum pellucidum
inferior frontal gyrus
choroid plexus of lateral ventricle
insular gyrus
body of fornix
claustrum
choroid membrane of third ventricle
superior temporal gyrus
lateral globus pallidus
amygdaloid body
medial globus pallidus
middle temporal gyrus
external capsule
hippocampus
third ventricle of cerebrum
inferior temporal gyrus
internal capsule
hippocampal gyrus
optic tract
lateral occipitotemporal gyrus
temporal horn of lateral ventricle of cerebrum
medial occipitotemporal gyrus
mammillary body of hippothalamus
pons
interpeduncular cistern
pontocerebellar cistern
A

FRONTAL SECTION at the HEIGHT of MAMMILARY BODIES

566

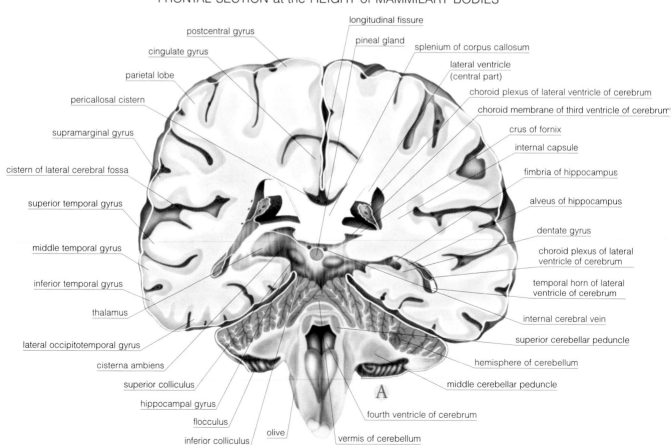

postcentral gyrus
longitudinal fissure
pineal gland
cingulate gyrus
splenium of corpus callosum
parietal lobe
lateral ventricle (central part)
pericallosal cistern
choroid plexus of lateral ventricle of cerebrum
supramarginal gyrus
choroid membrane of third ventricle of cerebrum
crus of fornix
cistern of lateral cerebral fossa
internal capsule
superior temporal gyrus
fimbria of hippocampus
middle temporal gyrus
alveus of hippocampus
inferior temporal gyrus
dentate gyrus
thalamus
choroid plexus of lateral ventricle of cerebrum
lateral occipitotemporal gyrus
temporal horn of lateral ventricle of cerebrum
cisterna ambiens
internal cerebral vein
superior colliculus
superior cerebellar peduncle
hippocampal gyrus
hemisphere of cerebellum
flocculus
middle cerebellar peduncle
inferior colliculus
olive
fourth ventricle of cerebrum
vermis of cerebellum
A

FRONTAL SECTION at the HEIGHT of PINEAL GLAND and FOURTH VENTRICLE

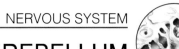

CEREBRUM (VIII). TRUNK of BRAIN and CEREBELLUM

INFERIOR VIEW

FRONTAL LOBE

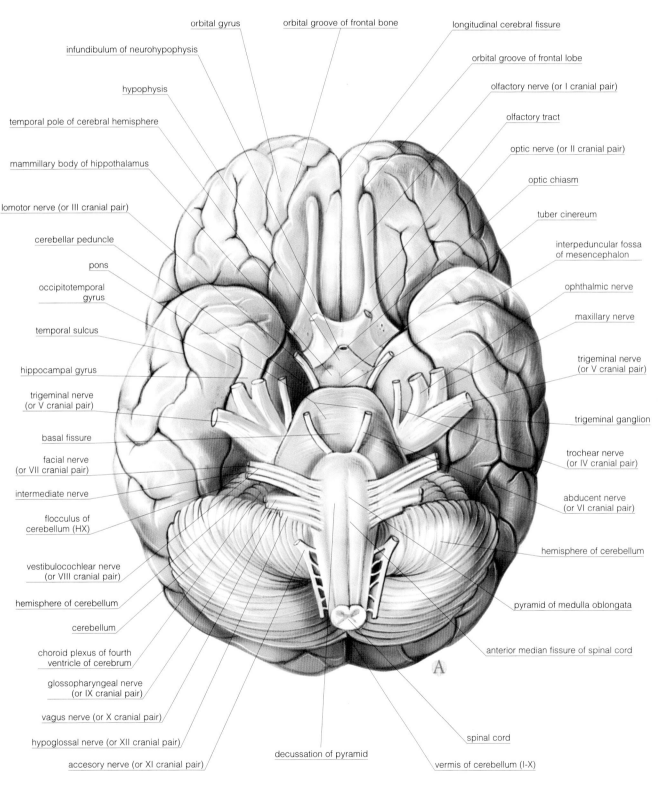

orbital gyrus

orbital groove of frontal bone

longitudinal cerebral fissure

infundibulum of neurohypophysis

orbital groove of frontal lobe

olfactory nerve (or I cranial pair)

hypophysis

olfactory tract

temporal pole of cerebral hemisphere

optic nerve (or II cranial pair)

mammillary body of hippothalamus

optic chiasm

lomotor nerve (or III cranial pair)

tuber cinereum

cerebellar peduncle

interpeduncular fossa of mesencephalon

pons

ophthalmic nerve

occipitotemporal gyrus

maxillary nerve

temporal sulcus

567

trigeminal nerve (or V cranial pair)

hippocampal gyrus

trigeminal nerve (or V cranial pair)

trigeminal ganglion

basal fissure

trochear nerve (or IV cranial pair)

facial nerve (or VII cranial pair)

intermediate nerve

abducent nerve (or VI cranial pair)

flocculus of cerebellum (HX)

hemisphere of cerebellum

vestibulocochlear nerve (or VIII cranial pair)

hemisphere of cerebellum

pyramid of medulla oblongata

cerebellum

choroid plexus of fourth ventricle of cerebrum

anterior median fissure of spinal cord

glossopharyngeal nerve (or IX cranial pair)

vagus nerve (or X cranial pair)

hypoglossal nerve (or XII cranial pair)

spinal cord

accesory nerve (or XI cranial pair)

decussation of pyramid

vermis of cerebellum (I-X)

A

OCCIPITAL LOBE

CEREBRUM (IX). BRAIN. TRUNK

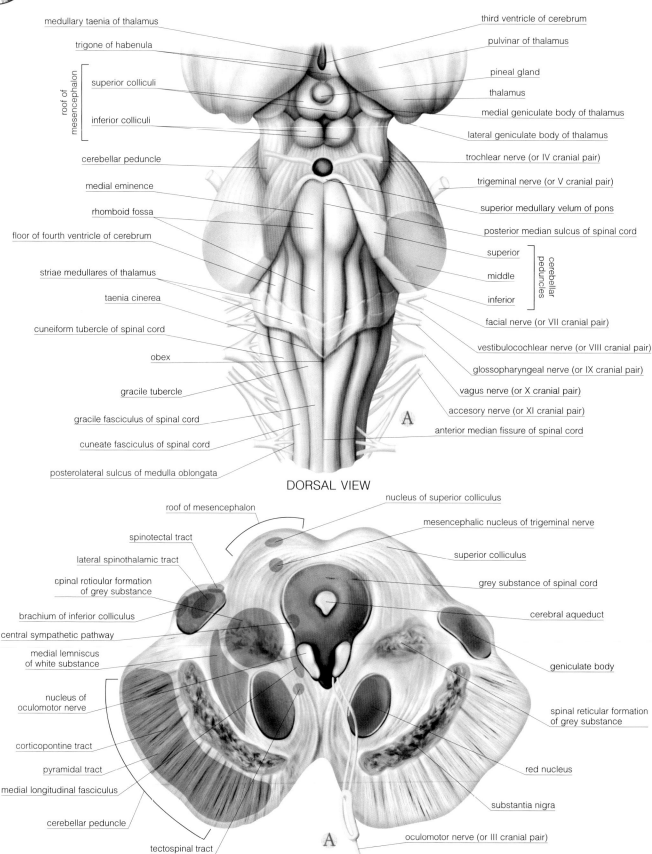

medullary taenia of thalamus

trigone of habenula

roof of mesencephalon

superior colliculi

inferior colliculi

cerebellar peduncle

medial eminence

rhomboid fossa

floor of fourth ventricle of cerebrum

striae medullares of thalamus

taenia cinerea

cuneiform tubercle of spinal cord

obex

gracile tubercle

gracile fasciculus of spinal cord

cuneate fasciculus of spinal cord

posterolateral sulcus of medulla oblongata

third ventricle of cerebrum

pulvinar of thalamus

pineal gland

thalamus

medial geniculate body of thalamus

lateral geniculate body of thalamus

trochlear nerve (or IV cranial pair)

trigeminal nerve (or V cranial pair)

superior medullary velum of pons

posterior median sulcus of spinal cord

superior
middle
inferior
cerebellar peduncles

facial nerve (or VII cranial pair)

vestibulocochlear nerve (or VIII cranial pair)

glossopharyngeal nerve (or IX cranial pair)

vagus nerve (or X cranial pair)

accesory nerve (or XI cranial pair)

anterior median fissure of spinal cord

DORSAL VIEW

roof of mesencephalon

spinotectal tract

lateral spinothalamic tract

spinal reticular formation of grey substance

brachium of inferior colliculus

central sympathetic pathway

medial lemniscus of white substance

nucleus of oculomotor nerve

corticopontine tract

pyramidal tract

medial longitudinal fasciculus

cerebellar peduncle

tectospinal tract

nucleus of superior colliculus

mesencephalic nucleus of trigeminal nerve

superior colliculus

grey substance of spinal cord

cerebral aqueduct

geniculate body

spinal reticular formation of grey substance

red nucleus

substantia nigra

oculomotor nerve (or III cranial pair)

TRANSVERSE SECTION

568

CEREBRUM (X). BRAIN and HYPOTHALAMUS

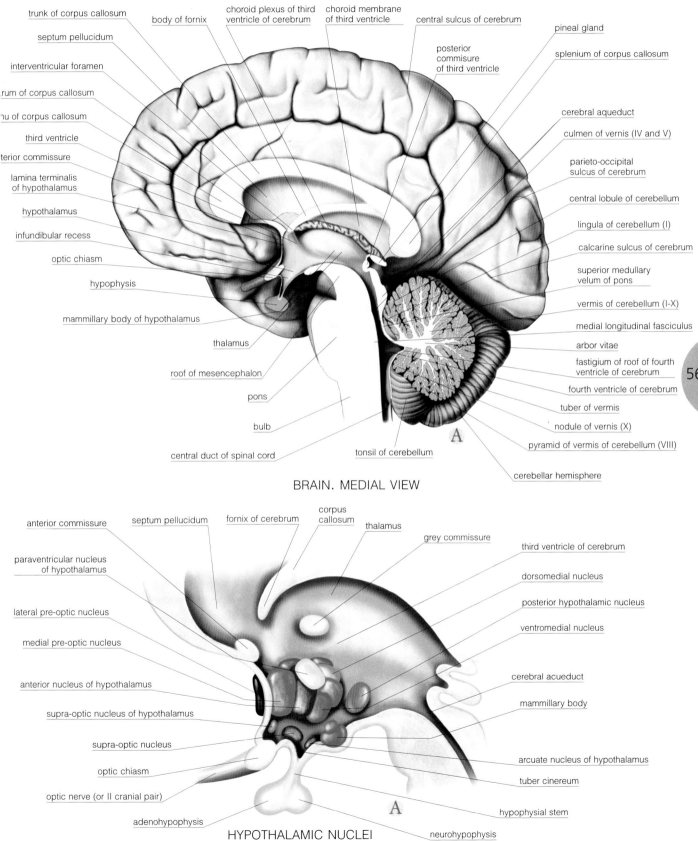

trunk of corpus callosum

septum pellucidum

interventricular foramen

rum of corpus callosum

nu of corpus callosum

third ventricle

terior commissure

lamina terminalis
of hypothalamus

hypothalamus

infundibular recess

optic chiasm

hypophysis

mammillary body of hypothalamus

thalamus

roof of mesencephalon

pons

bulb

central duct of spinal cord

body of fornix

choroid plexus of third
ventricle of cerebrum

choroid membrane
of third ventricle

central sulcus of cerebrum

posterior
commisure
of third ventricle

pineal gland

splenium of corpus callosum

cerebral aqueduct

culmen of vernis (IV and V)

parieto-occipital
sulcus of cerebrum

central lobule of cerebellum

lingula of cerebellum (I)

calcarine sulcus of cerebrum

superior medullary
velum of pons

vermis of cerebellum (I-X)

medial longitudinal fasciculus

arbor vitae

fastigium of roof of fourth
ventricle of cerebrum

fourth ventricle of cerebrum

tuber of vermis

nodule of vernis (X)

pyramid of vermis of cerebellum (VIII)

tonsil of cerebellum

cerebellar hemisphere

569

BRAIN. MEDIAL VIEW

anterior commissure

paraventricular nucleus
of hypothalamus

lateral pre-optic nucleus

medial pre-optic nucleus

anterior nucleus of hypothalamus

supra-optic nucleus of hypothalamus

supra-optic nucleus

optic chiasm

optic nerve (or II cranial pair)

adenohypophysis

septum pellucidum

fornix of cerebrum

corpus
callosum

thalamus

grey commissure

third ventricle of cerebrum

dorsomedial nucleus

posterior hypothalamic nucleus

ventromedial nucleus

cerebral acueduct

mammillary body

arcuate nucleus of hypothalamus

tuber cinereum

hypophysial stem

hypophysial stem

HYPOTHALAMIC NUCLEI

neurohypophysis

CRANIUM (I)
PROJECTION of MORE IMPORTANT STRUCTURES (I)

570

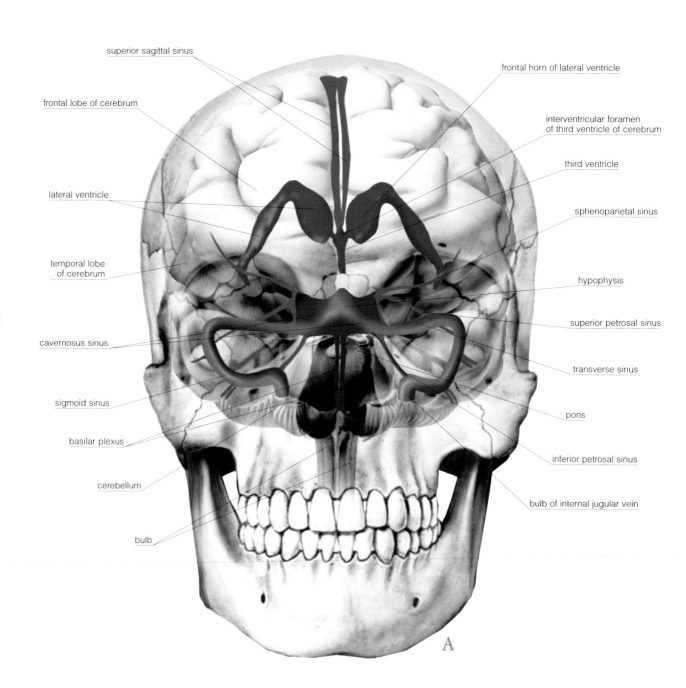

superior sagittal sinus

frontal horn of lateral ventricle

frontal lobe of cerebrum

interventricular foramen
of third ventricle of cerebrum

third ventricle

lateral ventricle

sphenoparietal sinus

temporal lobe
of cerebrum

hypophysis

cavernosus sinus

superior petrosal sinus

transverse sinus

sigmoid sinus

pons

basilar plexus

inferior petrosal sinus

cerebellum

bulb of internal jugular vein

bulb

A

CRANIUM (II)
PROJECTION of MORE IMPORTANT STRUCTURES (II)

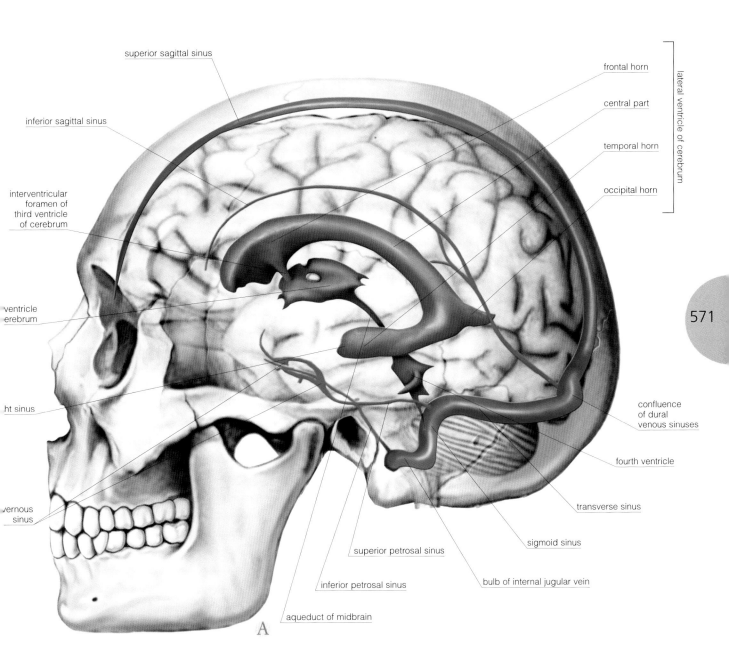

superior sagittal sinus

inferior sagittal sinus

interventricular foramen of third ventricle of cerebrum

ventricle erebrum

ht sinus

vernous sinus

frontal horn

central part

temporal horn

occipital horn

lateral ventricle of cerebrum

571

confluence of dural venous sinuses

fourth ventricle

transverse sinus

sigmoid sinus

bulb of internal jugular vein

superior petrosal sinus

inferior petrosal sinus

aqueduct of midbrain

A

RELATIONS of HYPOTHALAMUS and ADENOHYPOPHYSIS

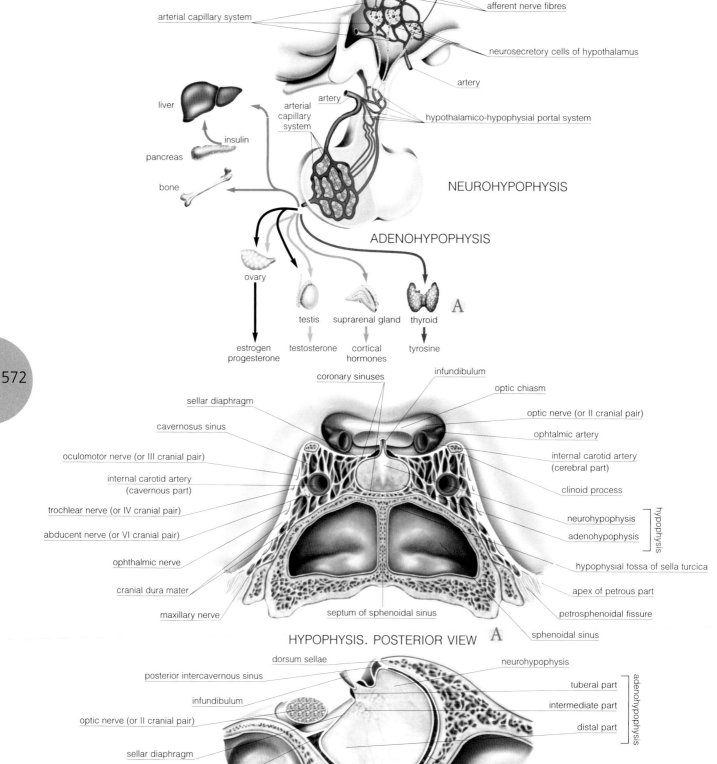

arterial capillary system

afferent nerve fibres

neurosecretory cells of hypothalamus

artery

liver

artery

arterial capillary system

hypothalamico-hypophysial portal system

insulin

pancreas

bone

NEUROHYPOPHYSIS

ADENOHYPOPHYSIS

ovary

testis

suprarenal gland

thyroid

estrogen progesterone

testosterone

cortical hormones

tyrosine

572

coronary sinuses

infundibulum

sellar diaphragm

optic chiasm

optic nerve (or II cranial pair)

cavernosus sinus

ophtalmic artery

oculomotor nerve (or III cranial pair)

internal carotid artery (cerebral part)

internal carotid artery (cavernous part)

clinoid process

trochlear nerve (or IV cranial pair)

neurohypophysis

hypophysis

adenohypophysis

abducent nerve (or VI cranial pair)

ophthalmic nerve

hypophysial fossa of sella turcica

cranial dura mater

apex of petrous part

maxillary nerve

septum of sphenoidal sinus

petrosphenoidal fissure

sphenoidal sinus

HYPOPHYSIS. POSTERIOR VIEW

dorsum sellae

neurohypophysis

posterior intercavernous sinus

tuberal part

adenohypophysis

infundibulum

intermediate part

optic nerve (or II cranial pair)

distal part

sellar diaphragm

anterior intercavernous sinus

sella turcica

sphenoidal sinus

sphenoidal bone

HYPOPHYSIS. MEDIOSAGITTAL SECTION

CENTRAL NERVOUS SYSTEM
HYPOTHALAMUS and HYPOPHYSIS

hypothalamus

Part of the central nervous system, which is, formed, from the development of the ventral portion of the diencephalon and that forms the floor and part of the lateral wall of the third ventricle. Has a conic form with the lower vortex and is found under the thalamus and beside the subthalamic areas. Involves the tuber cinereum, the infundibulum, the optic chiasm, the mammillary bodies and the neurohypophysis and contains different nucleus. Is the center of integration and exteriorization of the motor impulses that produce the emotional expression. In there is produced the hormonal liberation factors that act on the adenohypophysis and the neurohypophysis. Stimulating in them the production of multiple and important hormones and take part in different functions of the human body: corporal temperature regulation, hidrosaline metabolism and the immediate principles, sexual activity, food ingestion (provoking the sensation of hanger), etc. The hypothalamus constitutes a determinant center for the integration of the sympathetic and parasympathetic activities of the organism.

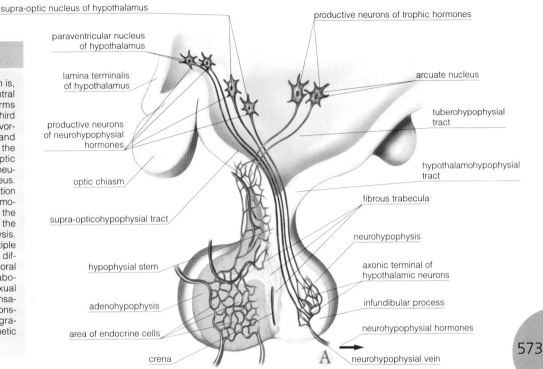

HYPOTHALAMIC-PITUITARY AXIS

573

hypophysis

Unique structure, small and ovoid shape, located in the interior of the cranium, in the cavity of the sphenoid bone known as sella turcica. Consists in two parts or lobes: anterior (or adenohypophysis), that comes from the hypofyseal diverticle (or Ratke's bag), and posterior (or neurohypophysis) formed by the nervous tissue of the infundibular stalk. Measures about 1.3cm long,1cm wide and 0.5cm thick and weights about 0.6g. Is called master gland of the body because of the great variety of hormones that segregates and, for the influence that they have in the whole set of the organism. The adenohypohysis segregate the hormones somatotropin (regulates the cellular division and the synthesis of proteins for the growth), adenocorticotropic (regulates the function of the suprarenal cortex). Thyrotropic (regulates the function of the thyroid), prolactin (induces the production of maternal milk), gonadotropic (follicle-stimulating and luteinizing that affects the gonads). The neurohypophysis segregates the hormones oxitocine (acts on the smooth muscle of the uterus) and the antidiuretic (increases the reabsorption of water by the renal tubules).

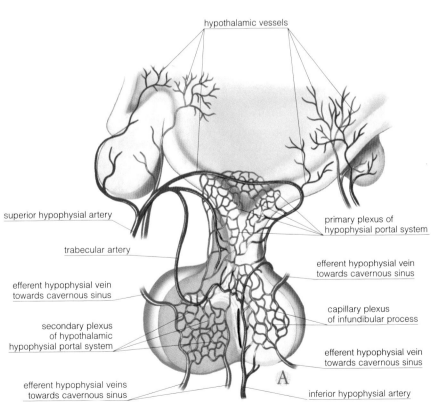

VASCULAR NETWORK

BASAL NUCLEI

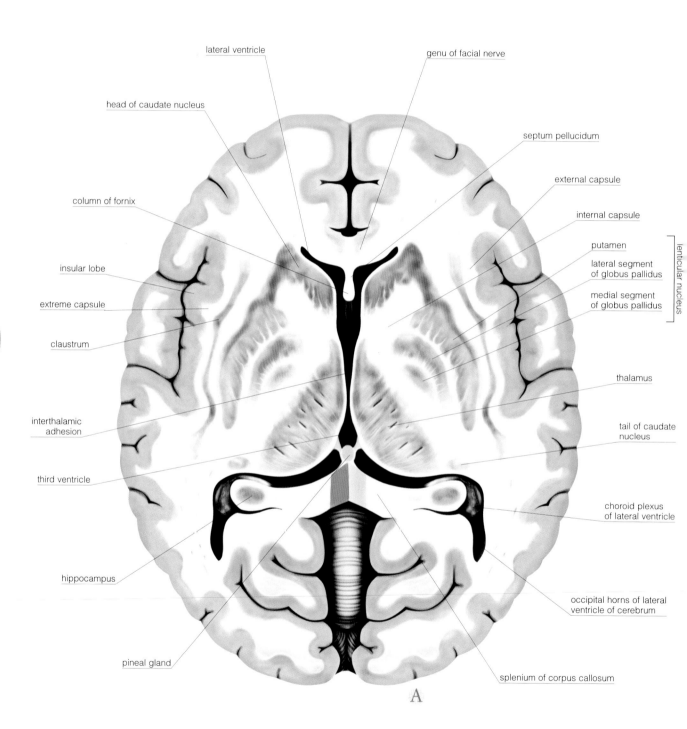

lateral ventricle

genu of facial nerve

head of caudate nucleus

septum pellucidum

external capsule

column of fornix

internal capsule

putamen

lateral segment of globus pallidus

medial segment of globus pallidus

lenticular nucleus

insular lobe

extreme capsule

claustrum

thalamus

interthalamic adhesion

tail of caudate nucleus

third ventricle

choroid plexus of lateral ventricle

hippocampus

occipital horns of lateral ventricle of cerebrum

pineal gland

splenium of corpus callosum

A

574

FORNIX and BASAL NUCLEI

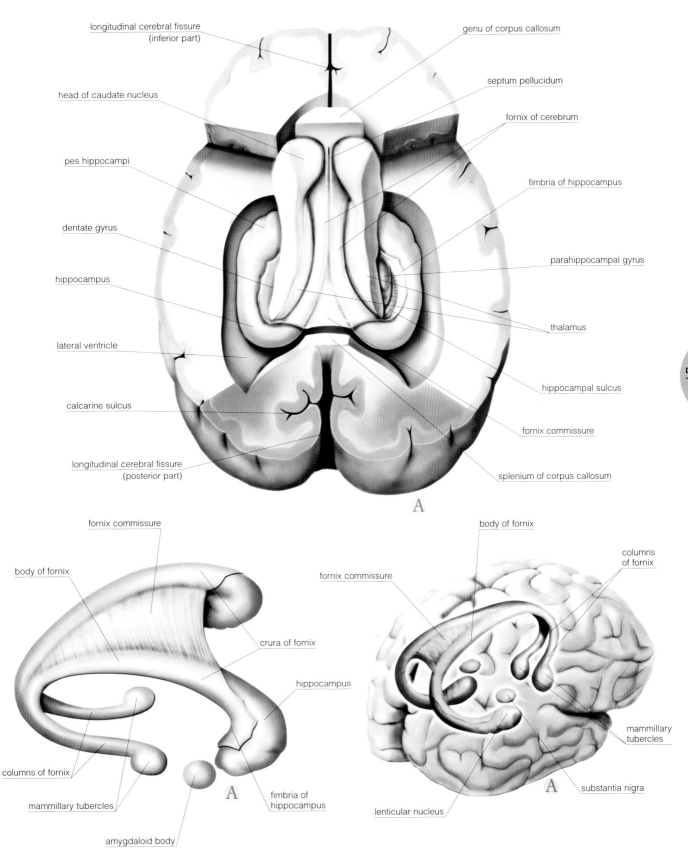

longitudinal cerebral fissure
(inferior part)

genu of corpus callosum

head of caudate nucleus

septum pellucidum

fornix of cerebrum

pes hippocampi

fimbria of hippocampus

dentate gyrus

parahippocampal gyrus

hippocampus

thalamus

lateral ventricle

hippocampal sulcus

calcarine sulcus

fornix commissure

longitudinal cerebral fissure
(posterior part)

splenium of corpus callosum

A

fornix commissure

body of fornix

body of fornix

columns
of fornix

fornix commissure

crura of fornix

hippocampus

columns of fornix

mammillary
tubercles

mammillary tubercles

A

fimbria of
hippocampus

lenticular nucleus

substantia nigra

A

amygdaloid body

575

THALAMUS

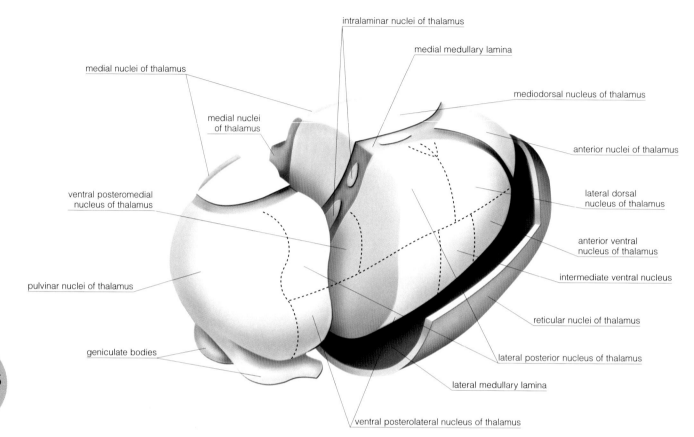

intralaminar nuclei of thalamus

medial medullary lamina

medial nuclei of thalamus

mediodorsal nucleus of thalamus

medial nuclei
of thalamus

anterior nuclei of thalamus

ventral posteromedial
nucleus of thalamus

lateral dorsal
nucleus of thalamus

anterior ventral
nucleus of thalamus

intermediate ventral nucleus

pulvinar nuclei of thalamus

reticular nuclei of thalamus

lateral posterior nucleus of thalamus

geniculate bodies

lateral medullary lamina

ventral posterolateral nucleus of thalamus

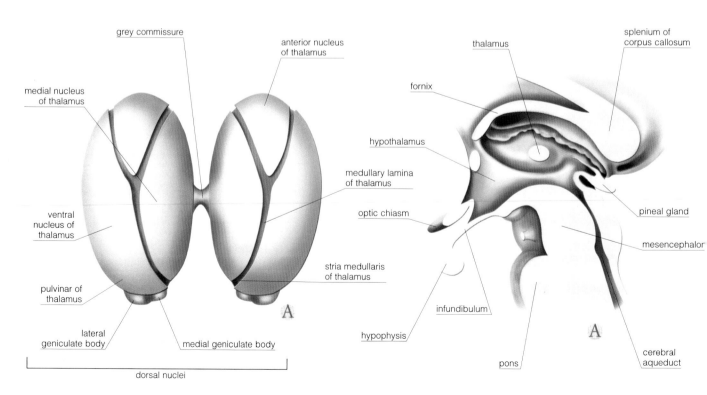

grey commissure

anterior nucleus
of thalamus

splenium of
corpus callosum

thalamus

medial nucleus
of thalamus

fornix

hypothalamus

medullary lamina
of thalamus

ventral
nucleus of
thalamus

optic chiasm

pineal gland

stria medullaris
of thalamus

mesencephalor

pulvinar of
thalamus

infundibulum

cerebral
aqueduct

lateral
geniculate body

medial geniculate body

hypophysis

pons

A

dorsal nuclei

A

HYPOPHYSIS. HYPOPHYSIAL HORMONES
and TARGET ORGANS

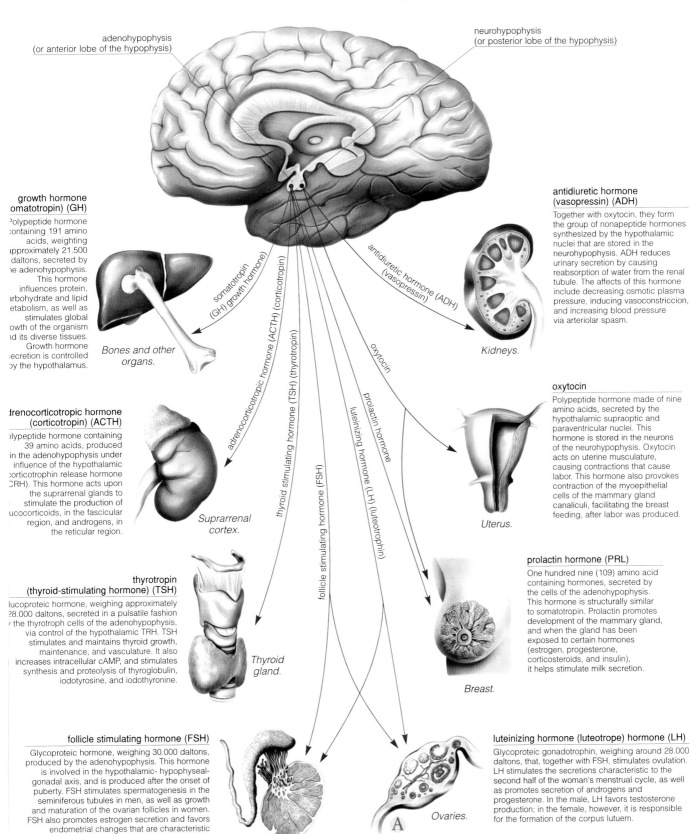

adenohypophysis
(or anterior lobe of the hypophysis)

neurohypophysis
(or posterior lobe of the hypophysis)

growth hormone (somatotropin) (GH)

Polypeptide hormone containing 191 amino acids, weighting approximately 21.500 daltons, secreted by the adenohypophysis. This hormone influences protein, carbohydrate and lipid metabolism, as well as stimulates global growth of the organism and its diverse tissues.
Growth hormone secretion is controlled by the hypothalamus.

Bones and other organs.

adrenocorticotropic hormone (corticotropin) (ACTH)

Polypeptide hormone containing 39 amino acids, produced in the adenohypophysis under influence of the hypothalamic corticotrophin release hormone CRH). This hormone acts upon the suprarrenal glands to stimulate the production of glucocorticoids, in the fascicular region, and androgens, in the reticular region.

Suprarrenal cortex.

thyrotropin (thyroid-stimulating hormone) (TSH)

Glucoproteic hormone, weighing approximately 28.000 daltons, secreted in a pulsatile fashion by the thyrotroph cells of the adenohypophysis, via control of the hypothalamic TRH. TSH stimulates and maintains thyroid growth, maintenance, and vasculature. It also increases intracellular cAMP, and stimulates synthesis and proteolysis of thyroglobulin, iodotyrosine, and iodothyronine.

Thyroid gland.

follicle stimulating hormone (FSH)

Glycoproteic hormone, weighing 30.000 daltons, produced by the adenohypophysis. This hormone is involved in the hypothalamic- hypophyseal-gonadal axis, and is produced after the onset of puberty. FSH stimulates spermatogenesis in the seminiferous tubules in men, as well as growth and maturation of the ovarian follicles in women. FSH also promotes estrogen secretion and favors endometrial changes that are characteristic of the first half of a woman's menstrual cycle.

Testes.

somatotropin (GH) growth hormone)

adrenocorticotropic hormone (ACTH) (corticotropin)

thyroid stimulating hormone (TSH) (thyrotropin)

antidiuretic hormone (ADH) (vasopressin)

oxytocin

prolactin hormone

luteinizing hormone (LH) (luteotrophin)

follicle stimulating hormone (FSH)

antidiuretic hormone (vasopressin) (ADH)

Together with oxytocin, they form the group of nonapeptide hormones synthesized by the hypothalamic nuclei that are stored in the neurohypophysis. ADH reduces urinary secretion by causing reabsorption of water from the renal tubule. The affects of this hormone include decreasing osmotic plasma pressure, inducing vasoconstriccion, and increasing blood pressure via arteriolar spasm.

Kidneys.

577

oxytocin

Polypeptide hormone made of nine amino acids, secreted by the hypothalamic supraoptic and paraventricular nuclei. This hormone is stored in the neurons of the neurohypophysis. Oxytocin acts on uterine musculature, causing contractions that cause labor. This hormone also provokes contraction of the myoepithelial cells of the mammary gland canaliculi, facilitating the breast feeding, after labor was produced.

Uterus.

prolactin hormone (PRL)

One hundred nine (109) amino acid containing hormones, secreted by the cells of the adenohypophysis. This hormone is structurally similar to somatotropin. Prolactin promotes development of the mammary gland, and when the gland has been exposed to certain hormones (estrogen, progesterone, corticosteroids, and insulin), it helps stimulate milk secretion.

Breast.

luteinizing hormone (luteotrope) hormone (LH)

Glycoproteic gonadotrophin, weighing around 28.000 daltons, that, together with FSH, stimulates ovulation. LH stimulates the secretions characteristic to the second half of the woman's menstrual cycle, as well as promotes secretion of androgens and progesterone. In the male, LH favors testosterone production; in the female, however, it is responsible for the formation of the corpus lutuem.

Ovaries.

CEREBRAL CORTEX
MOTOR and SENSORY FUNCTIONAL AREAS

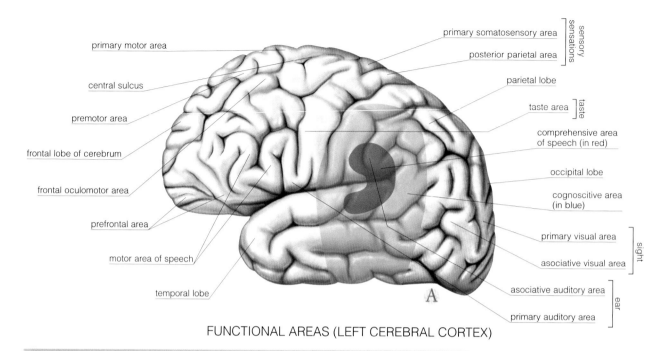

primary motor area

central sulcus

premotor area

frontal lobe of cerebrum

frontal oculomotor area

prefrontal area

motor area of speech

temporal lobe

primary somatosensory area — sensory sensations

posterior parietal area

parietal lobe

taste area — taste

comprehensive area of speech (in red)

occipital lobe

cognoscitive area (in blue)

primary visual area — sight

asociative visual area

asociative auditory area — ear

primary auditory area

A

FUNCTIONAL AREAS (LEFT CEREBRAL CORTEX)

cerebral cortex

Superficial layer of gray matter, about 3mm thick, which covers the entire surface of each cerebral hemisphere. It is folded, forming gyri delimited by sulci and consists mainly of cell bodies of neurons. The neocortex (newest portion) has a laminar organization composed of six layers of fibers (molecular, external granular -or small pyramids layer-, external pyramidal, internal granular, internal pyramidal or nodal, and multiform layers). The allocortex or heterotypic cortex (original and oldest part), contains fewer layers. According to local differences of this structure, the German neuro-

logist Korbinian Brodmann (1869-1918) distinguished 47 areas in the cerebral cortex, which can classified into three great categories: motor area (low development of the internal granular layer -agranular area- and prominent pyramidal layers), sensitive area (important development of the internal granular layer; includes the granular and somatosensory areas, auditory and visual) and association area. The cerebral cortex is responsible for the higher mental functions and behavioral movements as well as the association and integration of these functions.

motor areas (motor cortex)

The primary motor area is located in the procentral gyrus of the frontal lobe, in front of the central sulcus. The secondary motor area includes the premotor cortex and supplementary motor area.

sensory areas (somatosensory cortex)

Include the primary and secondary somatosensory areas, located in the anterior portion of the parietal lobe.

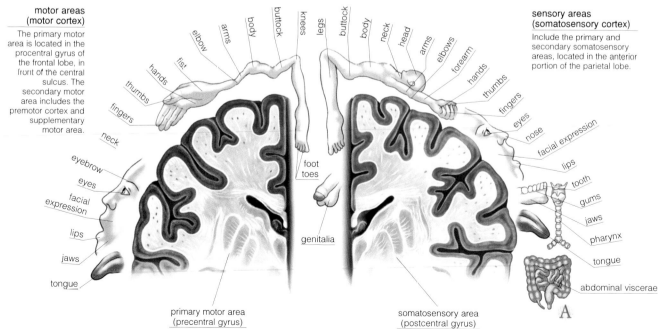

elbow, arms, body, buttock, knees, legs, buttock, body, neck, head, arms, elbows, forearm, hands, thumbs, fingers, eyes, nose, facial expression, lips, tooth, gums, jaws, pharynx, tongue, abdominal viscerae

fist, hands, thumbs, fingers, neck, eyebrow, eyes, facial expression, lips, jaws, tongue, foot, toes, genitalia

primary motor area (precentral gyrus)

somatosensory area (postcentral gyrus)

A

MOTOR and SENSITIVE AREAS of the CEREBRAL CORTEX

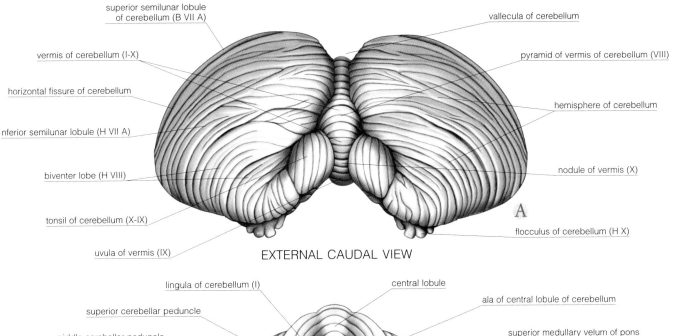

superior semilunar lobule of cerebellum (B VII A)

vermis of cerebellum (I-X)

horizontal fissure of cerebellum

nferior semilunar lobule (H VII A)

biventer lobe (H VIII)

tonsil of cerebellum (X-IX)

uvula of vermis (IX)

vallecula of cerebellum

pyramid of vermis of cerebellum (VIII)

hemisphere of cerebellum

nodule of vermis (X)

flocculus of cerebellum (H X)

EXTERNAL CAUDAL VIEW

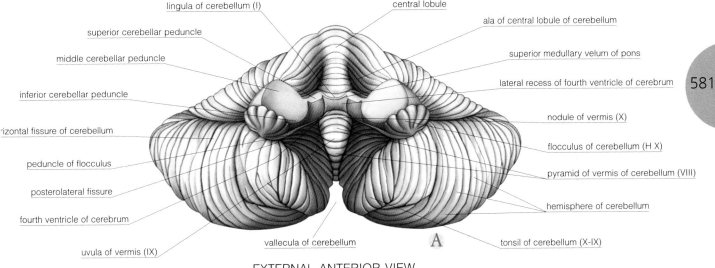

lingula of cerebellum (I)

central lobule

superior cerebellar peduncle

ala of central lobule of cerebellum

middle cerebellar peduncle

superior medullary velum of pons

inferior cerebellar peduncle

lateral recess of fourth ventricle of cerebrum

rizontal fissure of cerebellum

nodule of vermis (X)

peduncle of flocculus

flocculus of cerebellum (H X)

posterolateral fissure

pyramid of vermis of cerebellum (VIII)

fourth ventricle of cerebrum

hemisphere of cerebellum

uvula of vermis (IX)

vallecula of cerebellum

tonsil of cerebellum (X-IX)

EXTERNAL ANTERIOR VIEW

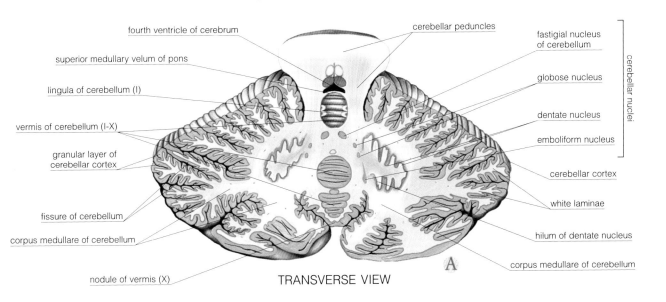

fourth ventricle of cerebrum

cerebellar peduncles

fastigial nucleus of cerebellum

superior medullary velum of pons

globose nucleus

lingula of cerebellum (I)

dentate nucleus

vermis of cerebellum (I-X)

emboliform nucleus

granular layer of cerebellar cortex

cerebellar nuclei

cerebellar cortex

fissure of cerebellum

white laminae

corpus medullare of cerebellum

hilum of dentate nucleus

nodule of vermis (X)

corpus medullare of cerebellum

TRANSVERSE VIEW

NUCLEI of CRANIAL NERVES
NUCLEI of ENCEPHALIC TRUNKS (I)
POSTERIOR VIEW

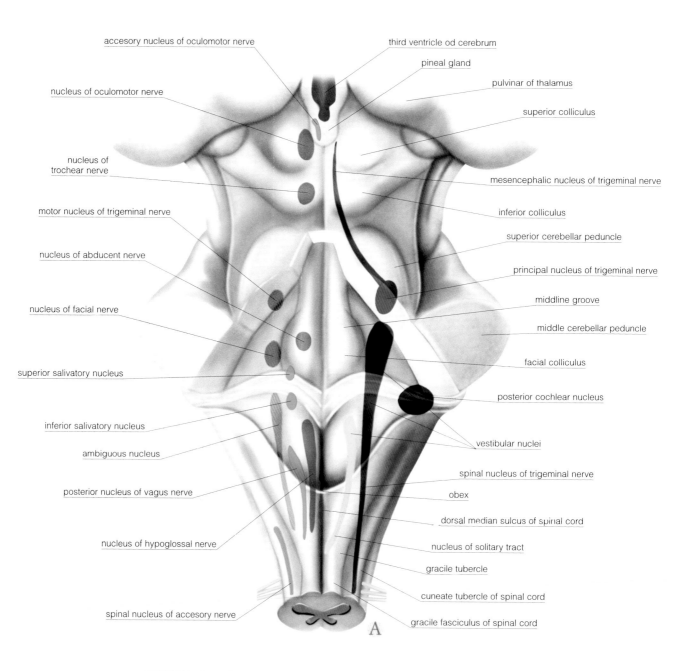

accesory nucleus of oculomotor nerve

third ventricle od cerebrum

pineal gland

pulvinar of thalamus

nucleus of oculomotor nerve

superior colliculus

nucleus of trochear nerve

mesencephalic nucleus of trigeminal nerve

inferior colliculus

motor nucleus of trigeminal nerve

superior cerebellar peduncle

principal nucleus of trigeminal nerve

nucleus of abducent nerve

middline groove

middle cerebellar peduncle

nucleus of facial nerve

facial colliculus

superior salivatory nucleus

posterior cochlear nucleus

inferior salivatory nucleus

vestibular nuclei

ambiguous nucleus

spinal nucleus of trigeminal nerve

posterior nucleus of vagus nerve

obex

dorsal median sulcus of spinal cord

nucleus of hypoglossal nerve

nucleus of solitary tract

gracile tubercle

cuneate tubercle of spinal cord

spinal nucleus of accesory nerve

gracile fasciculus of spinal cord

A

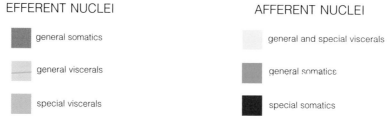

EFFERENT NUCLEI

general somatics

general viscerals

special viscerals

AFFERENT NUCLEI

general and special viscerals

general somatics

special somatics

NUCLEI of CRANIAL NERVES
NUCLEI of ENCEPHALIC TRUNKS (II)
MEDIAL VIEW

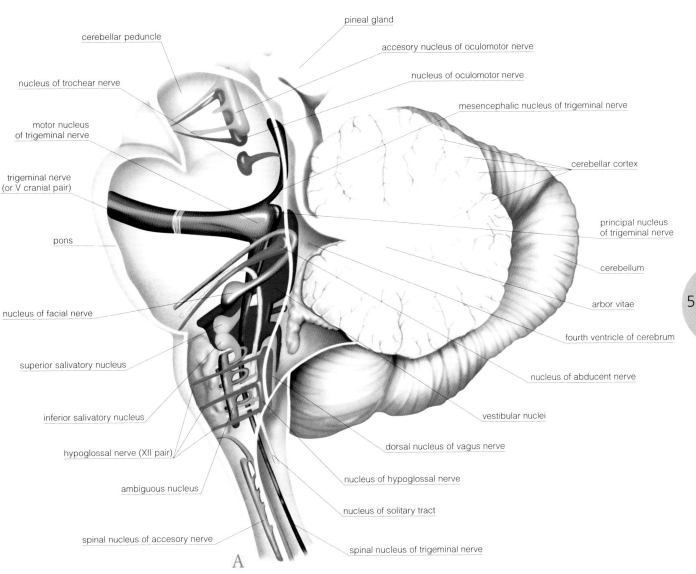

pineal gland

cerebellar peduncle

accesory nucleus of oculomotor nerve

nucleus of trochear nerve

nucleus of oculomotor nerve

mesencephalic nucleus of trigeminal nerve

motor nucleus of trigeminal nerve

cerebellar cortex

trigeminal nerve (or V cranial pair)

principal nucleus of trigeminal nerve

pons

cerebellum

nucleus of facial nerve

arbor vitae

583

fourth ventricle of cerebrum

superior salivatory nucleus

nucleus of abducent nerve

inferior salivatory nucleus

vestibular nuclei

hypoglossal nerve (XII pair)

dorsal nucleus of vagus nerve

ambiguous nucleus

nucleus of hypoglossal nerve

nucleus of solitary tract

spinal nucleus of accesory nerve

spinal nucleus of trigeminal nerve

A

EFFERENT NUCLEI

general somatics

general viscerals

special viscerals

AFFERENT NUCLEI

general and special viscerals

general somatics

special somatics

AUTONOMIC PLEXUS

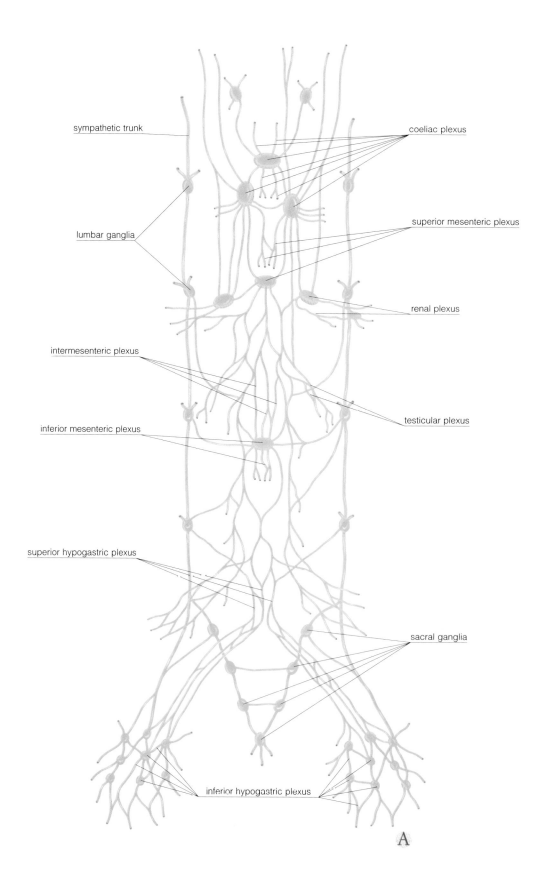

sympathetic trunk

coeliac plexus

lumbar ganglia

superior mesenteric plexus

renal plexus

intermesenteric plexus

inferior mesenteric plexus

testicular plexus

superior hypogastric plexus

sacral ganglia

inferior hypogastric plexus

A

CRANIAL PAIRS (I). DISTRIBUTION

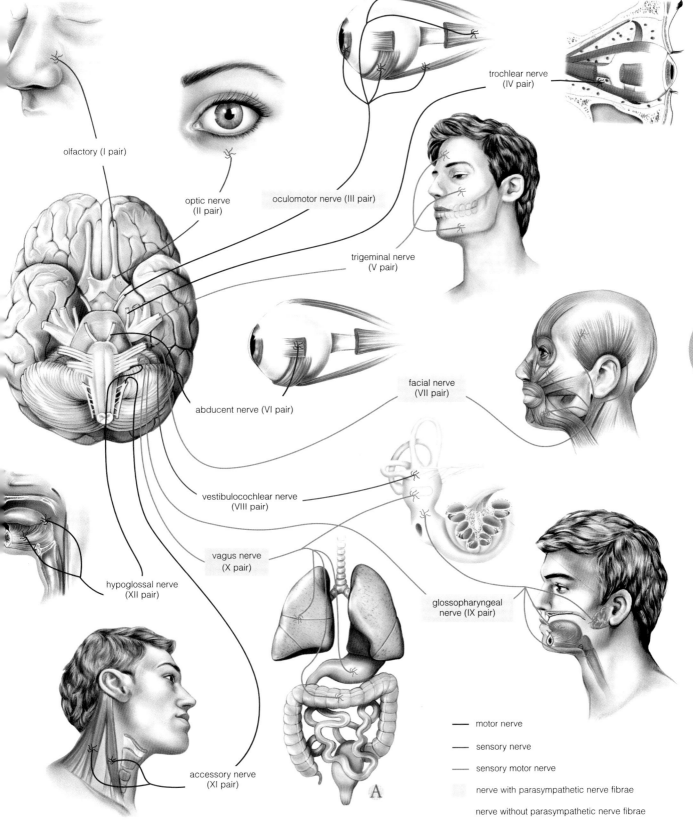

olfactory (I pair)

optic nerve (II pair)

oculomotor nerve (III pair)

trochlear nerve (IV pair)

trigeminal nerve (V pair)

abducent nerve (VI pair)

facial nerve (VII pair)

vestibulocochlear nerve (VIII pair)

vagus nerve (X pair)

glossopharyngeal nerve (IX pair)

hypoglossal nerve (XII pair)

accessory nerve (XI pair)

A

— motor nerve

— sensory nerve

— sensory motor nerve

nerve with parasympathetic nerve fibrae

nerve without parasympathetic nerve fibrae

585

CRANIAL PAIRS (II). OLFACTORY NERVE (I PAIR)

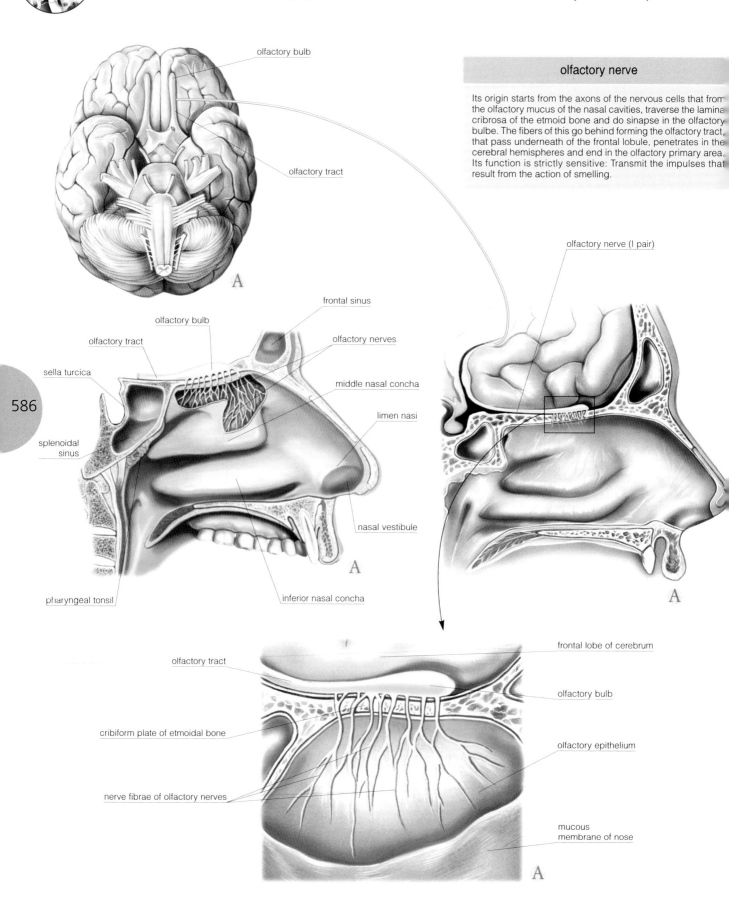

olfactory bulb

olfactory tract

A

olfactory nerve

Its origin starts from the axons of the nervous cells that from
the olfactory mucus of the nasal cavities, traverse the lamina
cribrosa of the etmoid bone and do sinapse in the olfactory
bulbe. The fibers of this go behind forming the olfactory tract,
that pass underneath of the frontal lobule, penetrates in the
cerebral hemispheres and end in the olfactory primary area.
Its function is strictly sensitive: Transmit the impulses that
result from the action of smelling.

olfactory nerve (I pair)

frontal sinus

olfactory bulb

olfactory nerves

olfactory tract

middle nasal concha

sella turcica

limen nasi

splenoidal
sinus

nasal vestibule

pharyngeal tonsil

inferior nasal concha

A

A

frontal lobe of cerebrum

olfactory tract

olfactory bulb

cribiform plate of etmoidal bone

olfactory epithelium

nerve fibrae of olfactory nerves

mucous
membrane of nose

A

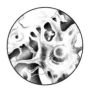

CRANIAL PAIRS (III). OPTIC NERVE (II PAIR)

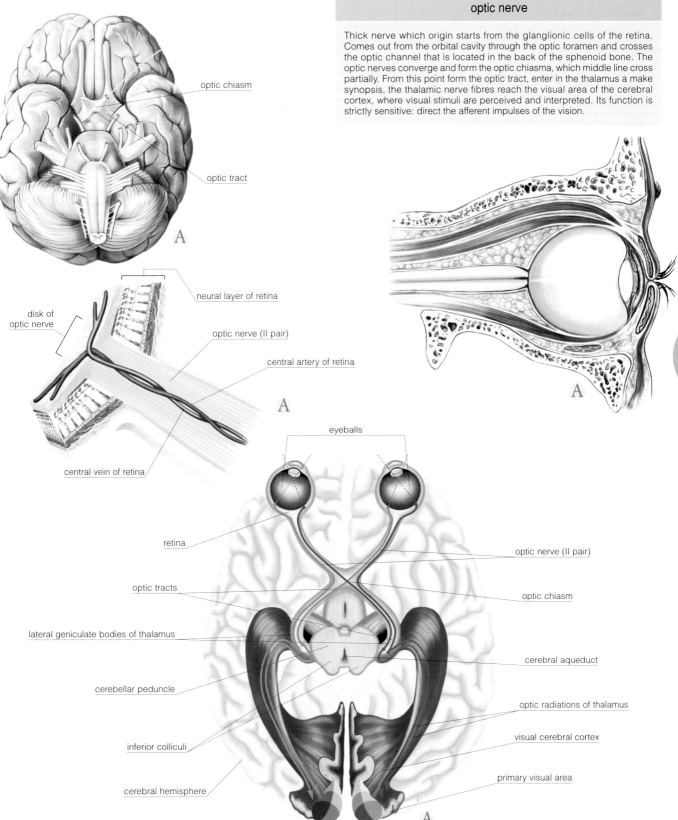

optic chiasm

optic tract

A

optic nerve

Thick nerve which origin starts from the glanglionic cells of the retina. Comes out from the orbital cavity through the optic foramen and crosses the optic channel that is located in the back of the sphenoid bone. The optic nerves converge and form the optic chiasma, which middle line cross partially. From this point form the optic tract, enter in the thalamus a make synopsis, the thalamic nerve fibres reach the visual area of the cerebral cortex, where visual stimuli are perceived and interpreted. Its function is strictly sensitive: direct the afferent impulses of the vision.

neural layer of retina

disk of optic nerve

optic nerve (II pair)

central artery of retina

A

central vein of retina

A

587

eyeballs

retina

optic nerve (II pair)

optic tracts

optic chiasm

lateral geniculate bodies of thalamus

cerebral aqueduct

cerebellar peduncle

optic radiations of thalamus

inferior colliculi

visual cerebral cortex

cerebral hemisphere

primary visual area

A

CRANIAL PAIRS (IV). OCULOMOTOR NERVE (III PAIR)

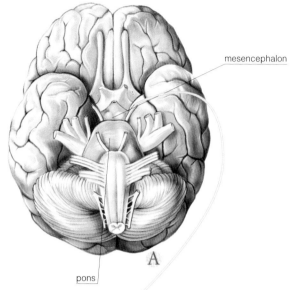

mesencephalon

pons

A

oculomotor nerve (or motor ocular common nerve)

The nerve fibres that originate it start from the anterior part of the mesencephalon, close to its union with the bridge. Cross the groove existing between the cerebral peduncles and such bridge, pass over the sphenoid bone and enters in the upper orbital cavity through the sphenoid cleft. The two branches in which are divided (upper and lower) reaches the majority of the eye muscles. Its function is mixed, although contains some afferent proprioceptive, these are specially motors. Transmit the motor commands to all the ciliary muscles of the pupi that control the ciliary muscles and constrictor of the pupil.

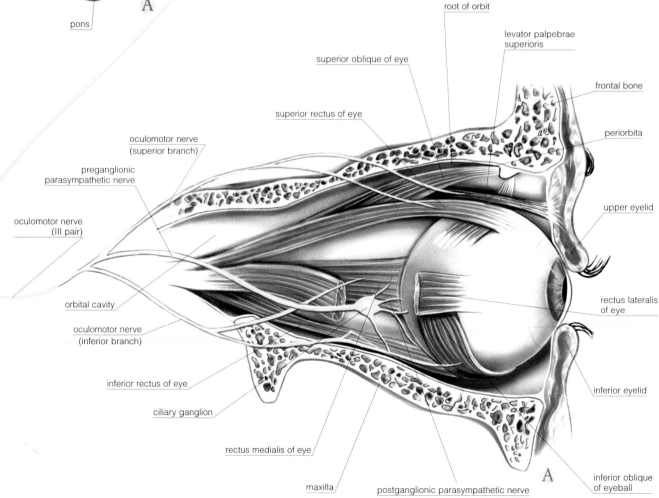

root of orbit

levator palpebrae superioris

superior oblique of eye

frontal bone

superior rectus of eye

periorbita

oculomotor nerve
(superior branch)

preganglionic
parasympathetic nerve

upper eyelid

oculomotor nerve
(III pair)

orbital cavity

rectus lateralis
of eye

oculomotor nerve
(inferior branch)

inferior rectus of eye

inferior eyelid

ciliary ganglion

rectus medialis of eye

A

maxilla

postganglionic parasympathetic nerve

inferior oblique
of eyeball

CRANIAL PAIRS (V). TROCHLEAR NERVE (IV PAIR)

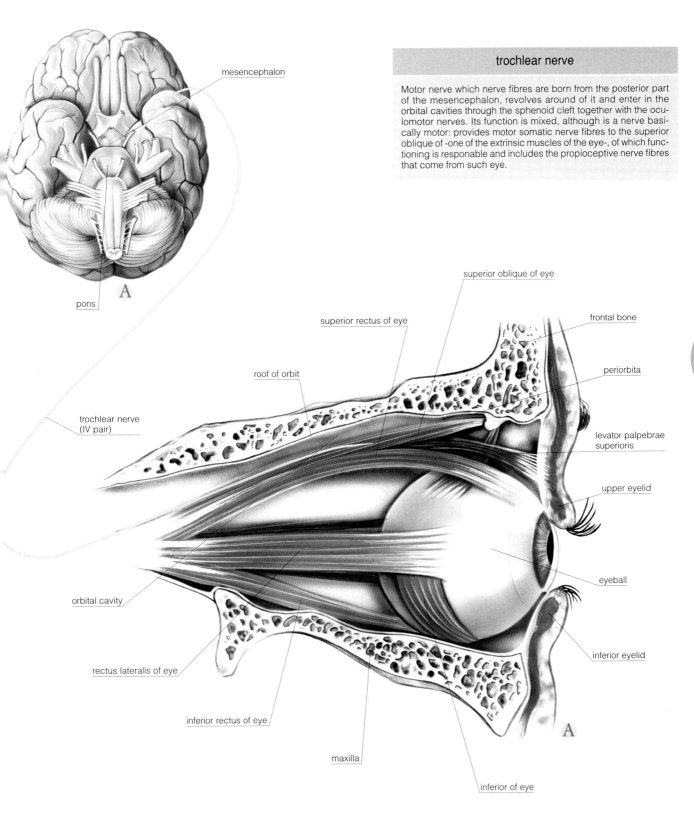

mesencephalon

pons

A

trochlear nerve

Motor nerve which nerve fibres are born from the posterior part of the mesencephalon, revolves around of it and enter in the orbital cavities through the sphenoid cleft together with the ocu-lomotor nerves. Its function is mixed, although is a nerve basi-cally motor: provides motor somatic nerve fibres to the superior oblique of -one of the extrinsic muscles of the eye-, of which func-tioning is responable and includes the propioceptive nerve fibres that come from such eye.

superior oblique of eye

superior rectus of eye

frontal bone

roof of orbit

periorbita

589

trochlear nerve
(IV pair)

levator palpebrae
superioris

upper eyelid

eyeball

orbital cavity

inferior eyelid

rectus lateralis of eye

inferior rectus of eye

maxilla

inferior of eye

A

CRANIAL PAIRS (VI). TRIGEMINAL NERVE (V PAIR) (I)

trigeminal nerve

Nerve consisting in two roots (one sensitive and other motor), has its origin in the bridge un soon after divides in three branches (ophthalmic, maxillary and mandibular nerves), that constitute the most important sensitive nerves of the sight. Transmit their afferent impulses associated to the tact, to the temperature and the pain. The cellular bodies of the sensitive neurons of the three branches are located in the node of the trigeminal that is located near the origin point of the nerve. The mandibular nerves contain also some motor neural-fibers that innervate the skin of the face, the mastication muscle, teeth, mouth and nasal cavity.

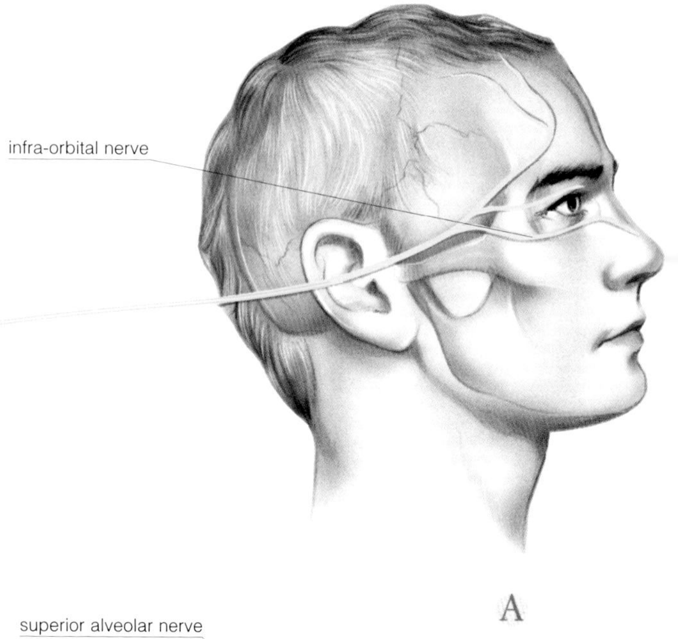

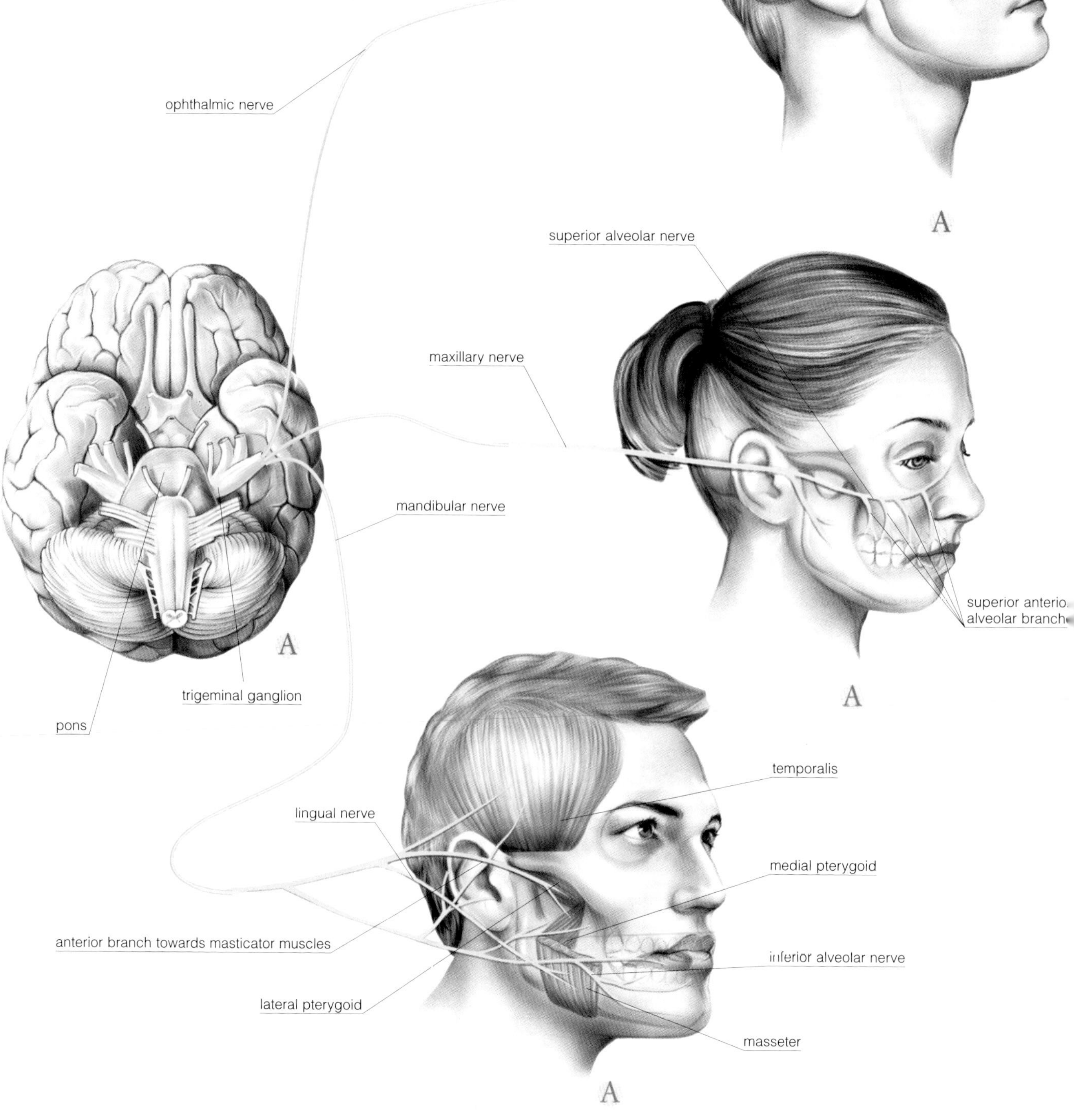

infra-orbital nerve

ophthalmic nerve

A

superior alveolar nerve

maxillary nerve

mandibular nerve

A

trigeminal ganglion

pons

superior anterio
alveolar branch

A

temporalis

lingual nerve

medial pterygoid

inferior alveolar nerve

anterior branch towards masticator muscles

lateral pterygoid

masseter

A

CRANIAL PAIRS (VII). TRIGEMINAL NERVE (V PAIR) (II)

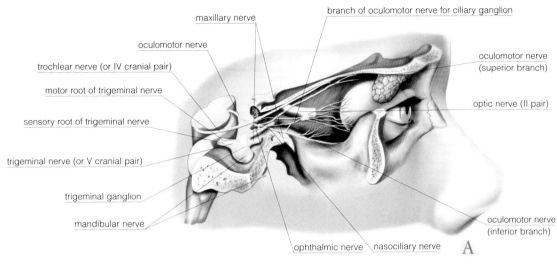

maxillary nerve

branch of oculomotor nerve for ciliary ganglion

oculomotor nerve

trochlear nerve (or IV cranial pair)

motor root of trigeminal nerve

sensory root of trigeminal nerve

trigeminal nerve (or V cranial pair)

trigeminal ganglion

mandibular nerve

oculomotor nerve (superior branch)

optic nerve (II pair)

oculomotor nerve (inferior branch)

ophthalmic nerve   nasociliary nerve   A

OCULOMOTOR and TROCHLEAR NERVES

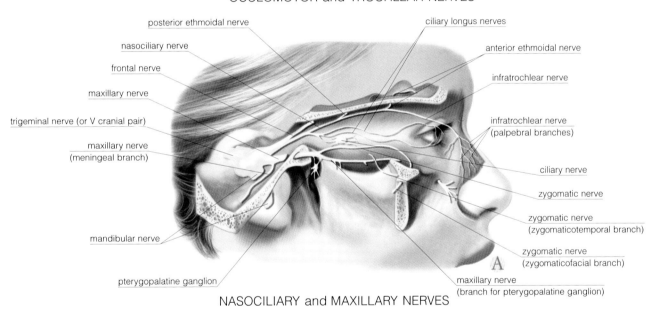

posterior ethmoidal nerve

nasociliary nerve

frontal nerve

maxillary nerve

trigeminal nerve (or V cranial pair)

maxillary nerve (meningeal branch)

mandibular nerve

pterygopalatine ganglion

ciliary longus nerves

anterior ethmoidal nerve

infratrochlear nerve

infratrochlear nerve (palpebral branches)

ciliary nerve

zygomatic nerve

zygomatic nerve (zygomaticotemporal branch)

zygomatic nerve (zygomaticofacial branch)

maxillary nerve (branch for pterygopalatine ganglion)

A

NASOCILIARY and MAXILLARY NERVES

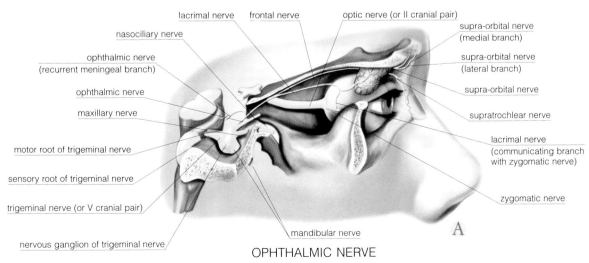

lacrimal nerve   frontal nerve   optic nerve (or II cranial pair)

nasociliary nerve

ophthalmic nerve (recurrent meningeal branch)

ophthalmic nerve

maxillary nerve

motor root of trigeminal nerve

sensory root of trigeminal nerve

trigeminal nerve (or V cranial pair)

nervous ganglion of trigeminal nerve

supra-orbital nerve (medial branch)

supra-orbital nerve (lateral branch)

supra-orbital nerve

supratrochlear nerve

lacrimal nerve (communicating branch with zygomatic nerve)

zygomatic nerve

mandibular nerve   A

OPHTHALMIC NERVE

CRANIAL PAIRS (VIII). ABDUCENT NERVE (VI PAIR)

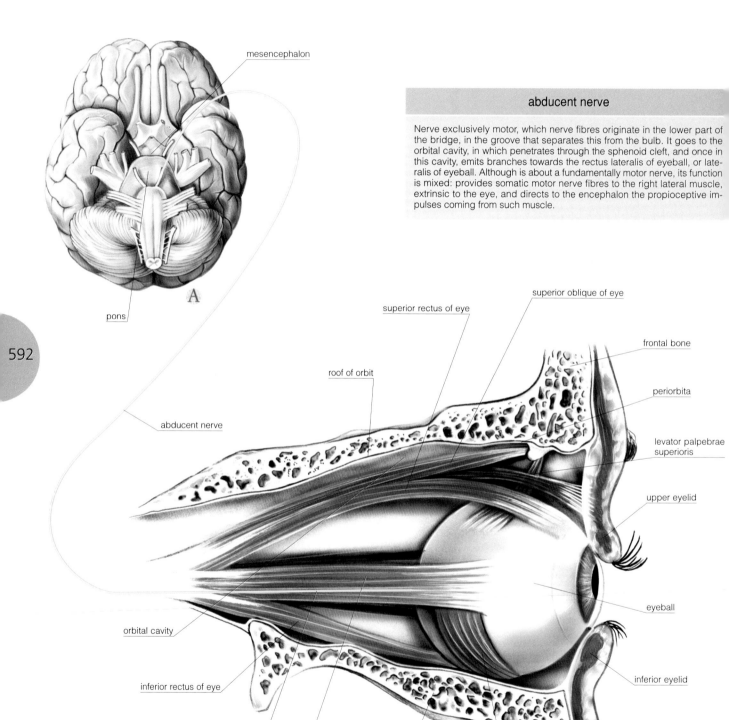

mesencephalon

pons

A

abducent nerve

Nerve exclusively motor, which nerve fibres originate in the lower part of the bridge, in the groove that separates this from the bulb. It goes to the orbital cavity, in which penetrates through the sphenoid cleft, and once in this cavity, emits branches towards the rectus lateralis of eyeball, or lateralis of eyeball. Although is about a fundamentally motor nerve, its function is mixed: provides somatic motor nerve fibres to the right lateral muscle, extrinsic to the eye, and directs to the encephalon the propioceptive impulses coming from such muscle.

superior oblique of eye

superior rectus of eye

frontal bone

roof of orbit

periorbita

abducent nerve

levator palpebrae superioris

upper eyelid

eyeball

orbital cavity

inferior rectus of eye

inferior eyelid

rectus lateralis of eye

rectus medialis of eye

maxillary

inferior oblique of eye

A

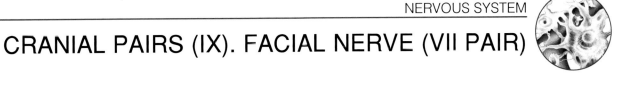

CRANIAL PAIRS (IX). FACIAL NERVE (VII PAIR)

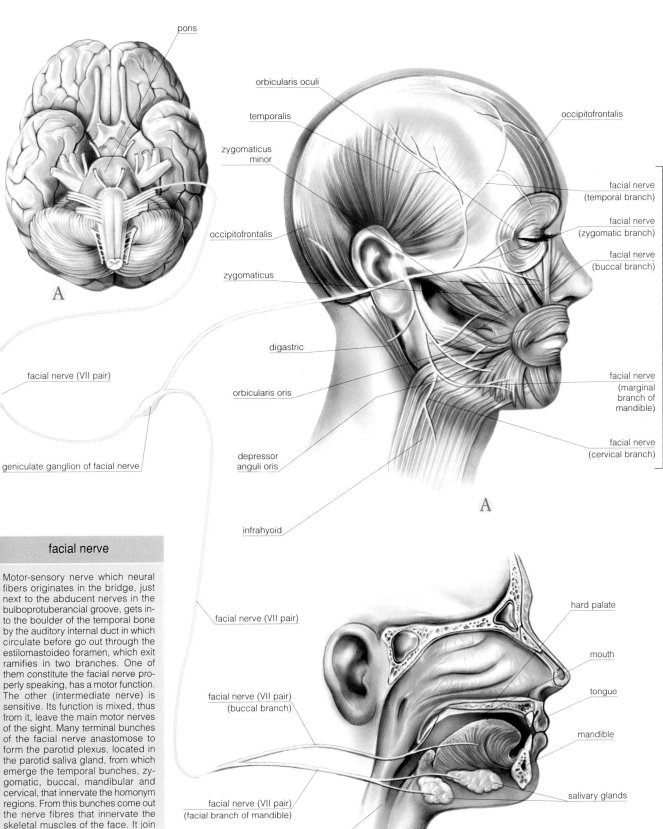

pons

orbicularis oculi

temporalis

zygomaticus minor

occipitofrontalis

occipitofrontalis

zygomaticus

digastric

facial nerve (VII pair)

orbicularis oris

geniculate ganglion of facial nerve

depressor anguli oris

infrahyoid

occipitofrontalis

facial nerve (temporal branch)

facial nerve (zygomatic branch)

facial nerve (buccal branch)

facial nerve (marginal branch of mandible)

facial nerve (cervical branch)

motor branches for muscles of scalp and of visual expression

593

A

A

facial nerve

Motor-sensory nerve which neural fibers originates in the bridge, just next to the abducent nerves in the bulboprotuberancial groove, gets into the boulder of the temporal bone by the auditory internal duct in which circulate before go out through the estilomastoideo foramen, which exit ramifies in two branches. One of them constitute the facial nerve properly speaking, has a motor function. The other (intermediate nerve) is sensitive. Its function is mixed, thus from it, leave the main motor nerves of the sight. Many terminal bunches of the facial nerve anastomose to form the parotid plexus, located in the parotid saliva gland, from which emerge the temporal bunches, zygomatic, buccal, mandibular and cervical, that innervate the homonym regions. From this bunches come out the nerve fibres that innervate the skeletal muscles of the face. It join with the glossopharyngeal nerve through loop of Haller.

facial nerve (VII pair)

facial nerve (VII pair) (buccal branch)

facial nerve (VII pair) (facial branch of mandible)

hypopharynx

hard palate

mouth

tongue

mandible

salivary glands

A

CRANIAL PAIRS (X)
VESTIBULOCOCHLEAR NERVE (VIII PAIR)

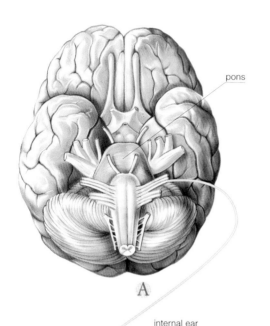

pons

A

vestibulocochlear nerve

Sensitive nerve which nerve fibres are originated in the audition and balance system, located in the boulder of the temporal bone, pass through the internal auditory duct and penetrates in the cerebral trunk in the lateral part of the bulboprotuberancial groove. The afferent nerve fibres that comes from the receptors of audition of the cochlea (external) form the cochlear nerve and the afferent neural-fibers coming from the balance receptors of the semicircular channels and of the vestibule (internal) form the vestibular nerve. These two nerves, or bunches, merge and form the vestibulecoclhear nerve. The vestibular nerve transmits the afferent stimuli of the balance sense and the cellular bodies of sensitive neurons locate in the vestibular nodes. The cochlear nerves transmit the afferent impulses of the hearing sense and the cellular bodies of the sensitive neurons locate in the spiral organs, found in the interior of the cochlea.

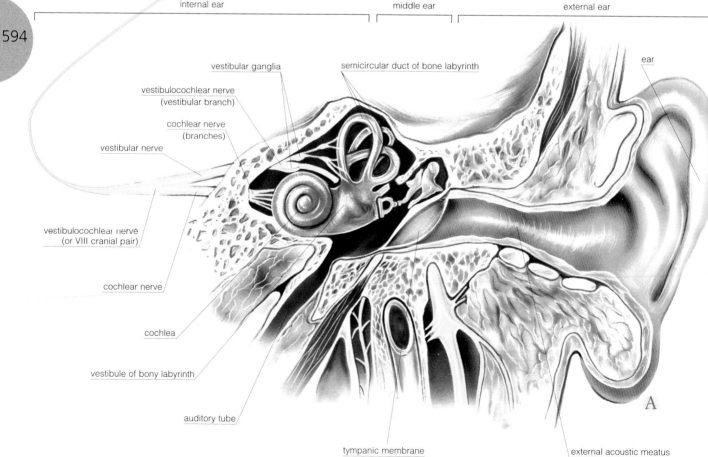

internal ear   middle ear   external ear

594

vestibular ganglia

vestibulocochlear nerve
(vestibular branch)

cochlear nerve
(branches)

vestibular nerve

semicircular duct of bone labyrinth

ear

vestibulocochlear nerve
(or VIII cranial pair)

cochlear nerve

cochlea

vestibule of bony labyrinth

auditory tube

tympanic membrane

external acoustic meatus

A

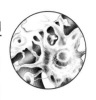

CRANIAL PAIRS (XI)
GLOSSOPHARYNGEAL NERVE (IX PAIR)

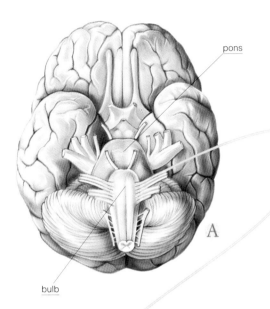

pons

bulb

A

glossopharyngeal nerve

Sensory-motor nerve which nerve fibres originates in the lateral region of the bulb, in the collateral posterior groove, above the vagus nerve. Together with this nerve and the accessory, comes out from the cranium through the jugular foramen and emits nervous terminations, some of which join to the facial nerve and others go to the tympanic cavity, penetrating in the cleft towards the carotid, lingual and pharyngeal regions, where innervates the muscles of that region. Provides the motor neural fibers to the skeletal muscles of the upper part of the pharynx, important in the deglutition and the reflex of the nausea, and includes propioceptive nerve fibres that come from this region. Also provides parasymphatetic motor neural fibrils to the parotid glands. The sensitive nerve fibres transport the impulses associated to the taste, tact, to the pressure and to the pain coming from the pharynx and from the posterior part of the tongue, the impulses of the chemoreceptors of the carotid corpuscle and the impulses coming from the baroreceptors of the carotid sinus. The cellular bodies of the sensory neurons are found in the upper and lower ganglia of the glossopharyngeal nerve.

595

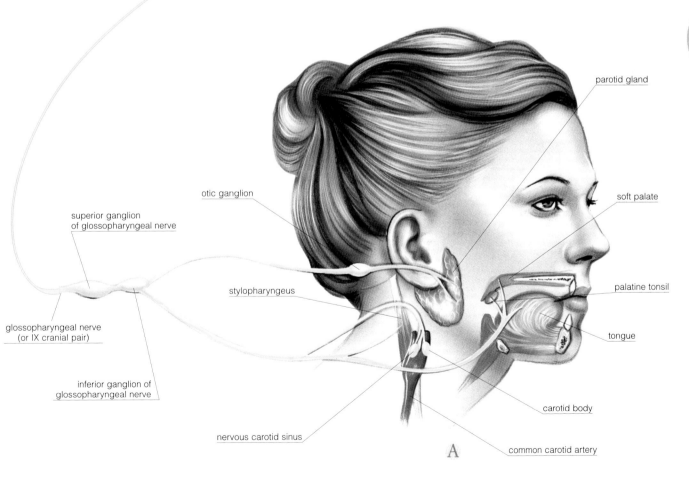

parotid gland

soft palate

otic ganglion

superior ganglion
of glossopharyngeal nerve

palatine tonsil

stylopharyngeus

tongue

glossopharyngeal nerve
(or IX cranial pair)

inferior ganglion of
glossopharyngeal nerve

carotid body

nervous carotid sinus

common carotid artery

A

CRANIAL PAIRS (XII). VAGUS NERVE (X PAIR)

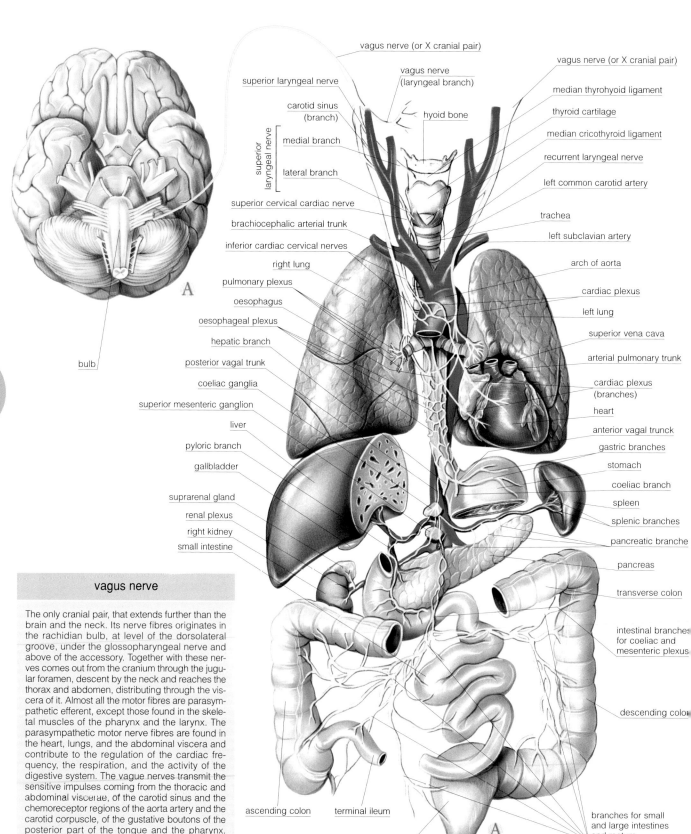

vagus nerve (or X cranial pair)

vagus nerve (or X cranial pair)

vagus nerve
(laryngeal branch)

superior laryngeal nerve

median thyrohyoid ligament

carotid sinus
(branch)

hyoid bone

thyroid cartilage

median cricothyroid ligament

medial branch

superior laryngeal nerve

recurrent laryngeal nerve

lateral branch

left common carotid artery

superior cervical cardiac nerve

trachea

brachiocephalic arterial trunk

left subclavian artery

inferior cardiac cervical nerves

arch of aorta

right lung

cardiac plexus

pulmonary plexus

left lung

oesophagus

superior vena cava

oesophageal plexus

arterial pulmonary trunk

hepatic branch

cardiac plexus
(branches)

bulb

posterior vagal trunk

heart

coeliac ganglia

anterior vagal trunck

superior mesenteric ganglion

gastric branches

liver

stomach

pyloric branch

coeliac branch

gallbladder

spleen

splenic branches

suprarenal gland

pancreatic branche

renal plexus

pancreas

right kidney

transverse colon

small intestine

intestinal branches
for coeliac and
mesenteric plexus

descending color

ascending colon

terminal ileum

branches for small
and large intestines
and rectum

rectum

anus

596

vagus nerve

The only cranial pair, that extends further than the brain and the neck. Its nerve fibres originates in the rachidian bulb, at level of the dorsolateral groove, under the glossopharyngeal nerve and above of the accessory. Together with these nerves comes out from the cranium through the jugular foramen, descent by the neck and reaches the thorax and abdomen, distributing through the viscera of it. Almost all the motor fibres are parasympathetic efferent, except those found in the skeletal muscles of the pharynx and the larynx. The parasympathetic motor nerve fibres are found in the heart, lungs, and the abdominal viscera and contribute to the regulation of the cardiac frequency, the respiration, and the activity of the digestive system. The vague nerves transmit the sensitive impulses coming from the thoracic and abdominal viscerae, of the carotid sinus and the chemoreceptor regions of the aorta artery and the carotid corpuscle, of the gustative boutons of the posterior part of the tongue and the pharynx. Contains propioceptive nerve fibres coming from the muscles, the larynx and the pharynx.

CRANIAL PAIRS (XIII). ACCESSORY NERVE (XI PAIR)

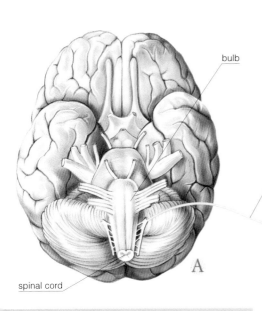

bulb

accessory nerve
(or XI cranial pair)

spinal cord

A

accessory nerve

Nerve that results from the union of two roots: cranial, o bulbar (vagal portion, that originates in the lateral part of the bulb and the spinal root, (spinal portion, that is born from the upper region of the spinal cord, by whose journey goes up, enters the cranium through the occipital foramen and rapidly joins to the cranial root). The accessory nerve comes out from the cranium through by the jugular foramen and a little after its cranial and spinal neural fibers separate. Those join to the nerve fibres of the vagus nerve, while those reach the big skeletal of the neck, is about a sensory-motor, but especially motor. The cranial roots join to the vagus nerve and distribute its motor nerve fibres to the pharynx, the larynx and the soft palate. The spinal root after join to motor bunches of the cervical spinal nerves, distribute its motor nerve fibres to the trapezoid and esternocleidomastoid, that allow the movements of the head and the neck; this one, also, transmits to the brain the propioceptive impulses that come from these muscles. Also emit a bunch that joins with the vagus nerve.

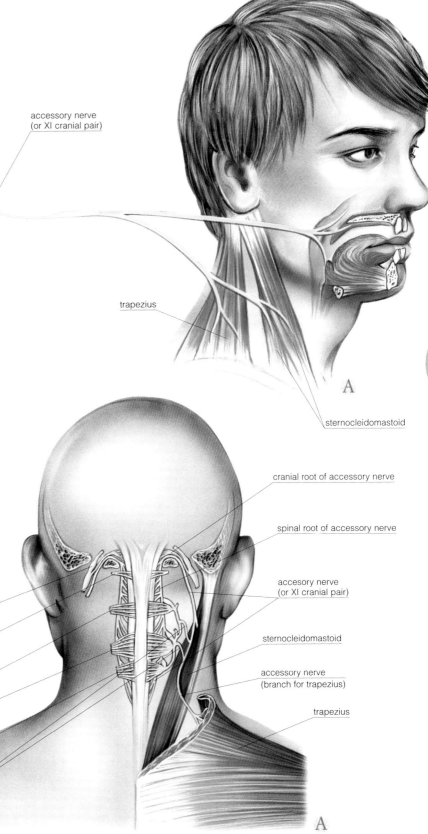

trapezius

sternocleidomastoid

A

597

cranial root of accessory nerve

spinal root of accessory nerve

accesory nerve
(or XI cranial pair)

sternocleidomastoid

accessory nerve
(branch for trapezius)

trapezius

vagus nerve (or X cranial pair)

posterior roots of C1 nerve

posterior roots of C2 nerve

posterior roots of C3 nerve

posterior roots of C4 nerve

cervical plexus C2-C4
(branches with sensory
fibrae of accessory nerve)

A

CRANIAL PAIRS (XIV)
HYPOGLOSSAL NERVE (XII PAIR)

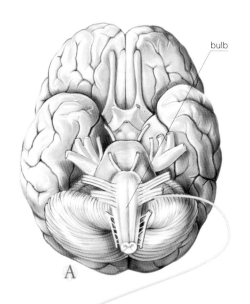

bulb

A

hypoglossal nerve

Is found under the tongue to which innervates. Its nerve fibres have its origin in the lateral region of the bulb, of the posterior collateral groove, above the vagus nerve. Together with this and the accessory nerve, comes out from the cranium through the jugular foramen and emit nervous terminals, some of which go to join to the facial nerve and other reach the tympanic cavity, penetrating the in the boulder of the temporal bone and the carotid, lingual and pharyngeal regions. Is a sensory-motor nerve, although especially motor. Their somatic nerve fibres reach until the intrinsic and extrinsic muscles of the tongue and transmit to the brain the propioceptive impulses that come from those muscles. Allows the movement of the tongue necessary for the mastication, deglutition and phonation.

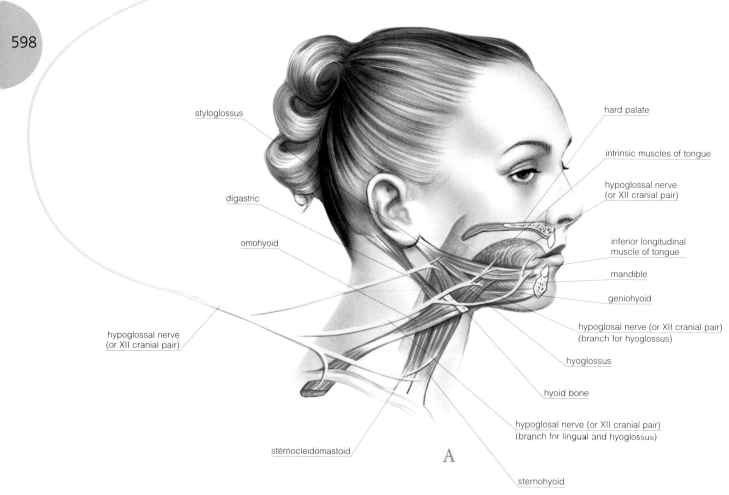

styloglossus

digastric

omohyoid

hypoglossal nerve
(or XII cranial pair)

sternocleidomastoid

hard palate

intrinsic muscles of tongue

hypoglossal nerve
(or XII cranial pair)

inferior longitudinal
muscle of tongue

mandible

geniohyoid

hypoglosal nerve (or XII cranial pair)
(branch for hyoglossus)

hyoglossus

hyoid bone

hypoglosal nerve (or XII cranial pair)
(branch for lingual and hyoglossus)

sternohyoid

A

MEDULLA and SPINAL NERVES

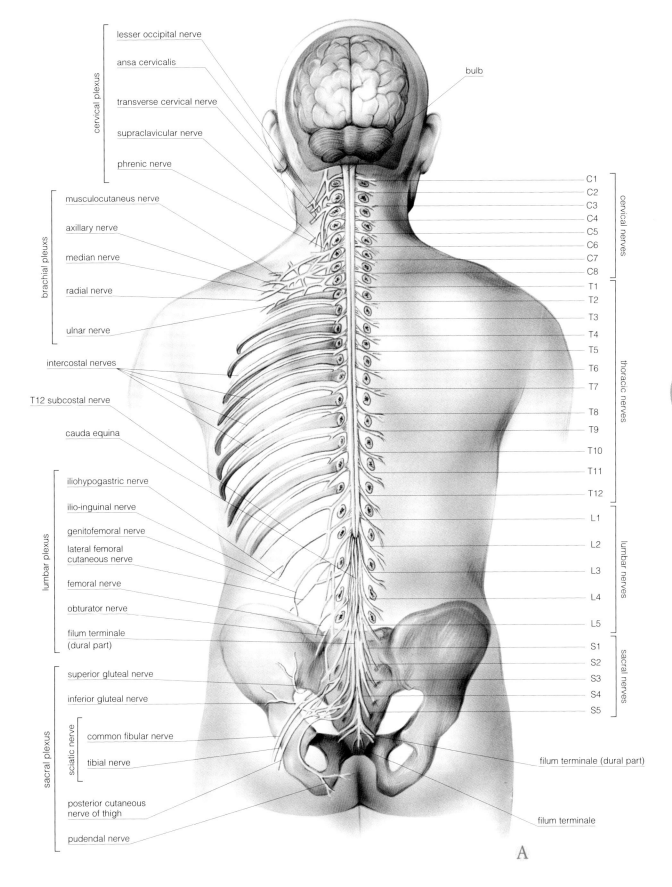

lesser occipital nerve

ansa cervicalis

transverse cervical nerve

supraclavicular nerve

phrenic nerve

cervical plexus

bulb

musculocutaneus nerve

axillary nerve

median nerve

radial nerve

ulnar nerve

brachial pleuxs

intercostal nerves

T12 subcostal nerve

cauda equina

iliohypogastric nerve

ilio-inguinal nerve

genitofemoral nerve

lateral femoral
cutaneous nerve

femoral nerve

obturator nerve

filum terminale
(dural part)

lumbar plexus

superior gluteal nerve

inferior gluteal nerve

common fibular nerve

tibial nerve

sciatic nerve

sacral plexus

posterior cutaneous
nerve of thigh

pudendal nerve

C1
C2
C3
C4
C5
C6
C7
C8

cervical nerves

T1
T2
T3
T4
T5
T6
T7
T8
T9
T10
T11
T12

thoracic nerves

L1
L2
L3
L4
L5

lumbar nerves

S1
S2
S3
S4
S5

sacral nerves

filum terminale (dural part)

filum terminale

599

A

SPINAL NERVES

spinal nerve

One of the types in which nerves are classified, the spinal nerves are lateral bunches that emit the spinal cord along its route for the backbone. Come out from it for the vertebral foramen and immediately group in anterior and posterior bunches, forming plexus of which originates collateral and terminal bunches through which comes the innervation to the different territories of the organism. There are 31 pairs of spinal nerves: eight cervical, twelve dorsal, five lumbar, five sacral and one coccygeal.

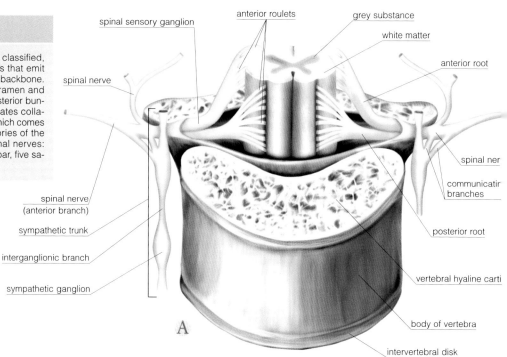

- spinal sensory ganglion
- anterior roulets
- grey substance
- white matter
- anterior root
- spinal nerve
- spinal ner
- communicatir branches
- posterior root
- spinal nerve (anterior branch)
- sympathetic trunk
- interganglionic branch
- sympathetic ganglion
- vertebral hyaline carti
- body of vertebra
- intervertebral disk

A

FORMATION of the PAIR of SPINAL NERVES

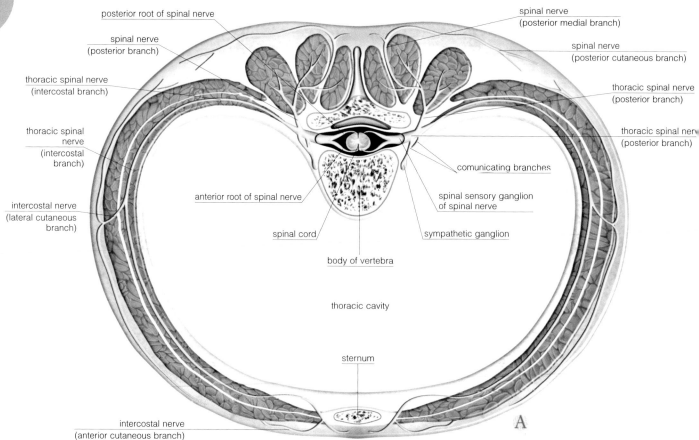

- posterior root of spinal nerve
- spinal nerve (posterior medial branch)
- spinal nerve (posterior branch)
- spinal nerve (posterior cutaneous branch)
- thoracic spinal nerve (intercostal branch)
- thoracic spinal nerve (posterior branch)
- thoracic spinal nerve (intercostal branch)
- thoracic spinal ner (posterior branch)
- comunicating branches
- intercostal nerve (lateral cutaneous branch)
- anterior root of spinal nerve
- spinal sensory ganglion of spinal nerve
- spinal cord
- sympathetic ganglion
- body of vertebra
- thoracic cavity
- sternum
- intercostal nerve (anterior cutaneous branch)

A

THORACIC CAVITY. INTERCOSTAL NERVES

PLEXUS (I). CERVICAL PLEXUS

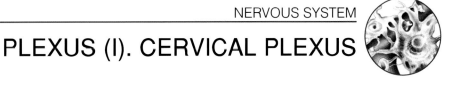

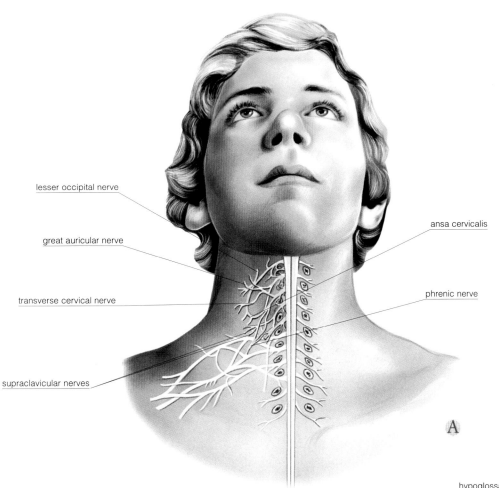

lesser occipital nerve

great auricular nerve

transverse cervical nerve

supraclavicular nerves

ansa cervicalis

phrenic nerve

A

601

cervical plexus

Set of nerves that before its peripheral distribution are found at deep level in the neck, under and behind of the posterior edge of esternocleidomastoideo muscle, between the pre-vertebral muscles and the insertions of the splenius and angular nerves. Is formed by the ventral bunches of the four upper cervical nerves. Is arranged as irregular loops and from there leave superficial bunches (occipital, minor, auricular major, transverse cervical, and supraclavicular nerves) and deep (phrenic, accessory phrenic, asa cervical and muscular nerves).The numerous efferent bunches are cutaneous (superficial cervical plexus) and transport the sensitive impulses of the skin and the neck of the ear and back's region, while the motor bunches (cervical deep plexus), together with the phrenic nerves, innervate the muscles of the anterior part of the neck.

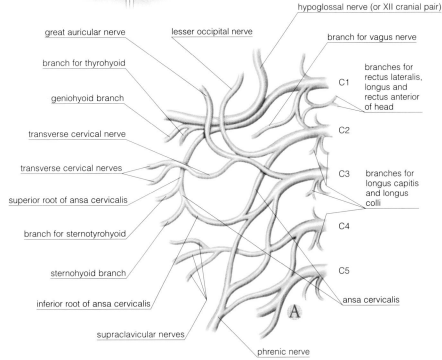

great auricular nerve

branch for thyrohyoid

geniohyoid branch

transverse cervical nerve

transverse cervical nerves

superior root of ansa cervicalis

branch for sternotyrohyoid

sternohyoid branch

inferior root of ansa cervicalis

supraclavicular nerves

lesser occipital nerve

hypoglossal nerve (or XII cranial pair)

branch for vagus nerve

branches for rectus lateralis, longus and rectus anterior of head

C1

C2

C3   branches for longus capitis and longus colli

C4

C5

ansa cervicalis

phrenic nerve

A

PLEXUS (II). BRACHIAL PLEXUS (I)

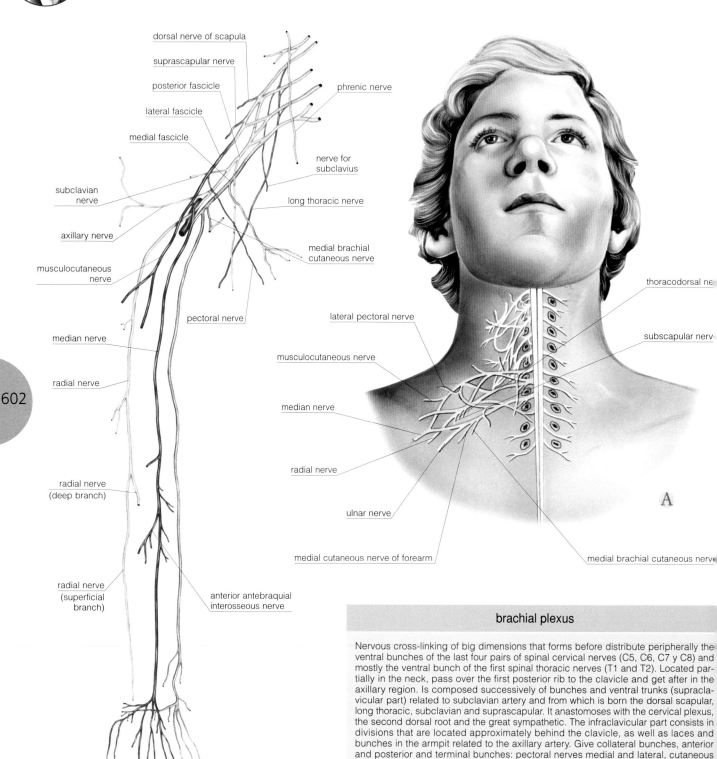

dorsal nerve of scapula

suprascapular nerve

posterior fascicle

lateral fascicle

medial fascicle

phrenic nerve

nerve for subclavius

subclavian nerve

long thoracic nerve

axillary nerve

medial brachial cutaneous nerve

musculocutaneous nerve

pectoral nerve

median nerve

lateral pectoral nerve

radial nerve

musculocutaneous nerve

median nerve

radial nerve (deep branch)

radial nerve

radial nerve (superficial branch)

anterior antebraquial interosseous nerve

ulnar nerve

medial cutaneous nerve of forearm

thoracodorsal ne

subscapular nerv

medial brachial cutaneous nerv

602

RIGHT UPPER LIMB
ANTERIOR VIEW

brachial plexus

Nervous cross-linking of big dimensions that forms before distribute peripherally the ventral bunches of the last four pairs of spinal cervical nerves (C5, C6, C7 y C8) and mostly the ventral bunch of the first spinal thoracic nerves (T1 and T2). Located partially in the neck, pass over the first posterior rib to the clavicle and get after in the axillary region. Is composed successively of bunches and ventral trunks (supraclavicular part) related to subclavian artery and from which is born the dorsal scapular, long thoracic, subclavian and suprascapular. It anastomoses with the cervical plexus, the second dorsal root and the great sympathetic. The infraclavicular part consists in divisions that are located approximately behind the clavicle, as well as laces and bunches in the armpit related to the axillary artery. Give collateral bunches, anterior and posterior and terminal bunches: pectoral nerves medial and lateral, cutaneous brachial medial, cutaneous antebrachial medial, median, ulnar, radial, subscapular, thoracodorsal and axillary. Its importance comes from the fact that groups practically all the nerves that goes to the superior nerve. Its complexity complicate its study; that's why usually we find three parts: roots (anterior bunches of the spinal nerves), trunks (located in the inferior part of the neck are three: upper, medium and lower, and in the posterior part of the clavicle divides in two: anterior and posterior) and fascicles (are the reunions that form the divisions anterior and posterior; according to its relation to the axillary artery, divided in lateral, medial and posterior). The most important nerves of the brachial plexus (axillary, musculocutaneous, radial, medial and cubital) are bunches of the fascicles.

PLEXUS (III). BRACHIAL PLEXUS (II)

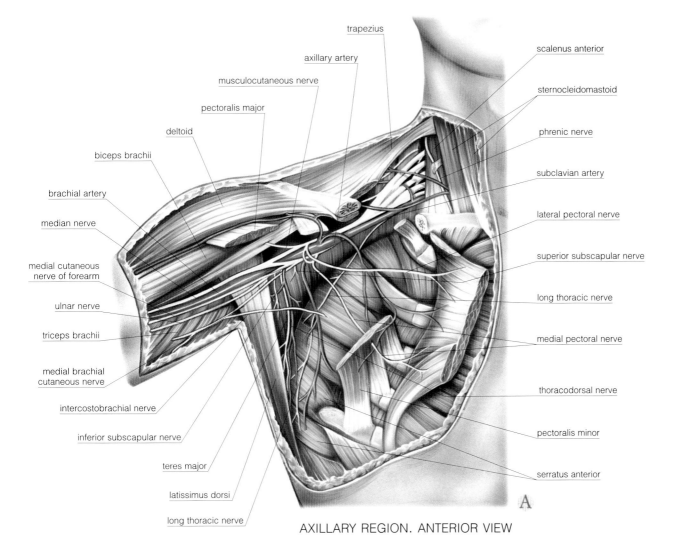

trapezius

axillary artery

musculocutaneous nerve

pectoralis major

deltoid

biceps brachii

brachial artery

median nerve

medial cutaneous
nerve of forearm

ulnar nerve

triceps brachii

medial brachial
cutaneous nerve

intercostobrachial nerve

inferior subscapular nerve

teres major

latissimus dorsi

long thoracic nerve

scalenus anterior

sternocleidomastoid

phrenic nerve

subclavian artery

lateral pectoral nerve

superior subscapular nerve

long thoracic nerve

medial pectoral nerve

thoracodorsal nerve

pectoralis minor

serratus anterior

AXILLARY REGION. ANTERIOR VIEW

A

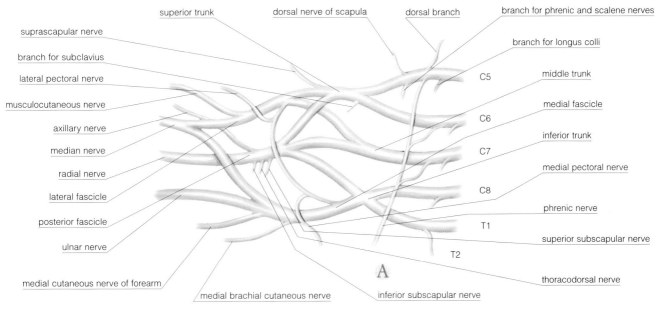

superior trunk

dorsal nerve of scapula

dorsal branch

branch for phrenic and scalene nerves

suprascapular nerve

branch for subclavius

lateral pectoral nerve

musculocutaneous nerve

axillary nerve

median nerve

radial nerve

lateral fascicle

posterior fascicle

ulnar nerve

medial cutaneous nerve of forearm

branch for longus colli

C5

middle trunk

C6

medial fascicle

C7

inferior trunk

C8

medial pectoral nerve

phrenic nerve

T1

superior subscapular nerve

T2

thoracodorsal nerve

medial brachial cutaneous nerve

inferior subscapular nerve

A

PLEXUS (IV). LUMBAR PLEXUS

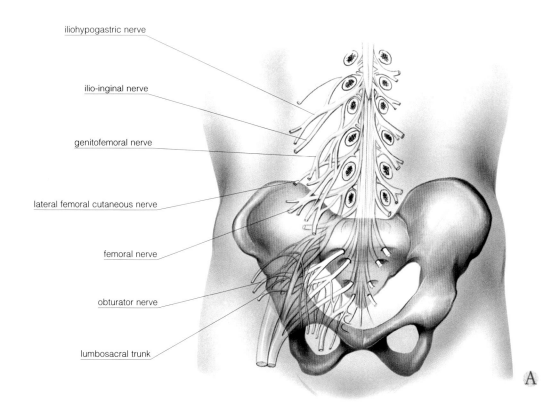

iliohypogastric nerve

ilio-inginal nerve

genitofemoral nerve

lateral femoral cutaneous nerve

femoral nerve

obturator nerve

lumbosacral trunk

A

lumbar plexus

Group of anastomoses which, before their peripheral distribution, jointly comprise the ventral branches of L1 (not always included), L2, L3, L4, and L5 lumbar nerves in the major psoas muscle. It is deeply located in the dihedral which forms the vertebral bodies and their transverse processes. The plexus passes obliquely and outwardly through both sides of the four lumbar vertebrae and in front of the quadratus lumborum muscle. Subsequently, it gives rise to the peripheral nerves. The inferior division of the fourth lumbar nerve joins with the fifth and the lumbosacral trunk, thus formed, becomes a part of the sacral plexus. In the psoas, it creates anastomoses with the 12th intercostal nerve, the sacral plexus and the sympathetic plexus. The branches of the first lumbar plexus are the ilioinguinal and the iliohypogastric nerves, and the branches of the plexus proper are the genitofemoral, lateral femoral cutaneous, obturator and femoral nerves. It innervates the anterolateral wall of the abdomen, the external genitalia and the lower extremities.

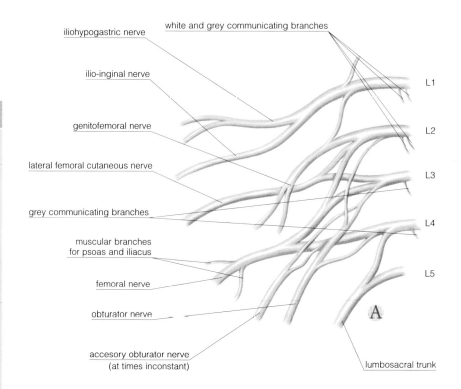

iliohypogastric nerve

white and grey communicating branches

ilio-inginal nerve

genitofemoral nerve

lateral femoral cutaneous nerve

grey communicating branches

muscular branches
for psoas and iliacus

femoral nerve

obturator nerve

accesory obturator nerve
(at times inconstant)

L1

L2

L3

L4

L5

A

lumbosacral trunk

PLEXUS (V). SACRAL PLEXUS

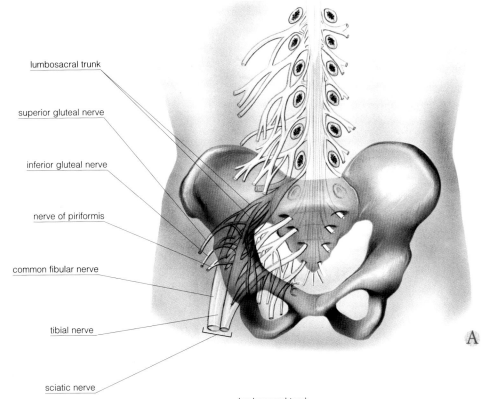

lumbosacral trunk

superior gluteal nerve

inferior gluteal nerve

nerve of piriformis

common fibular nerve

tibial nerve

sciatic nerve

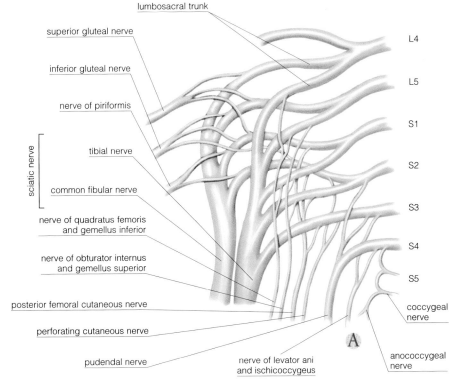

lumbosacral trunk

superior gluteal nerve

inferior gluteal nerve

nerve of piriformis

tibial nerve

sciatic nerve

common fibular nerve

nerve of quadratus femoris
and gemellus inferior

nerve of obturator internus
and gemellus superior

posterior femoral cutaneous nerve

perforating cutaneous nerve

pudendal nerve

nerve of levator ani
and ischicoccygeus

L4

L5

S1

S2

S3

S4

S5

coccygeal
nerve

anococcygeal
nerve

sacral plexus

Nervous cross-linking that before its peripheral distribution, form the lumbosacral trunk and the anterior bunches of the four first sacral pairs and origins in front of the piriform. Is found in a deep plane in the minor pelvis, immediately following the lumbar plexus, in which forms anastomosis, the same as with the sacrococcigeal and the great sympathetic, Has twelve collateral bunches, five of which, anterior or intrapelvic innervate the pelvical structures (nerves of the piriform, levator ani and coccygeal, and also the anal sphincters, splanchnic nerves, pelvic and pudental) and seven posterior or extrapelvic that help to innervate the buttocks and the lower extremities (gluteal nerves upper and lower, femorocutaneous posterior, perforating cutaneous and sciatic and nerves of the muscles square femoral and internal obturator). The anterior roots of the spinal nerves S4 and S5 and the coccigeous nerve form a small plexus called coccygeal plexus, that innervate a reduced area of the homonymous region.

HEAD and NECK (I)

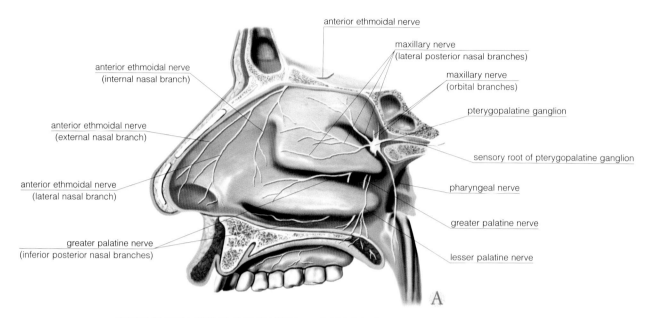

anterior ethmoidal nerve

maxillary nerve
(lateral posterior nasal branches)

anterior ethmoidal nerve
(internal nasal branch)

maxillary nerve
(orbital branches)

pterygopalatine ganglion

anterior ethmoidal nerve
(external nasal branch)

sensory root of pterygopalatine ganglion

anterior ethmoidal nerve
(lateral nasal branch)

pharyngeal nerve

greater palatine nerve

greater palatine nerve
(inferior posterior nasal branches)

lesser palatine nerve

PTERYGOPALATINE GANGLION and ANTERIOR ETHMOIDAL NERVE

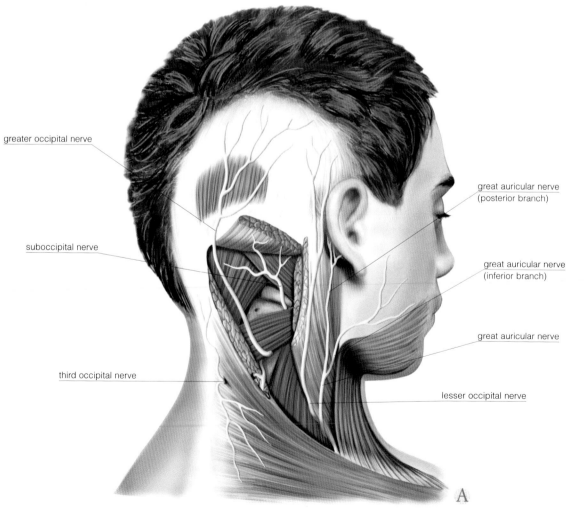

greater occipital nerve

great auricular nerve
(posterior branch)

suboccipital nerve

great auricular nerve
(inferior branch)

great auricular nerve

third occipital nerve

lesser occipital nerve

NAPE of NECK

HEAD and NECK (II)

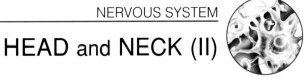

pharynx

The glossopharyngeal nerve innervates the stylopharyngeal muscle derived from the third brachial arch while the rest of muscles are innervated by the pharyngeal bunch of vague nerve. The mucus receives most of the sensory nerves of the glossopharyngeal, but the upper extreme of the pharynx is also innervated by the correspondent bunches of the maxillary division, of the trigeminal nerve, and on the tonsillar region of the soft palate the descendent palate bunches of the same nerve. The mucus is also innervated by the sympathetic nervous system through the cervical superior node. The 9th and 10th nerves and bunches of the node (pharyngeal plexus) cervical superior form a plexus over the medial constrictor of the pharynx.

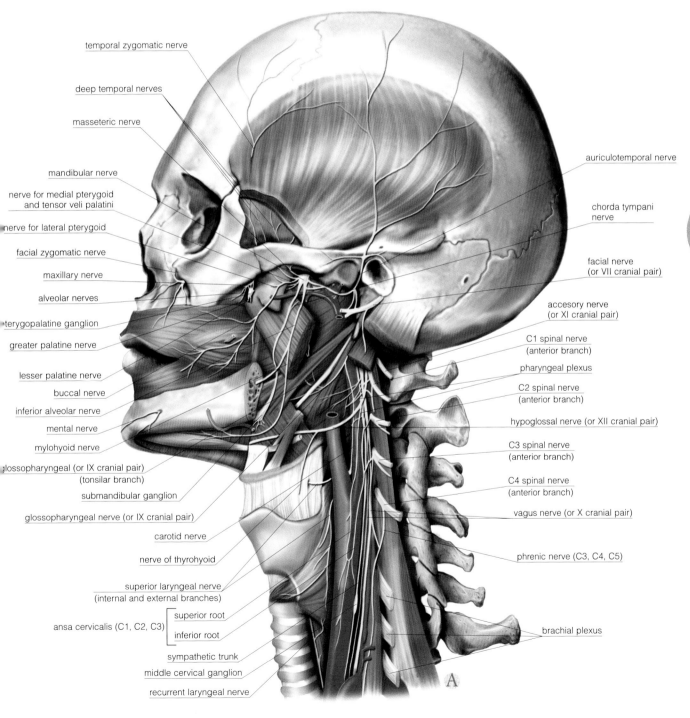

temporal zygomatic nerve

deep temporal nerves

masseteric nerve

mandibular nerve

nerve for medial pterygoid
and tensor veli palatini

nerve for lateral pterygoid

facial zygomatic nerve

maxillary nerve

alveolar nerves

terygopalatine ganglion

greater palatine nerve

lesser palatine nerve

buccal nerve

inferior alveolar nerve

mental nerve

mylohyoid nerve

glossopharyngeal (or IX cranial pair)
(tonsilar branch)

submandibular ganglion

glossopharyngeal nerve (or IX cranial pair)

carotid nerve

nerve of thyrohyoid

superior laryngeal nerve
(internal and external branches)

ansa cervicalis (C1, C2, C3)
superior root
inferior root

sympathetic trunk

middle cervical ganglion

recurrent laryngeal nerve

auriculotemporal nerve

chorda tympani
nerve

facial nerve
(or VII cranial pair)

accesory nerve
(or XI cranial pair)

C1 spinal nerve
(anterior branch)

pharyngeal plexus

C2 spinal nerve
(anterior branch)

hypoglossal nerve (or XII cranial pair)

C3 spinal nerve
(anterior branch)

C4 spinal nerve
(anterior branch)

vagus nerve (or X cranial pair)

phrenic nerve (C3, C4, C5)

brachial plexus

A

607

HEAD and NECK (III).
POSTERIOR CERVICAL REGION (I)

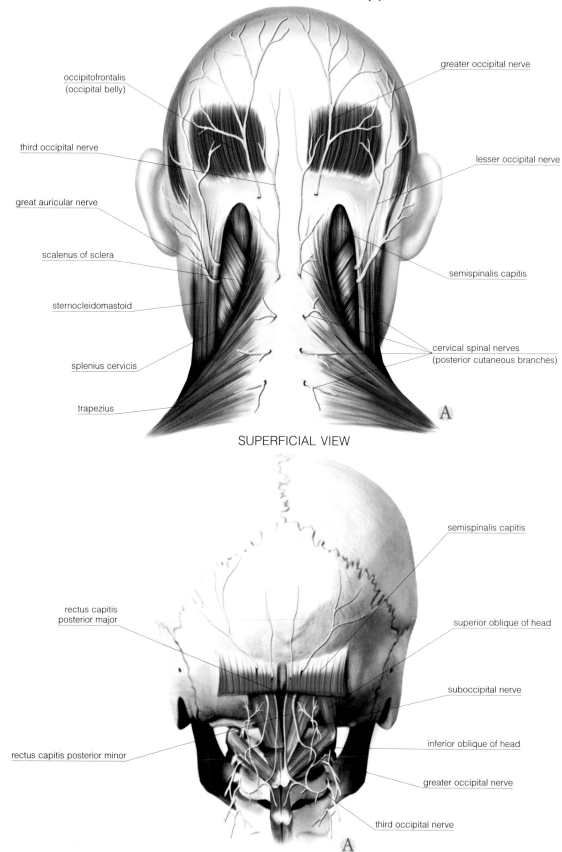

occipitofrontalis
(occipital belly)

greater occipital nerve

third occipital nerve

lesser occipital nerve

great auricular nerve

scalenus of sclera

semispinalis capitis

sternocleidomastoid

cervical spinal nerves
(posterior cutaneous branches)

splenius cervicis

trapezius

SUPERFICIAL VIEW

semispinalis capitis

rectus capitis
posterior major

superior oblique of head

suboccipital nerve

inferior oblique of head

rectus capitis posterior minor

greater occipital nerve

third occipital nerve

DEEP VIEW

HEAD and NECK (IV)
POSTERIOR CERVICAL REGION (II)
LATERAL VIEW

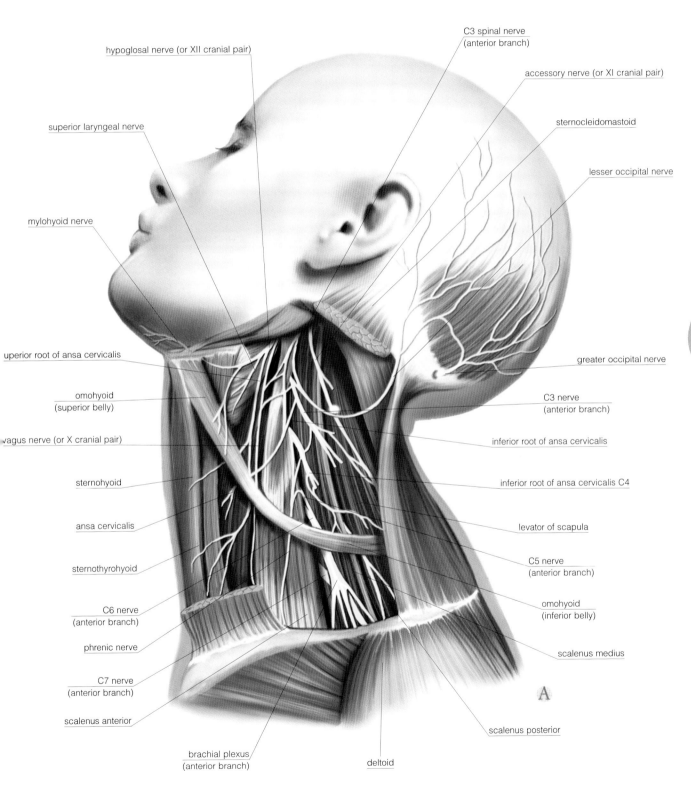

hypoglosal nerve (or XII cranial pair)

C3 spinal nerve
(anterior branch)

accessory nerve (or XI cranial pair)

superior laryngeal nerve

sternocleidomastoid

lesser occipital nerve

mylohyoid nerve

uperior root of ansa cervicalis

greater occipital nerve

omohyoid
(superior belly)

C3 nerve
(anterior branch)

vagus nerve (or X cranial pair)

inferior root of ansa cervicalis

sternohyoid

inferior root of ansa cervicalis C4

ansa cervicalis

levator of scapula

sternothyrohyoid

C5 nerve
(anterior branch)

C6 nerve
(anterior branch)

omohyoid
(inferior belly)

phrenic nerve

scalenus medius

C7 nerve
(anterior branch)

scalenus anterior

scalenus posterior

brachial plexus
(anterior branch)

deltoid

A

609

HEAD and NECK (V). MUSCLES and NERVES
LEFT SUPERFICIAL LATERAL VIEW

610

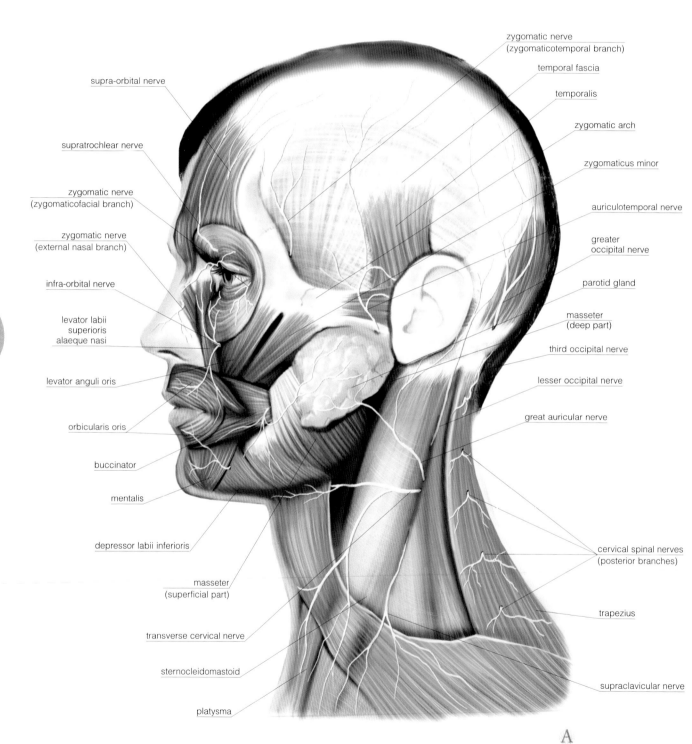

zygomatic nerve
(zygomaticotemporal branch)

temporal fascia

temporalis

zygomatic arch

zygomaticus minor

auriculotemporal nerve

greater
occipital nerve

parotid gland

masseter
(deep part)

third occipital nerve

lesser occipital nerve

great auricular nerve

cervical spinal nerves
(posterior branches)

trapezius

supraclavicular nerve

supra-orbital nerve

supratrochlear nerve

zygomatic nerve
(zygomaticofacial branch)

zygomatic nerve
(external nasal branch)

infra-orbital nerve

levator labii
superioris
alaeque nasi

levator anguli oris

orbicularis oris

buccinator

mentalis

depressor labii inferioris

masseter
(superficial part)

transverse cervical nerve

sternocleidomastoid

platysma

A

HEAD and NECK (VI). FACIAL and CERVICAL REGIONS
LEFT DEEP LATERAL VIEW

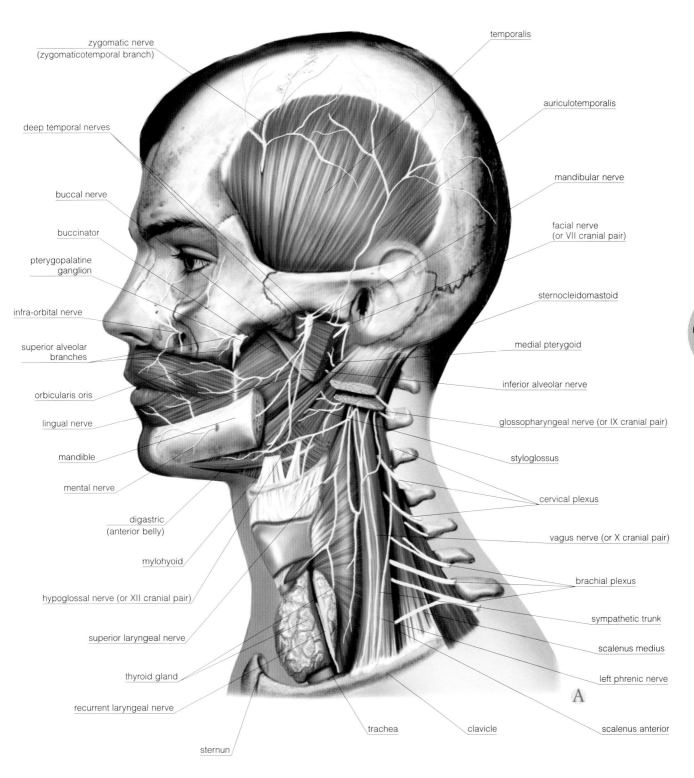

zygomatic nerve
(zygomaticotemporal branch)

deep temporal nerves

buccal nerve

buccinator

pterygopalatine
ganglion

infra-orbital nerve

superior alveolar
branches

orbicularis oris

lingual nerve

mandible

mental nerve

digastric
(anterior belly)

mylohyoid

hypoglossal nerve (or XII cranial pair)

superior laryngeal nerve

thyroid gland

recurrent laryngeal nerve

sternun

trachea

temporalis

auriculotemporalis

mandibular nerve

facial nerve
(or VII cranial pair)

sternocleidomastoid

medial pterygoid

inferior alveolar nerve

glossopharyngeal nerve (or IX cranial pair)

styloglossus

cervical plexus

vagus nerve (or X cranial pair)

brachial plexus

sympathetic trunk

scalenus medius

left phrenic nerve

clavicle

scalenus anterior

A

HEAD and NECK (VII). PHARYNX
POSTERIOR VIEW

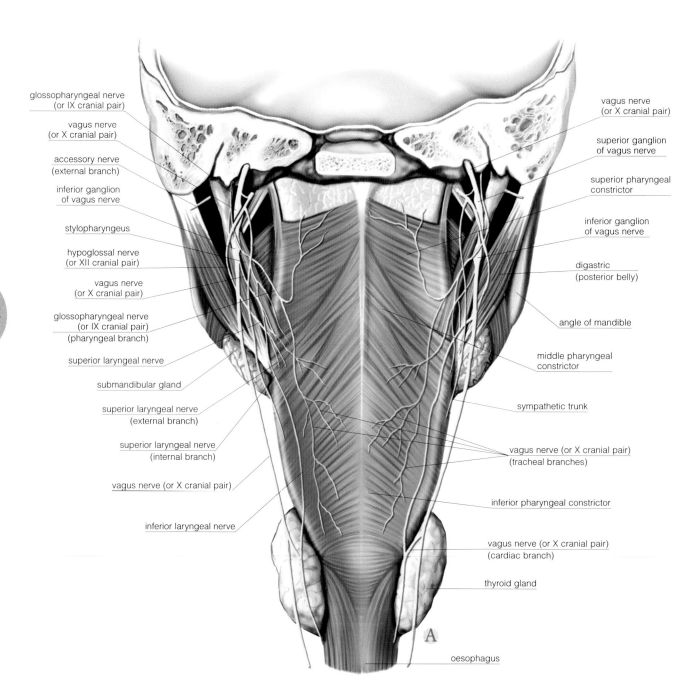

glossopharyngeal nerve
(or IX cranial pair)

vagus nerve
(or X cranial pair)

accessory nerve
(external branch)

inferior ganglion
of vagus nerve

stylopharyngeus

hypoglossal nerve
(or XII cranial pair)

vagus nerve
(or X cranial pair)

glossopharyngeal nerve
(or IX cranial pair)
(pharyngeal branch)

superior laryngeal nerve

submandibular gland

superior laryngeal nerve
(external branch)

superior laryngeal nerve
(internal branch)

vagus nerve (or X cranial pair)

inferior laryngeal nerve

vagus nerve
(or X cranial pair)

superior ganglion
of vagus nerve

superior pharyngeal
constrictor

inferior ganglion
of vagus nerve

digastric
(posterior belly)

angle of mandible

middle pharyngeal
constrictor

sympathetic trunk

vagus nerve (or X cranial pair)
(tracheal branches)

inferior pharyngeal constrictor

vagus nerve (or X cranial pair)
(cardiac branch)

thyroid gland

oesophagus

612

A

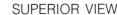

HEAD and NECK (VIII). LARYNX

SUPERIOR VIEW

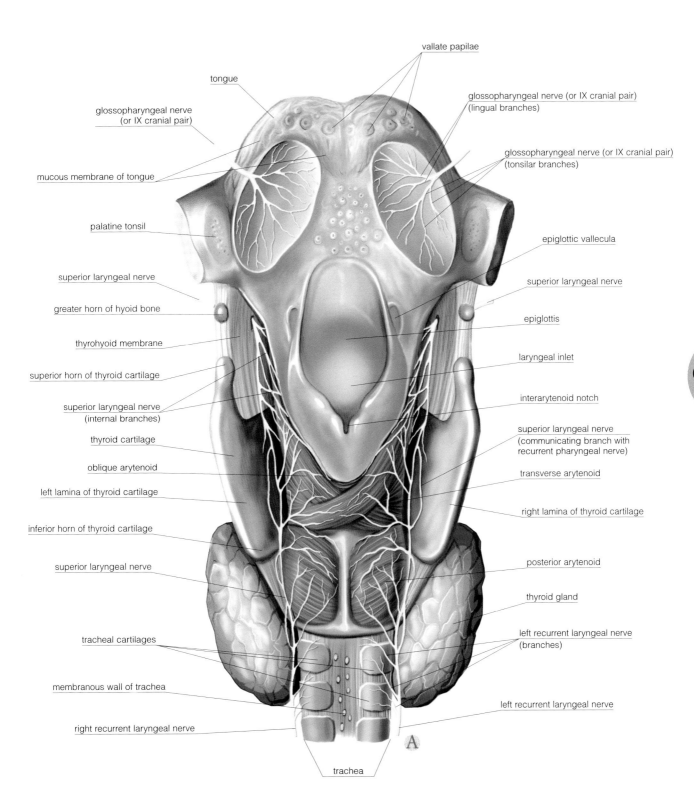

vallate papilae

tongue

glossopharyngeal nerve (or IX cranial pair)
(lingual branches)

glossopharyngeal nerve
(or IX cranial pair)

glossopharyngeal nerve (or IX cranial pair)
(tonsilar branches)

mucous membrane of tongue

palatine tonsil

epiglottic vallecula

superior laryngeal nerve

superior laryngeal nerve

greater horn of hyoid bone

epiglottis

thyrohyoid membrane

laryngeal inlet

superior horn of thyroid cartilage

interarytenoid notch

superior laryngeal nerve
(internal branches)

superior laryngeal nerve
(communicating branch with
recurrent pharyngeal nerve)

thyroid cartilage

transverse arytenoid

oblique arytenoid

left lamina of thyroid cartilage

right lamina of thyroid cartilage

inferior horn of thyroid cartilage

superior laryngeal nerve

posterior arytenoid

thyroid gland

tracheal cartilages

left recurrent laryngeal nerve
(branches)

membranous wall of trachea

left recurrent laryngeal nerve

right recurrent laryngeal nerve

A

trachea

CARDIAC NERVES

ANTERIOR VIEW

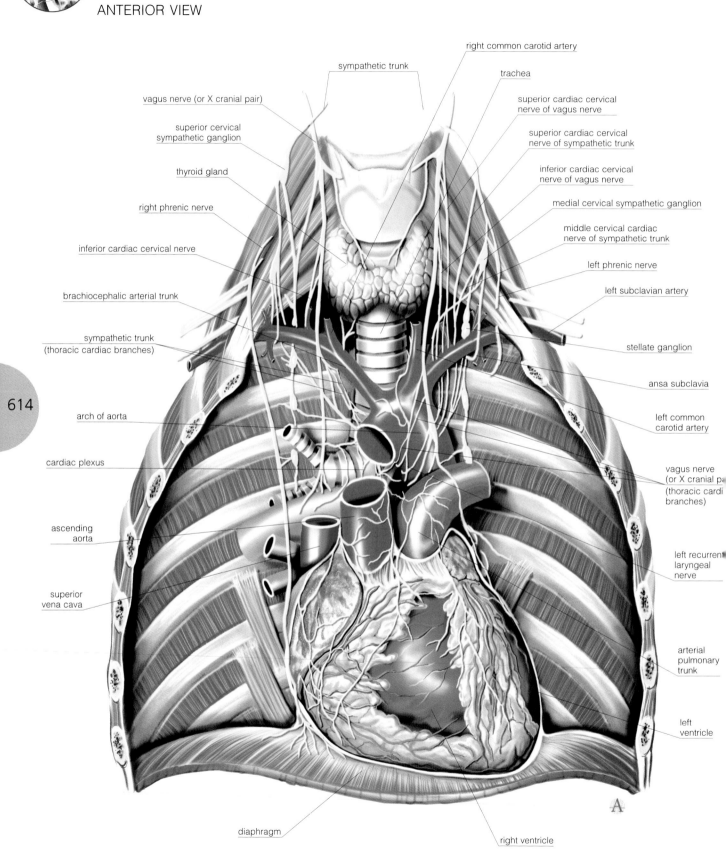

right common carotid artery

sympathetic trunk

trachea

vagus nerve (or X cranial pair)

superior cardiac cervical
nerve of vagus nerve

superior cervical
sympathetic ganglion

superior cardiac cervical
nerve of sympathetic trunk

thyroid gland

inferior cardiac cervical
nerve of vagus nerve

right phrenic nerve

medial cervical sympathetic ganglion

inferior cardiac cervical nerve

middle cervical cardiac
nerve of sympathetic trunk

left phrenic nerve

brachiocephalic arterial trunk

left subclavian artery

sympathetic trunk
(thoracic cardiac branches)

stellate ganglion

ansa subclavia

614

arch of aorta

left common
carotid artery

cardiac plexus

vagus nerve
(or X cranial pa
(thoracic cardi
branches)

ascending
aorta

left recurren
laryngeal
nerve

superior
vena cava

arterial
pulmonary
trunk

left
ventricle

diaphragm

right ventricle

A

ABDOMINAL CAVITY (I)
MALE SEX. ANTERIOR VIEW

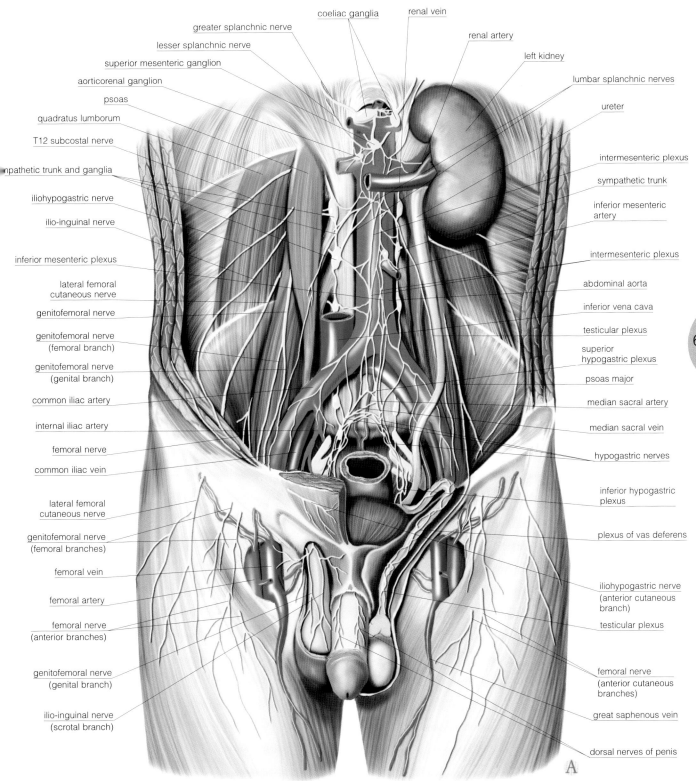

coeliac ganglia

renal vein

greater splanchnic nerve

renal artery

lesser splanchnic nerve

left kidney

superior mesenteric ganglion

lumbar splanchnic nerves

aorticorenal ganglion

ureter

psoas

quadratus lumborum

intermesenteric plexus

T12 subcostal nerve

sympathetic trunk

sympathetic trunk and ganglia

inferior mesenteric artery

iliohypogastric nerve

ilio-inguinal nerve

intermesenteric plexus

inferior mesenteric plexus

abdominal aorta

lateral femoral cutaneous nerve

inferior vena cava

genitofemoral nerve

testicular plexus

genitofemoral nerve (femoral branch)

superior hypogastric plexus

genitofemoral nerve (genital branch)

psoas major

common iliac artery

median sacral artery

internal iliac artery

median sacral vein

femoral nerve

hypogastric nerves

common iliac vein

lateral femoral cutaneous nerve

inferior hypogastric plexus

genitofemoral nerve (femoral branches)

plexus of vas deferens

femoral vein

femoral artery

iliohypogastric nerve (anterior cutaneous branch)

femoral nerve (anterior branches)

testicular plexus

genitofemoral nerve (genital branch)

femoral nerve (anterior cutaneous branches)

ilio-inguinal nerve (scrotal branch)

great saphenous vein

dorsal nerves of penis

615

A

ABDOMINAL CAVITY (II). ABDOMINAL WALL (I)
ANTERIOR VIEW

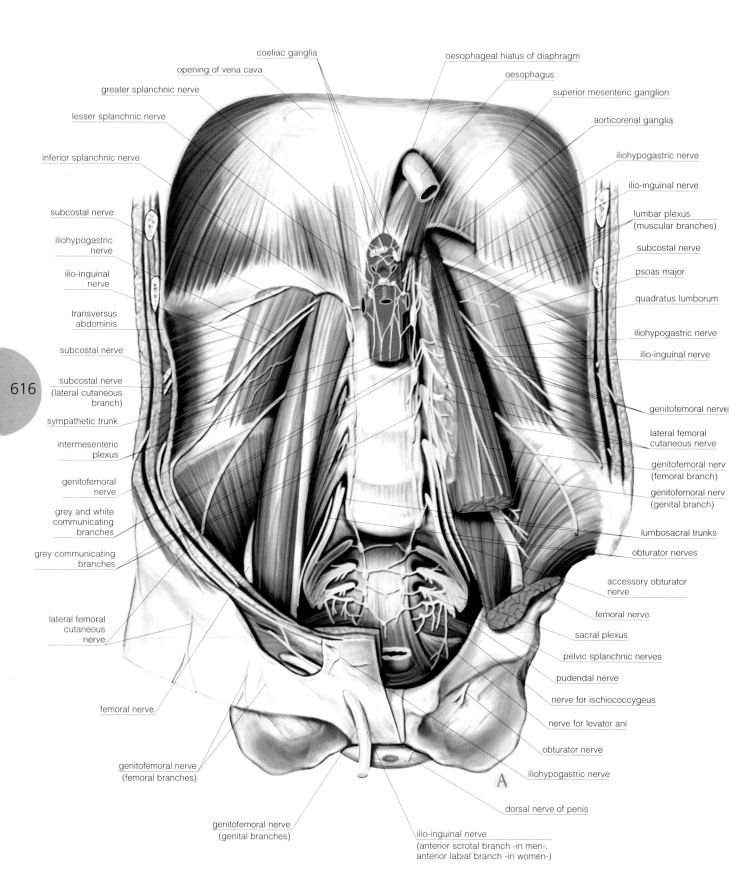

coeliac ganglia

opening of vena cava

greater splanchnic nerve

lesser splanchnic nerve

inferior splanchnic nerve

subcostal nerve

iliohypogastric nerve

ilio-inguinal nerve

transversus abdominis

subcostal nerve

subcostal nerve (lateral cutaneous branch)

sympathetic trunk

intermesenteric plexus

genitofemoral nerve

grey and white communicating branches

grey communicating branches

lateral femoral cutaneous nerve

femoral nerve

genitofemoral nerve (femoral branches)

genitofemoral nerve (genital branches)

oesophageal hiatus of diaphragm

oesophagus

superior mesenteric ganglion

aorticorenal ganglia

iliohypogastric nerve

ilio-inguinal nerve

lumbar plexus (muscular branches)

subcostal nerve

psoas major

quadratus lumborum

iliohypogastric nerve

ilio-inguinal nerve

genitofemoral nerve

lateral femoral cutaneous nerve

genitofemoral nerve (femoral branch)

genitofemoral nerve (genital branch)

lumbosacral trunks

obturator nerves

accessory obturator nerve

femoral nerve

sacral plexus

pelvic splanchnic nerves

pudendal nerve

nerve for ischiococcygeus

nerve for levator ani

obturator nerve

iliohypogastric nerve

dorsal nerve of penis

ilio-inguinal nerve (anterior scrotal branch -in men-, anterior labial branch -in women-)

A

616

ABDOMINAL CAVITY (III). ABDOMINAL WALL (II)

ANTERIOR VIEW

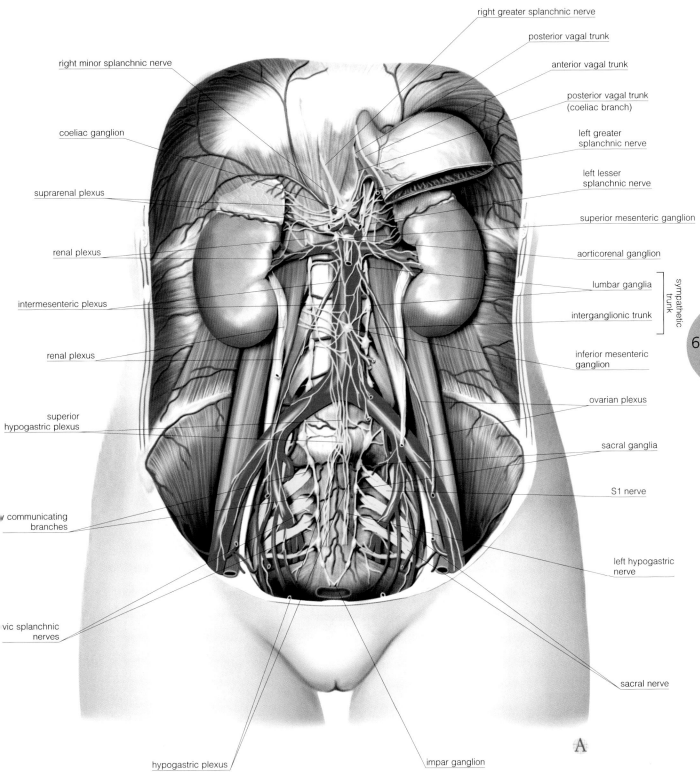

right greater splanchnic nerve

posterior vagal trunk

anterior vagal trunk

posterior vagal trunk
(coeliac branch)

left greater
splanchnic nerve

left lesser
splanchnic nerve

superior mesenteric ganglion

aorticorenal ganglion

lumbar ganglia

interganglionic trunk

sympathetic trunk

inferior mesenteric
ganglion

ovarian plexus

sacral ganglia

S1 nerve

left hypogastric
nerve

sacral nerve

right minor splanchnic nerve

coeliac ganglion

suprarenal plexus

renal plexus

intermesenteric plexus

renal plexus

superior
hypogastric plexus

communicating
branches

vic splanchnic
nerves

hypogastric plexus

impar ganglion

617

A

ABDOMINAL CAVITY (IV). ABDOMINAL WALL (III)
ANTERIOR VIEW

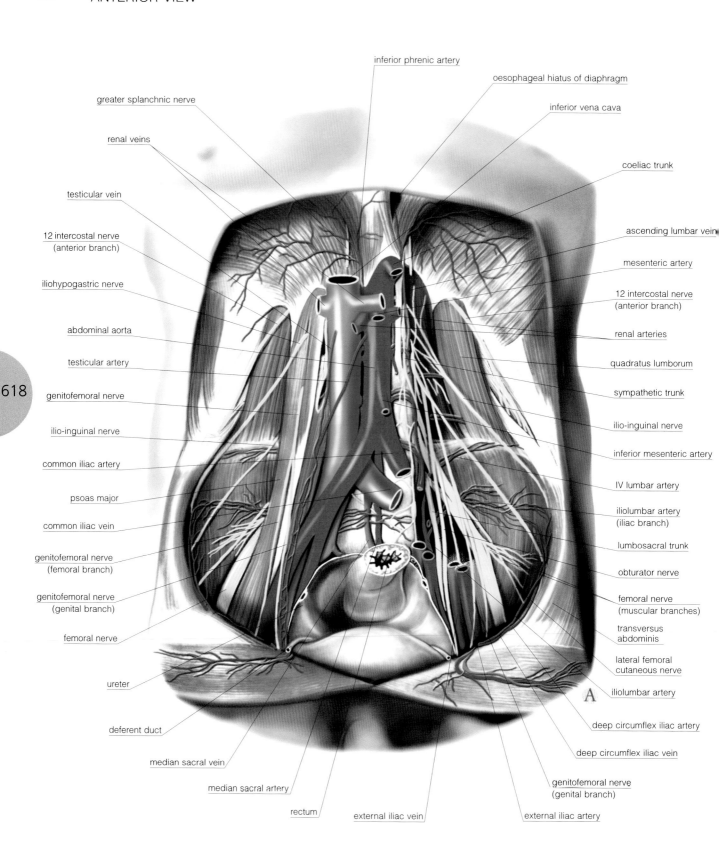

inferior phrenic artery

oesophageal hiatus of diaphragm

inferior vena cava

greater splanchnic nerve

renal veins

coeliac trunk

testicular vein

ascending lumbar vein

12 intercostal nerve
(anterior branch)

mesenteric artery

iliohypogastric nerve

12 intercostal nerve
(anterior branch)

renal arteries

abdominal aorta

quadratus lumborum

testicular artery

sympathetic trunk

genitofemoral nerve

ilio-inguinal nerve

ilio-inguinal nerve

inferior mesenteric artery

common iliac artery

IV lumbar artery

psoas major

iliolumbar artery
(iliac branch)

common iliac vein

lumbosacral trunk

genitofemoral nerve
(femoral branch)

obturator nerve

genitofemoral nerve
(genital branch)

femoral nerve
(muscular branches)

femoral nerve

transversus
abdominis

ureter

lateral femoral
cutaneous nerve

A iliolumbar artery

deferent duct

deep circumflex iliac artery

median sacral vein

deep circumflex iliac vein

median sacral artery

genitofemoral nerve
(genital branch)

rectum

external iliac vein

external iliac artery

618

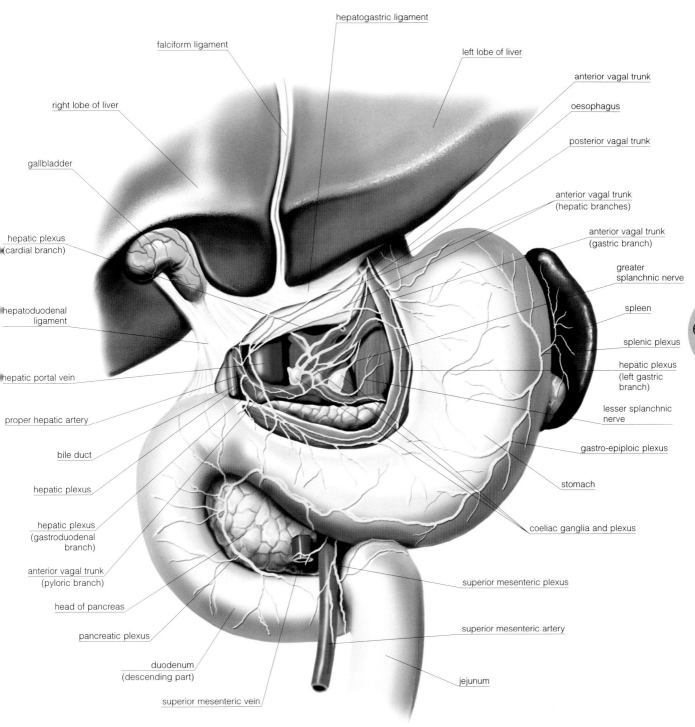

hepatogastric ligament

falciform ligament

left lobe of liver

anterior vagal trunk

oesophagus

right lobe of liver

posterior vagal trunk

gallbladder

anterior vagal trunk
(hepatic branches)

hepatic plexus
(cardial branch)

anterior vagal trunk
(gastric branch)

greater
splanchnic nerve

hepatoduodenal
ligament

spleen

splenic plexus

hepatic portal vein

hepatic plexus
(left gastric
branch)

proper hepatic artery

lesser splanchnic
nerve

bile duct

gastro-epiploic plexus

hepatic plexus

stomach

hepatic plexus
(gastroduodenal
branch)

coeliac ganglia and plexus

anterior vagal trunk
(pyloric branch)

superior mesenteric plexus

head of pancreas

pancreatic plexus

superior mesenteric artery

duodenum
(descending part)

jejunum

superior mesenteric vein

A

KIDNEY and URINARY TRACTS

MALE SEX. ANTERIOR VIEW

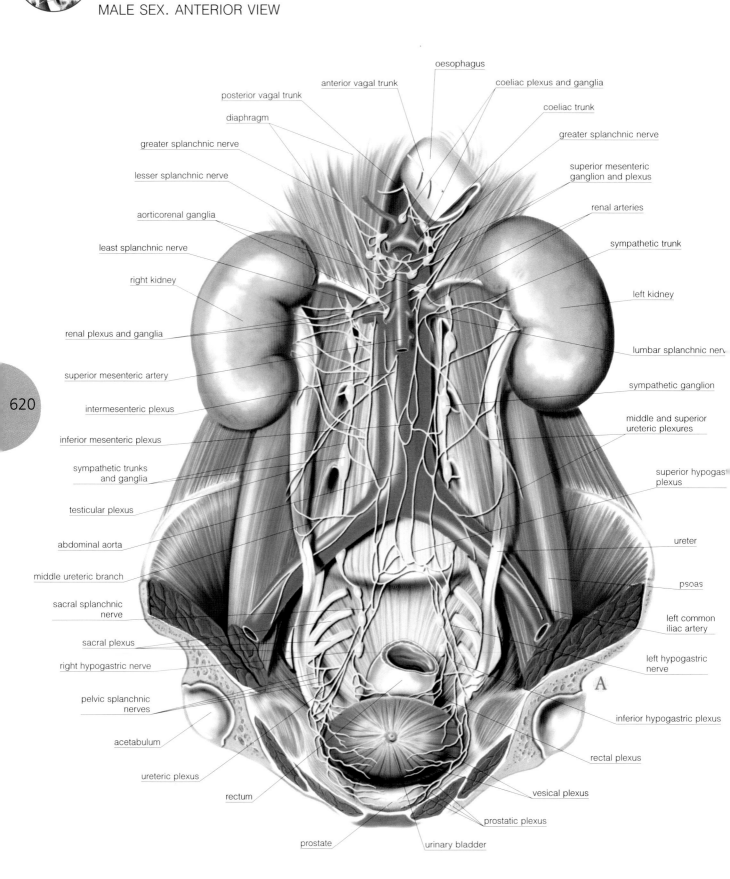

oesophagus

anterior vagal trunk

coeliac plexus and ganglia

posterior vagal trunk

coeliac trunk

diaphragm

greater splanchnic nerve

greater splanchnic nerve

lesser splanchnic nerve

superior mesenteric ganglion and plexus

aorticorenal ganglia

renal arteries

least splanchnic nerve

sympathetic trunk

right kidney

left kidney

renal plexus and ganglia

lumbar splanchnic nerv

superior mesenteric artery

sympathetic ganglion

intermesenteric plexus

middle and superior ureteric plexures

inferior mesenteric plexus

sympathetic trunks and ganglia

superior hypogas plexus

testicular plexus

abdominal aorta

ureter

middle ureteric branch

psoas

sacral splanchnic nerve

left common iliac artery

sacral plexus

left hypogastric nerve

right hypogastric nerve

A

pelvic splanchnic nerves

inferior hypogastric plexus

acetabulum

rectal plexus

ureteric plexus

vesical plexus

rectum

prostatic plexus

prostate

urinary bladder

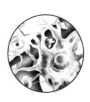

COELIAC and SUPERIOR MESENTERIC PLEXURES, SMALL INTESTINE and ASCENDING COLON

ANTERIOR VIEW

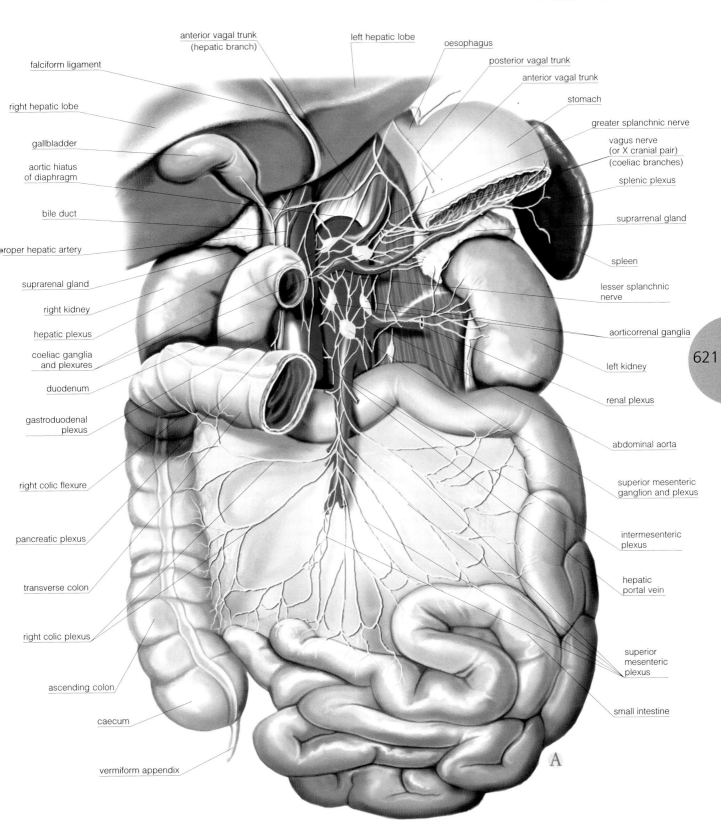

anterior vagal trunk (hepatic branch)

left hepatic lobe

oesophagus

posterior vagal trunk

anterior vagal trunk

stomach

greater splanchnic nerve

vagus nerve (or X cranial pair) (coeliac branches)

splenic plexus

suprarrenal gland

spleen

lesser splanchnic nerve

aorticorrenal ganglia

left kidney

renal plexus

abdominal aorta

superior mesenteric ganglion and plexus

intermesenteric plexus

hepatic portal vein

superior mesenteric plexus

small intestine

falciform ligament

right hepatic lobe

gallbladder

aortic hiatus of diaphragm

bile duct

roper hepatic artery

suprarenal gland

right kidney

hepatic plexus

coeliac ganglia and plexures

duodenum

gastroduodenal plexus

right colic flexure

pancreatic plexus

transverse colon

right colic plexus

ascending colon

caecum

vermiform appendix

621

A

LARGE INTESTINE (I)

ANTERIOR VIEW

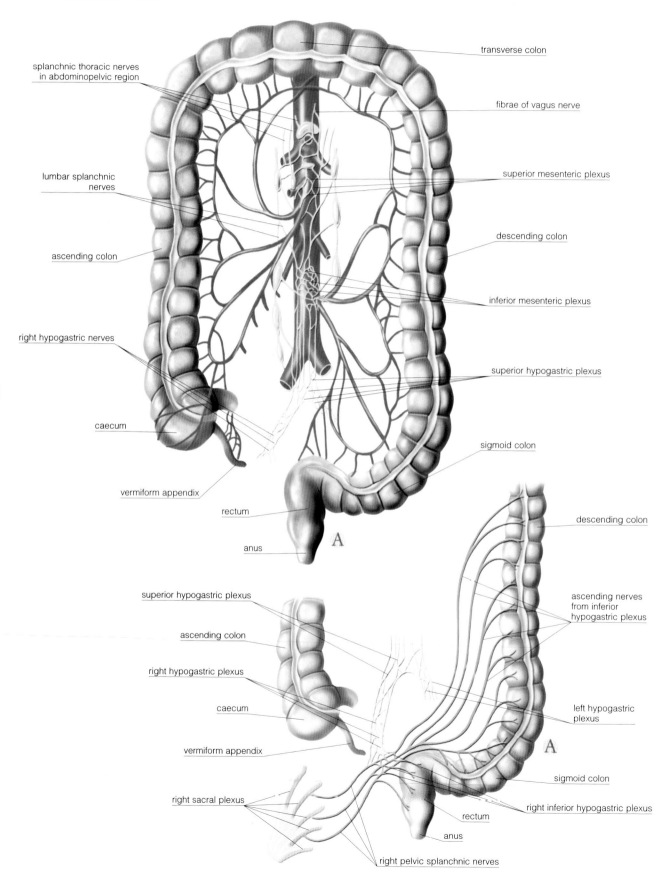

transverse colon

splanchnic thoracic nerves in abdominopelvic region

fibrae of vagus nerve

lumbar splanchnic nerves

superior mesenteric plexus

descending colon

ascending colon

inferior mesenteric plexus

right hypogastric nerves

superior hypogastric plexus

caecum

sigmoid colon

vermiform appendix

rectum

A

anus

superior hypogastric plexus

descending colon

ascending colon

ascending nerves from inferior hypogastric plexus

right hypogastric plexus

caecum

left hypogastric plexus

vermiform appendix

A

sigmoid colon

right sacral plexus

right inferior hypogastric plexus

rectum

anus

right pelvic splanchnic nerves

622

LARGE INTESTINE (II)
ANTERIOR VIEW

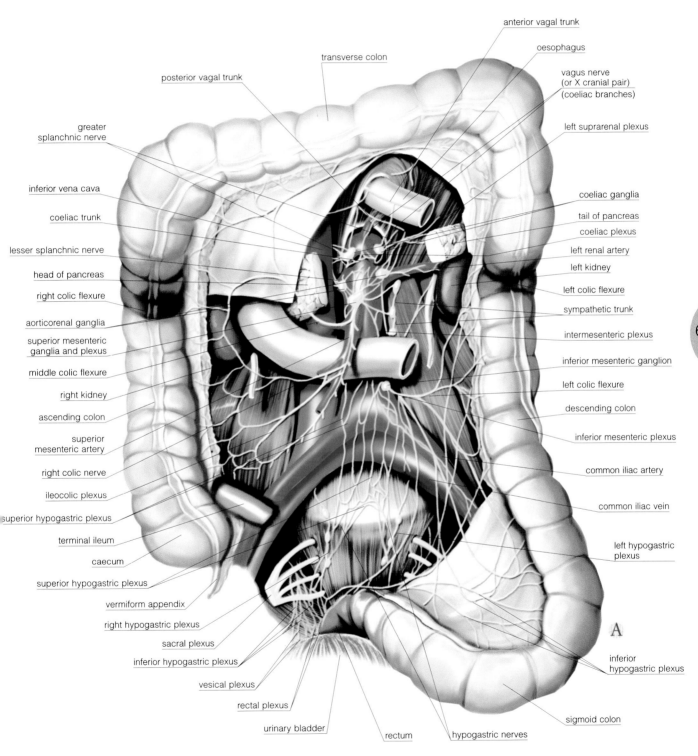

anterior vagal trunk

oesophagus

vagus nerve
(or X cranial pair)
(coeliac branches)

transverse colon

posterior vagal trunk

left suprarenal plexus

greater
splanchnic nerve

coeliac ganglia

inferior vena cava

tail of pancreas

coeliac trunk

coeliac plexus

lesser splanchnic nerve

left renal artery

head of pancreas

left kidney

right colic flexure

left colic flexure

aorticorenal ganglia

sympathetic trunk

superior mesenteric
ganglia and plexus

intermesenteric plexus

middle colic flexure

inferior mesenteric ganglion

right kidney

left colic flexure

ascending colon

descending colon

superior
mesenteric artery

inferior mesenteric plexus

right colic nerve

common iliac artery

ileocolic plexus

common iliac vein

superior hypogastric plexus

terminal ileum

left hypogastric
plexus

caecum

superior hypogastric plexus

vermiform appendix

right hypogastric plexus

inferior
hypogastric plexus

sacral plexus

inferior hypogastric plexus

vesical plexus

rectal plexus

sigmoid colon

urinary bladder

rectum

hypogastric nerves

A

623

TRUNK (I)
FEMALE SEX. ANTERIOR SUPERFICIAL VIEW

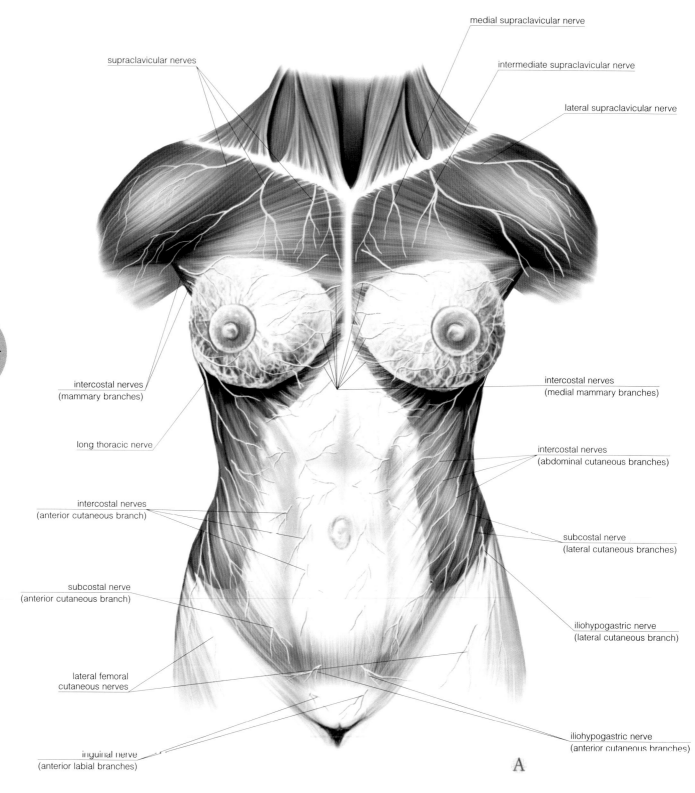

medial supraclavicular nerve

intermediate supraclavicular nerve

lateral supraclavicular nerve

supraclavicular nerves

intercostal nerves
(mammary branches)

long thoracic nerve

intercostal nerves
(anterior cutaneous branch)

subcostal nerve
(anterior cutaneous branch)

lateral femoral
cutaneous nerves

inguinal nerve
(anterior labial branches)

intercostal nerves
(medial mammary branches)

intercostal nerves
(abdominal cutaneous branches)

subcostal nerve
(lateral cutaneous branches)

iliohypogastric nerve
(lateral cutaneous branch)

iliohypogastric nerve
(anterior cutaneous branches)

A

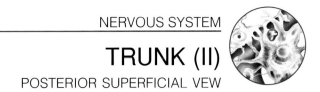

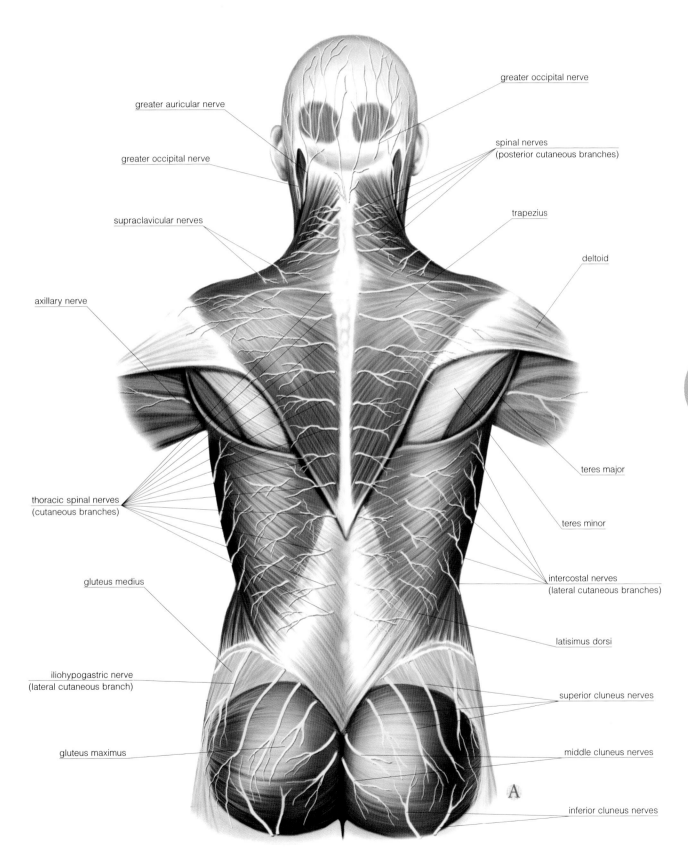

greater occipital nerve

greater auricular nerve

spinal nerves
(posterior cutaneous branches)

greater occipital nerve

trapezius

supraclavicular nerves

deltoid

axillary nerve

625

teres major

thoracic spinal nerves
(cutaneous branches)

teres minor

intercostal nerves
(lateral cutaneous branches)

gluteus medius

latisimus dorsi

iliohypogastric nerve
(lateral cutaneous branch)

superior cluneus nerves

gluteus maximus

middle cluneus nerves

A

inferior cluneus nerves

THORAX, OESOPHAGUS and BRONCHI
ANTERIOR VIEW

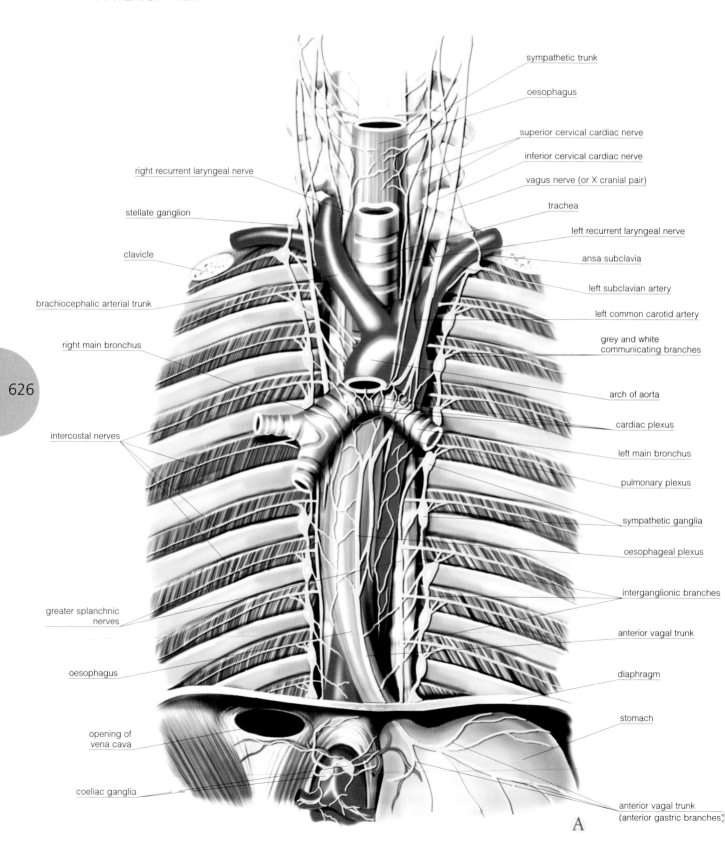

sympathetic trunk

oesophagus

superior cervical cardiac nerve

inferior cervical cardiac nerve

vagus nerve (or X cranial pair)

right recurrent laryngeal nerve

trachea

stellate ganglion

left recurrent laryngeal nerve

clavicle

ansa subclavia

left subclavian artery

brachiocephalic arterial trunk

left common carotid artery

grey and white
communicating branches

right main bronchus

arch of aorta

cardiac plexus

intercostal nerves

left main bronchus

pulmonary plexus

sympathetic ganglia

oesophageal plexus

interganglionic branches

greater splanchnic
nerves

anterior vagal trunk

oesophagus

diaphragm

stomach

opening of
vena cava

coeliac ganglia

anterior vagal trunk
(anterior gastric branches)

626

A

PELVIC CAVITY (I)
FEMALE SEX. LEFT HEMIPELVIS. SAGITTAL SECTION

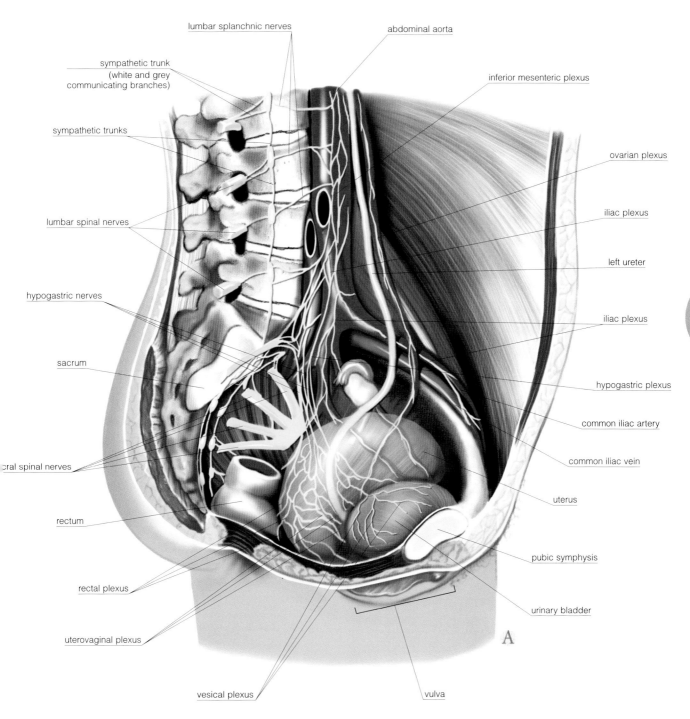

lumbar splanchnic nerves

sympathetic trunk
(white and grey
communicating branches)

sympathetic trunks

lumbar spinal nerves

hypogastric nerves

sacrum

cral spinal nerves

rectum

rectal plexus

uterovaginal plexus

vesical plexus

abdominal aorta

inferior mesenteric plexus

ovarian plexus

iliac plexus

left ureter

iliac plexus

hypogastric plexus

common iliac artery

common iliac vein

uterus

pubic symphysis

urinary bladder

vulva

627

A

PELVIC CAVITY (II)

MALE SEX. LATERAL VIEWS

628

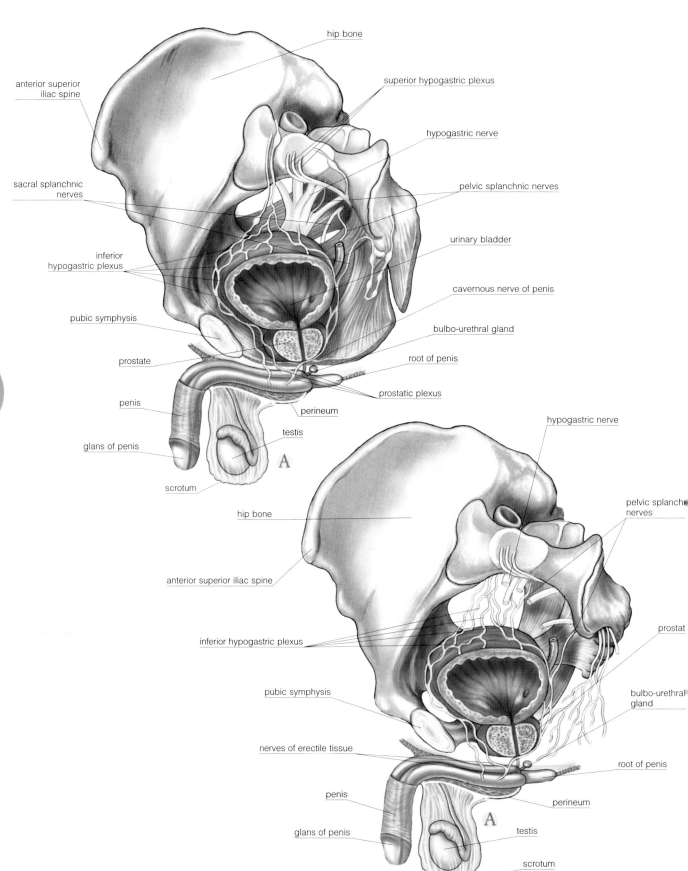

hip bone

superior hypogastric plexus

hypogastric nerve

anterior superior
iliac spine

pelvic splanchnic nerves

sacral splanchnic
nerves

urinary bladder

inferior
hypogastric plexus

cavernous nerve of penis

pubic symphysis

bulbo-urethral gland

prostate

root of penis

penis

prostatic plexus

perineum

testis

glans of penis

A

scrotum

hypogastric nerve

hip bone

pelvic splanch
nerves

anterior superior iliac spine

prostat

inferior hypogastric plexus

pubic symphysis

bulbo-urethral
gland

nerves of erectile tissue

root of penis

penis

perineum

A

glans of penis

testis

scrotum

PELVIC CAVITY (III)

FEMALE SEX. ANTERIOR VIEW

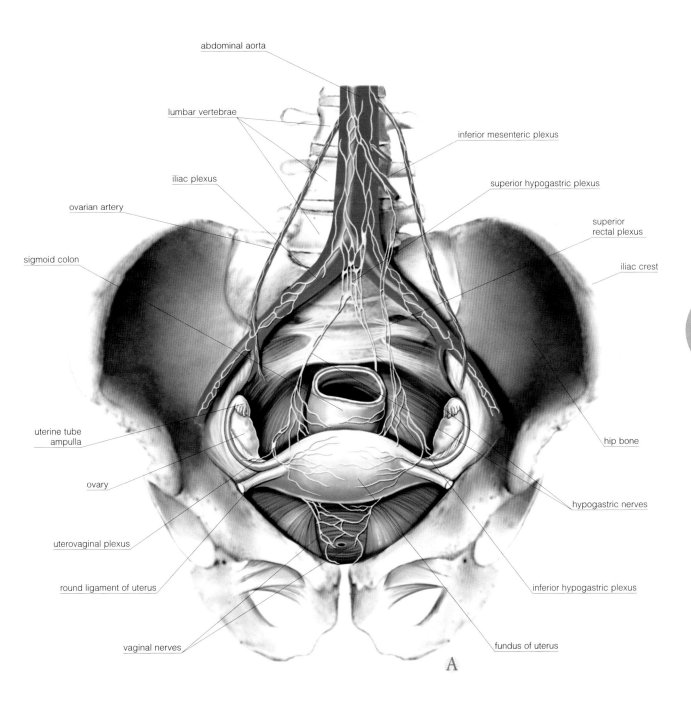

abdominal aorta

lumbar vertebrae

iliac plexus

ovarian artery

sigmoid colon

uterine tube
ampulla

ovary

uterovaginal plexus

round ligament of uterus

vaginal nerves

inferior mesenteric plexus

superior hypogastric plexus

superior
rectal plexus

iliac crest

hip bone

hypogastric nerves

inferior hypogastric plexus

fundus of uterus

A

629

LUMBOSACRAL PLEXUS (I)
MALE SEX. ANTERIOR VIEW

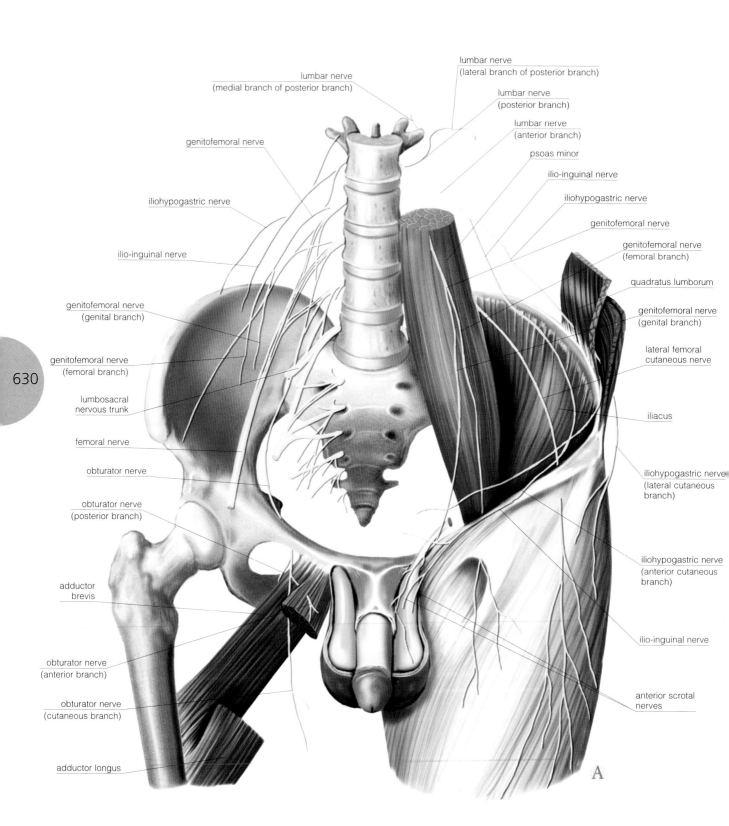

lumbar nerve
(medial branch of posterior branch)

lumbar nerve
(lateral branch of posterior branch)

lumbar nerve
(posterior branch)

lumbar nerve
(anterior branch)

genitofemoral nerve

psoas minor

ilio-inguinal nerve

iliohypogastric nerve

iliohypogastric nerve

ilio-inguinal nerve

genitofemoral nerve

genitofemoral nerve
(femoral branch)

genitofemoral nerve
(genital branch)

quadratus lumborum

genitofemoral nerve
(femoral branch)

genitofemoral nerve
(genital branch)

lateral femoral
cutaneous nerve

lumbosacral
nervous trunk

iliacus

femoral nerve

obturator nerve

iliohypogastric nerve
(lateral cutaneous
branch)

obturator nerve
(posterior branch)

iliohypogastric nerve
(anterior cutaneous
branch)

adductor
brevis

obturator nerve
(anterior branch)

ilio-inguinal nerve

obturator nerve
(cutaneous branch)

anterior scrotal
nerves

adductor longus

A

LUMBOSACRAL PLEXUS (II)
ANTERIOR VIEW

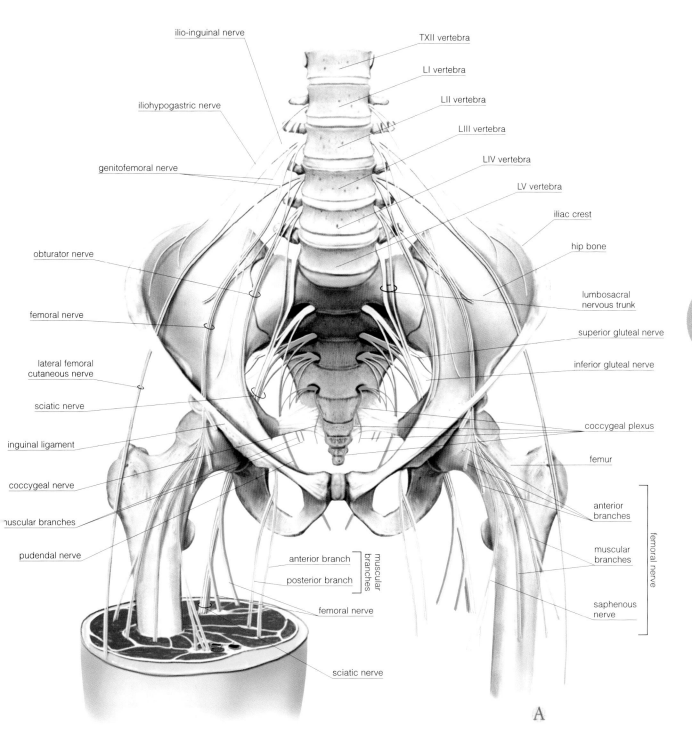

ilio-inguinal nerve

iliohypogastric nerve

genitofemoral nerve

obturator nerve

femoral nerve

lateral femoral
cutaneous nerve

sciatic nerve

inguinal ligament

coccygeal nerve

muscular branches

pudendal nerve

TXII vertebra

LI vertebra

LII vertebra

LIII vertebra

LIV vertebra

LV vertebra

iliac crest

hip bone

lumbosacral
nervous trunk

superior gluteal nerve

inferior gluteal nerve

coccygeal plexus

femur

anterior
branches

muscular
branches

saphenous
nerve

femoral nerve

anterior branch

posterior branch

muscular
branches

femoral nerve

sciatic nerve

A

GLUTEAL REGION (I)

RIGHT LOWER LIMB. MALE SEX. DEEP VIEW

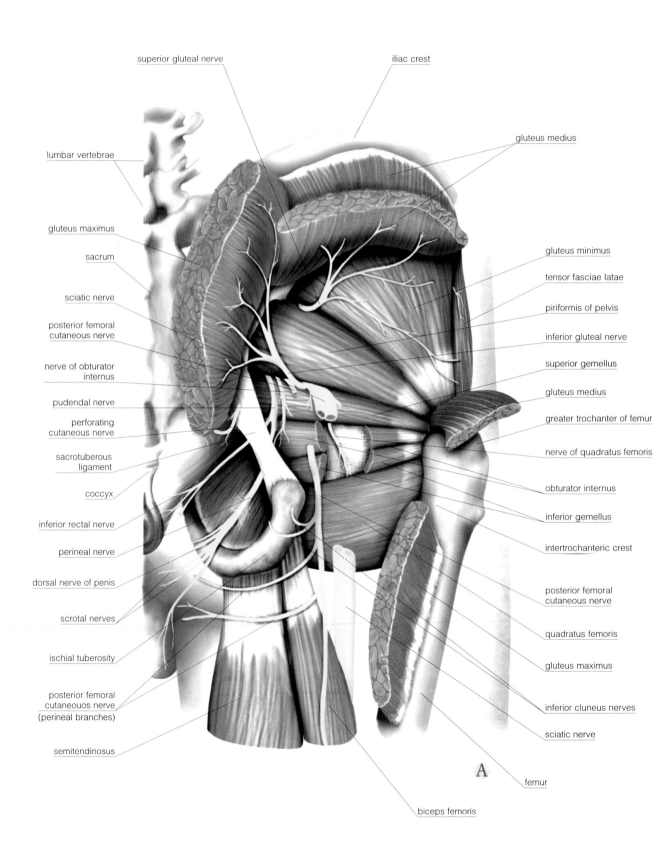

superior gluteal nerve

iliac crest

gluteus medius

lumbar vertebrae

gluteus maximus

sacrum

gluteus minimus

tensor fasciae latae

sciatic nerve

piriformis of pelvis

posterior femoral
cutaneous nerve

inferior gluteal nerve

nerve of obturator
internus

superior gemellus

pudendal nerve

gluteus medius

greater trochanter of femur

perforating
cutaneous nerve

nerve of quadratus femoris

sacrotuberous
ligament

obturator internus

coccyx

inferior gemellus

inferior rectal nerve

intertrochanteric crest

perineal nerve

dorsal nerve of penis

posterior femoral
cutaneous nerve

scrotal nerves

quadratus femoris

ischial tuberosity

gluteus maximus

posterior femoral
cutaneouos nerve
(perineal branches)

inferior cluneus nerves

sciatic nerve

semitendinosus

A

femur

biceps femoris

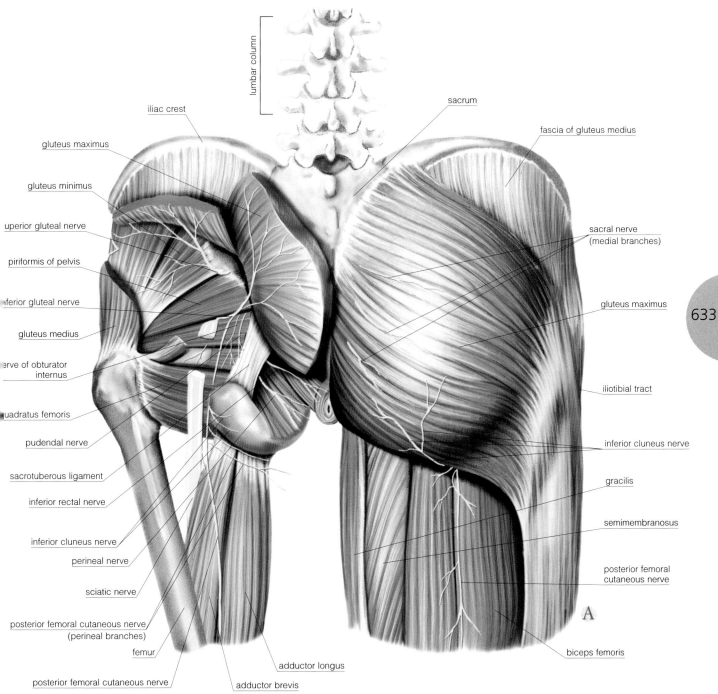

lumbar column

iliac crest

gluteus maximus

gluteus minimus

uperior gluteal nerve

piriformis of pelvis

ferior gluteal nerve

gluteus medius

erve of obturator internus

uadratus femoris

pudendal nerve

sacrotuberous ligament

inferior rectal nerve

inferior cluneus nerve

perineal nerve

sciatic nerve

posterior femoral cutaneous nerve (perineal branches)

femur

posterior femoral cutaneous nerve

adductor longus

adductor brevis

sacrum

fascia of gluteus medius

sacral nerve (medial branches)

gluteus maximus

iliotibial tract

inferior cluneus nerve

gracilis

semimembranosus

posterior femoral cutaneous nerve

biceps femoris

A

LEFT SIDE. DEEP VIEW

RIGHT SIDE. SUPERFICIAL VIEW

633

UPPER LIMB (I)
RIGHT UPPER LIMB. PALMAR VIEW

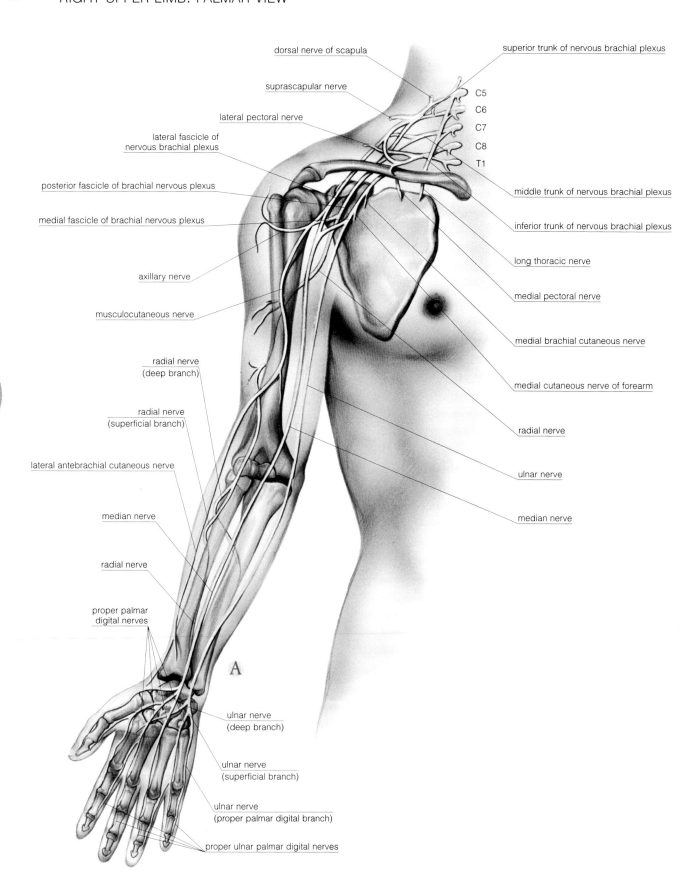

dorsal nerve of scapula

superior trunk of nervous brachial plexus

suprascapular nerve

lateral pectoral nerve

C5
C6
C7
C8
T1

lateral fascicle of
nervous brachial plexus

posterior fascicle of brachial nervous plexus

middle trunk of nervous brachial plexus

medial fascicle of brachial nervous plexus

inferior trunk of nervous brachial plexus

axillary nerve

long thoracic nerve

medial pectoral nerve

musculocutaneous nerve

medial brachial cutaneous nerve

radial nerve
(deep branch)

medial cutaneous nerve of forearm

radial nerve
(superficial branch)

radial nerve

lateral antebrachial cutaneous nerve

ulnar nerve

median nerve

median nerve

radial nerve

proper palmar
digital nerves

A

ulnar nerve
(deep branch)

ulnar nerve
(superficial branch)

ulnar nerve
(proper palmar digital branch)

proper ulnar palmar digital nerves

634

UPPER LIMB (II). AXILLARY FOSSA and SHOULDER

LEFT UPPER LIMB. ANTERIOR VIEW

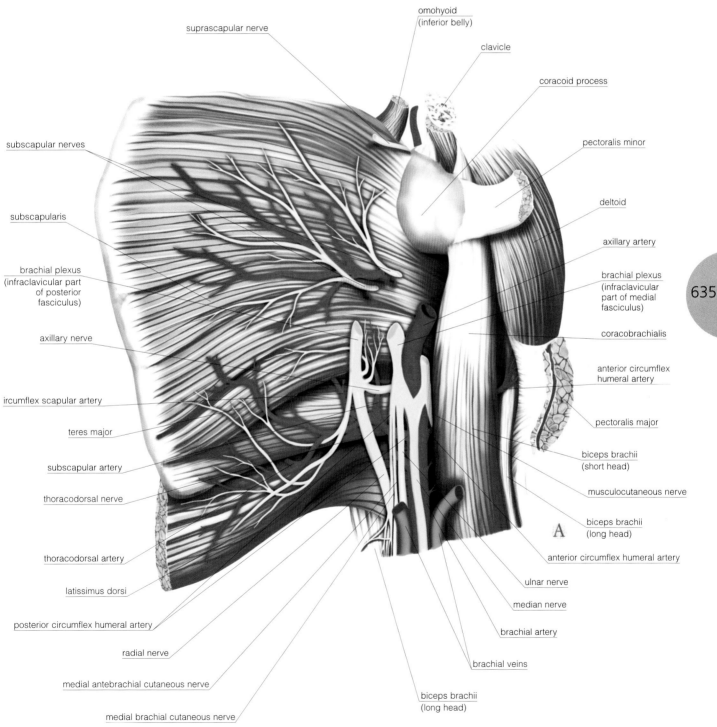

suprascapular nerve

omohyoid (inferior belly)

clavicle

coracoid process

pectoralis minor

deltoid

subscapular nerves

subscapularis

axillary artery

brachial plexus (infraclavicular part of posterior fasciculus)

brachial plexus (infraclavicular part of medial fasciculus)

635

axillary nerve

coracobrachialis

anterior circumflex humeral artery

ircumflex scapular artery

teres major

pectoralis major

subscapular artery

biceps brachii (short head)

thoracodorsal nerve

musculocutaneous nerve

biceps brachii (long head)

thoracodorsal artery

A

anterior circumflex humeral artery

latissimus dorsi

ulnar nerve

posterior circumflex humeral artery

median nerve

radial nerve

brachial artery

medial antebrachial cutaneous nerve

brachial veins

medial brachial cutaneous nerve

biceps brachii (long head)

UPPER LIMB (III). FACIAL and AXILLARY NERVES

RIGHT UPPER LIMB. POSTERIOR VIEW

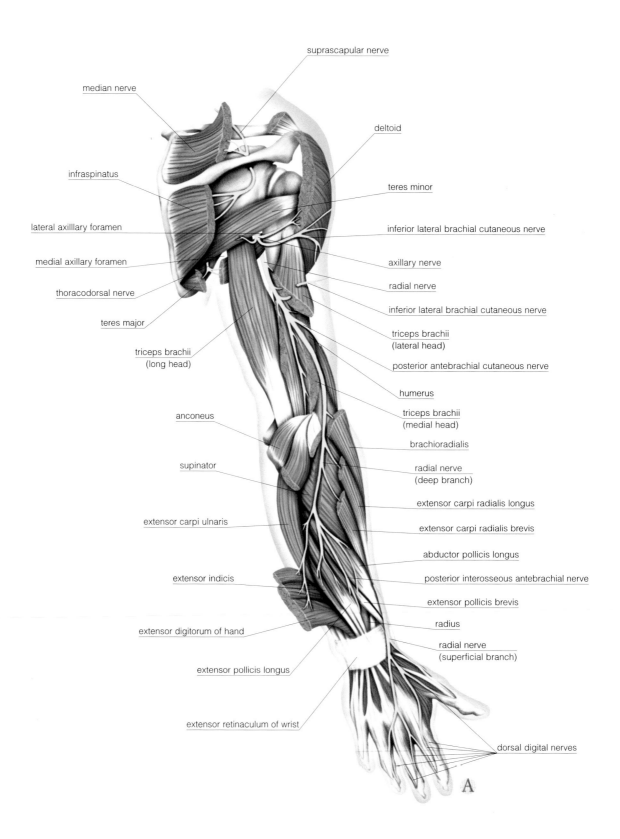

suprascapular nerve

median nerve

deltoid

infraspinatus

teres minor

lateral axilllary foramen

inferior lateral brachial cutaneous nerve

medial axillary foramen

axillary nerve

thoracodorsal nerve

radial nerve

inferior lateral brachial cutaneous nerve

teres major

triceps brachii
(lateral head)

triceps brachii
(long head)

posterior antebrachial cutaneous nerve

humerus

anconeus

triceps brachii
(medial head)

brachioradialis

supinator

radial nerve
(deep branch)

extensor carpi radialis longus

extensor carpi radialis brevis

extensor carpi ulnaris

abductor pollicis longus

extensor indicis

posterior interosseous antebrachial nerve

extensor pollicis brevis

radius

extensor digitorum of hand

radial nerve
(superficial branch)

extensor pollicis longus

extensor retinaculum of wrist

dorsal digital nerves

A

UPPER LIMB (IV). MEDIAN NERVE
RIGHT UPPER LIMB. ANTERIOR VIEW

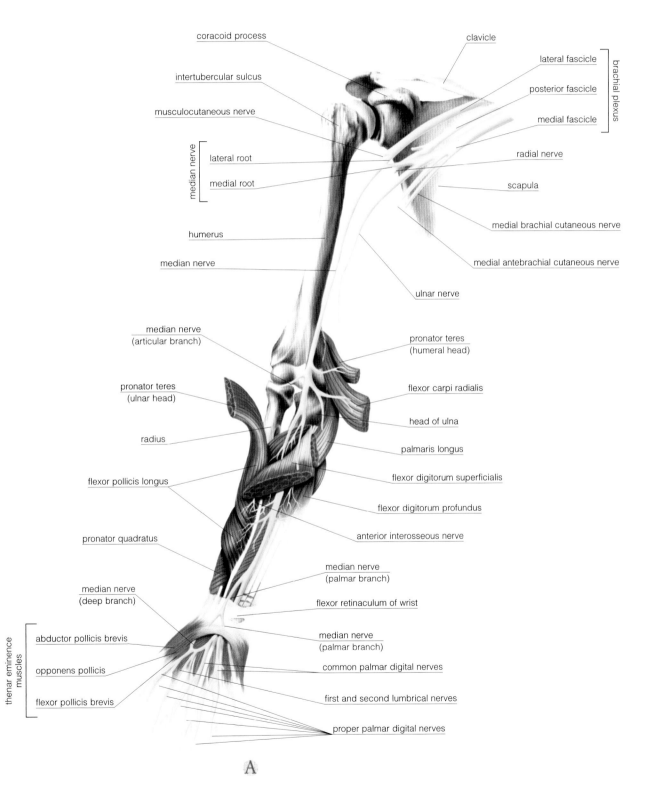

coracoid process

clavicle

lateral fascicle

brachial plexus

intertubercular sulcus

posterior fascicle

musculocutaneous nerve

medial fascicle

median nerve

lateral root

radial nerve

medial root

scapula

humerus

medial brachial cutaneous nerve

median nerve

medial antebrachial cutaneous nerve

ulnar nerve

median nerve
(articular branch)

pronator teres
(humeral head)

pronator teres
(ulnar head)

flexor carpi radialis

head of ulna

radius

palmaris longus

flexor pollicis longus

flexor digitorum superficialis

flexor digitorum profundus

anterior interosseous nerve

pronator quadratus

median nerve
(palmar branch)

median nerve
(deep branch)

flexor retinaculum of wrist

thenar eminence muscles

abductor pollicis brevis

median nerve
(palmar branch)

opponens pollicis

common palmar digital nerves

first and second lumbrical nerves

flexor pollicis brevis

proper palmar digital nerves

A

637

UPPER LIMB (V). BRACHIAL REGION (I)

LEFT UPPER LIMB. ANTERIOR SUPERFICIAL VIEW

638

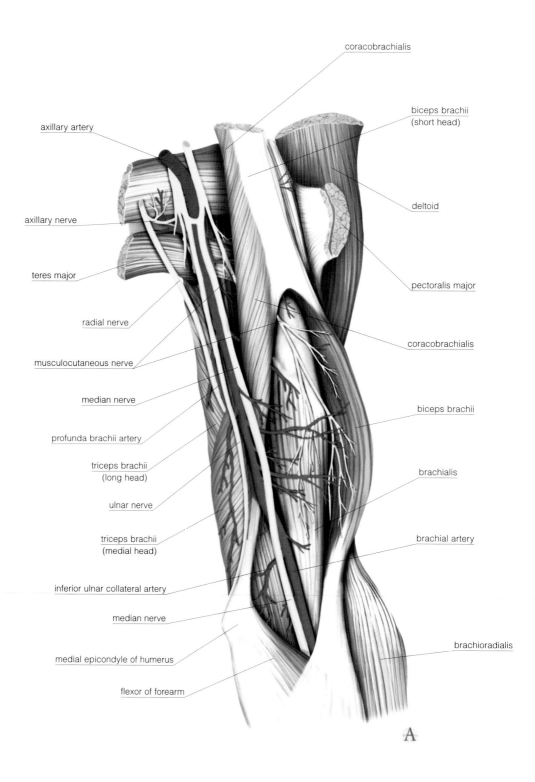

coracobrachialis

biceps brachii
(short head)

axillary artery

deltoid

axillary nerve

teres major

pectoralis major

radial nerve

coracobrachialis

musculocutaneous nerve

median nerve

biceps brachii

profunda brachii artery

triceps brachii
(long head)

brachialis

ulnar nerve

triceps brachii
(medial head)

brachial artery

inferior ulnar collateral artery

median nerve

brachioradialis

medial epicondyle of humerus

flexor of forearm

A

UPPER LIMB (VI). BRACHIAL REGION (II)

LEFT UPPER LIMB. POSTERIOR DEEP VIEW

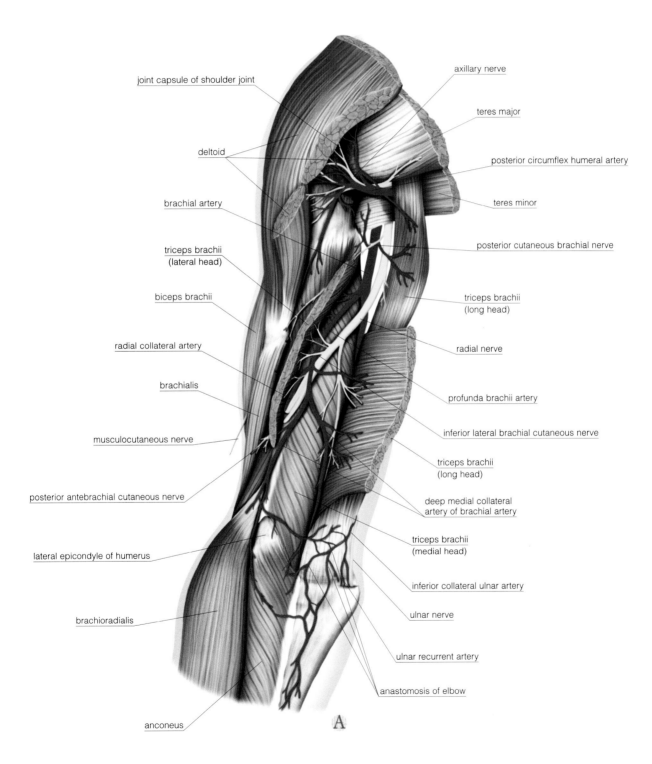

joint capsule of shoulder joint

axillary nerve

teres major

deltoid

posterior circumflex humeral artery

brachial artery

teres minor

triceps brachii
(lateral head)

posterior cutaneous brachial nerve

biceps brachii

triceps brachii
(long head)

radial collateral artery

radial nerve

brachialis

profunda brachii artery

musculocutaneous nerve

inferior lateral brachial cutaneous nerve

triceps brachii
(long head)

posterior antebrachial cutaneous nerve

deep medial collateral
artery of brachial artery

triceps brachii
(medial head)

lateral epicondyle of humerus

inferior collateral ulnar artery

ulnar nerve

brachioradialis

ulnar recurrent artery

anastomosis of elbow

anconeus

A

UPPER LIMB (VII). ANTEBRACHIAL REGION (I)

LEFT UPPER LIMB. ANTERIOR SUPERFICIAL VIEW

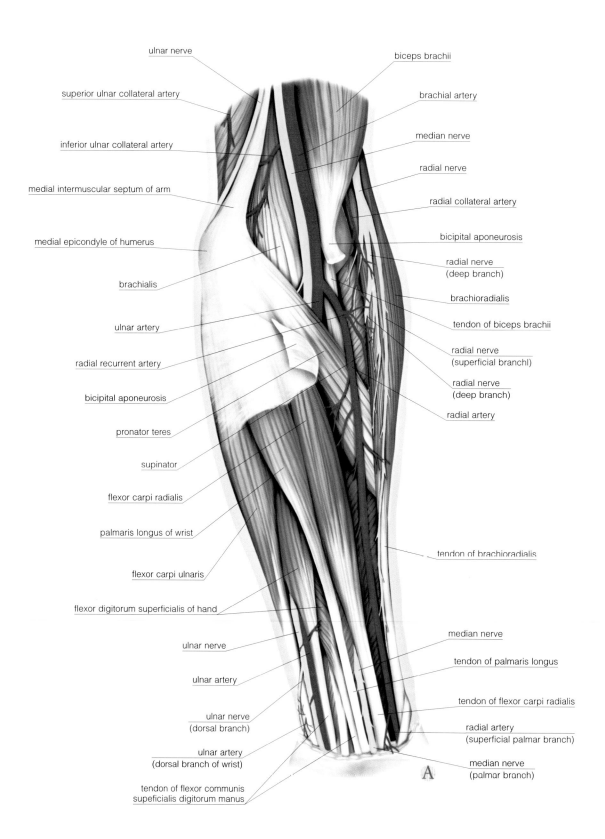

ulnar nerve

superior ulnar collateral artery

inferior ulnar collateral artery

medial intermuscular septum of arm

medial epicondyle of humerus

brachialis

ulnar artery

radial recurrent artery

bicipital aponeurosis

pronator teres

supinator

flexor carpi radialis

palmaris longus of wrist

flexor carpi ulnaris

flexor digitorum superficialis of hand

ulnar nerve

ulnar artery

ulnar nerve
(dorsal branch)

ulnar artery
(dorsal branch of wrist)

tendon of flexor communis
supeficialis digitorum manus

biceps brachii

brachial artery

median nerve

radial nerve

radial collateral artery

bicipital aponeurosis

radial nerve
(deep branch)

brachioradialis

tendon of biceps brachii

radial nerve
(superficial branchl)

radial nerve
(deep branch)

radial artery

tendon of brachioradialis

median nerve

tendon of palmaris longus

tendon of flexor carpi radialis

radial artery
(superficial palmar branch)

median nerve
(palmar branch)

A

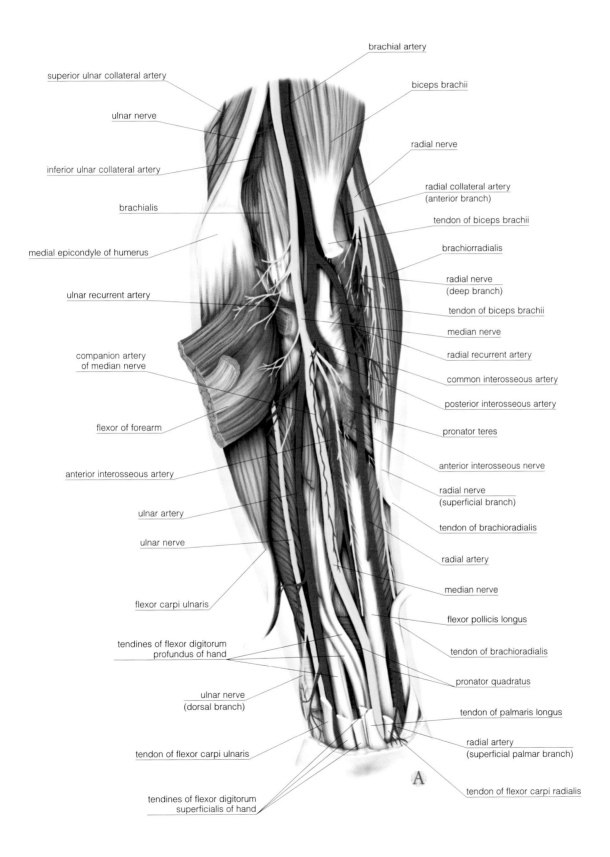

brachial artery

superior ulnar collateral artery

biceps brachii

ulnar nerve

radial nerve

inferior ulnar collateral artery

radial collateral artery
(anterior branch)

brachialis

tendon of biceps brachii

medial epicondyle of humerus

brachioradialis

radial nerve
(deep branch)

ulnar recurrent artery

tendon of biceps brachii

median nerve

companion artery
of median nerve

radial recurrent artery

common interosseous artery

posterior interosseous artery

flexor of forearm

pronator teres

anterior interosseous artery

anterior interosseous nerve

radial nerve
(superficial branch)

ulnar artery

tendon of brachioradialis

ulnar nerve

radial artery

flexor carpi ulnaris

median nerve

flexor pollicis longus

tendines of flexor digitorum
profundus of hand

tendon of brachioradialis

pronator quadratus

ulnar nerve
(dorsal branch)

tendon of palmaris longus

radial artery
(superficial palmar branch)

tendon of flexor carpi ulnaris

tendon of flexor carpi radialis

tendines of flexor digitorum
superficialis of hand

A

LOWER LIMB (I)

RIGHT LOWER LIMB. GENERAL SUPERFICIAL SCHEMA

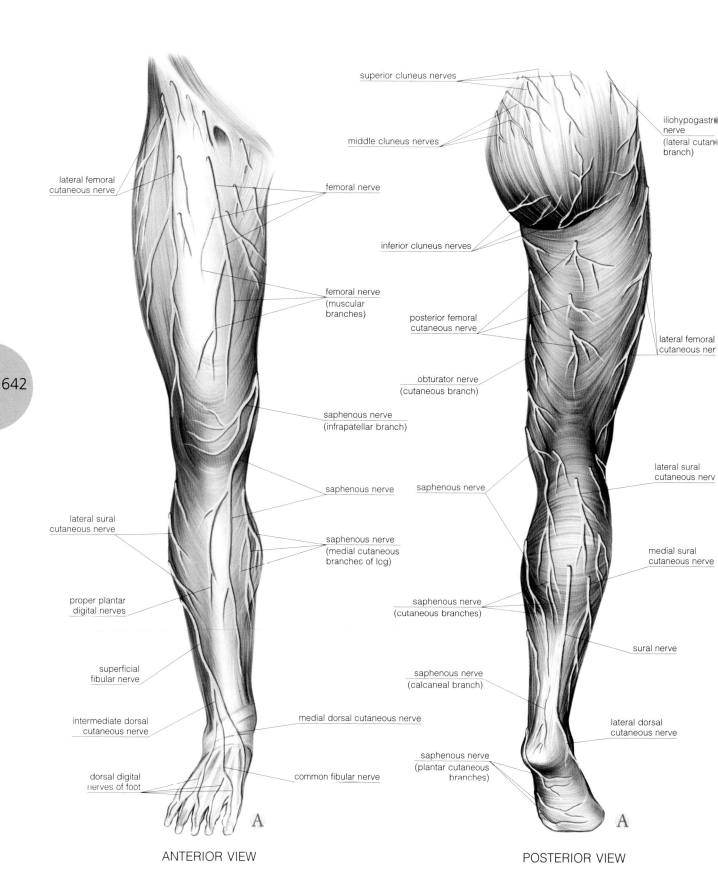

superior cluneus nerves

middle cluneus nerves

iliohypogastric nerve (lateral cutaneous branch)

lateral femoral cutaneous nerve

femoral nerve

inferior cluneus nerves

femoral nerve (muscular branches)

posterior femoral cutaneous nerve

lateral femoral cutaneous nerve

obturator nerve (cutaneous branch)

saphenous nerve (infrapatellar branch)

saphenous nerve

saphenous nerve

lateral sural cutaneous nerve

lateral sural cutaneous nerve

saphenous nerve (medial cutaneous branches of leg)

medial sural cutaneous nerve

proper plantar digital nerves

saphenous nerve (cutaneous branches)

sural nerve

superficial fibular nerve

saphenous nerve (calcaneal branch)

intermediate dorsal cutaneous nerve

medial dorsal cutaneous nerve

lateral dorsal cutaneous nerve

dorsal digital nerves of foot

common fibular nerve

saphenous nerve (plantar cutaneous branches)

ANTERIOR VIEW

POSTERIOR VIEW

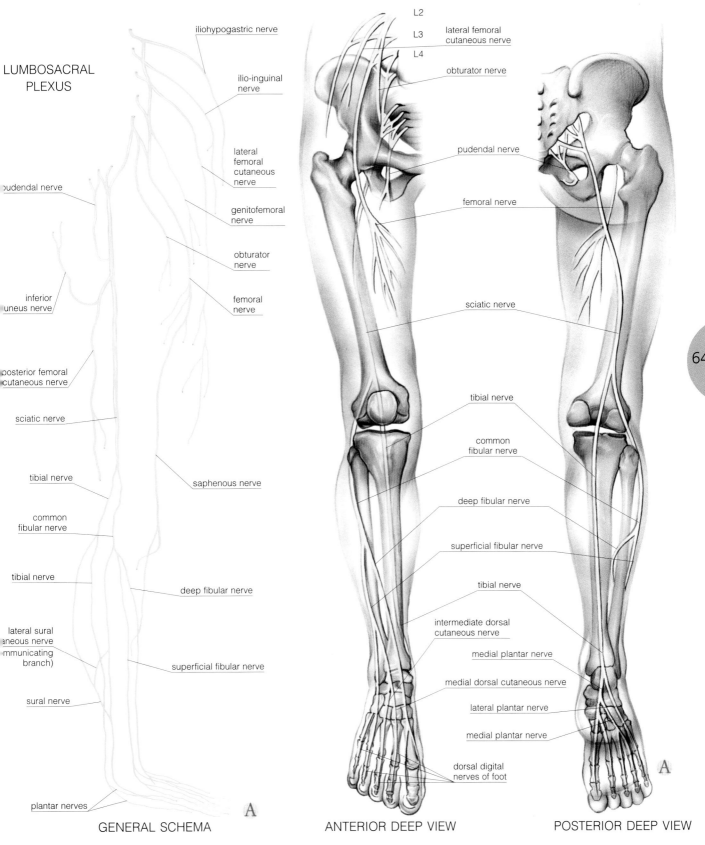

LUMBOSACRAL
PLEXUS

iliohypogastric nerve

ilio-inguinal
nerve

lateral
femoral
cutaneous
nerve

genitofemoral
nerve

obturator
nerve

femoral
nerve

pudendal nerve

inferior
gluteus nerve

posterior femoral
cutaneous nerve

sciatic nerve

tibial nerve

saphenous nerve

common
fibular nerve

tibial nerve

deep fibular nerve

lateral sural
cutaneous nerve
(communicating
branch)

superficial fibular nerve

sural nerve

plantar nerves

GENERAL SCHEMA

L2
L3
L4

lateral femoral
cutaneous nerve

obturator nerve

pudendal nerve

femoral nerve

sciatic nerve

tibial nerve

common
fibular nerve

deep fibular nerve

superficial fibular nerve

tibial nerve

intermediate dorsal
cutaneous nerve

medial plantar nerve

medial dorsal cutaneous nerve

lateral plantar nerve

medial plantar nerve

dorsal digital
nerves of foot

ANTERIOR DEEP VIEW

POSTERIOR DEEP VIEW

643

UPPER LIMB (III). FEMORAL and LATERAL FEMORAL CUTANEOUS NERVES

RIGHT INFERIOR LIMB. ANTERIOR VIEW

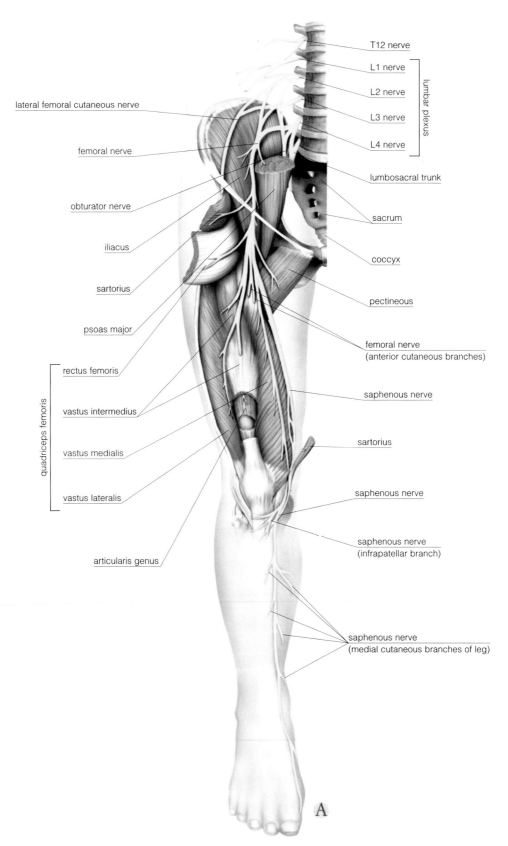

T12 nerve

L1 nerve

L2 nerve

lumbar plexus

L3 nerve

L4 nerve

lateral femoral cutaneous nerve

femoral nerve

lumbosacral trunk

obturator nerve

sacrum

iliacus

coccyx

sartorius

pectineous

psoas major

femoral nerve
(anterior cutaneous branches)

rectus femoris

saphenous nerve

quadriceps femoris

vastus intermedius

sartorius

vastus medialis

saphenous nerve

vastus lateralis

saphenous nerve
(infrapatellar branch)

articularis genus

saphenous nerve
(medial cutaneous branches of leg)

A

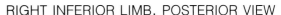

LOWER LIMB (IV). SCIATIC NERVE

RIGHT INFERIOR LIMB. POSTERIOR VIEW

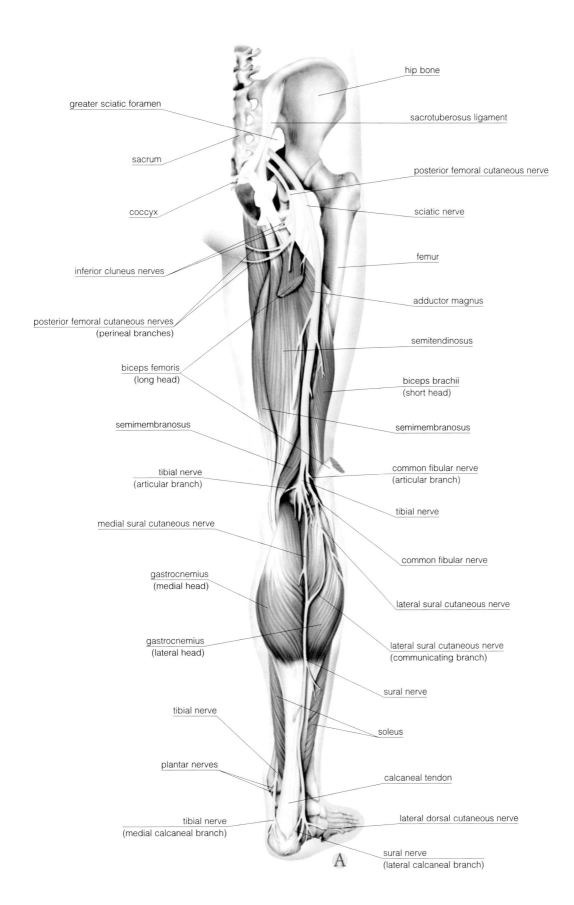

greater sciatic foramen

sacrum

coccyx

inferior cluneus nerves

posterior femoral cutaneous nerves
(perineal branches)

biceps femoris
(long head)

semimembranosus

tibial nerve
(articular branch)

medial sural cutaneous nerve

gastrocnemius
(medial head)

gastrocnemius
(lateral head)

tibial nerve

plantar nerves

tibial nerve
(medial calcaneal branch)

hip bone

sacrotuberosus ligament

posterior femoral cutaneous nerve

sciatic nerve

femur

adductor magnus

semitendinosus

biceps brachii
(short head)

semimembranosus

common fibular nerve
(articular branch)

tibial nerve

common fibular nerve

lateral sural cutaneous nerve

lateral sural cutaneous nerve
(communicating branch)

sural nerve

soleus

calcaneal tendon

lateral dorsal cutaneous nerve

sural nerve
(lateral calcaneal branch)

A

645

LOWER LIMB (V). FEMORAL and OBTURATOR NERVES
RIGHT LOWER LIMB. ANTERIOR DEEP VIEW

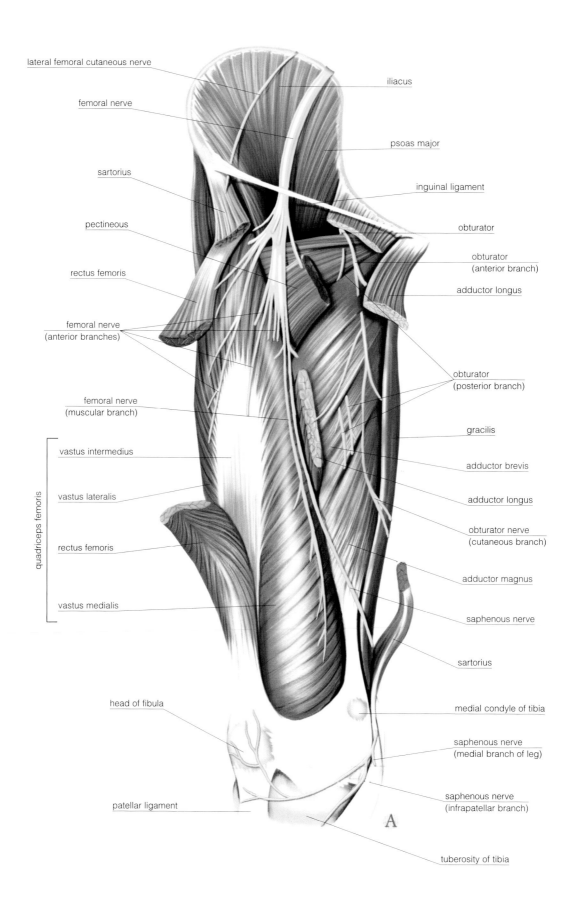

lateral femoral cutaneous nerve

femoral nerve

sartorius

pectineous

rectus femoris

femoral nerve
(anterior branches)

femoral nerve
(muscular branch)

quadriceps femoris

vastus intermedius

vastus lateralis

rectus femoris

vastus medialis

head of fibula

patellar ligament

iliacus

psoas major

inguinal ligament

obturator

obturator
(anterior branch)

adductor longus

obturator
(posterior branch)

gracilis

adductor brevis

adductor longus

obturator nerve
(cutaneous branch)

adductor magnus

saphenous nerve

sartorius

medial condyle of tibia

saphenous nerve
(medial branch of leg)

saphenous nerve
(infrapatellar branch)

A

tuberosity of tibia

646

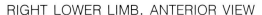

LOWER LIMB (VI). OBTURATOR NERVE

RIGHT LOWER LIMB. ANTERIOR VIEW

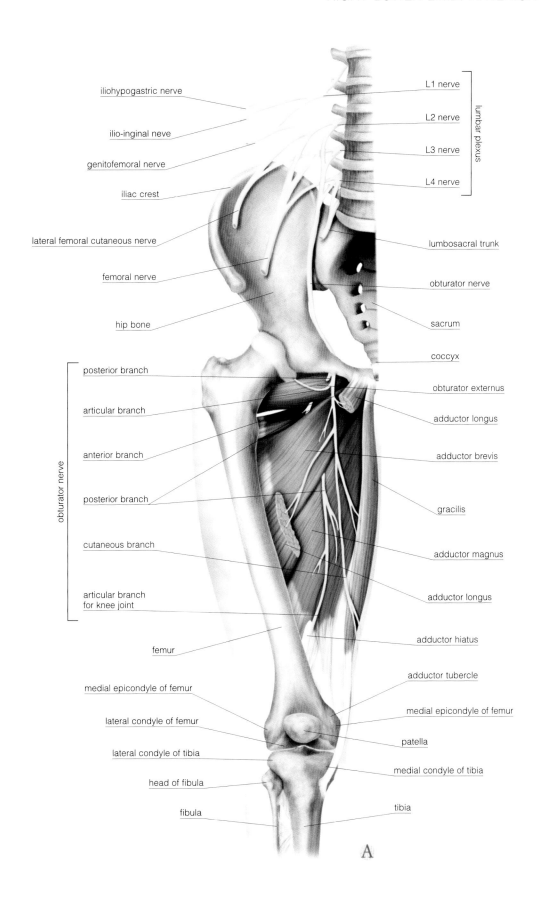

iliohypogastric nerve

ilio-inginal neve

genitofemoral nerve

iliac crest

lateral femoral cutaneous nerve

femoral nerve

hip bone

posterior branch

articular branch

anterior branch

posterior branch

cutaneous branch

articular branch
for knee joint

obturator nerve

femur

medial epicondyle of femur

lateral condyle of femur

lateral condyle of tibia

head of fibula

fibula

L1 nerve

L2 nerve

L3 nerve

L4 nerve

lumbar plexus

lumbosacral trunk

obturator nerve

sacrum

coccyx

obturator externus

adductor longus

adductor brevis

gracilis

adductor magnus

adductor longus

adductor hiatus

adductor tubercle

medial epicondyle of femur

patella

medial condyle of tibia

tibia

647

A

LOWER LIMB (VII). COMMON FIBULAR NERVE

RIGHT LOWER LIMB. ANTERIOR VIEW

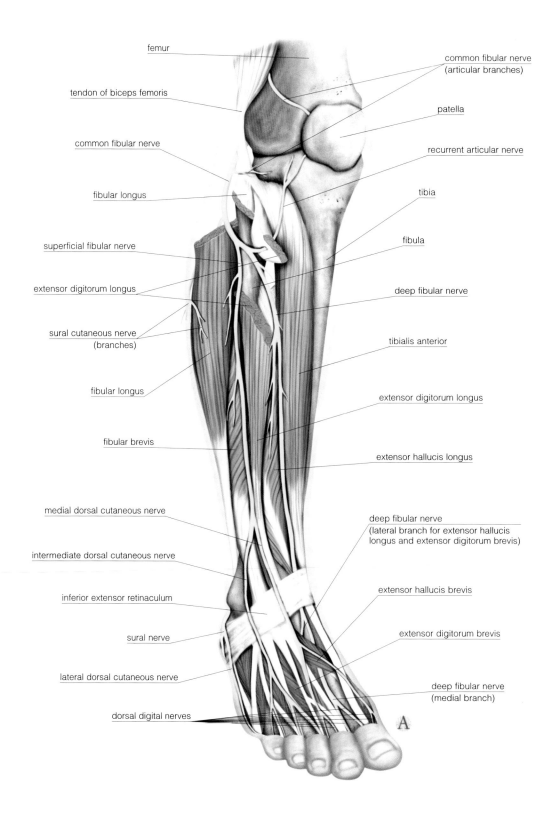

femur

common fibular nerve (articular branches)

tendon of biceps femoris

patella

common fibular nerve

recurrent articular nerve

fibular longus

tibia

superficial fibular nerve

fibula

extensor digitorum longus

deep fibular nerve

sural cutaneous nerve (branches)

tibialis anterior

fibular longus

extensor digitorum longus

fibular brevis

extensor hallucis longus

medial dorsal cutaneous nerve

deep fibular nerve (lateral branch for extensor hallucis longus and extensor digitorum brevis)

intermediate dorsal cutaneous nerve

inferior extensor retinaculum

extensor hallucis brevis

sural nerve

extensor digitorum brevis

lateral dorsal cutaneous nerve

deep fibular nerve (medial branch)

dorsal digital nerves

A

648

LOWER LIMB (VIII). TIBIAL NERVE

RIGHT LOWER LIMB. POSTERIOR VIEW

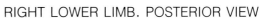

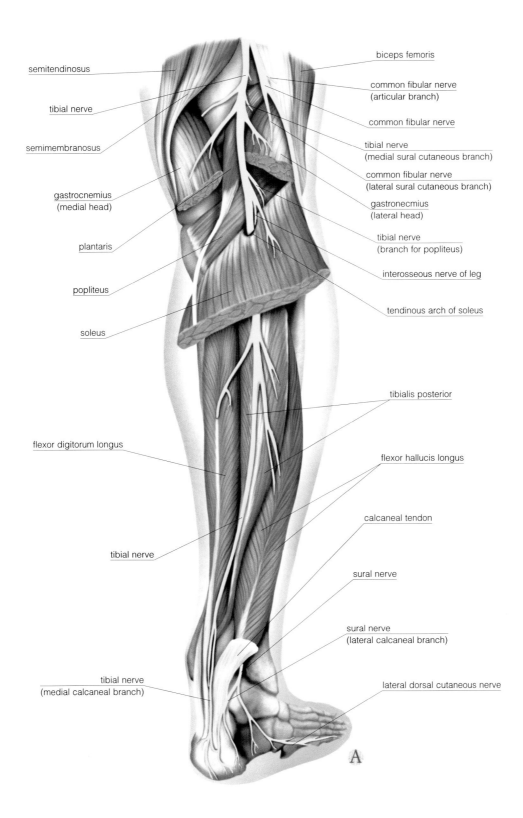

semitendinosus

tibial nerve

semimembranosus

gastrocnemius
(medial head)

plantaris

popliteus

soleus

flexor digitorum longus

tibial nerve

tibial nerve
(medial calcaneal branch)

biceps femoris

common fibular nerve
(articular branch)

common fibular nerve

tibial nerve
(medial sural cutaneous branch)

common fibular nerve
(lateral sural cutaneous branch)

gastronecmius
(lateral head)

tibial nerve
(branch for popliteus)

interosseous nerve of leg

tendinous arch of soleus

tibialis posterior

flexor hallucis longus

calcaneal tendon

sural nerve

sural nerve
(lateral calcaneal branch)

lateral dorsal cutaneous nerve

A

649

LOWER LIMB (IX). FOOT (I)

RIGHT LOWER LIMB. PLANTAR VIEW

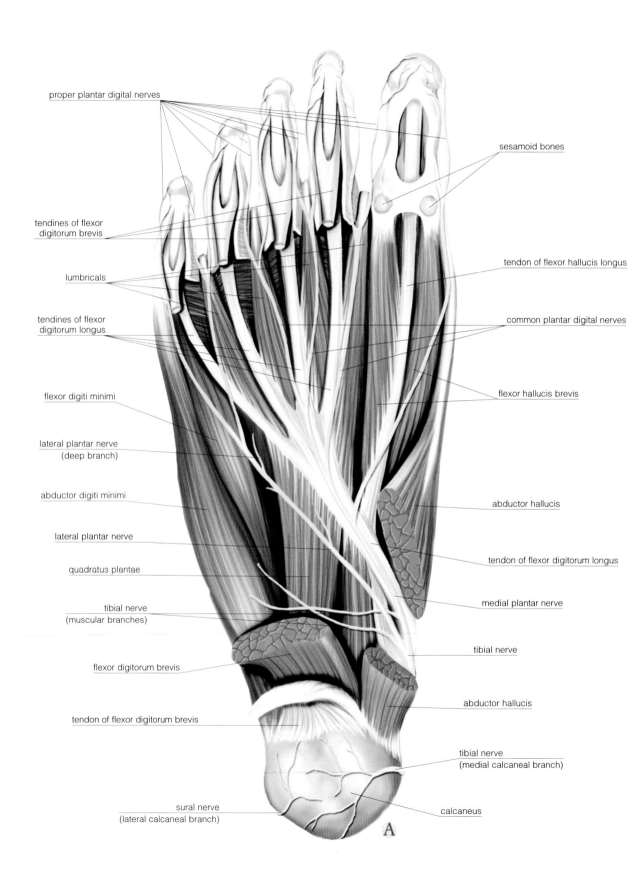

proper plantar digital nerves

sesamoid bones

tendines of flexor
digitorum brevis

tendon of flexor hallucis longus

lumbricals

common plantar digital nerves

tendines of flexor
digitorum longus

flexor digiti minimi

flexor hallucis brevis

lateral plantar nerve
(deep branch)

abductor digiti minimi

abductor hallucis

lateral plantar nerve

tendon of flexor digitorum longus

quadratus plantae

medial plantar nerve

tibial nerve
(muscular branches)

tibial nerve

flexor digitorum brevis

abductor hallucis

tendon of flexor digitorum brevis

tibial nerve
(medial calcaneal branch)

sural nerve
(lateral calcaneal branch)

calcaneus

A

LOWER LIMB (X). FOOT (II)
LEFT LOWER LIMB. DORSAL VIEW

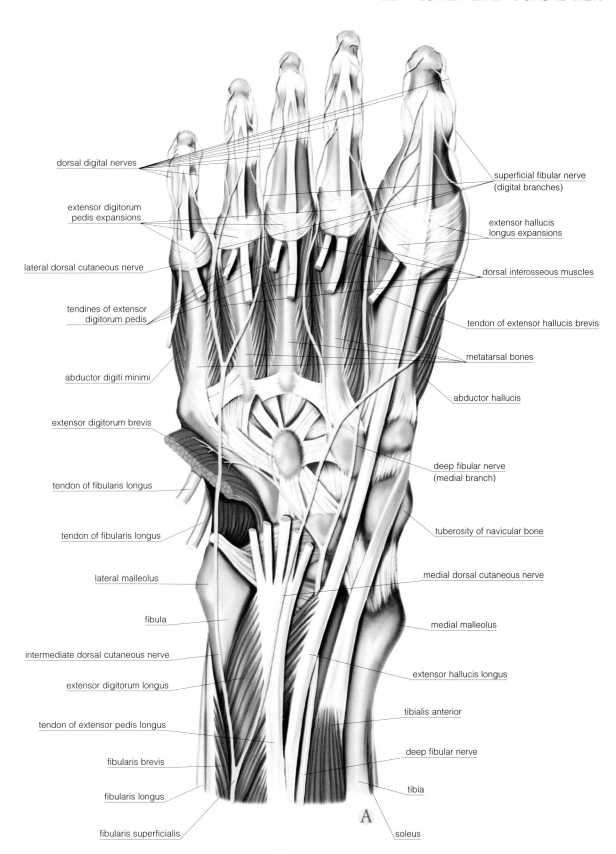

dorsal digital nerves

superficial fibular nerve
(digital branches)

extensor digitorum
pedis expansions

extensor hallucis
longus expansions

lateral dorsal cutaneous nerve

dorsal interosseous muscles

tendines of extensor
digitorum pedis

tendon of extensor hallucis brevis

metatarsal bones

abductor digiti minimi

abductor hallucis

extensor digitorum brevis

deep fibular nerve
(medial branch)

tendon of fibularis longus

tendon of fibularis longus

tuberosity of navicular bone

lateral malleolus

medial dorsal cutaneous nerve

fibula

medial malleolus

intermediate dorsal cutaneous nerve

extensor digitorum longus

extensor hallucis longus

tendon of extensor pedis longus

tibialis anterior

fibularis brevis

deep fibular nerve

fibularis longus

tibia

fibularis superficialis

soleus

A

651

AUTONOMIC NERVOUS SYSTEM (I)
SYMPATHETIC PART

sympathetic part of the autonomic nervous system

Thoracolumbar division of the autonomic nervous system its preganglionic fibres originate in the thoracic and lumbar segments of the spinal cord and make synapses with the postganglionic neurons in the sympathetic ganglia. Most of these sympathetic ganglia are found in two chains that located in lateral position with respect to the spinal column and others, in the interior of the trunk. The postganglionic fibres extend up to the innervated organs. Some effects of the sympathetic stimulation are: increasing of cardiac frequency and th intensity of the heartbeat, dilatation of the bronchioles to increase the ventilation of the lungs and of the pupils, cutaneous and visceral vasoconstriction, vasodilatation of the cardiac muscle and the skeletal muscles to increase the irrigation of these organs and the supply of oxygen to its cells, reduction of the peristalsis and the gastrointestinal secretions, transformation of glycogen into glucose in the liver, that is liberated to the blood flow to give energy to the cells and secretion of epinephrine and norepinephrine by the suprarenal medulla, temporal deceleration of different

functions: (for example, digestives and urinary) to favor a better development of others (for example, practice sport, do some work when tired, etc.), increasing of the activity of sweat glands, secretion of little quantities of thick saliva by the saliva glands, bristling of hair, (chicken skin/goosebumps), in situations of cold, fear, etc. In brief, the parasympathetic nervous system slows down a series of functions that allow the organism to adapt quickly and efficiently to situations that might damage the homeostasis. The sympathetic effects are more general than specific and prepare the organism raising reactions of fighting or escaping in front of situations of stress (surprise, excitement, anger, fear, etc.), such as that the heart is triggered, the respiration is faster and more intense, chills, etc. The modifications of the electroencephalographic waves and the cutaneous electric resistant, characteristics of these situations, are not very visible, although the polygraph detector of lies, register them. Most of sympathetic neurons liberate the neurotransmitter norepinephrine in the visceral effector.

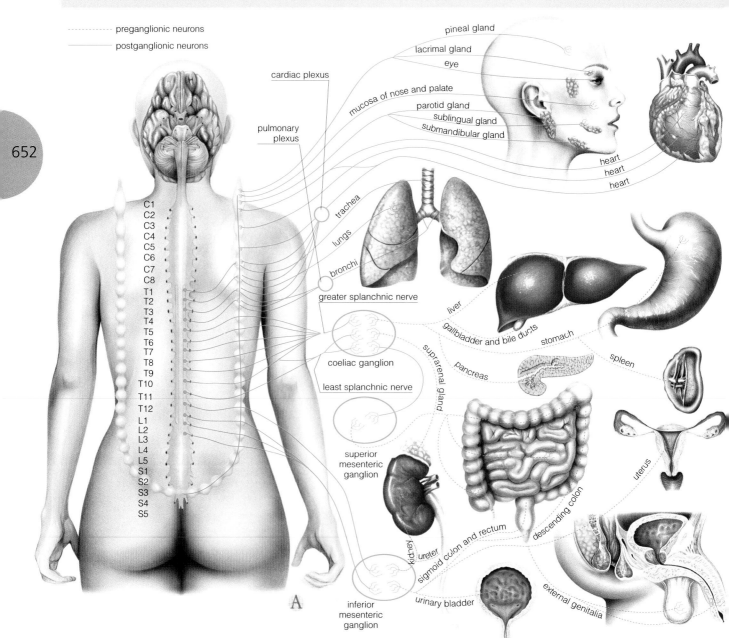

- - - - - - preganglionic neurons
———— postganglionic neurons

pineal gland
lacrimal gland
eye
mucosa of nose and palate
parotid gland
sublingual gland
submandibular gland
heart
heart
heart

cardiac plexus
pulmonary plexus

trachea
lungs
bronchi

greater splanchnic nerve

coeliac ganglion

least splanchnic nerve

superior mesenteric ganglion

liver
gallbladder and bile ducts
stomach
spleen
pancreas
suprarenal gland

uterus

descending colon

kidney
ureter
sigmoid colon and rectum

external genitalia

A

inferior mesenteric ganglion

urinary bladder

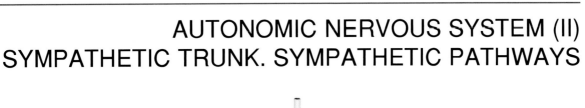

AUTONOMIC NERVOUS SYSTEM (II)
SYMPATHETIC TRUNK. SYMPATHETIC PATHWAYS

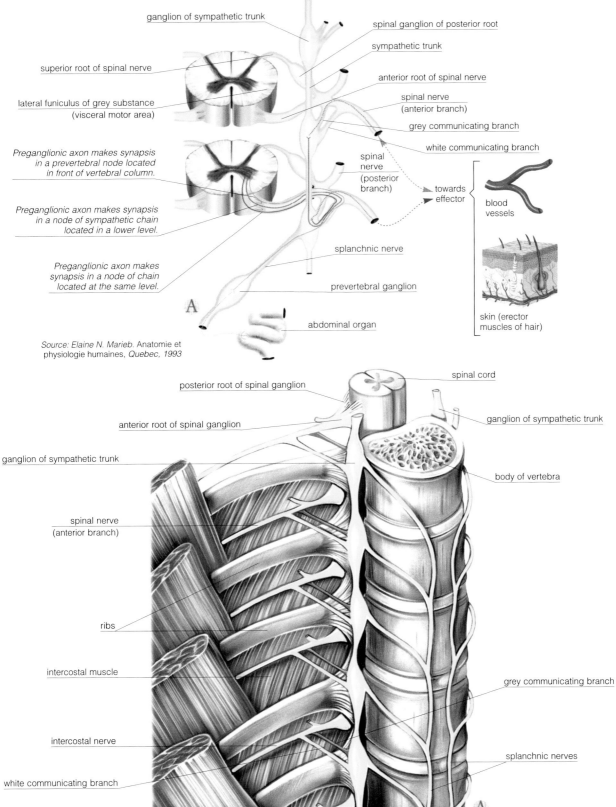

ganglion of sympathetic trunk

spinal ganglion of posterior root

sympathetic trunk

superior root of spinal nerve

anterior root of spinal nerve

lateral funiculus of grey substance
(visceral motor area)

spinal nerve
(anterior branch)

grey communicating branch

white communicating branch

Preganglionic axon makes synapsis
in a prevertebral node located
in front of vertebral column.

spinal
nerve
(posterior
branch)

towards
effector

blood
vessels

Preganglionic axon makes synapsis
in a node of sympathetic chain
located in a lower level.

Preganglionic axon makes
synapsis in a node of chain
located at the same level.

splanchnic nerve

prevertebral ganglion

skin (erector
muscles of hair)

A

abdominal organ

Source: Elaine N. Marieb. Anatomie et
physiologie humaines, *Quebec, 1993*

653

posterior root of spinal ganglion

spinal cord

anterior root of spinal ganglion

ganglion of sympathetic trunk

ganglion of sympathetic trunk

body of vertebra

spinal nerve
(anterior branch)

ribs

intercostal muscle

grey communicating branch

intercostal nerve

splanchnic nerves

white communicating branch

A

AUTONOMIC NERVOUS SYSTEM (III) PARASYMPATHETIC PART

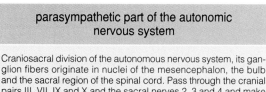

parasympathetic part of the autonomic nervous system

Craniosacral division of the autonomous nervous system, its ganglion fibers originate in nuclei of the mesencephalon, the bulb and the sacral region of the spinal cord. Pass through the cranial pairs III, VII, IX and X and the sacral nerves 2, 3 and 4 and make synapses with neurons of the autonomous ganglia (terminal) that are found in the walls of the innervated organs or close to them. Some of the effects of the parasympathetic stimulation are the contraction of bronchi, of the pupil, of the smooth muscle of the digestive tube and of the bladder to its normal state, the constriction of the bronquioles, normalization of the heart rate, the increasing of peristalsis, and secretion of gastrointestinal glands. Its main function is to reduce the consumption of energy during the realization of certain activities like the digestion, and the elimination of waste, that if an individual carries out them at the same time than other where is not stress (for example, read, watch T.V., make some handcraft, etc.), does not need an supplementary sanguineous supply, because the parasympathetic portion takes care of the heart rate, the respiratory frequency, etc. keep themselves normally. The parasympathetic neurons liberate acetylcholine transmitter in the visceral effector.

654

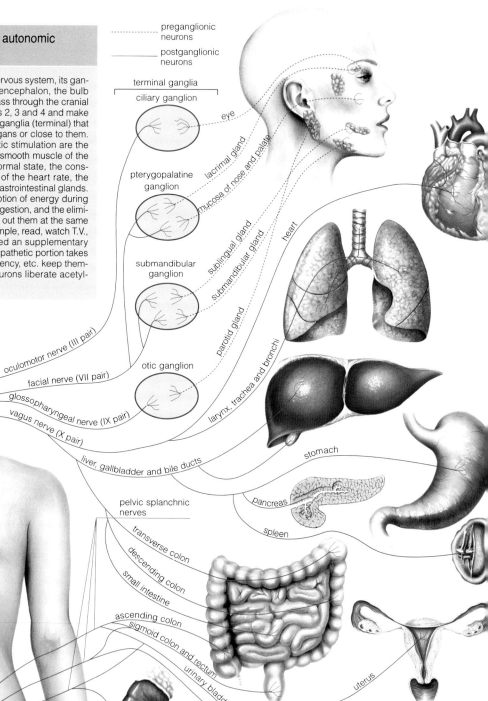

ORGANS
of the SENSES

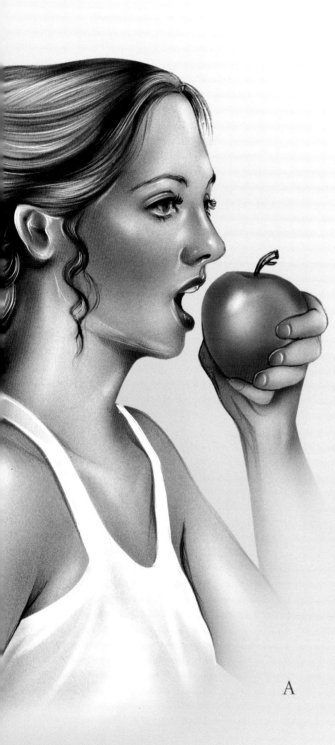

A

The senses come to be an extension of the nervous system and constitute themselves in the organs of relation of the body with the environment that surround it, for that the body is endowed with millions of sensorial receptors capable of perceive all kind of stimuli and of a set nervous ducts through of which such stimuli is transmitted to the central nervous system to be processed and give the appropriate orders that constitute the answer or reaction correspondent.

The receptor of tact are disseminated for the whole surface of the skin, while the sensory receptors specific of the taste, the smell, the sight and the hearing are found in concrete areas of the head either in the organs of sense (eyes and ears), or in structures epithelial perfectly delimitated (taste buds or epithelium of the olfactory region) reference may be also made to the sense of balance which receptor are found in the internal ear.

Through the photoreceptor of the retina, and a system of lens the eye captures the images from the exterior, that by the optic ways reach the visual brain cortex found in the occipital lobes, where acquire awareness of them.

The external sound waves introduce in the medial ear, where in the Corti s organ, transform themselves in bioelectric impulses, that through the nervous ways reach the auditory brain cortex, located in the temporal lobes of the brain.

In the internal ear, in the semicircular conducts of the labyrinth there are some receptors capable of capture the spatial situation of the body. Its information is transmitted to the brain and the cerebellum and once processed the body adopts automatically the necessary posture to keep in balance.

The dermis is full of sensory receptors or tactile corpuscles of several types, capable of detect any sensation (temperature, pressure, pain, etc.). these receptor through the peripheral nerves, send their stimuli to the spinal cord that in a reflex manner, activates the pertinent reaction and then is transmitted to the brain.

The receptors of taste and smell are denominated chemoreceptors, because they react, stimulated by chemical substances dissolved in an aqueous medium. In the tasting receptors the chemical substances are found in the food and are dissolved in the saliva: In the olfactory receptors the chemical substances are suspended in the air and dissolve in the liquids of the nasal mucus.

Although each sensory function requires an specific type of receptor the basic functioning is always the same: Caption of an stimulus, send of the pertinent information, to the brain to process and transmission of the command that in each case dictates the brain, for the body to act in a determinate way.

VISION (I). EYEBALL (I)

HORIZONTAL SECTION

ora serrata

anterior ciliary artery

palpebral conjunctiva

ciliary body

greater circulus
arteriosus of iris

corneoscleral junction

iridocorneal angle

ciliary zonule

iris

cornea

corneal
epithelium

anterior chamber
of eyeball

pupil

lens

posterior chamber of eyeball

orbiculus ciliaris

superior rectus of eye

retina

sclera

vorticose vein

choroid

vascular lamina
of choroid

posterior ciliary arter

posterior long
ciliary artery

posterior short
ciliary arteries

central
retinal vein

central
rctinal artery

optic nerve
(or II cranial pair)

inferior rectus of eye

depression of optic disk

blood vessels of retina

656

sight

Refers to one of the five senses, comprised of very diverse organs in terms of their constitution and purpose, capable of capturing light and its intensity and also to reproduce an image of an object which emits its own light or a reflection, which in turn stimulates the photo transmitters of the retina. This sense allows for the perception of light, color, shape and contrast. The sight of exterior objects is performed by the eyes. The eyes contain a series of cells which are sensitive to light. When these cells are stimulated by light, they transform to nervous impulses which are sent to the brain through the optic nerve. The brain process and interprets these impulses. The ocular globe is a sphere with a 24mm diameter, which is comprised of three membranes: sclera, choroid, and retina.

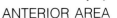

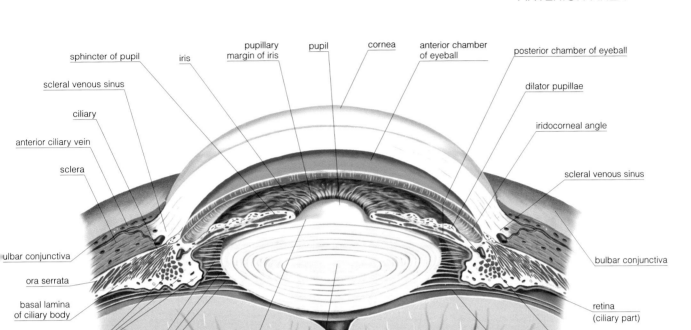

sphincter of pupil

iris

pupillary margin of iris

pupil

cornea

anterior chamber of eyeball

posterior chamber of eyeball

scleral venous sinus

dilator pupillae

ciliary

iridocorneal angle

anterior ciliary vein

sclera

scleral venous sinus

bulbar conjunctiva

bulbar conjunctiva

ora serrata

retina (ciliary part)

basal lamina of ciliary body

ciliary process

root of iris

zonular fibres

lens capsule

lens

hyaloid duct

vitreous chamber

A

HORIZONTAL SECTION at the LEVEL of the MIDDLE AREA of PUPIL

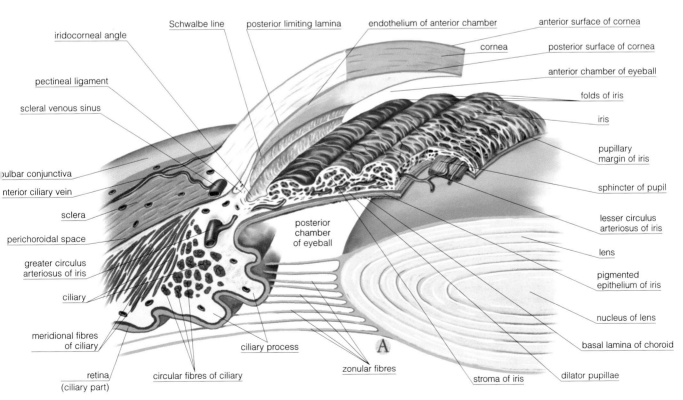

iridocorneal angle

Schwalbe line

posterior limiting lamina

endothelium of anterior chamber

anterior surface of cornea

cornea

posterior surface of cornea

anterior chamber of eyeball

folds of iris

pectineal ligament

iris

scleral venous sinus

pupillary margin of iris

bulbar conjunctiva

sphincter of pupil

anterior ciliary vein

sclera

lesser circulus arteriosus of iris

posterior chamber of eyeball

lens

perichoroidal space

pigmented epithelium of iris

greater circulus arteriosus of iris

ciliary

nucleus of lens

meridional fibres of ciliary

basal lamina of choroid

retina (ciliary part)

ciliary process

circular fibres of ciliary

zonular fibres

A

stroma of iris

dilator pupillae

IRIS. BASIC STRUCTURE

VISION (III). EYEBALL (III)

658

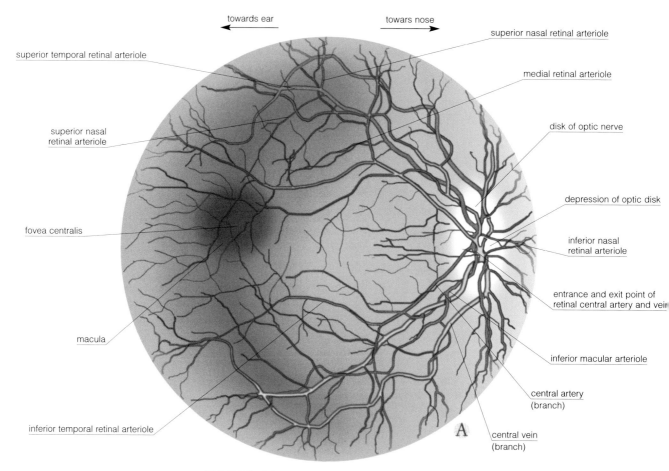

towards ear · towars nose

superior temporal retinal arteriole

superior nasal retinal arteriole

superior nasal retinal arteriole

medial retinal arteriole

disk of optic nerve

depression of optic disk

inferior nasal retinal arteriole

entrance and exit point of retinal central artery and vein

fovea centralis

macula

inferior macular arteriole

central artery (branch)

inferior temporal retinal arteriole

central vein (branch)

A

FUNDUS OCULI. OPHTHALMOSCOPIC VIEW

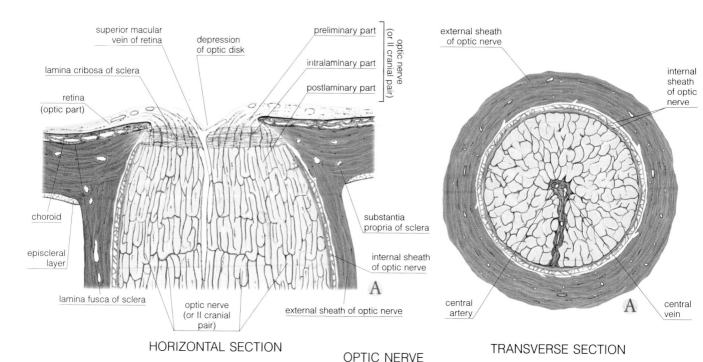

superior macular vein of retina

depression of optic disk

preliminary part

intralaminary part

postlaminary part

optic nerve (or II cranial pair)

external sheath of optic nerve

internal sheath of optic nerve

lamina cribosa of sclera

retina (optic part)

choroid

episcleral layer

lamina fusca of sclera

optic nerve (or II cranial pair)

substantia propria of sclera

internal sheath of optic nerve

external sheath of optic nerve

central artery

central vein

A

A

HORIZONTAL SECTION

OPTIC NERVE

TRANSVERSE SECTION

VISION (IV). EYEBALL (IV)
MUSCLES and LACRIMAL SYSTEM

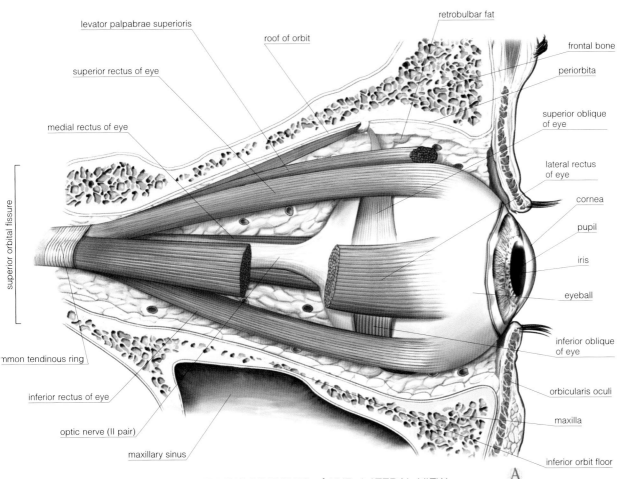

levator palpabrae superioris

roof of orbit

retrobulbar fat

frontal bone

periorbita

superior rectus of eye

superior oblique of eye

medial rectus of eye

lateral rectus of eye

cornea

pupil

iris

eyeball

superior orbital fissure

inferior oblique of eye

common tendinous ring

orbicularis oculi

inferior rectus of eye

maxilla

optic nerve (II pair)

maxillary sinus

inferior orbit floor

EXTRINSIC MUSCLES of EYE. LATERAL VIEW

A

659

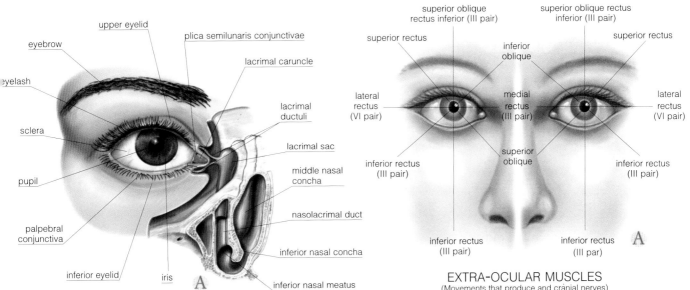

upper eyelid

plica semilunaris conjunctivae

eyebrow

lacrimal caruncle

eyelash

lacrimal ductuli

sclera

lacrimal sac

pupil

middle nasal concha

palpebral conjunctiva

nasolacrimal duct

inferior eyelid

iris

inferior nasal concha

inferior nasal meatus

A

RIGHT LACRIMAL SYSTEM. ANTERIOR VIEW

superior oblique rectus inferior (III pair)

superior oblique rectus inferior (III pair)

superior rectus

inferior oblique

superior rectus

lateral rectus (VI pair)

medial rectus (III pair)

lateral rectus (VI pair)

inferior rectus (III pair)

superior oblique

inferior rectus (III pair)

inferior rectus (III pair)

inferior rectus (III par)

A

EXTRA-OCULAR MUSCLES
(Movements that produce and crànial nerves)

Extra-oculars muscles are stuck muscles to eyeball which control the coordination and ocular movements. It is about six muscles which move the eyeball: muscles, superior straight, lower, inner and external and superior and lower oblique muscles.

VISION (V). RETINA (I)

cones

The extensions oriented towards the exterior of the cells are known as cones or canes, each of which consists of internal segment and other external. The pigmentary epithelium engulfs the detached portions of the external segments. Between the sensory cells and the muller's are form the adherent zonules, which set corresponds to the external limiting membrane. The membrane of Bruch is composed by a basal lamina, collagen fibers and a dense net of elastic fibers. Against this it supports fenestrated capillaries.

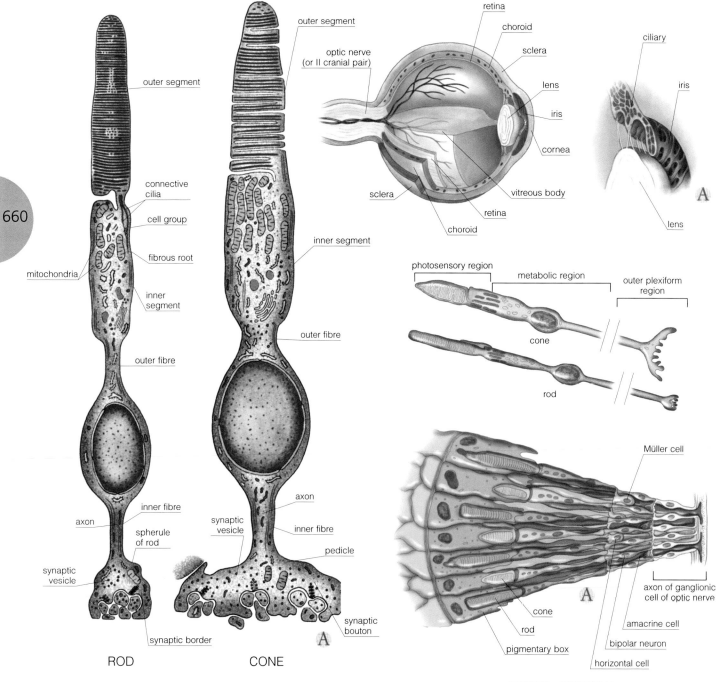

660

ROD

CONE

RETINA. SECTION

VISION (VI). RETINA (II)

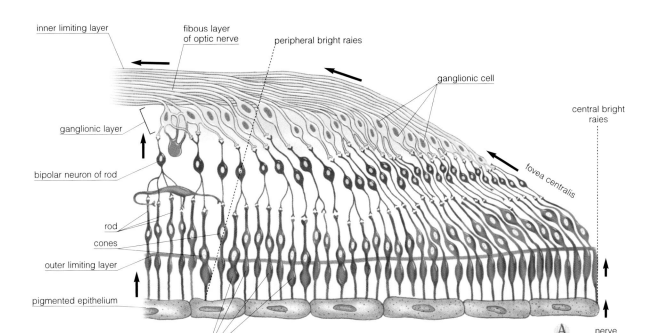

inner limiting layer

fibous layer
of optic nerve

peripheral bright raies

ganglionic cell

central bright
raies

ganglionic layer

bipolar neuron of rod

rod

cones

outer limiting layer

pigmented epithelium

fovea centralis

cones and rods

STRUCTURE

A

nerve
impulse

661

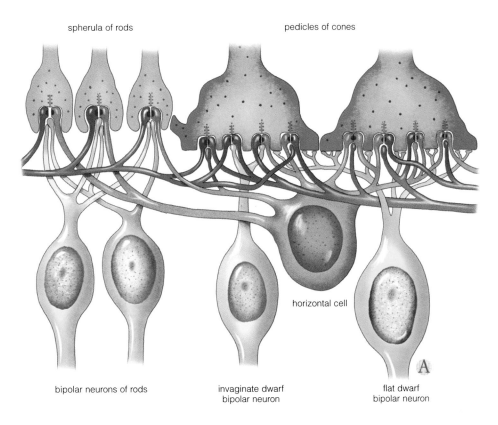

spherula of rods

pedicles of cones

horizontal cell

A

bipolar neurons of rods

invaginate dwarf
bipolar neuron

flat dwarf
bipolar neuron

OPTIC RELATIONS

VISION (VII). IRIS. VISUAL FIELD

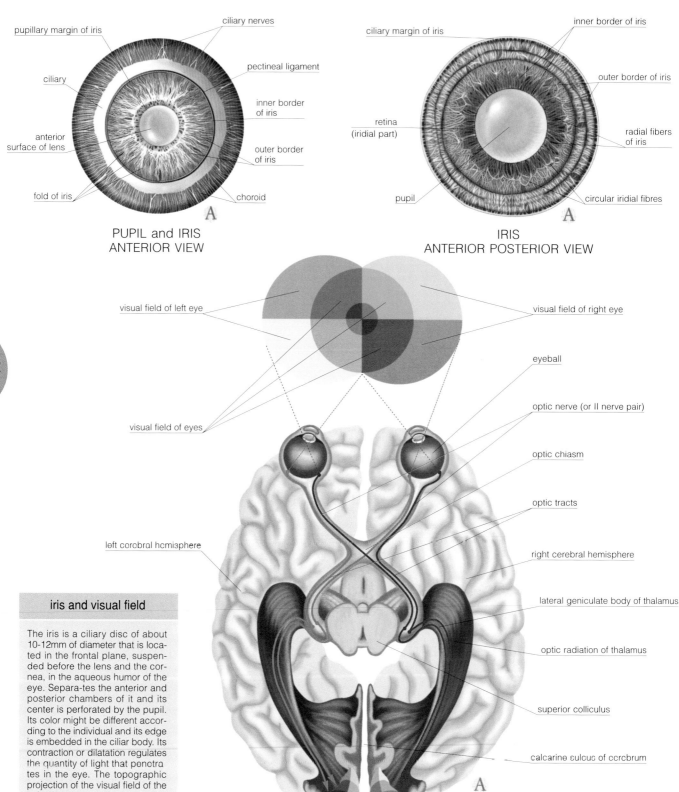

PUPIL and IRIS
ANTERIOR VIEW

- pupillary margin of iris
- ciliary nerves
- ciliary
- pectineal ligament
- inner border of iris
- anterior surface of lens
- outer border of iris
- fold of iris
- choroid

IRIS
ANTERIOR POSTERIOR VIEW

- ciliary margin of iris
- inner border of iris
- outer border of iris
- retina (iridial part)
- radial fibers of iris
- pupil
- circular iridial fibres

- visual field of left eye
- visual field of right eye
- eyeball
- optic nerve (or II nerve pair)
- visual field of eyes
- optic chiasm
- optic tracts
- left cerebral hemisphere
- right cerebral hemisphere
- lateral geniculate body of thalamus
- optic radiation of thalamus
- superior colliculus
- calcarine sulcus of cerebrum
- primary visual área of cerebral cortex

TOPOGRAPHIC PROJECTION of VISUAL FIELD
SUPERIOR VIEW

iris and visual field

The iris is a ciliary disc of about 10-12mm of diameter that is located in the frontal plane, suspended before the lens and the cornea, in the aqueous humor of the eye. Separa-tes the anterior and posterior chambers of it and its center is perforated by the pupil. Its color might be different according to the individual and its edge is embedded in the ciliar body. Its contraction or dilatation regulates the quantity of light that penetra tes in the eye. The topographic projection of the visual field of the retina is product of the crosslink of the fibers of the half nasal of each optic nerve that is produce in the chiasmatic area.

662

HEARING (I)
FRONTAL GENERAL VIEW

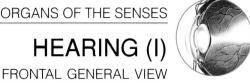

ear
Sense for which the human being, perceive the noise, this perception constitutes the audition, and the corresponding organ is the ear. The ear is divided in three parts: external, medial and internal. And is innervated by the facial nerve (VII cranial pair) The human ear corresponds to a variety of sounds with frequency that goes from the 20 to the 20.000Hz. This sensibility is high especially the sound that are found between the frequency 500 and 4.000Hz, that corresponds to the frequency of the human speech.

663

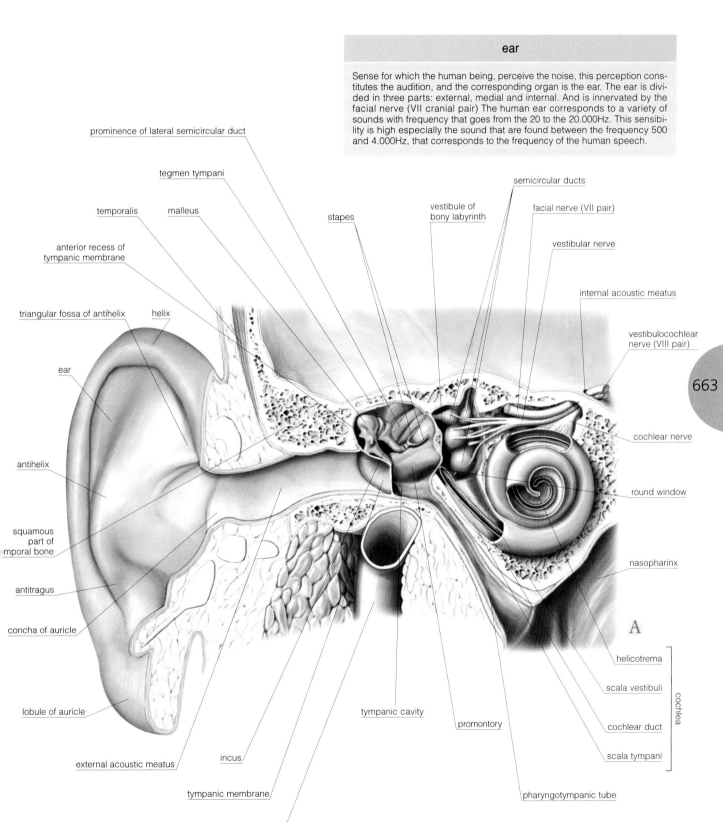

prominence of lateral semicircular duct

tegmen tympani

temporalis   malleus

anterior recess of tympanic membrane

triangular fossa of antihelix   helix

ear

antihelix

squamous part of mporal bone

antitragus

concha of auricle

lobule of auricle

external acoustic meatus

incus

tympanic membrane

internal jugular vein

stapes

semicircular ducts

vestibule of bony labyrinth

facial nerve (VII pair)

vestibular nerve

internal acoustic meatus

vestibulocochlear nerve (VIII pair)

cochlear nerve

round window

nasopharinx

A

helicotrema

scala vestibuli

cochlear duct

scala tympani

cochlea

tympanic cavity

promontory

pharyngotympanic tube

HEARING (II). COCHLEA. BONY LABYRINTH

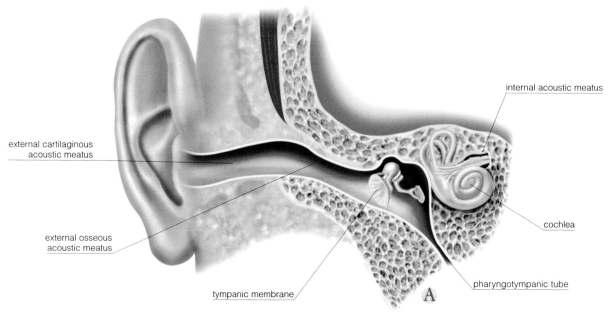

internal acoustic meatus

external cartilaginous
acoustic meatus

cochlea

external osseous
acoustic meatus

pharyngotympanic tube

tympanic membrane

A

ACOUSTIC MEATUS

664

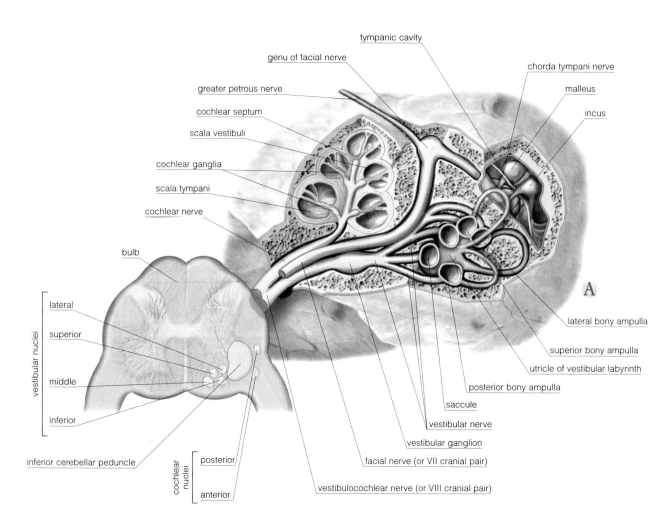

tympanic cavity

genu of facial nerve

chorda tympani nerve

greater petrous nerve

malleus

cochlear septum

incus

scala vestibuli

cochlear ganglia

scala tympani

cochlear nerve

bulb

A

lateral

superior

vestibular nuclei

middle

lateral bony ampulla

superior bony ampulla

utricle of vestibular labyrinth

posterior bony ampulla

inferior

saccule

vestibular nerve

vestibular ganglion

inferior cerebellar peduncle

posterior

cochlear nuclei

facial nerve (or VII cranial pair)

anterior

vestibulocochlear nerve (or VIII cranial pair)

HEARING (III). BONY LABYRINTH

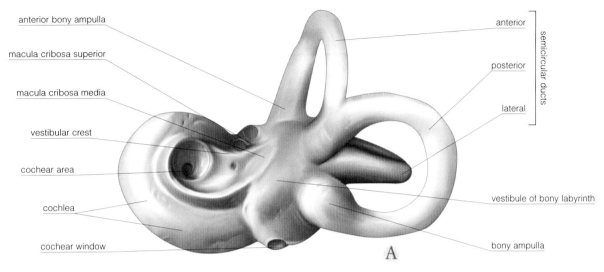

anterior bony ampulla

macula cribosa superior

macula cribosa media

vestibular crest

cochear area

cochlea

cochear window

anterior

posterior

lateral

semicircular ducts

vestibule of bony labyrinth

bony ampulla

POSTERIOR SUPERIOR VIEW

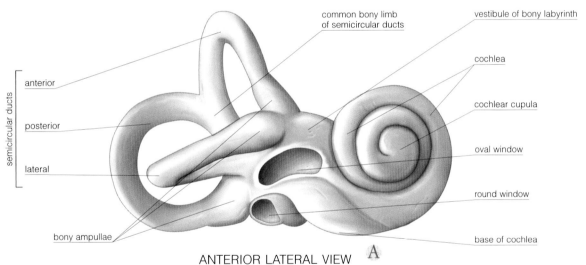

common bony limb
of semicircular ducts

vestibule of bony labyrinth

anterior

posterior

lateral

semicircular ducts

cochlea

cochlear cupula

oval window

round window

bony ampullae

base of cochlea

ANTERIOR LATERAL VIEW

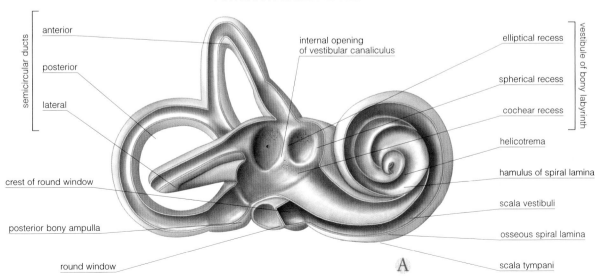

anterior

posterior

lateral

semicircular ducts

internal opening
of vestibular canaliculus

crest of round window

posterior bony ampulla

round window

elliptical recess

spherical recess

cochear recess

vestibule of bony labyrinth

helicotrema

hamulus of spiral lamina

scala vestibuli

osseous spiral lamina

scala tympani

ANTERIOR LATERAL SECTION

665

HEARING (IV). AUDITORY OSSICLES

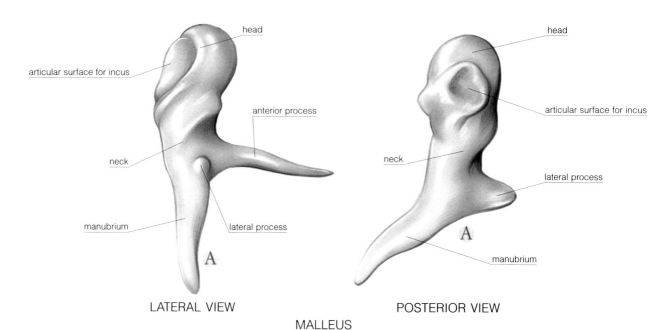

head

articular surface for incus

anterior process

neck

manubrium

lateral process

A

LATERAL VIEW

head

articular surface for incus

neck

lateral process

A

manubrium

POSTERIOR VIEW

MALLEUS

ossicles of the medial ear

The ossicles of the medial ear are three little bones: (hammer, anvil and stirrup) that are disposed forming a little chain that extends transversely from the tympanic membrane until the oval window. Form an articulate set and fixes to the walls of the tympanic cavity through ligaments. Are provided with own muscles that give them great mobility. Their function is to transmit to the liquid of the labyrinth of the internal ear the vibrations that due to the sound waves that have reach it, have remain impressed in the tympanic membrane, for which put in movement its articulation through a system of arms of lever.

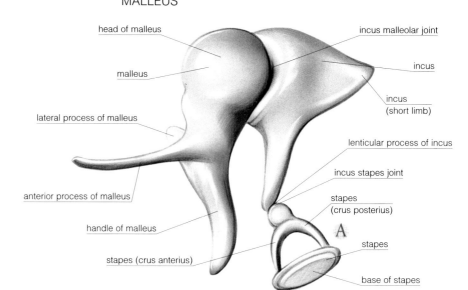

head of malleus

incus malleolar joint

incus

malleus

incus
(short limb)

lateral process of malleus

lenticular process of incus

incus stapes joint

stapes
(crus posterius)

anterior process of malleus

A

handle of malleus

stapes

stapes (crus anterius)

base of stapes

ARTICULATE BONES. POSTERIOR VIEW

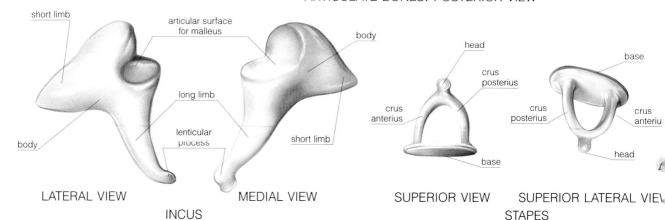

short limb

articular surface
for malleus

body

head

base

crus
posterius

long limb

body

lenticular
process

short limb

crus
anterius

crus
posterius

crus
anteriu

base

head

LATERAL VIEW

MEDIAL VIEW

SUPERIOR VIEW

SUPERIOR LATERAL VIEW

INCUS

STAPES

HEARING (V). EAR. TYMPANIC MEMBRANE

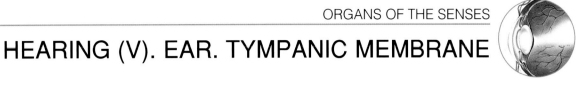

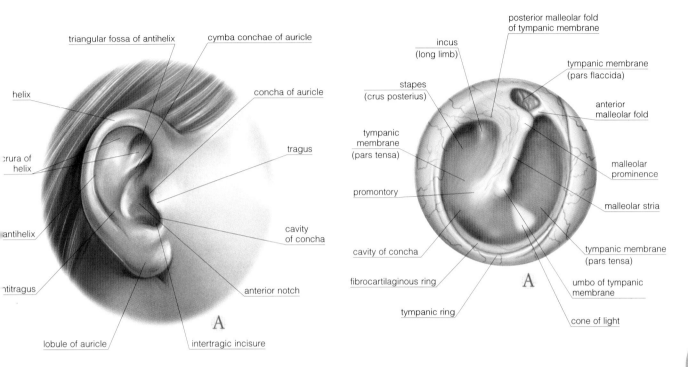

triangular fossa of antihelix

cymba conchae of auricle

helix

concha of auricle

crura of helix

tragus

antihelix

cavity of concha

antitragus

anterior notch

lobule of auricle

intertragic incisure

EAR

posterior malleolar fold of tympanic membrane

incus (long limb)

tympanic membrane (pars flaccida)

stapes (crus posterius)

anterior malleolar fold

tympanic membrane (pars tensa)

malleolar prominence

promontory

malleolar stria

cavity of concha

tympanic membrane (pars tensa)

fibrocartilaginous ring

umbo of tympanic membrane

tympanic ring

cone of light

A

TYMPANIC MEMBRANE

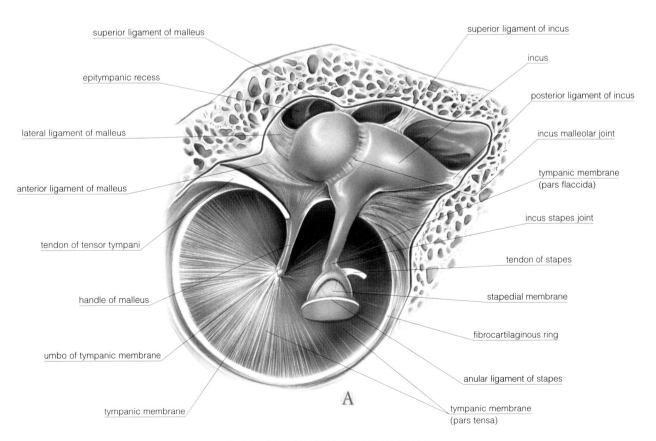

superior ligament of malleus

superior ligament of incus

epitympanic recess

incus

posterior ligament of incus

lateral ligament of malleus

incus malleolar joint

anterior ligament of malleus

tympanic membrane (pars flaccida)

tendon of tensor tympani

incus stapes joint

tendon of stapes

handle of malleus

stapedial membrane

umbo of tympanic membrane

fibrocartilaginous ring

anular ligament of stapes

tympanic membrane

tympanic membrane (pars tensa)

A

TYMPANIC CAVITY. LATERAL WALL

HEARING (VI). AUDITORY STRUCTURES (I)

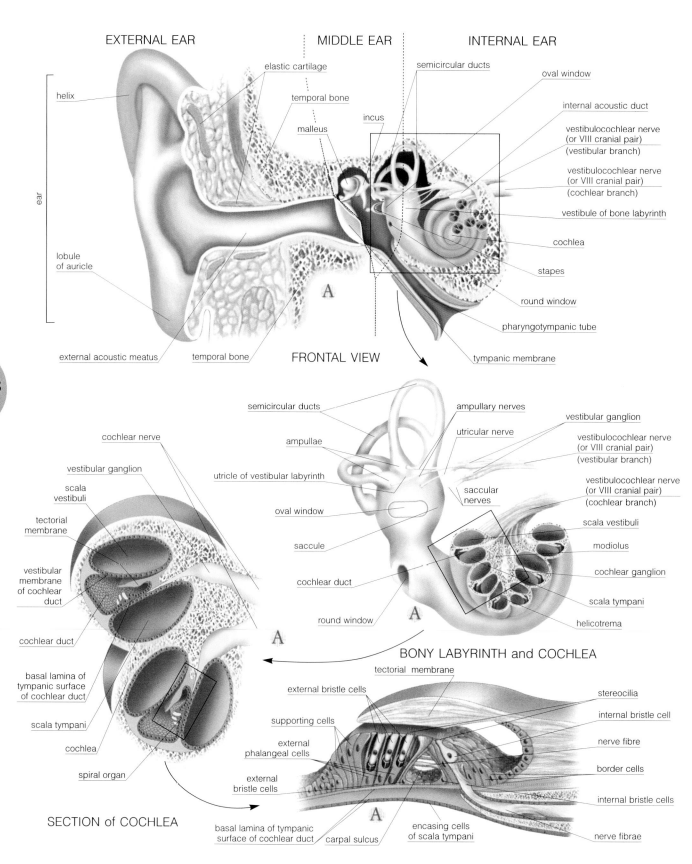

EXTERNAL EAR   MIDDLE EAR   INTERNAL EAR

helix

elastic cartilage

temporal bone

malleus

incus

semicircular ducts

oval window

internal acoustic duct

vestibulocochlear nerve (or VIII cranial pair) (vestibular branch)

vestibulocochlear nerve (or VIII cranial pair) (cochlear branch)

vestibule of bone labyrinth

cochlea

stapes

round window

pharyngotympanic tube

tympanic membrane

ear

lobule of auricle

external acoustic meatus

temporal bone

A

FRONTAL VIEW

668

cochlear nerve

vestibular ganglion

scala vestibuli

tectorial membrane

vestibular membrane of cochlear duct

cochlear duct

basal lamina of tympanic surface of cochlear duct

scala tympani

cochlea

spiral organ

A

SECTION of COCHLEA

semicircular ducts

ampullae

utricle of vestibular labyrinth

oval window

saccule

cochlear duct

round window

ampullary nerves

utricular nerve

saccular nerves

vestibular ganglion

vestibulocochlear nerve (or VIII cranial pair) (vestibular branch)

vestibulocochlear nerve (or VIII cranial pair) (cochlear branch)

scala vestibuli

modiolus

cochlear ganglion

scala tympani

helicotrema

A

BONY LABYRINTH and COCHLEA

tectorial membrane

external bristle cells

supporting cells

external phalangeal cells

external bristle cells

basal lamina of tympanic surface of cochlear duct

carpal sulcus

encasing cells of scala tympani

stereocilia

internal bristle cell

nerve fibre

border cells

internal bristle cells

nerve fibres

A

HEARING (VII). AUDITORY STRUCTURES (II)

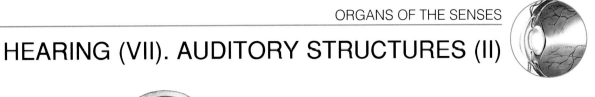

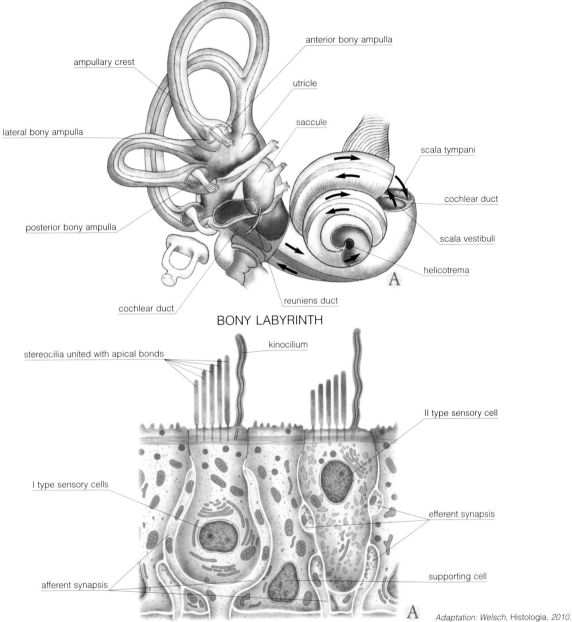

anterior bony ampulla

ampullary crest

utricle

saccule

lateral bony ampulla

scala tympani

cochlear duct

scala vestibuli

posterior bony ampulla

helicotrema

cochlear duct

reuniens duct

BONY LABYRINTH

stereocilia united with apical bonds

kinocilium

II type sensory cell

I type sensory cells

efferent synapsis

afferent synapsis

supporting cell

Adaptation: Welsch, Histología, 2010.

SENSORY CELLS of BALANCE SENSE

669

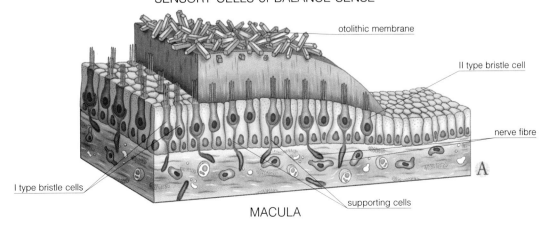

otolithic membrane

II type bristle cell

nerve fibre

I type bristle cells

supporting cells

MACULA

HEARING (VIII). AUDITORY STRUCTURES (III)
BONY LABYRINTH and COCHLEA
VASCULAR and NERVOUS NETWORKS

internal ear (or labyrinth)

Part of the auditory organ that is found in the interior of the boulder, bone wrought by a complex system of membranous channels denominated labyrinth that is divided in two: Osseous labyrinth (set of cavities excavated in the temporal bone, that form the circular conducts, the vestibule and the cochlea, in which is staying the receptor for the balance) and membranous labyrinth (wrapped by the osseous labyrinth and constitute like this one, by a complex system of sacs and ducts). The osseous labyrinth is covered by peristeum and contains the perilymph, liquid which chemical composition is similar to the cerebrospinal fluid, while the membranous is covered by the epithelium and contains the endolymph.

cochlea

Conduct that like a snail rolls over itself, around a central osseous nucleus (columella), giving almost three laps, consist in two parts one osseous or peripheral part, carved in the bone and other membranous, constituted by the internal ducts. In the interior contains three conducts (vestibular ramp, cochlear conduct or medial ramp, and tympanic ramp) for which circulate a liquid through which the sound waves are transmitted that in the cochlear duct transform in nervous impulses. In the cochlear duct, or central channel, is found the spiral organ or organ of ear properly said.

670

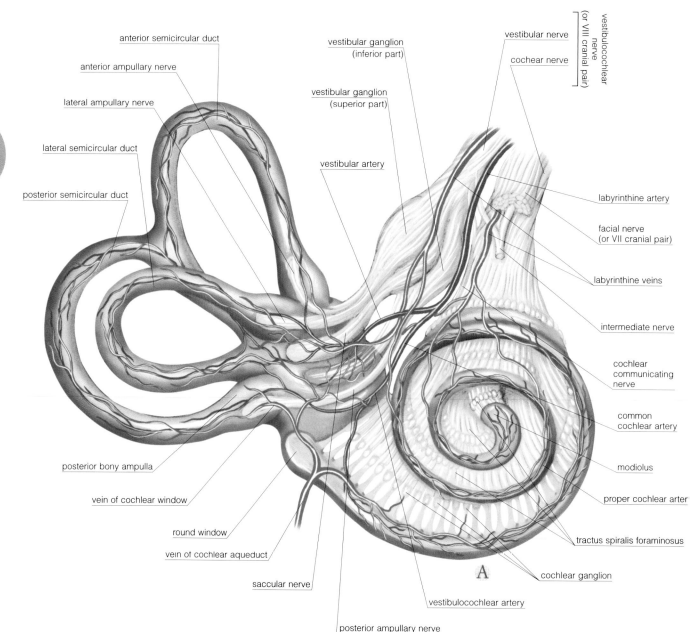

anterior semicircular duct

anterior ampullary nerve

lateral ampullary nerve

lateral semicircular duct

posterior semicircular duct

posterior bony ampulla

vein of cochlear window

round window

vein of cochlear aqueduct

saccular nerve

posterior ampullary nerve

vestibular ganglion (inferior part)

vestibular ganglion (superior part)

vestibular artery

vestibular nerve

cochear nerve

vestibulocochlear nerve (or VIII cranial pair)

labyrinthine artery

facial nerve (or VII cranial pair)

labyrinthine veins

intermediate nerve

cochlear communicating nerve

common cochlear artery

modiolus

proper cochlear arter

tractus spiralis foraminosus

cochlear ganglion

vestibulocochlear artery

A

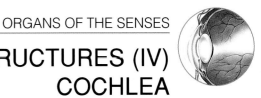

HEARING (IX). AUDITORY STRUCTURES (IV)
COCHLEA

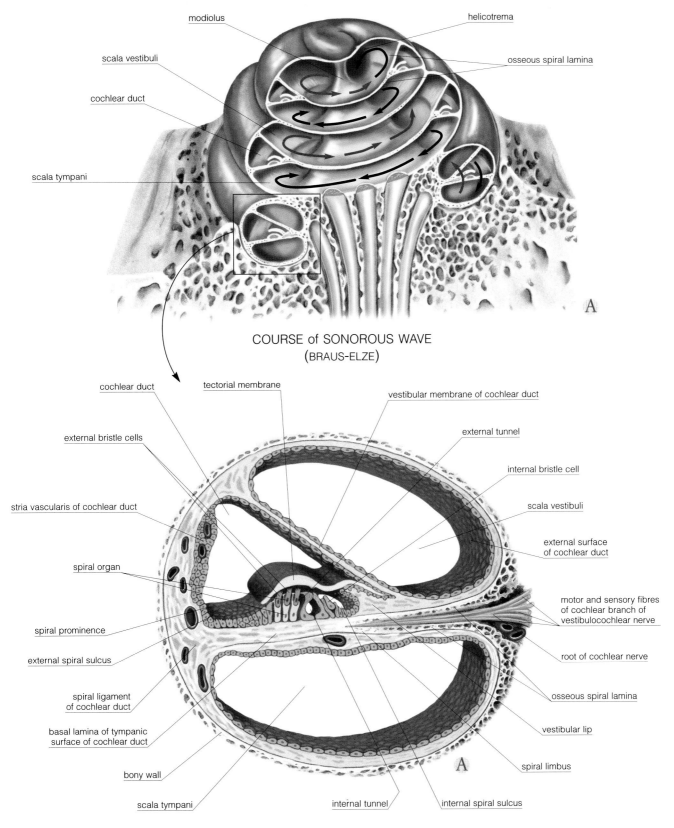

modiolus

helicotrema

scala vestibuli

osseous spiral lamina

cochlear duct

scala tympani

A

COURSE of SONOROUS WAVE
(BRAUS-ELZE)

671

cochlear duct

tectorial membrane

vestibular membrane of cochlear duct

external bristle cells

external tunnel

internal bristle cell

stria vascularis of cochlear duct

scala vestibuli

spiral organ

external surface
of cochlear duct

spiral prominence

motor and sensory fibres
of cochlear branch of
vestibulocochlear nerve

external spiral sulcus

root of cochlear nerve

spiral ligament
of cochlear duct

osseous spiral lamina

basal lamina of tympanic
surface of cochlear duct

vestibular lip

bony wall

spiral limbus

scala tympani

internal tunnel

internal spiral sulcus

A

COCHLEA and SPIRAL ORGAN

HEARING (X). CENTRAL MECHANISMS and AUDITORY TRACT

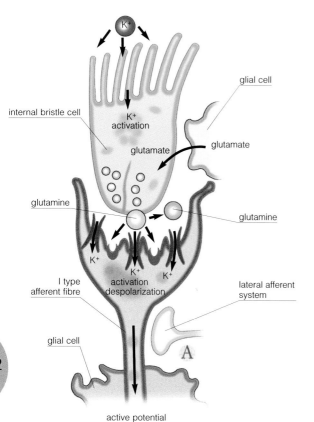

internal bristle cell

glial cell

K+

K+ activation

glutamate

glutamate

glutamine

glutamine

I type afferent fibre

K+

K+ activation despolarization

K+

lateral afferent system

glial cell

A

active potential

LIKELY NEUROBIOCHEMISTRY MECHANISM
of PRODUCTION, TRANSMISSION
and MODULATION of AUDIBLE SIGNAL

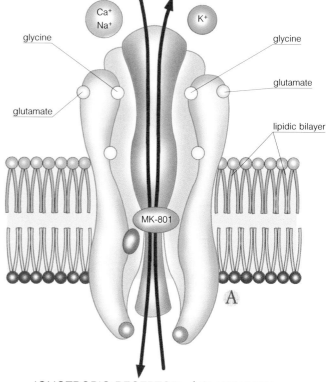

Ca+ Na+

K+

glycine

glutamate

glycine

glutamate

lipidic bilayer

MK-801

A

IONOTROPIC RECEPTOR of GLUTAMATE
and IONIC DUCT

672

auditory pathway

The primary auditory signal is transmitted through the internal ciliated cells through synapses with afferent fibers of type I, such signal is modulated by the external ciliated cells that feed back by efferent fibers of the brain stalk. The centripetal fiber of the neurons of the spiral ganglion conform the auditory component of the VIII cranial pair (vestibulocochlear nerve) which next synaptic station is the cochlear nuclear complex, from this goes to the lower colliculus of the mesencephalon, and after to the lower colliculus. From this point some additional neurons goes to the medial geniculated nucleus of the thalamus and towards other areas of secondary association. In all the levels of brain stalk the auditory signals are bilateral and keeps the tonotopia, which means a spatial disposition that allows the transmission of some determined frequencies of tone.

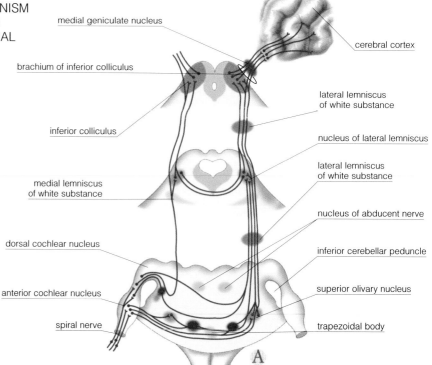

medial geniculate nucleus

cerebral cortex

brachium of inferior colliculus

lateral lemniscus of white substance

inferior colliculus

nucleus of lateral lemniscus

lateral lemniscus of white substance

medial lemniscus of white substance

nucleus of abducent nerve

dorsal cochlear nucleus

inferior cerebellar peduncle

anterior cochlear nucleus

superior olivary nucleus

spiral nerve

trapezoidal body

A

AUDITORY TRACT SCHEMA
(PREDOMINANCE of CONTRALATERAL TRANSMISSION)

HEARING (XI). BALANCE ORGAN

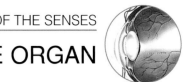

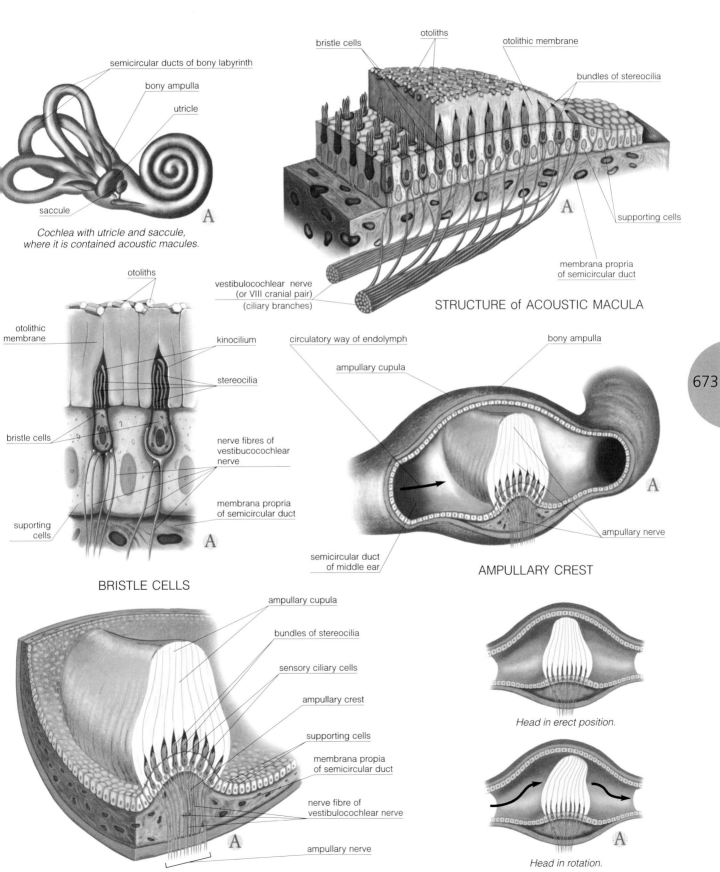

semicircular ducts of bony labyrinth

bony ampulla

utricle

saccule

*Cochlea with utricle and saccule,
where it is contained acoustic macules.*

bristle cells

otoliths

otolithic membrane

bundles of stereocilia

supporting cells

membrana propria
of semicircular duct

vestibulocochlear nerve
(or VIII cranial pair)
(ciliary branches)

STRUCTURE of ACOUSTIC MACULA

otoliths

otolithic
membrane

kinocilium

stereocilia

bristle cells

nerve fibres of
vestibucocochlear
nerve

membrana propria
of semicircular duct

suporting
cells

BRISTLE CELLS

circulatory way of endolymph

ampullary cupula

bony ampulla

semicircular duct
of middle ear

ampullary nerve

AMPULLARY CREST

ampullary cupula

bundles of stereocilia

sensory ciliary cells

ampullary crest

supporting cells

membrana propia
of semicircular duct

nerve fibre of
vestibulocochlear nerve

ampullary nerve

Head in erect position.

Head in rotation.

673

OLFACTION (I). NASAL REGION. LATERAL WALL

smell

Chemical sense that allows to detect the presence of volatile substances in the environment. In the human being consist in two nasal pits or nostrils, located in the middle of the face and opend to the exterior through the nose. The olfactory region of mankind is located in the upper part of the nasal cavity, occupies a surface of 240mm², equivalent to one fingernail and consist of 1.5 million of olfactory cells. Stimulated the hair of its surface, the cells transmit through the axons the sensory excitement to the brain center to process the information and emit the pertinent commands. The human being has less olfactory capacity than many animals.

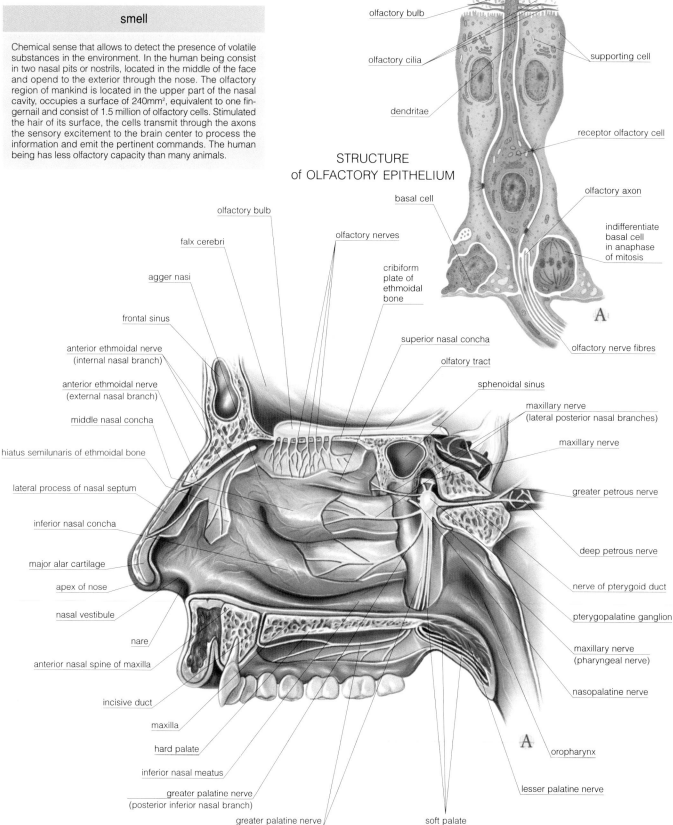

sheath mucus

olfactory bulb

olfactory cilia

supporting cell

dendritae

receptor olfactory cell

STRUCTURE
of OLFACTORY EPITHELIUM

basal cell

olfactory axon

indifferentiate
basal cell
in anaphase
of mitosis

olfactory bulb

olfactory nerves

falx cerebri

cribiform
plate of
ethmoidal
bone

agger nasi

superior nasal concha

frontal sinus

olfatory tract

olfactory nerve fibres

anterior ethmoidal nerve
(internal nasal branch)

sphenoidal sinus

anterior ethmoidal nerve
(external nasal branch)

maxillary nerve
(lateral posterior nasal branches)

middle nasal concha

maxillary nerve

hiatus semilunaris of ethmoidal bone

greater petrous nerve

lateral process of nasal septum

inferior nasal concha

deep petrous nerve

major alar cartilage

nerve of pterygoid duct

apex of nose

pterygopalatine ganglion

nasal vestibule

maxillary nerve
(pharyngeal nerve)

nare

anterior nasal spine of maxilla

nasopalatine nerve

incisive duct

maxilla

hard palate

oropharynx

inferior nasal meatus

greater palatine nerve
(posterior inferior nasal branch)

lesser palatine nerve

greater palatine nerve

soft palate

OLFACTION (II). OLFACTORY TRACT

olfactory tract

From the three chemical senses (taste, smell and the trigeminal) the smell is the most developed, although the fact that counting with an important subjective component becomes in especially complex, the olfactory via or sensory via for the smell, transport the olfactory stimuli from the osmo-receptors until the brain cortex. Begins in the olfactory mucus that is found in the upper portion of each nasal pit, Is formed by the olfactory cells, or bipolar neurons with regenerative capacity that are the truly olfactory receptors. Its thin unmyelinated axons, grouped in about 20 beams on each side of the nose, extend through the cribrosa lamina of the ethmoid bone, forming the olfactory nerves (1 cranial pair) that end in a pair of structures of gray substance (olfactory bulbs) that are found under the front lobules and lateral to the apophyses crista galli of the ethmoid bone. In the olfactory bulb, the axonic terminal of the olfactory receptors, make synapses with the dendrites and the cellular bodies of second order. The axons of the neurons of the olfactory bulb extend towards the rear part to form the olfactory tract. Some of this axons goes to the primary olfactory area, in the surface superomedial of the temporal lobule, that is where the conscious olfactory perception begins. Other axons goes to the limbic system and to the hypothalamus, where under the influx of the olfactory memory, promote the corresponding emotional answer.

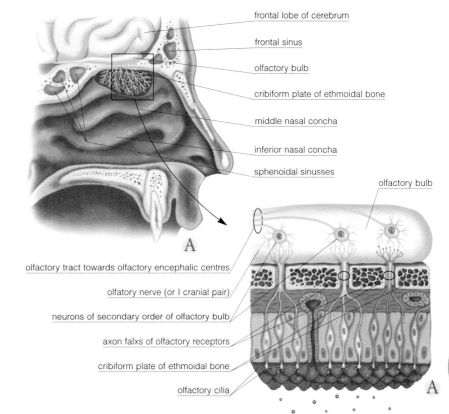

frontal lobe of cerebrum

frontal sinus

olfactory bulb

cribiform plate of ethmoidal bone

middle nasal concha

inferior nasal concha

sphenoidal sinusses

olfactory bulb

olfactory tract towards olfactory encephalic centres

olfatory nerve (or I cranial pair)

neurons of secondary order of olfactory bulb

axon falxs of olfactory receptors

cribiform plate of ethmoidal bone

olfactory cilia

675

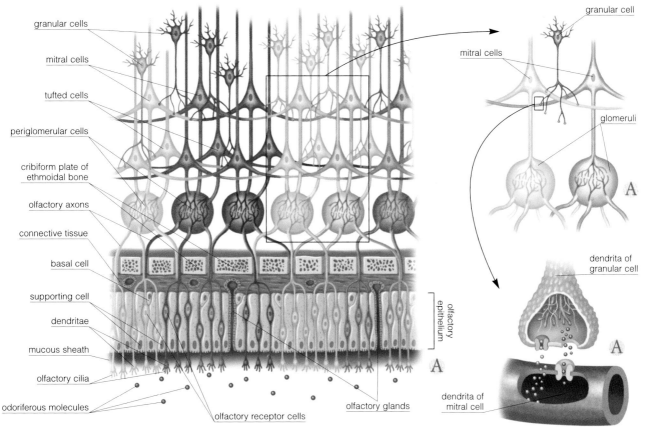

granular cells

mitral cells

tufted cells

periglomerular cells

cribiform plate of ethmoidal bone

olfactory axons

connective tissue

basal cell

supporting cell

dendritae

mucous sheath

olfactory cilia

odoriferous molecules

olfactory receptor cells

olfactory glands

olfactory epithelium

granular cell

mitral cells

glomeruli

dendrita of granular cell

dendrita of mitral cell

TASTE. GUSTATIVE STRUCTURES

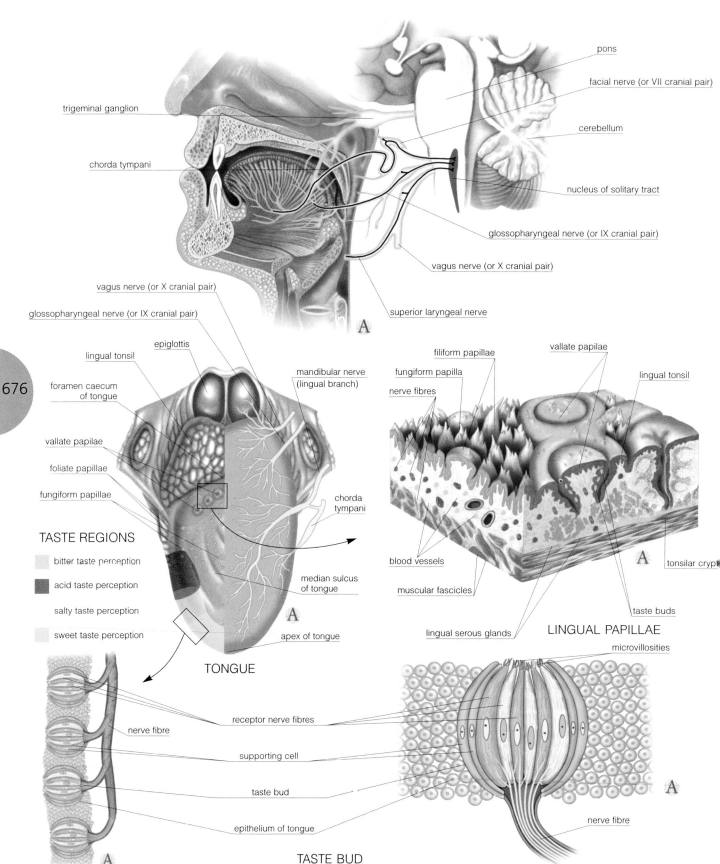

trigeminal ganglion

chorda tympani

pons

facial nerve (or VII cranial pair)

cerebellum

nucleus of solitary tract

glossopharyngeal nerve (or IX cranial pair)

vagus nerve (or X cranial pair)

superior laryngeal nerve

A

vagus nerve (or X cranial pair)

glossopharyngeal nerve (or IX cranial pair)

epiglottis

lingual tonsil

foramen caecum
of tongue

vallate papilae

foliate papillae

fungiform papillae

mandibular nerve
(lingual branch)

chorda
tympani

median sulcus
of tongue

apex of tongue

A

TASTE REGIONS

bitter taste perception

acid taste perception

salty taste perception

sweet taste perception

TONGUE

filiform papillae

fungiform papilla

nerve fibres

vallate papilae

lingual tonsil

blood vessels

muscular fascicles

lingual serous glands

taste buds

tonsilar crypt

A

LINGUAL PAPILLAE

microvillosities

receptor nerve fibres

nerve fibre

supporting cell

taste bud

epithelium of tongue

nerve fibre

A

A

TASTE BUD

TOUCH. TACTILE RECEPTORS
and MECHANISM of TRANSMISSION

TACTILE SKIN RECEPTORS

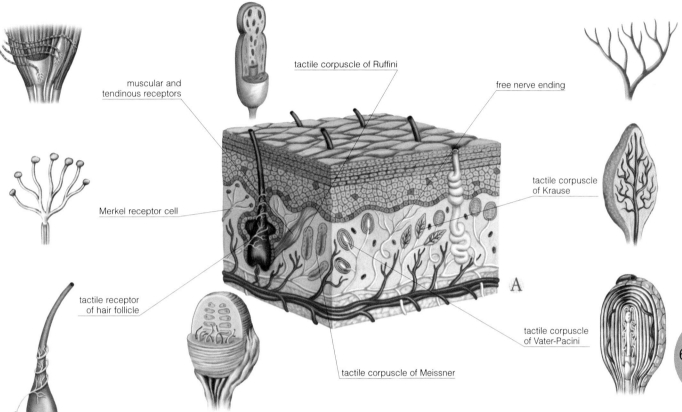

tactile corpuscle of Ruffini

free nerve ending

muscular and tendinous receptors

tactile corpuscle of Krause

Merkel receptor cell

tactile receptor of hair follicle

tactile corpuscle of Vater-Pacini

A

677

tactile corpuscle of Meissner

MECHANISM of PERCEPTION and SENSORY TRANSMISSION

Sensations which are originated on face, lips and tongue are straight directed to brain through trigeminal nerve, without passing through vertebral column.

Fibers are projected in specific regions of cerebral cortex and conduct the corresponding impulses.

Fibers information is projected to specific regions of cerebral cortex and conduct the corresponding impulses.

tactile sensations

The tactile sensations are the results of some nervous mechanisms that collect the sensory information of the body, are classified in: exteroceptive, mechano-receptive, thermo-receptive and painful. Are perceived through seven types of receptors, each one of them different and specialized in the catchment of specific sensations. from these the sensations are transmitted through the spinal medulla until the central nervous system, where they are received, processed and from is generate an adequate answer in every case, in order, for the human being, to be conscious of a determinate sensation (cold, pain, pressure, etc.). It must have gone previously through a two-way journey from the point where the sensation originated until the central nervous system.

In spin cord, fibers of column dorsal medial-lemniscus system cross to opposite side and are directed to thalamus. It means that sensations from right side are perceived in left side of brain and viceversa.

Spinal-thalamus way fibers cross the opposite side, cross briefly vertebral column and dorsal rods of gray spinal matter and reach to thalamus.

Sign, received basically by mechanoreceptors is transmitted through column dorsal medial-lemniscus system.

Sign, received by free nervous terminations, is transmitted through spinal-thalamus way.

Skin receiver tactile perceives a sign. This sign is transmitted to spinal cord. If it deals about pressure, tension or vibration, is used a fast way, and if signal is thermic or painful, is transmitted through slower way.

fast way

slow way

DERMATOMES

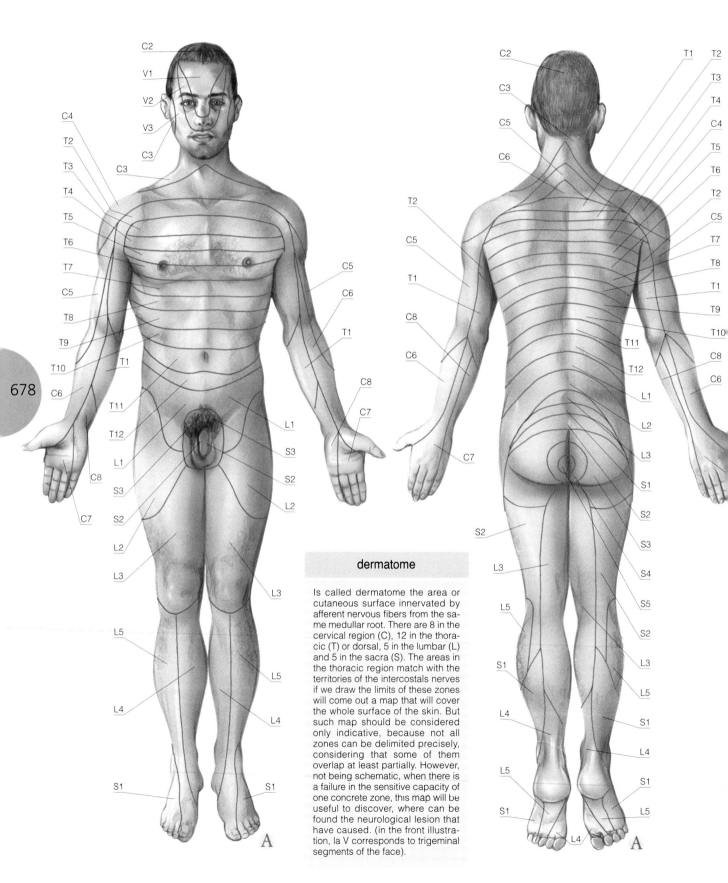

678

dermatome

Is called dermatome the area or cutaneous surface innervated by afferent nervous fibers from the same medullar root. There are 8 in the cervical region (C), 12 in the thoracic (T) or dorsal, 5 in the lumbar (L) and 5 in the sacra (S). The areas in the thoracic region match with the territories of the intercostals nerves if we draw the limits of these zones will come out a map that will cover the whole surface of the skin. But such map should be considered only indicative, because not all zones can be delimited precisely, considering that some of them overlap at least partially. However, not being schematic, when there is a failure in the sensitive capacity of one concrete zone, this map will be useful to discover, where can be found the neurological lesion that have caused. (in the front illustration, la V corresponds to trigeminal segments of the face).

BIBLIOGRAPHY

Feneis H: Feneis *Bild-Lexikon der Anatomie*, Georg Thieme Verlag KG, Suttgart 1967.

Testut I, Latarjet A: *Tratado de Anatomía Humana*, Ed. Salvat, Barcelona 1975.

Orts Llorca F: *Anatomía Humana*, Ed. Científica Médica, 8ª ed, Barcelona 1985.

Romanes GJ: Cunningham. *Tratado de Anatomía*, Ed McGraw-Hill Interamericana, 12ª ed, Madrid 1987.

Rohen JW, Yokochi Ch: *Atlas Fotográfico de Anatomía Humana*, Ed. Doyma, Barcelona 1989.

McMinn-Hut Chings: *Atlas de Anatomía Humana*, Ed Océano, Barcelona 1991.

Marieb EN, Laurendeau G: *Anatomie et Physiologie Humaines*, The Benjamin/Cummings Publishing Company Inc, Quebec 1992.

Latarjet M, Ruíz Liard A: *Anatomía Humana*, Ed Médica. Panamericana, Barcelona 1993.

Sobotta J: *Atlas de Anatomía Humana* (2 vols.), Ed. Médica Panamericana, 20ª ed, Madrid 1994.

Agur AMR: *Gran Atlas de Anatomía*, Ed. Médica Panamericana-Sans Tache, Williams et Wilkins, 9ª ed, Buenos Aires 1994.

Di Fiori MSH: *Atlas de Histología Normal*, El Ateneo, 7ª ed, Buenos Aires 1994.

Kahle-Leonhart-Platzer: *Atlas de Anatomía*, 3 vols, Ed. Omega, Barcelona 1997.

Williams PL, Bannister LH, Berry MM, Collins P, Dyson M, Dussek JE, Fergusson MWJ: *Anatomía de Gray. Bases anatómicas de Medicina y Cirugía*, Churchill Livingstone-Harcourt Brace de España SA, Madrid 1998.

Panski B: *Anatomía Humana*, Ed. McGraw-Hill Interamericana, 6ª ed, México 1998.

Rouvière H; Delmas A: *Anatomía Humana Descriptiva, Topográfica y Funcional*, Masson S.A. 10ª ed, Barcelona 1999.

VV.AA.: *Diccionari Enciclopèdic de Medicina*, Enciclopèdia Catalana, Barcelona 2000.

Geneser F: *Histología*, Ed. Médica Panamericana, 3ª ed, Barcelona 2000.

FCAT Comité Federal sobre Terminología Anatómica:*Terminología Anatómica*, Ed. Médica Panamericana, Madrid 2001.

Clascá F, Bover R, Burón JA, Castro A: *Anatomía seccional*, Ed. Masson, Barcelona 2002.

Espín J, Mérida JA, Sánchez-Montesinos I: Lecciones de Anatomía Humana, Librería Fleming, Granada 2003.

Diccionario Mosby (2 vols.), Elsevier, Madrid 2003.

Netter FH: *Atlas de Anatomía Humana*, Masson, 3ª ed, Barcelona 2004.

Vigué J, Martín Orte E: *Atlas del Cuerpo Humano*, Gorg Blanc, Barcelona 2004.

Cochard LR, Netter FH: *Atlas de Embriología Humana*, Masson, Barcelona 2005.

Dorland, *Diccionario Enciclopédico Ilustrado de Medicina*, Elsevier, 30ª ed, Madrid 2005.

Drake R, Vogl W, Mitchell AWM: *Anatomía para estudiantes*, Elsevier, Madrid 2005.

Carlson BA: *Embriología Humana y Biología del Desarrollo*, Elsevier, Madrid 2005.

Gilroy AM, Schünke M, MacPherson BR, Schulte E, Ross LM, Schumacher U: *Prometheus. Texto y Atlas de Anatomía* (3 vols.), Thieme Medical Publisher, Suttgart 2005-2008.

Tortora GJ, Derrikson B: *Principios de Anatomía y Fisiología*, Ed. Médica Panamericana, Madrid 2006.

Buja LM, Krueger GRF, Netter FH: *Anatomía Patológica*, Masson, Barcelona 2006.

Moore KL, Arthur F. Dalley AF: *Anatomía con orientación clínica*, Elsevier, 5ª ed, México 2007.

Vigué J, Martín Orte E: *Atlas del Cuerpo Humano, Anatomía, Histología, Patologías*, Barcelona 2007.

Atlas de Anatomía con correlación clínica (3 vols):
Platzer W: t. 1: *Aparato locomotor*, Ed. Médica Panamericana, 9ª ed, Madrid 2007.
Fritsch H, Kühnel W: t. 2: *Órganos internos*, Ed. Médica Panamericana, 9ª ed, Madrid 2007.
Kohle W, Frotcher M: t. 3: *Sistema nervioso y órganos de los sentidos*, Ed. Médica Panamericana, 9ª ed, Madrid 2007.

Langman S: *Embriología Médica con orientación clínica*, Ed. Panamericana, Buenos Aires 2007.

Diccionario Médico Taber de Ciencias de la Salud, DAE, Madrid 2007.

Vigué J, Martín Orte E, *Atlas de Anatomía Humana*, Barcelona 2008.

Atlas Ilustrado de Anatomía, Giunti Gruppo Editoriale, Florencia 2008.

Gartner LP, Hiatt JL: Atlas de Color de Histología, Ed. Panamericana, 3ª ed, Buenos Aires 2008.

Wesh U: *Histología*, Ed. Panamericana, Madrid 2009.

Barrett K, Barman SM, Boitano S, Brooks HL: *Fisiología Moderna*, Mc Graw-Hill, 23ª ed, México 2010.

Vigué J: *Vocabulario de Anatomía Humana* (en prensa).

ONOMASTIC INDEX

a

- A band 42
- abdomen 4, 5, 15, 34, 76, 77, 78, 79, 282, 308, 314, 369, 370, 371, 377, 380, 420, 421, 446, 447, 448
- abdomen (anterior surface) 34
- abdominal aorta 21, 281, 282, 283, 300, 301, 303, 304, 305, 307, 308, 309, 310, 311, 312, 313, 314, 326, 328, 332, 393, 394, 395, 417, 418, 420, 439, 441, 442, 447, 465, 468, 485, 506, 526, 615, 618, 620, 621, 627, 629
- abdominal artery 315
- abdominal cavity 615, 616, 617, 618
- abdominal entrail 422
- abdominal fold 32
- abdominal layer of urogenital region 504
- abdominal organ 653
- abdominal ostium of uterine tube 520
- abdominal region
- abdominal viscera 580
- abdominal wall 307, 494, 616, 617, 618
- abdominal wall musculature 445
- abdominal wall of epigastrium 426
- abdominogenital region 394, 395
- abducent nerve (or VI cranial pair) 290, 567, 572, 585, 592
- abductor digiti minimi of foot 50, 145, 148, 150, 154, 254, 255, 337, 339, 650, 651
- abductor digiti minimi of hand 50, 93, 115, 116, 117, 119, 121
- abductor hallucis 50, 122, 127, 145, 151, 153, 154, 155, 156, 254, 255, 337, 339, 650, 651
- abductor hallucis (oblique head) 155, 339
- abductor hallucis (transverse head) 155, 339
- abductor of fifth metatarsal bone 149, 151, 153
- abductor of fifth toe 155, 156
- abductor of hip muscle 51
- abductor pollicis 92, 114, 115, 117, 323
- adductor pollicis (oblique head) 117
- abductor pollicis (transverse head) 115
- abductor pollicis brevis 40, 93, 114, 115, 116, 117, 121, 323, 637

- abductor pollicis longus 45, 50, 92, 94, 95, 96, 97, 112, 114, 636
- acanthion 167
- accessory cephalic vein 356, 357, 358
- accessory hemi-azygos vein 354, 366, 370, 371, 372, 373, 374, 375, 467
- accessory nerve (or XI cranial pair) 567, 568, 585, 597, 607, 609, 612
- accessory nerve (or XI cranial pair) (branch for trapezius) 597
- accessory nerve (or XI cranial pair) (external branch) 612
- accessory nucleus of oculomotor nerve 582, 583
- accessory obturator nerve 604, 616
- accessory organ of the skin 35, 36
- accessory pancreatic duct 428, 443, 543
- accessory parotid gland 411
- accessory saphenous vein 146, 361, 362, 363
- acetabular fossa 218, 249
- acetabular labrum 248, 249
- acetabular margin 214, 217, 218
- acetabular notch 218
- acetabulum 214, 218, 249, 505, 620
- acid taste perception 676
- acinus 479
- acoustic meatus 664
- acoustic structure of hearing 668, 669
- acromial angle of scapula 204, 205
- acromioclavicular joint 99, 232, 233, 238, 239
- acromioclavicular ligament 101, 238
- acromion 61, 68, 73, 80, 81, 98, 99, 100, 101, 102, 103, 104, 105, 106, 164, 200, 201, 204, 205, 238, 239
- acrosomal granule of spermatid 511
- acrosomal hood of spermatid 511
- acrosomal vesicle 511
- acrosome of spermatozoid 511
- ACTH (or adrenocorticotropic hormone or corticotropin) 540, 544, 577
- action of pancreatic the exocrine secretion 401
- activin 545
- adductor 50, 51
- adductor brevis 50, 51, 123, 125, 131, 132, 135, 330, 331, 448, 630, 633, 646, 647
- adductor hallucis 50, 156, 339
- adductor hallucis (oblique head) 339

- adductor hiatus 123, 131, 132, 330, 331, 647
- adductor longus 21, 44, 50, 51, 122, 123, 127, 130, 131, 132, 137, 146, 330, 331, 448, 630, 633, 646, 647
- adductor magnus 45, 50, 51, 122, 123, 124, 125, 127, 129, 131, 132, 133, 134, 135, 137, 146, 329, 330, 331, 645, 646, 647
- adductor magnus (anterior part) 51
- adductor pollicis 50, 116, 117, 119, 121
- adductor pollicis (oblique head) 119
- adductor tubercle 220, 647
- adenohypophysis (or anterior lobe of pituitary gland) 540, 541, 544, 569, 572, 577
- adenohypophysis (or anterior lobe of pituitary gland) (distal part) 572
- adenohypophysis (or anterior lobe of pituitary gland) (intermediate part) 572
- adenohypophysis (or anterior lobe of pituitary gland) (tuberal part) 572, 573, 577
- ADH (or antidiuretic hormone, or vasopressin) 540, 544, 577
- adhering fascia 42
- adipose capsule 541
- adipose tissue 35, 504, 546
- adipose tissue of lymph node 536
- adipose tissue of mouth 56
- adjacent organs of kidney 487
- adjacent structures of uterus 525
- adjacent structures of vagina 525
- adrenaline 545
- adrenocorticotropic hormone (or corticotropin) (ACTH) 540, 544, 577
- adult 412
- adventitia of artery 279, 280
- adventitia of great vein 278, 280
- adventitia of muscular artery 278
- adventitia of tracheal wall 43
- adventitita of ureter 485
- adventitia of vein 279
- afferent glomerular artery 488
- afferent hypophysial vein towards cavernous sinus 573
- afferent lymph vessel 384, 385, 536, 537
- afferent nerve fibre 572
- afferent neuron 555
- afferent nucleus 582, 583
- afferent synapsis 669

683

684

b

687

688

689

d

690

e

692

f

693

695

698

701

703

707

709

710

712

O

713

715

719

724

725

728

729

731

W